REVIEW OF
OPHTHALMOLOGY

FOURTH EDITION

REVIEW OF
OPHTHALMOLOGY

Neil J. Friedman, MD
Adjunct Clinical Professor,
Department of Ophthalmology, Stanford University School of Medicine
Partner, Mid-Peninsula Ophthalmology Medical Group
Menlo Park, CA, USA

William B. Trattler, MD
Director of Cornea, Center for Excellence in Eye Care
Vice Chair of Research for the Department of Ophthalmology
Florida International University Wertheim College of Medicine
Miami, FL, USA

Peter K. Kaiser, MD
Chaney Family Endowed Chair for Ophthalmology Research
Professor of Ophthalmology
Cleveland Clinic Lerner College of Medicine
Cole Eye Institute, Cleveland Clinic
Cleveland, OH, USA

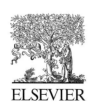

ELSEVIER

Elsevier
1600 John F. Kennedy Blvd.
Ste 1800
Philadelphia, PA 19103-2899

REVIEW OF OPHTHALMOLOGY, FOURTH EDITION   ISBN: 978-0-323-79418-3

Notice

Practitioners and researchers must always rely on their own experience and knowledge in evaluating and using any information, methods, compounds, or experiments described herein. Because of rapid advances in the medical sciences, in particular, independent verification of diagnoses and drug dosages should be made. To the fullest extent of the law, no responsibility is assumed by Elsevier, authors, editors, or contributors for any injury and/or damage to persons or property as a matter of products liability, negligence or otherwise, or from any use or operation of any methods, products, instructions, or ideas contained in the material herein.

Previous editions copyrighted 2018, 2012, and 2004.

Senior Content Strategist: Kayla Wolfe
Content Development Manager: Somodatta Roy Choudhury
Senior Content Development Specialist: Shweta Pant
Publishing Services Manager: Shereen Jameel
Senior Project Manager: Manikandan Chandrasekaran
Design Direction: Ryan Cook

Printed in India

Last digit is the print number: 9 8 7 6 5 4 3 2

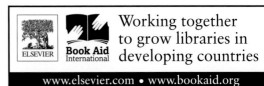

Preface

It gives us great pleasure to introduce the fourth edition of *Review of Ophthalmology*. The book retains its outline format and multiple-choice questions organized into chapters based on common written exam sections. In this edition, we have expanded the content with new topics and questions, rewritten large sections, and updated disease management with the latest treatments. We are committed to providing you with essential information in the most concise and user-friendly manner. We hope that we have met this goal and you continue to find *Review of Ophthalmology* a valuable book.

We wish you the best of luck on your exams and in your future careers!

Neil J. Friedman, MD
William B. Trattler, MD
Peter K. Kaiser, MD

Acknowledgments

We owe thanks to our colleagues, family, and friends who supported us with the fourth edition of *Review of Ophthalmology*; we are grateful for all your assistance.

We appreciate the time and effort of Dr. Sruthi Arepalli for her diligent chapter review.

We continue to work with a wonderful editorial team at Elsevier: thank you, Kayla Wolfe, Laura Klein, Shweta Pant, Manikandan Chandrasekaran and your staff for all your hard work and dedication.

Finally, a special thank-you to our families for their love and understanding: Mae, Jake, Dawn, Peter Jr., Stephanie, Jennifer, Ali, Jeremy, Josh, and Danny.

Neil J. Friedman, MD
William B. Trattler, MD
Peter K. Kaiser, MD

Contents

1

Optics

PROPERTIES OF LIGHT

Basic ideas of optics from camera obscura ("dark chamber"; pinhole camera): small dark room or box with a small hole to capture image of an outside scene or object (projected onto opposite side from aperture); 3 observations:

1. Image is inverted (light rays travel in straight line, intersect at aperture)
2. Image is dim (small aperture limits amount of light)
3. Depth of field is infinite (small aperture only allows entering light from 1 direction)

Enlarging aperture makes image brighter but blurry

Adding lens makes image sharp but lose depth of field

Challenge of optics: manipulate light from aperture to create sharp enough and bright enough image for a specific application

Geometric Optics

Describes macroscopic behavior of light; uses artificial construct of light rays, ignores wave characteristics

Basic principles of geometric optics:

1. Light rays travel in straight lines through uniform media
2. Light rays deviated by reflection or refraction
3. When light rays encounter multiple refractive surfaces, image formed at each becomes object for next
4. Paths of light rays are reversible

Fermat's principle: light travels along fastest path between 2 points

Physical Optics

Describes microscopic wave and particle (photon) properties of light

Speed (velocity) (v) is directly proportional to **wavelength (λ)** and **frequency (ν):** $v = \lambda \nu$

In any given medium, speed of light is constant ($v_{vacuum} = c = 3.0 \times 10^{10}$ cm/s); therefore, wavelength and frequency are inversely proportional

Light slows down in any substance other than air or vacuum; amount of slowing depends on medium; frequency of light remains unchanged, but wavelength changes (becomes shorter) (Fig. 1.1)

Energy is directly proportional to frequency and inversely proportional to wavelength: $E = h\nu = h(c/\lambda)$

Index of refraction (n): ratio of speed of light in a vacuum to speed of light in specific material ($n = c/v$)

Air = 1.00, water = 1.33, aqueous and vitreous = 1.34, cornea = 1.37, crystalline lens = 1.42, intraocular

1

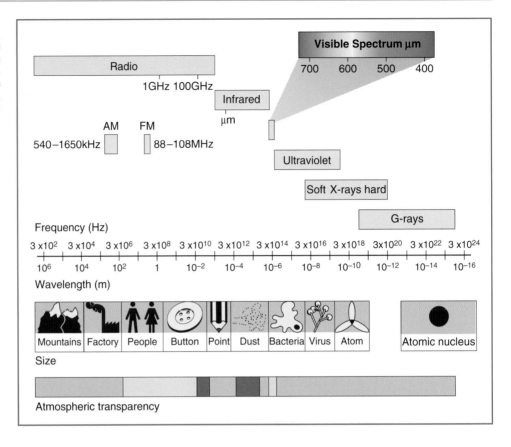

Figure 1.1 The electromagnetic spectrum. The pictures of mountains, people, buttons, viruses, and so forth are used to produce a real (i.e., visceral) feeling of the size of some of the wavelengths. (With permission from Miller D, Burns SK. Visible light. In: Yanoff M, Duker JS, eds. *Ophthalmology,* 2nd ed. St Louis: Mosby; 2004.)

lens (IOL; silicone = 1.41; polymethyl methacrylate 1.49; acrylic = 1.55), glass = 1.52, high-index lenses = 1.6-1.8

Interference: overlapping of light waves; may be constructive or destructive

Constructive (additive): peaks of two waves overlap, resulting in maximum intensity at that wavelength

Destructive (subtractive): peak of one wave overlaps with trough of another, obliterating both waves

Example: antireflective coatings (destructive interference, 1/4 wavelength apart); interference filters (allow only green light out of the eye during fluorescein angiography); laser interferometry (retinal function test; optical coherence tomography [OCT])

Coherence: ability of two light beams to cause interference (large white source has a coherence close to zero)

Example: OCT

Polarization: each light wave has an electrical field with a particular orientation

Nonpolarized light: electrical field of each wave has a random orientation

Polarized light: all electrical fields have same orientation

Example: Haidinger brushes (polarizing filter rotated in front of blue background produces rotating image like a double-ended brush or propeller; type of entopic phenomenon; test of macular function), Titmus stereo testing, polarized microscopy, polarizing sunglasses

Diffraction: bending/spreading of light waves around edges; change in direction of light wave is related to wavelength (the shorter the wavelength, the less the change in direction); amount of diffraction is related to size of aperture (the smaller the aperture, the greater the diffraction); interference of new waves with original rays forms a diffraction pattern

Example: Airy disc (diffraction pattern produced by a small, circular aperture; occurs when pupil size is <2.5 mm; diameter of central disc increases as pupil size decreases); pinhole (reduces refractive error and improves vision by increasing depth of focus, but limited by diffraction; optimal size is 1.2 mm; may correct for as much as 5 D; smaller aperture limits visual acuity; squinting is method of creating a natural pinhole to improve vision; pinhole can also improve vision in eyes with corneal or lenticular irregularities; pinhole can reduce vision in eyes with dense cataracts and macular disease)

Scattering: disruption of light by irregularities in light path; 3 types depending on size of particles in scattering compared with wavelength of light:

Rayleigh scattering: caused by particles smaller than the light wavelength; strong dependence on wavelength (shorter scatter more than longer)

Example: blue light from sun scattered most in atmosphere (sky appears blue)

Mei scattering: caused by particles similar in size to light wavelength; little dependence on wavelength; direction of scatter is mostly forward

Example: sunlight scattered equally by water droplets in sky (clouds appear white); light scattered by corneal scar or cataract makes opacity appear white, and forward scatter causes increased glare, decreased contrast, and image degradation

Geometric scattering: caused by particles larger than the light wavelength; refraction and reflection as described by geometric optics

Example: sunlight refracted and reflected by surface of raindrops (rainbow)

Reflection: bouncing of light off optical interfaces; the greater the refractive index difference between the two media, the greater is the reflection; also varies with angle of incidence

> **Example:** Asteroid hyalosis (asteroids reflect light back into examiner's eye, creating glare; patient is asymptomatic)

Transmission: percentage of light penetrating a substance (%*T*); can vary with wavelength

Absorption: expressed as optical density (OD) = $\log 1/T$

Illumination: measure of incident light

Luminance: measure of reflected or emitted light (lumen/m^2); apostilb = diffusing surface with luminance of 1 lumen/m^2 (used in Humphrey and Goldmann visual field testing)

> **Example:** contrast sensitivity is the ability to detect small changes in luminance

Laser: light amplification by stimulated emission of radiation; excited material releases photons of same wavelength and frequency; process is amplified so that released photons are in phase (constructive interference); produces monochromatic, coherent, high-intensity polarized light; power can be increased by increasing energy or decreasing time ($P = E/t$); Q switching and mode locking (types of shutters that synchronize light phase) are methods of increasing laser power by compressing output in time

REFRACTION

Light changes direction when it travels from one material to another of different refractive index (e.g., across an optical interface); direction of refraction is toward the normal when light passes from a medium with a lower index of refraction to a medium with a higher one and away from the normal when light passes from a more dense to a less dense medium (higher-refractive-index materials are more difficult for light to travel through, so light takes a shorter path [closer to the normal]); light does not deviate if it is perpendicular to interface (parallel to the normal)

Snell's law: $n_1 \sin (i) = n_2 \sin (r)$; n = refractive index of material; i = angle of incidence (measured from the normal); r = angle of refraction (measured from the normal) (Fig. 1.2)

Critical angle: angle at which incident light is bent exactly 90° away from the normal (when going from medium of higher to lower n) and after which all light is reflected

> **Example:** Glass–air interface has a critical angle of 41°; critical angle of cornea = 46.5°

Total internal reflection: angle of incidence exceeds critical angle, so light is reflected back into material with higher index of refraction; $n \sin (i_c) = n' \sin (90°)$; $\sin (i_c) = (n'/n) \times 1$

> **Example:** Gonioscopy lens is necessary to view angle structures because of total internal reflection of the cornea

PRISMS

Prisms displace and deviate light (because their surfaces are nonparallel); light rays are deviated toward the base; image is displaced toward the apex (Fig. 1.3)

Prism diopter (PD, Δ): displacement (in cm) of light ray passing through a prism, measured 100 cm (1 m) from prism

> **Example:** 15 Δ = ray displaced 15 cm at a distance of 1 m (1 Δ = 1 cm displacement/1 m); 1° ≈ 2 Δ (this approximation is useful for angles smaller than 45°)

Angle of minimum deviation: total angle of deviation is least when there is equal bending at both surfaces of prism

Plastic prisms are calibrated by angle of minimum deviation: back surface parallel to frontal plane

Glass prisms are calibrated in **Prentice position:** back surface perpendicular to visual axis

Prism placed in front of the eye creates a phoria in the direction of the base

> **Example:** Base-out (BO) prism induces exophoria; to correct, use prism with apex in the opposite direction

Apex is always pointed in direction of deviation: base-out for esotropia, base-in for exotropia, base-down (BD) for hypertropia

Stacking prisms is not additive; 1 prism in front of each eye is additive

Risley prism: two right-angle prisms positioned back to back, which can be rotated to yield variable prism diopters

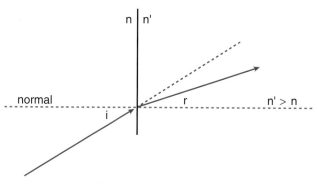

Figure 1.2 Refraction of light ray.

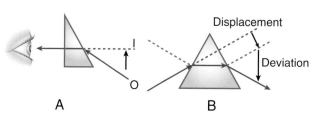

Figure 1.3 (A) Displacement of image toward apex. (B) Displacement and deviation of light by prism.

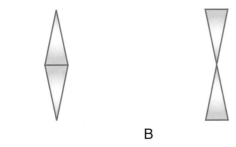

Figure 1.4 (A) Plus lenses act like two prisms base to base. (B) Minus lenses act like two prisms apex to apex.

from 0-30 Δ; used to measure prismatic correction for tropias

Fresnel prisms: composed of side-by-side strips of small prisms; prism power is related to apex angle, not the size of the prism; available as lightweight, thin press-on prism to reduce base thickness of the spectacle prism; disadvantage is reflection and scatter at prism interface, causing decreased visual acuity

Prismatic effect of lenses (Fig. 1.4): spectacles induce prism; all off-axis rays are bent toward or away from axis, depending on lens vergence

Perceived movement of fixation target when lens moves in front of the eye:
  Plus lenses: produce "against" motion (target moves in opposite direction from lens)
  Minus lenses: produce "with" motion (target moves in same direction as lens)
Amount of motion is proportional to the power of the lens

Prismatic effect of glasses on strabismic deviations:
$2.5 \times D$ = percent difference; minus lenses make deviation appear larger ("minus measures more"); plus lenses decrease measured deviation

Prentice rule: prismatic power of lens = $\Delta = hD$
(h = distance from optical axis of lens [cm], D = power of lens [D])

Prismatic power of a lens increases as one moves farther away from optical center (vs. power of prism, which is constant)
  Example: Reading 1 cm below optical center: oculus dexter (OD) – 3.00; oculus sinister (OS) + 1.00 + 3.00 × 90
  OD – right eye: prism power = 1 cm × 3 D = 3 Δ BD
  OS – left eye: prism power vertical meridian: 1 cm + 1 D = 1 Δ base-up (BU)
  (Note: power of cylinder in 90° meridian is zero)
  Net prismatic effect = 4 Δ (either BD over OD, or BU over OS)

Treatment of anisophoria (reduce vertical prismatic effect of anisometropia):
  1. Contact lenses (CL) (optical center moves with eyes)
  2. Lower optical centers of lenses (reduce amount of induced prism)
  3. Slab-off prism (technique of grinding lens [done to the more minus lens] to remove BD prism [to reduce amount of induced prism])
  4. Separate single vision distance and reading glasses
  5. Bifocals with dissimilar segment styles

Prismatic effect of bifocal glasses:
  Image jump: produced by sudden prismatic power at top of bifocal segment; not influenced by type of underlying lens; as line of sight crosses from optical center of lens to bifocal segment, image position suddenly shifts up owing to BD prismatic effect of bifocal segment (more bothersome than image displacement; therefore, choose segment type to minimize image jump)
  Image displacement: displacement of image by total prismatic effect of lens and bifocal segment; minimized when prismatic effect of bifocal segment and distance lens are in opposite directions
  Prismatic effect of underlying lens:
    Hyperopic lenses induce BU prism, causing image to move progressively downward in downgaze
    Myopic lenses induce BD prism, causing image to move progressively upward in downgaze
  Prismatic effect of bifocal segment:
    Round top (acts like BD prism): maximum image jump; image displacement less for hyperope than for myope
    Flat top (acts like BU prism): minimum image jump; image displacement more for hyperope than for myope
    Executive type or progressive lenses: no image jump (optical centers at top of segment)
  Plus lens: choose round top
  Minus lens: choose flat top or executive type (for myopes, image jump is very difficult to ignore because it is in same direction as image displacement, so avoid round tops in myopes)

Chromatic effects: prismatic effect varies with wavelength
  Shorter wavelengths are bent farther, causing chromatic aberration
  White light shines through prism: blue rays closer to base (bend farthest), red rays closer to apex
  In the eye, blue rays come to focus closer to lens than do red rays; difference between blue and red is 1.5-3 D

Duochrome test: red and green filters create 0.5 D difference; use to check accuracy of refraction
  If letters on red side are clearer, focal point is in front of retina (eye is "fogged" or myopic)
  If letters on green side are clearer, focal point is behind retina (eye is overminused or hyperopic)
  Technique: start with red side clearer and add minus sphere in 0.25 D steps until red and green sides are

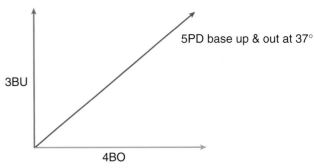

Figure 1.5 Addition of base-up and base-out prisms.

equal (focal point on retina; mnemonic **RAM-GAP** [**R**ed **A**dd **M**inus – **G**reen **A**dd **P**lus]); works in color blind patients because it is based on chromatic aberration rather than color discrimination

Vector addition of prisms: prismatic deviations in different directions are additive, based on Pythagorean theorem ($a^2 + b^2 = c^2$) (Fig. 1.5)

VERGENCE

The amount of spreading of a bundle of light rays (wavefront) emerging from a point source

Direction of light travel must be specified (by convention, left to right)

Convergence (converging rays): plus vergence; rare in nature; must be produced by an optical system (convex lens)

Divergence (diverging rays): minus vergence (from concave lens)

Parallel rays: zero vergence

Diopter: unit of vergence; reciprocal of distance (in meters) to point at which rays intersect; reciprocal of focal length of lens

Lens: adds vergence to light (amount of vergence = power of lens [in diopters])
　　Plus (convex) lens adds vergence (Fig. 1.6)
　　Minus (concave) lens subtracts vergence (Fig. 1.7)

Objects and images:
　　Object rays: rays that define the object; always on incoming (left) side of lens
　　Image rays: rays that define the image; always on outgoing (right) side of lens
　　Objects and images can be on either side of lens: real if on same side as respective rays; virtual if on opposite side from rays (locate by imaginary extension of rays through lens)
　　If object is moved, image moves in same direction relative to light
　　Adding power to system also moves image: plus power pulls image against light; minus power pushes image with light (lens system uses minus lens to shift image away [farther to right] from another lens)
　　Power of lens system (adjacent lenses) is sum of individual lens powers: $P = P_1 + P_2$

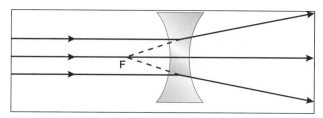

Figure 1.7 Concave lens produces divergence and virtual image.

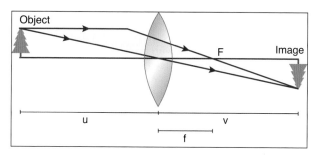

Figure 1.8 Object and image distances.

Vergence equation: power of a thin lens
　　$n_1/u + P = n_2/v$
　　(n_1 and n_2 = refractive indices to left and right of refracting surface; u = object distance; v = image distance)
　　Basic lens formula: $U + P = V$
　　　　Simple form of vergence equation (in air, $n = 1$, terms become simple reciprocals [object and image vergences])
　　　　$U = 1/u$ = vergence of light entering lens; P = power of lens; $V = 1/v$ = vergence of light leaving lens (Fig. 1.8)

Lensmaker's equation: power of a curved surface separating regions of different refractive index; $P = (n_2 - n_1)/r$
　　($n_2 - n_1$ = difference in refractive indices; r = radius of curvature of surface [in meters])
　　Example: power of corneal surface: back = –5.7 D; front = +52.9 D
　　(front: $n_2 = 1.37$, $n_1 = 1.00$; back: $n_2 = 1.33$, $n_1 = 1.37$; $r = 0.007$)
　　Power of a thin lens immersed in fluid: $P_{air}/P_{fluid} = (n_{lens} - n_{air})/(n_{lens} - n_{fluid})$
　　Refracting power of a thin lens is proportional to difference in refractive indices between lens and medium

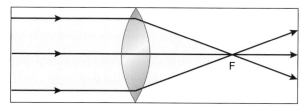

Figure 1.6 Convex lens produces convergence and real image.

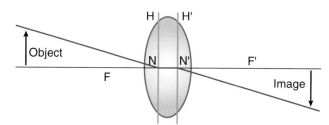

Figure 1.9 Conjugate points of real lens: each pair of object–image points in an optical system is conjugate; if direction of light is reversed, positions of object and image are exactly reversed.

Lenses:

Real (thick) lenses (Fig. 1.9): 2-sided, have front and back refractive surface

THICK LENS FORMULA: $P = P_1 + P_2 - (t/n)P_1P_2$
(P_1 = front surface power; P_2 = back surface power; t = lens thickness in meters; n = lens refractive index)

6 CARDINAL POINTS: 2 principal planes (H_1 and H_2); 2 nodal points (N_1 and N_2); 2 focal points (F_1 and F_2)

Refraction occurs at principal planes (U is measured from H_1; V is measured from H_2)

Focal lengths are also measured from principal planes

Nodal points coincide with principal planes (exception: if different refractive media are on opposite sides of the lens, then nodal points are both displaced toward the medium with the higher refractive index)

Central ray: passes through both nodal points (tip of object to N_1, across to N_2; then emerges parallel to original direction)

MENISCUS LENSES: difference between anterior and posterior curvature determines power

Steeper anterior curvature = convergent lens (+ power); principal planes displaced anteriorly

Steeper posterior curvature = divergent lens (– power); principal planes displaced posteriorly

Power of lens is measured at posterior surface (posterior vertex power)

Conjugate points: each pair of object–image points in an optical system is conjugate; if direction of light is reversed, position of object and image is exactly reversed

Conjugate planes:

Example: Viewing a slide presentation (image of slide is formed on retina of each person in audience, and very faint image of each person's retina is projected on the screen), direct ophthalmoscope (patient's retina and examiner's retina are conjugate), indirect ophthalmoscope (three conjugate planes [patient's retina, aerial image plane, examiner's retina]; any object placed at far point [aerial image] will be imaged sharply in focus on patient's retina)

Ideal (thin) lenses: special case of thick lens; as lens gets thinner, principal planes move closer together; in an ideal lens, principal planes overlap at optical center

2 FOCAL POINTS (F):

PRIMARY (F_1): object point for image at infinity (point on optical axis at which object is placed so parallel rays emerge from lens)

SECONDARY (F_2): image point for object at infinity (point on optical axis at which incident parallel rays are focused)

FOCAL LENGTH (f): distance between lens and focal points; reciprocal of lens power ($f = 1/P$)

Example: Focal length of +20 D lens is 1/20 = 0.05 m

NODAL POINT (N): point through which light ray passes undeviated; located at center of thin lens (optical center)

RAY TRACING: use to determine image size, orientation, and position

3 PRINCIPAL RAYS:

1. Central ray: undeviated ray passing from tip of object through nodal point of lens (or center of curvature of mirror) to tip of image; gives size and

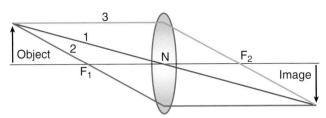

Figure 1.10 Three principal rays of ideal lens.

orientation of image (form similar triangles; thus, sizes of object and image are in same ratio as their distances from the lens)

2. Ray from tip of object through F_1 emerges from lens parallel to optical axis

3. Ray from tip of object parallel to optical axis emerges from lens and passes through F_2 (Fig. 1.10)

Depth of focus: region of best image focus; not a single point but a range of image locations in which object is in clear focus; pinhole has infinite depth of focus

Depth of field: range of object locations in clear focus for one image location; important for near-vision glasses to make depth of field large (near object locations) even though depth of focus small (image focused on retina)

Lens effectivity: function of lens power and distance from desired point of focus; depends on vertex distance and refractive index of media in which lens is placed ($P_{air} = [n_{IOL} - n_{air}]/[n_{IOL} - n_{aqueous}] \times P_{aqueous}$); moving a lens forward away from eye increases effective plus power, so plus lens becomes stronger and minus lens becomes weaker; when vertex distance decreases, a more plus lens is required to maintain the same distance correction (i.e., as desired point of focus is approached, more plus power is needed); the more powerful the lens, the more significant is the change in position

Vertex distance conversion:

1. Focal point of original lens = far point
2. Distance of new lens from far point = required focal length of new lens
3. Power of new lens = reciprocal of new focal length

Example: +12.50 D spectacle lens at vertex distance of 13 mm; calculate CL power:

1. +12.50 D lens has focal point of 0.08 m = 8 cm = far point
2. Distance of new lens (CL) from far point is 8 cm – 13 mm = 67 mm = required focal length of CL
3. Power of CL = 1/0.067 m = +15 D

Approximation: $P_2 = P + S(P_1)^2$ (S = vertex distance in meters)

Pure cylindrical lens: power only in 1 meridian (perpendicular to axis of lens); produces focal line parallel to axis

Spherocylindrical lens: power in 1 meridian greater than other; surface is toric (combination of sphere and cylinder)

Spherical equivalent: average spherical power of a spherocylindrical lens; equal to sphere plus 1/2 the cylinder; places circle of least confusion on retina

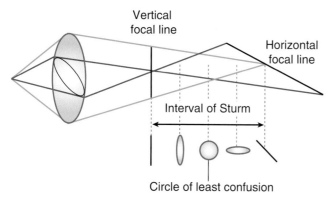

Figure 1.11 Conoid of Sturm.

Conoid of Sturm: 3-dimensional envelope of light rays refracted by a circular spherocylindrical lens; consists of vertical line → vertical ellipse → circle (of least confusion) → horizontal ellipse → horizontal line (Fig. 1.11)

Circle of least confusion: circular cross section of conoid of Sturm, which lies halfway (dioptrically) between the two focal lines at which image is least blurred; dioptrically calculated by spherical equivalent

Interval of Sturm: distance between anterior and posterior focal lines

Cylinder transposition: converting cylinder notation (plus → minus; minus → plus)
- New sphere = old sphere + old cylinder
- New cylinder = magnitude of old cylinder but with opposite power
- New axis = change old axis by 90°
- **Example:** +3.00 + 1.50 × 45 → +4.50 − 1.50 × 135

Power cross diagram: depicts two principal meridians of lens with the power acting in each meridian (90° from axis), rather than according to axis (Fig. 1.12)

Combining cylinders at oblique axis: complex calculation; therefore, measure with lensometer

Power of cylinder at oblique axis: power of the cylinder +1.00 × 180° is +1.00 @ 90°; +0.75 @ 60°; +0.50 @ 45°; +0.25 @ 30°; 0 @ 0°
  Example:
  JACKSON CROSS CYLINDER: special lens used for refraction to determine cylinder power and orientation; combination of plus cylinder in one axis and minus cylinder of equal magnitude in axis 90° away; spherical equivalent is zero (e.g., −1.00 + 2.00 × 180)
  Therefore, does not change the position of the circle of least confusion with respect to the retina; normally, have 0.25 D cross cylinder in phoropter; if patient's acuity is 20/40 or worse, must use larger power cross cylinder (i.e., 1.00 D) so that patient can discriminate difference
  TIGHT SUTURE AFTER CATARACT OR CORNEAL SURGERY: steepens cornea in meridian of suture, inducing astigmatism

Aberrations

Lenses behave ideally only near optical axis; peripheral to this paraxial region, aberrations occur; pupil size influences visual impact of aberrations (e.g., pinhole improves vision by reducing aberrations; night myopia caused by spherical aberration from larger pupil)

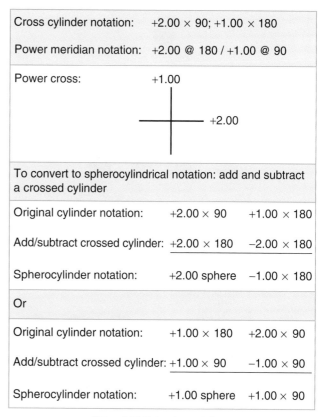

Cross cylinder notation:	+2.00 × 90; +1.00 × 180	
Power meridian notation:	+2.00 @ 180 / +1.00 @ 90	
Power cross:	+1.00 (vertical), +2.00 (horizontal)	
To convert to spherocylindrical notation: add and subtract a crossed cylinder		
Original cylinder notation:	+2.00 × 90	+1.00 × 180
Add/subtract crossed cylinder:	+2.00 × 180	−2.00 × 180
Spherocylinder notation:	+2.00 sphere	−1.00 × 180
Or		
Original cylinder notation:	+1.00 × 180	+2.00 × 90
Add/subtract crossed cylinder:	+1.00 × 90	−1.00 × 90
Spherocylinder notation:	+1.00 sphere	+1.00 × 90

Figure 1.12 Various lens notations.

Wavefront theory:
  Wavefront: physical representation of the optical quality of a monochromatic light beam; geometric surface representing location of isochronic (equal-time) light rays; can be constructed anywhere along group of rays from single object point. Ideal wavefront is plane or flat wave, but most wavefronts have irregular shape caused by disruption form imperfections in optical system (cornea and lens)

  Reference sphere: mathematical construct for wavefront comparison, surface represents arc centered on image point. If wavefront has same shape as reference sphere, then focused at center of sphere

  Wave aberration: difference between wavefront and reference sphere; smooth surface with irregular shape; described by multiple fundamental shapes. Measured with wavefront aberrometer (4 types: Hartmann-Shack, Tshering, thin-beam single-ray tracing, optical path difference); 2 algorithms to analyze data: Zernike polynomials and Fourier analysis

  Zernike polynomials: mathematical functions to describe complex shapes. Only uses subsample of Hartmann-Shack data points (usually to generate a 6th-order image), works well for the common lower-order shapes but loses precision in highly aberrated eyes. References shapes for wavefront aberrations (Zernike coefficients): lower-order aberrations (sphere and cylinder) and higher-order aberrations (HOAs; 3rd order and higher). Defocus, spherical aberration, coma, and secondary astigmatism affect quality of vision most. HOAs increase with increasing pupil size and age; corneal refractive surgery reduces lower-order

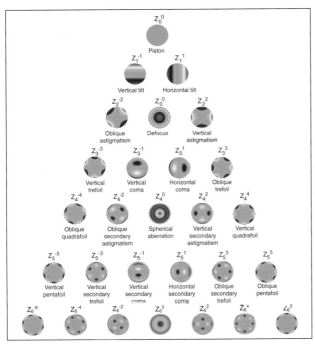

Figure 1.13 Zernike polynomials.

aberrations but often increases HOAs (especially spherical aberration and coma) (Fig. 1.13)

0 ORDER: piston

1ST ORDER: tilt (vertical and horizontal prism)

2ND ORDER: defocus and astigmatism (caused by spherocylindrical lenses; myopia [positive defocus], hyperopia [negative defocus], astigmatism)

3RD ORDER: coma (vertical and horizontal) and trefoil

4TH ORDER: spherical aberration, secondary astigmatism, tetrafoil

Root mean square (RMS) error: quantitative measure of optical aberrations; combines Zernike coefficients to determine total deviation of wavefront. More aberrations result in higher RMS value; dependent on pupil size; for 6-mm pupil, average RMS <0.3 μm. Most higher order aberrations have mean values near zero

Fourier analysis: sine waves derived transformations to reconstruct wavefront into complex shape; fully maps Hartmann-Shack data to derive more precise shape (equivalent to 20th order Zernike), can resolve highly aberrated patterns

Seidel aberrations: fundamental monochromatic aberrations caused by disparity in light ray focal lengths (spherical aberration, coma, astigmatism, curvature of field, and distortion)

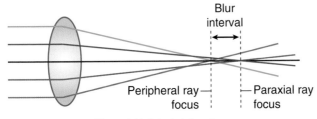

Figure 1.14 Spherical aberration.

Spherical aberration: rays from single axial object point refracted at different distances from center of lens (lens periphery has increasing prismatic effect); peripheral rays refracted more reaching axis closer than paraxial rays, producing a blur interval along the optical axis; increases depth of field, decreases contrast sensitivity (Fig. 1.14)

Positive spherical aberration (bowl-shaped wavefront) shifts focus point anteriorly

Increases with pupil dilation (i.e., night myopia; correct with additional −0.50 D distance lens)

Produces bull's-eye retinoscopic reflex

Reduce by avoiding biconvex lens shape; use plano-convex, meniscus, or aspheric lens surface

Eye has 3 mechanisms for reducing spherical aberration of lens:

1. Smaller pupil size eliminates a greater number of peripheral rays
2. Cornea progressively flattens in periphery
3. Nucleus of crystalline lens has higher index of refraction

Astigmatism: rays from single object point strike lens at different meridians; tilting spherical lens induces astigmatism (oblique rays encounter different curvatures at front and back lens surfaces)

Example: pantoscopic tilt (amount of induced sphere and cylinder depends on power of lens and amount of tilt)

Coma: rays from single off-axis object point refracted at different distances from center of lens; peripheral rays refracted farther from axis, producing comet-shaped image deformity; image appears smeared with sharp focus at one edge and fuzzy focus at other edge. Common in keratoconus, decentered corneal surgery (laser ablations, grafts)

Curvature of field: rays from object points at different distances from axis refracted at different distances from axis; spherical lens produces curved image of flat object

Distortion: rays from object points at different distances from axis have different transverse magnification; differential magnification from optical axis to lens periphery alters straight edges of square objects; shape of distortion is opposite of shape of lens (plus lens produces **pincushion** distortion; minus lens produces **barrel** distortion); effect increases with power of lens

Chromatic aberration: light of different wavelengths is refracted by different amounts; colors of white light spread apart (shorter wavelengths are bent farther; chromatic interval between blue and red is 1.5-3.0 D)

Example: at night with Purkinje shift, chromatic aberration moves focal point of eye anteriorly, producing myopia

MAGNIFICATION

Transverse (linear or lateral): magnification of image size (height perpendicular to optical axis); must be able to measure object and image size; ratio of image height to object height (or image distance to object distance); if image is inverted, magnification is negative $M_T = I/O$

Longitudinal (axial): magnification of depth (length along optical axis); equal to square of transverse magnification $M_L = M_T^2$

Angular: magnification of angle subtended by an image with respect to an object; useful when object or image size cannot be measured (afocal systems)
> **Example:** moon gazing with telescope
> $M_A = xP = P/4$ (standardized to 25 cm [1/4 m], the near point of the average eye)
> **Example:** with direct ophthalmoscope, eye acts as simple magnifier of retina: $M_A = 60/4 = 15 \times$ magnification

Size of image seen through glasses:
Shape factors: for any corrective lens, an increase in either front surface curvature or lens thickness will increase the image size (therefore, equalize the front surface curvatures and lens thickness for the 2 lenses)
> **FRONT SURFACE CURVATURE:** every D of change will change image size by 0.5% (magnification decreases while plus power decreases)
> **CENTER THICKNESS:** every mm of change in thickness will change image size by 0.5% (magnification decreases while lens thickness decreases)

Power factors:
> **VERTEX POWER (REFRACTIVE POWER):** minus power lenses produce smaller images than do plus lenses
> **VERTEX DISTANCE:** distance between front surface of cornea and back surface of lens; an increase in vertex distance will increase the magnification of plus lenses and decrease the magnification (increase the minification) of minus lenses
>> PLUS LENS: every mm increase in vertex distance will increase magnification by 0.1% per diopter of lens power
>> MINUS LENS: every mm increase in vertex distance will decrease magnification by 0.1% per D of lens power

Spectacle lens changes retinal image size by 2% per D of power at 12 mm vertex distance

Anisometropia: the difference in power between the two eyes; every 1 D produces approximately 2% of aniseikonia; prismatic effect of glasses varies in different directions of gaze, causing anisophoria (usually more problematic than aniseikonia)

Anisophoria: different ocular alignment in different positions of gaze

Aniseikonia: difference in image size between eyes from unequal magnification of correcting lenses
Up to 5%-8% is usually well tolerated; corresponds to approximately 3 D of spectacle anisometropia; children can adjust to much larger degrees
> **Example:** unilateral aphakia: 25% enlargement with spectacle lens; 7% with CL; 2.5% with IOL

Treatment of aniseikonia: decrease magnification
1. Reduce front surface power of lens
2. Decrease center thickness of lens
3. Decrease vertex distance (reduces magnifying effect of plus lens and minifying effect of minus lens)
4. CL (eliminate vertex distance)

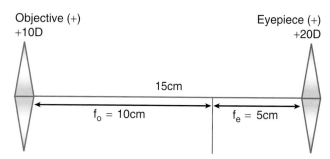

Figure 1.15 Astronomic telescope.

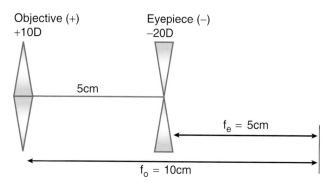

Figure 1.16 Galilean telescope.

Knapp's rule: when proper corrective lens is positioned at anterior focal point of eye, retinal image size will be equal in both eyes, no matter what the degree of anisometropia (applies only to axial ametropia)

Telescopes: magnify objects by increasing angle that object subtends on retina
> *Astronomical telescope (Keplerian):* combination of 2 plus lenses; focal points coincide in intermediate image plane; distance between lenses is sum of focal lengths; use higher power as eyepiece; inverted image (Fig. 1.15)
> *Galilean telescope:* combination of a weak plus lens (objective) and a strong minus lens (eyepiece); distance between lenses is difference of focal lengths; erect image (e.g., surgical loupe) (Fig. 1.16)

Angular magnification is the same for both telescopes (power of eyepiece/power of objective): $M_A = -P_e/P_o$

Accommodation through telescope: $A_T = A_N(M_A^2)$
(A_N = normal accommodation)
> **Example:** for monocular aphakia, overcorrect aphakic CL by + 3.00 D; then, correct induced myopic error with spectacle of −3.00 D. This produces an inverse Galilean telescope system that results in significantly smaller magnification difference between the two eyes than occurs with a CL alone

MIRRORS

Law of reflection: angle of incidence = angle of reflection (measured from the normal)

Objects and images: real if located on left side of mirror, virtual if on right side (inside) of mirror

Focal length: half the radius of curvature ($f = r/2$)

Reflecting power: reciprocal of focal length
($P = -1/f = -2/r$)

Convex: positive radius of curvature (R); adds minus vergence; produces virtual, **erect**, **min**ified image (mnemonic **VErMin**)
>   **Example:** rear view mirror; cornea (reflecting power of cornea = –1/f = –2/r = –2/0.0077 = –260 D [much stronger than refracting power])

Concave: negative r; adds plus vergence; image can be virtual or real, erect or inverted, magnified or minified, depending on object location with respect to center of curvature of mirror:
>   At twice focal length (center of curvature): real, inverted, same size
>   Between center and focal length: real, inverted, magnified
>   At focal length: at infinity
>   Inside focal length: virtual, erect, magnified

Plano: no change in vergence; image is virtual, erect, same size; field of view is double the size of the mirror
>   **Example:** dressing mirror needs to be only half of body length to provide view of entire self

Central ray: passes through center of curvature of mirror, not center of mirror
Primary and secondary focal points coincide
>   *Purkinje-Sanson images:* 4 images from reflecting surfaces of eye
>   1. Front surface of cornea (image of object at infinity is located at focal point of mirror = 1/–260 = –3.85 mm; thus, this is a virtual, erect, minified image 3.85 mm posterior to front surface of cornea)
>   **Example:** keratometry (see Fig. 1.28)
>
>   2. Back surface of cornea (virtual, erect, minified image)
>   3. Front surface of lens (virtual, erect, minified image)
>   4. Back surface of lens (real, inverted, minified image)
>   (If patient has IOL, Purkinje-Sanson images 3 and 4 are taken from front and back surfaces of the IOL, respectively; these are useful in assessment of mild degrees of pseudophacodonesis)

EYE AS OPTICAL SYSTEM

Model Eye

Gullstrand studied the eye's optical system and, based on average measurements (power = +58.64 D; F = 17.05 mm), he created a simplified model: the **"reduced"** or **"schematic" eye** (Fig. 1.17): power = +60 D; F = 17 mm; F' = 22.6 mm
>   **Example:** calculate the diameter of the blind spot projected 2 m in front of the eye (ON = 1.7 mm tall; thus, by similar triangles: 1.7/17 = x/2000; x = 2000(1.7/17) = 200 mm)

Vision Measurements

Minimum legible threshold: ability to distinguish progressively smaller forms; most commonly tested with Snellen visual acuity

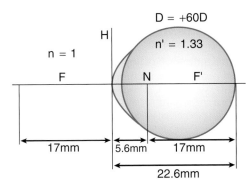
Figure 1.17 Schematic eye.

Minimum visible threshold: ability to distinguish lowest contrast of object from background; depends on amount of light striking photoreceptors

Minimum separable threshold: smallest angle at which two separate objects can be discriminated; detection of a break in a line

Vernier acuity: spatial discrimination; ability to detect smallest misalignment of two lines (8 seconds of arc; smaller than diameter of photoreceptor)

Snellen acuity: based on angle that smallest letter subtends on retina; each letter subtends 5 minutes of arc at a specific distance (represented by the denominator [i.e., 20/40 letter subtends 5 minutes at 40 feet, 20/20 letter subtends 5 minutes at 20 feet]; the numerator is the testing distance); each stroke width and space subtends 1 minute (Fig. 1.18)
>   **Example:** calculate the size of a 20/20 letter at 20 ft (6 m): tan = opposite/adjacent; tan 1' = 0.0003 therefore, tan 5' = 0.0015 = x/6000; x = 8.7 mm

Early Treatment Diabetic Retinopathy Study (ETDRS) chart: 5 letters per line; space between letters is equal to size of letter on that line; geometric proportion of optotype height (changes in 0.1 log unit increments)

Near acuity: must record testing distance

Acuity testing in children: optokinetic nystagmus (OKN); central, steady, maintain (CSM); preferential looking; Allen pictures; HOTV (letter symbols used in pediatric visual acuity testing); visual evoked potential (VEP)

Factors other than disease that reduce measured visual acuity: uncorrected refractive error, eccentric viewing, decreased contrast, smaller pupil size, older age

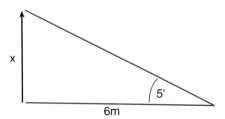
Figure 1.18 Calculation of Snellen letter size.

Legal blindness (in US): visual acuity (VA) ≤ 20/200 or visual field (VF) ≤20° in better-seeing eye

Visual acuity is influenced by pupil size: larger pupil limits vision owing to spherical and chromatic aberrations; smaller pupil limits vision owing to diffraction; optimal pupil size is 3 mm

Laser interferometer: helium-neon laser beam is split and projected onto retina, producing interference fringes; spacing of fringes can be varied; retinal function is estimated by narrowest fringes discernible

Contrast sensitivity: ability to detect difference in luminance between object and background. Snellen acuity tested at ~100% contrast (rare for daily tasks; 80% for most printed text).

Measured by modulation transfer function (MTF; Fourier transform of the point spread function): contrast degradation of a sinusoidal pattern at a spatial frequency relative to low frequencies; tested with targets of varying spatial frequency (light bands per unit length or per unit angle) and peak contrasts.

Contrast sensitivity is reciprocal of the contrast threshold, which is minimal resolvable target for a spatial frequency.

Contrast sensitivity function (CSF) is how contrast sensitivity changes in relation to spatial frequency; plotted to form a contrast sensitivity curve

Refractive Errors

Newborns have ~3 D of hyperopia, decreases to ~1 D by 2 years of age (changes in cornea and lens powers and axial length with eye growth)
At age 6 years, most children emmetropic, only 2% myopic (emmetropization; axial length increases 5 mm, power decreases in cornea 4 D and lens 2 D)

Myopia: increases with age; 3% in children 5-7 years old, 8% in children 8-10 years old, 14% in children 11-12 years old, 25% in children 12-17 years old; depends on ethnicity, higher rate of myopia in Chinese (12% in children 6 years old, 84% in children 16-18 years old)
  Juvenile-onset myopia: onset age is 7-16 years old, refractive error stable in ~75% by age 15-16 years; otherwise, progression into 20s and 30s
  Adult-onset myopia: onset in 20s, associated with extensive near work, incidence 20%-40%
  High myopia: −6 D or greater or axial length ≥26.5 mm; incidence 4%; increased risk retinal detachment, glaucoma, choroidal neovascularization

Hyperopia: increases with age (separate from cataract progression), ~20% of adults in 40s, ~60% adults in 70s-80s
  Total hyperopia = manifest hyperopia (absolute and facultative) + latent hyperopia (exposed with cycloplegia)

High ametropia, astigmatism, and anisometropia associated with poor nutrition
Refractive errors are described by focal point or far point

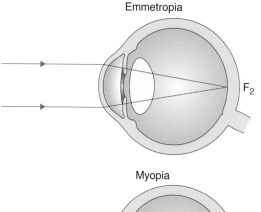

Emmetropia

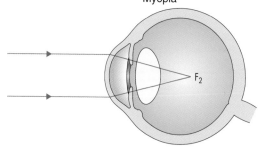

Myopia

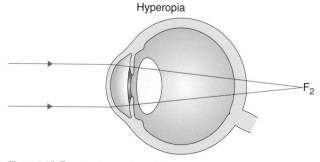

Hyperopia

Figure 1.19 Emmetropia, myopia, and hyperopia. In emmetropia, the focal point (F) is at the retina. In myopia, the focal point (F) is in the vitreous. In hyperopia, the focal point (F) is located behind the eye. (Modified with permission from Azar DT, Strauss L. Principles of applied clinical optics. In: Albert DM, Jakobiec FA, eds. *Principles and Practice of Ophthalmology,* vol 6, 2nd ed. Philadelphia: WB Saunders; 2000.)

Focal point: location of image formed by object at infinity through nonaccommodating eye (Fig. 1.19):
  Emmetropia: focal point on retina
  Myopia: focal point in front of retina
  Hyperopia: focal point behind retina

Far point: point in space conjugate to fovea in nonaccommodating eye. Farthest point eye can see clearly with accommodation completely relaxed (turn light around, start at retina, and trace rays backward through optics of eye; point at which rays intersect is far point)
  Emmetropia: far point is at infinity in front of eye
  Myopia: far point is centimeters to infinity in front of eye
  Hyperopia: far point is behind eye (virtual far point)

Axial vs. refractive:
  Axial myopia: length of eye too long (refractive power normal)
  Refractive myopia: refractive power too strong (length normal)
  Axial hyperopia: length too short (refractive power normal)

TABLE 1.1 Classification of astigmatism

Type	Location of focal lines	Corrective lens	
Compound myopic	Both in front of retina	– sph – cyl; – sph + cyl	(– sphere regardless of notation)
Simple myopic	1 in front, 1 on retina	– sph + cyl; plano – cyl	(– sphere or plano)
Mixed	1 in front, 1 behind	– sph + cyl; + sph – cyl	(– sphere or + sphere depending on notation)
Simple hyperopic	1 on retina, 1 behind	+ sph – cyl; plano + cyl	(+ sphere or plano)
Compound hyperopic	Both behind retina	+ sph + cyl; + sph – cyl	(+ sphere regardless of notation)

Refractive hyperopia: refractive power too weak (length normal)

Astigmatism: produces 2 focal lines rather than 1 focal point (Table 1.1)
   Classification: corneal or lenticular; regular (symmetric [mirror-image axis between eyes] or asymmetric) or irregular
   "With-the-rule": cornea is steepest in vertical meridian; axis of plus cylinder is 90° (±20°); usually young patients (elastic lids press on top and bottom of cornea)
   "Against-the-rule": cornea is steepest in horizontal meridian; axis of plus cylinder is 180° ± 20°; older patients

Correction of ametropia: choose lens with focal point that coincides with far point of patient's eye

Acquired hyperopia:
   Decreased effective axial length: retrobulbar tumor, choroidal tumor, central serous chorioretinopathy, posterior scleritis, serous retinal detachment
   Decreased refractive power: lens change (posterior lens dislocation, aphakia, diabetes), drugs (chloroquine, phenothiazines, antihistamines, benzodiazepines), poor accommodation (tonic pupil, drugs, trauma), flattening of cornea (contact lens, after radial keratotomy [RK] surgery), intraocular silicone oil

Acquired myopia:
   Increased lens power: osmotic effect (diabetes, galactosemia, uremia, sulfonamides), nuclear sclerotic cataracts, anterior lenticonus, change in lens position or shape (medication [miotics], anterior lens dislocation, excessive accommodation)
   Increased corneal power: keratoconus, congenital glaucoma, CL-induced corneal warpage
   Increased axial length: congenital glaucoma, posterior staphyloma, after scleral buckle, retinopathy of prematurity (ROP)

Night myopia: increased myopia in dark
   Pupil dilation: spherical aberration, irregular astigmatism uncovered
   Purkinje shift: spectral sensitivity shifts toward shorter wavelengths at lower light levels, and chromatic aberration moves the focal point anteriorly
   Dark focus: no accommodative target in dark; therefore, tend to overaccommodate for distance and underaccommodate for near
   Length of refraction lane: shorter than 20 feet produces 1/6 D undercorrection (add minus 0.25 D to final refraction)

Acquired astigmatism: lid lesion (tumor, chalazion, ptosis), pterygium, limbal dermoid, corneal degenerations and ectasias, surgery (corneal, cataract), lenticular, ciliary body (CB) tumor

Accommodation

Eye gains plus power when crystalline lens becomes more convex

Accommodation response can be described as:

Amplitude of accommodation: total dioptric amount eye can accommodate
   Near point: only for emmetropes
   Prince rule: combines reading card with a ruler calibrated in centimeters and diopters to measure amplitude of accommodation
   Technique: place +3.00 D lens in front of distance correction to bring far point to 1/3 m (33 cm); then, measure how near patient can read and convert into diopters; subtract far point from near point to determine amplitude
   Method of spheres: fixate on reading target (e.g., 40 cm), successively increase minus sphere until print blurs, then increase plus sphere until blurring occurs again; absolute difference between the spheres is the amplitude of accommodation
   Example: range of –4.00 D to +2.00 D = amplitude of 6 D

Range of accommodation: distance between far point and near point; measured with tape measure or accommodative rule
   Far point: point on visual axis conjugate to retina when accommodation is completely relaxed
   Near point: point on visual axis conjugate to retina when accommodation is fully active
      FOR MYOPIA: near point = amount of myopia + amplitude of accommodation
      FOR HYPEROPIA: near point = difference between amplitude of accommodation and amount of hyperopia

Presbyopia: loss of accommodation with age; becomes symptomatic in early 40s with asthenopic symptoms (i.e., eyestrain, fatigue, soreness, headache) and need for reading glasses

TABLE 1.2 Donder's table																
Age (years):	8	12	16	20	24	28	32	36	40	44	48	52	56	60	64	68
Accommodation (D):	14	13	12	11	10	9	8	7	6	4.5	3	2.5	2	1.5	1	0.5

Theories of accommodation:

Helmholtz: with accommodative effort ciliary muscle contracts, zonular tension decreases, outward tension on lens capsule decreases, lens becomes more convex, focusing power increases; presbyopia is caused by loss of lens elasticity

Coleman (catenary): zonules function as suspensory sling and lens curvature depends on opposing pressure between anterior and posterior chambers; ciliary muscle contracts, lens curvature steepens, and relative pressure between aqueous and vitreous causes central lens steepening and peripheral lens flattening

Schachar: equatorial zonular tension increases, lens diameter increases, central lens steepens, focusing power increases; lens grows throughout life, decreasing the working distance between lens and ciliary body; presbyopia is result of decreased ciliary muscle effectivity

Donder's table: average accommodative amplitudes for different ages (Table 1.2)

Up to age 40, accommodation decreases by 1 D every 4 years (starting at 14 D at age 8)

At age 40, accommodation is 6.0 D (±2 D)

Between ages 40 and 48, accommodation decreases by 1.5 D every 4 years

Above age 48, accommodation decreases by 0.5 D every 4 years

Conditions that cause asthenopia (eye fatigue with sustained near effort): hypothyroidism, anemia, pregnancy, nutritional deficiencies, chronic illness

Premature presbyopia (subnormal accommodation): debilitating illness, diphtheria, botulism, mercury toxicity, head injury, cranial nerve (CN) 3 palsy, Adie's tonic pupil, tranquilizers; treat with reading add, base-in prism (helps convergence)

Color Vision

3 components of color: hue, saturation, luminosity (lightness, brightness)

Hue: main component of color perception; depends on which wavelength is perceived as dominant; hue discrimination is the ability to distinguish between adjacent wavelengths

Saturation: richness of color; vivid colors are saturated; adding white desaturates color (paler) but does not change hue; saturation discrimination is measured by how much of a specific wavelength must be added to white before the mixture can be distinguished from white

Luminosity: sensation produced by retinal illumination; depends on relative luminous efficiency of the wavelengths; filters decrease brightness

Luminosity curve: illustrates sensitivity to different wavelengths

Constructed by asking observer to increase luminance of lights of various wavelengths until they appear equal in brightness to a yellow light of fixed luminance

Light-adapted eye: yellow, yellow-green, and orange appear brighter than blues, greens, and reds; peak sensitivity = 555 nm

Dark-adapted: peak sensitivity = 505 nm (blue)

Bezold-Brücke phenomenon: as brightness increases, most hues appear to change

At low intensities, blue-green, green, and yellow-green appear greener; at high intensities, they appear bluer

At low intensities, reds and oranges appear redder; at high intensities, they appear yellower

Exception: blue of 478 nm, green of 503 nm, and yellow of 578 nm do not change with changes in intensity

Abney effect: as white is added to any hue, desaturating it, the hue appears to change slightly in color; all colors (except yellow) appear yellower

Afterimages: after a color is stared at for 20 seconds, it begins to fade (desaturate)

Then, with gazing at white background, the complement of the color appears (afterimage)

Example: red is perceived when a greater number of red cones are stimulated than green or blue cones; after 20 seconds, red cones fatigue (cannot regenerate pigment fast enough), so color fades; when white background is looked at, there is a relatively greater response by green and blue cones; therefore, a blue-green afterimage is seen (complement of red)

Color perception: white wall appears white because white paint reflects all photons equally well

Charcoal appears black because it absorbs most of the light that strikes it

Blue flower appears blue because it best absorbs red, yellow, and green; blue is absorbed least, so a greater number of blue photons are reflected

Green leaf appears green because chlorophyll absorbs blue and red and reflects green

Incandescent/tungsten light emits a relatively greater number of photons of longer (red) wavelength than shorter (blue) wavelength; conversely, fluorescent light emits a relatively greater number of blue and green wavelengths; therefore, a purple dress may appear redder under incandescent light and bluer under fluorescent light

PRESCRIBING GLASSES

Use cycloplegia in children and hyperopes to uncover full refractive error

Children (Table 1.3): give full cycloplegic refraction

Adults: give manifest refraction; may not accept full astigmatic component, so if cylinder is decreased, adjust sphere to keep spherical equivalent constant; be careful about changing axis

Minus cylinder grinding: placing astigmatic correction on rear surface (closer to eye) is optically preferable

Astigmatic dial: 12 spokes corresponding to clock hours are projected on screen; spokes parallel to principal meridians of eye's astigmatism are sharp (corresponding with focal lines of conoid of Sturm); the others are blurred

Match base curves: when prescribing new glasses, keep base curve same as that of old lenses

Geneva lens clock: measures base curve of lens; direct dioptric power of convex, concave, or aspheric lens surface is read on the dial of the clock; calibration is based on the refractive index of crown glass (1.52)

Binocular balance: equally controls accommodation in both eyes (visual acuity must be equal)

Methods:

1. **PRISM DISSOCIATION:** 3 Δ BU over one eye and 3 Δ BD over the other (use Risley prism in phoropter)
2. **BALANCED FOGGING:** fog both eyes and alternate cover until equally fogged
3. **LANCASTER RED–GREEN (DUOCHROME) TEST:** red–green balance both eyes (vision must be ≥20/30); based on chromatic aberration

Bifocal add: place segments as high as practical in relation to optical centers of the distance lenses

Measure accommodation: perform monocularly, then binocularly

TABLE 1.3 Guidelines for prescribing glasses for children	
Hyperopia:	≥+5 D
Anisometropia:	≥1.5 D
Myopia:	
Up to age 1 year	≥−5 D
Ages 1–6 years	≥−3 D
Age >6 years	≥−1 D
Anisometropia	≥3 D
Astigmatism:	
Up to age 1 year	≥3 D
Ages 1–6 years	≥2 D
Age >6 years	≥1 D
Anisometropia	≥1.5 D

Near point of accommodation (use refractive correction)
Accommodative amplitude (use Prince rule)
Determine accommodative requirement for near vision task
Example: reading at 40 cm = 2.5 D
Hold 1/2 of measured accommodative amplitude in reserve to prevent asthenopic symptoms
Example: Prince rule measures 2.0 D of amplitude; thus 1.0 D is available to patient
Power of add is difference between accommodation (1.0 D) and total amount of accommodation required (2.5 D)
With calculated add in front of distance correction, measure accommodative range (near point to far point of accommodation); if range is too close, reduce add in steps of 0.25 D until correct range found

Kestenbaum rule: estimates strength of add power to read newspaper print (1.0 M, J5, 20/50, 8-pt font) without accommodation

Add power = reciprocal of best distance acuity
Reciprocal of add power = working distance (in meters)
Example: 20/80 vision; add = 80/20 = +4.00 D; working distance = 1/4 (0.25 m)

Aphakic spectacles: disadvantages include magnification of ~25%, altered depth perception, pincushion distortion, ring scotoma (prismatic effect at edge of lens causes visual field loss of 20% and "jack-in-the-box" phenomenon [peripherally invisible objects suddenly appear when gaze is shifted]), extreme sensitivity to lens position (vertex distance, tilt, height), problems with hand–eye coordination, cosmetic issues

Lens properties:

Index of refraction: higher index of refraction to reduce lens thickness for same power
Specific gravity: lower specific gravity to reduce lens weight
Abbe number: measure of chromatic aberration/distortion; higher number has better optical quality
Impact resistance: requirements by US Food and Drug Administration (FDA) and American National Standards Institute (ANSI) high-velocity impact standard (Z87.1)

Lens materials:

Glass: best optics and scratch resistant; low-impact resistance, thicker and heavier
Plastic: quality optics, lightweight, inexpensive, block 80% ultraviolet (UV) light; not thin, require coatings for scratch resistance and more UV blocking, not shatter resistant
Polycarbonate: plastic with higher index of refraction and lower specific gravity; thin, lightweight, high-velocity-impact resistant; high chromatic aberration, scratch easily (require coating)
Trivex: high-velocity-impact resistance, high optical quality, lightest weight, block all UV; not thin, scratch easily (require coating)
High index: index of refraction ≥1.60, glass or plastic, enables thinner lens for higher-power prescriptions, but increases weight and decreases optical quality, not

high-impact resistant, plastic scratches easily (require coating)

Absorptive lenses (sunglasses): advantages in high-illumination conditions include improve contrast sensitivity, preserve dark adaptation, reduce glare sensitivity (polarized lenses), photochromic lenses (short-wavelength light of 300–400 nm darken lens by reversibly converting silver ions to elemental silver), absorb UV light (5% sunlight is UV [90% UVA and 10% UVB]; UVA = 400–320 nm, UVB = 320–290 nm, UVC = <290 nm [absorbed by ozone])

CONTACT LENSES (CL)

Toric lens: lenses with different radii of curvature in each meridian
Front toric: anterior surface with two different radii of curvature, posterior surface spherical; corrects lenticular astigmatism
Back toric: cylinder on back surface only; corrects corneal astigmatism
Bitoric: minus cylinder on posterior surface, plus cylinder on anterior surface; corrects corneal and lenticular astigmatism

Ballasted lens: heavier base to orient lens by gravity; 2 types:
Prism: 1.5-2 Δ BD prism added
Truncated: flat along inferior edge

Sagittal depth/apical height: distance between back surface of lens center and a flat surface

Radius of curvature (base curve): curvature of posterior lens surface for a given diameter; the shorter the radius of curvature, the greater is the sagittal depth (the steeper the lens)

Overall diameter: for a given base curve, increasing diameter increases the sagittal depth
> **Example:** to tighten a lens, reduce radius of curvature (steeper base curve) or increase diameter

Oxygen transmission: *DK* (relative gas permeability) value; *D* = diffusion coefficient; *K* = solubility of oxygen in material; oxygen transmissibility – *DK/L* (*L* – lens thickness)

Accommodative demand: depends on magnification, which varies with different lens powers and vertex distances
Hyperopes: decreased accommodative demand when CL are worn compared with spectacles (presbyopic symptoms appear earlier with spectacles)
Myopes: increased accommodative demand when CL are used (presbyopic symptoms appear earlier with CL). In high myopia, spectacles induce base-in prism with near convergence, lessening requirement for convergence

Fitting rigid CL: SAM-FAP rule ("steeper add minus, flatter add plus")
Fit steeper than corneal surface (forms a plus tear meniscus between cornea and CL, which alters required power of CL). Therefore, need to subtract power (add minus) at end of calculation; for each diopter, the base curve is made steeper than *K*; subtract 1 D from the final CL power; if lens is fit flatter than *K*, a minus tear meniscus is formed, so must add plus power
Remember, a rigid lens with base curve of 44 D does not have a power of 44 D; rather, the radius of the CL's central posterior curve is equal to the radius of curvature of a cornea with a calculated power of 44 D

Power calculation: if trial lens not available for overrefraction
1. Measure refraction and keratometry
2. Choose base curve steeper than low *K* (usually +0.50 D steeper to form a tear lens; tear lens prevents apical touch)
3. Convert refraction to minus cylinder form and zero vertex distance; disregard the cylinder (minus cylinder is formed by the tears)
4. Power of CL is sphere from refraction adjusted for tear lens (subtract + 0.50); "SAM-FAP"

Evaluating fit:
Soft lens: evaluate movement (poor movement = too tight [too steep], excessive movement = too flat); choose power based on spherical equivalent
Rigid lens: assess fluorescein pattern (Figs. 1.20–1.22)

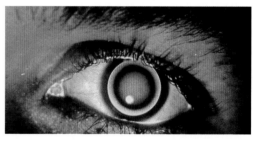

Figure 1.20 Fluorescein pattern of corneal contact lens fitted 1 D steeper than "flat K." Note the central clearance. (With permission from White P, Scott C. Contact lenses. In: Yanoff M, Duker JS, eds. *Ophthalmology.* London: Mosby; 1999.)

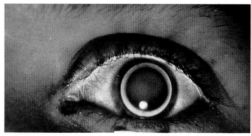

Figure 1.21 Fluorescein pattern of corneal contact lens fitted "on K." Note the central alignment. (With permission from White P, Scott C. Contact lenses. In: Yanoff M, Duker JS, eds. *Ophthalmology.* London: Mosby; 1999.)

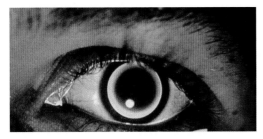

Figure 1.22 Fluorescein pattern of corneal contact lens fitted 1 D flatter than "flat K." Note the central touch. (With permission from White P, Scott C. Contact lenses. In: Yanoff M, Duker JS, eds. *Ophthalmology*. London: Mosby; 1999.)

VISION REHABILITATION

Vision impairment is visual acuity <20/40, blindness is best-corrected vision ≤20/200 or visual field ≤20°. Up to 1/3 have **Charles Bonnet syndrome** (vivid recurrent hallucinations in areas of visual loss, aware images are not real, normal cognitive status, no other neurologic symptoms [see Chapter 4, Neuro-Ophthalmology])

Low-vision evaluation for acuity <20/40, scotoma, field loss, reduced contrast sensitivity; multidisciplinary approach assessing magnification requirements for near work, daily activities, safety, driving, well-being, occupational therapy

Low-Vision Aids

Near devices:
High bifocal add or single-vision reading glasses (up to +20 D): large field of view but short reading distance; add power estimated as inverse of best-corrected distance visual acuity (Kestenbaum rule; see above)
Magnifiers: handheld (up to +20 D; small field of view) or stand (up to +50 D; bulky), illuminated or nonilluminated. For high-power stand magnifier, reference distance is 25 cm, magnification is lens power divided by 4 (for simple magnifier, $M_A = xP = P/4$)
Loupes: spectacle-mounted close-focusing telescopes; longer working distance but smaller field of view and depth of field
Electronic devices: video magnifiers (closed-circuit televisions [CCTVs]), computers, tablets; range of magnification, adjustable contrast, more comfortable reading distances, text-to-speech capability but expensive

Distance devices:
Telescopes: handheld monoculars, binoculars, and spectacle-mounted telescopes; provide magnification at longer distance but reduced contrast and smaller field of view and depth of field

Prosthetic devices:
Retinal implants: vision restoration; contrast and outlines with current technology

Field loss: rehabilitation for hemianopia (neurologic may have processing deficits) includes sector prisms (displace image from scotoma to area of sight), scanning and computer training

Nonoptical devices: many items for daily activities, including large-format devices (phones, watches, remote controls, playing cards, etc.), audio books, talking clocks and scales

INTRAOCULAR LENSES (IOL)

Formulas for IOL power calculation (see Chapter 10, Anterior Segment)

Requires accurate biometric measurements (axial length *[AL]* and central corneal power *[K]*), estimated (or effective) lens position (ELP), and desired/target postoperative refraction

ELP was originally a constant, the anterior chamber depth (ACD), because most IOLs were anterior chamber lenses. ELP became incorporated into the A constant and in newer generation formulas has been improved based on additional variables

Historical formulas: first formulas, based on refraction, obsolete

Theoretical formulas: based on theoretical optics
Regression: empiric based on data analysis, simple but frequent power errors
 FIRST GENERATION: Sanders-Retzlaff-Kraff (SRK), Gills-Lloyd
 SECOND GENERATION: SRK II, Thompson-M, Donzis
Vergence: based on geometric optics, more accurately predict ELP
 FIRST GENERATION: Binkhorst I, Fyodorov, Colenbrander
 SECOND GENERATION: Binkhorst II, Shamas
 THIRD GENERATION: Hoffer Q, Holladay 1, SRK/T
 FOURTH GENERATION: Holladay 2, Haigis, Barrett, Olsen
 FIFTH GENERATION: Barrett Universal II, Hoffer H-5
Other formulas: Hill-RBF (artificial intelligence, pattern recognition algorithm), Ladas Super Formula (amalgam of existing formulas)
A rough estimation of lens power can be quickly obtained with the SRK formula:
IOL power for emmetropia = $P = A - 2.5 L - 0.9 K$
 A = A constant (related to lens type); lens position important, 1 mm error = 1.0 D change in power
 L = axial length in mm; 1 mm error = 2.5 D error in IOL power
 K = average keratometry value in D; 1.0 D error = 1.0 D error in IOL power

IOL power adjustment for sulcus placement: power calculated for in-the-bag placement must be reduced when IOL placed in sulcus because of change in ELP (more anterior).
General rule is to reduce IOL power by 1.00 D, but adjustment depends on axial length (i.e., IOL power: higher power requires more adjustment with change in position)

IOL +28.5 – +30.0	subtract 1.5 D
+17.5 – +28.0	subtract 1.0 D
+9.5 – +17.0	subtract 0.5 D
+5.0 – +9.0	no change in power

When sulcus IOL optic is captured posteriorly through an intact capsulorhexis, no power change is necessary

Calculate IOL power for refractive target other than emmetropia: $D_{IOL} = P - (R/1.5)$ (R = desired refractive error)

IOL power for a different lens = original IOL power $\pm$ difference in A constants

Example: if instead of +20.0 D IOL with A constant of 118, you want to use a different style IOL with A constant of 118.5, equivalent power of the new IOL is +20.5 D

OPHTHALMIC INSTRUMENTS

Direct ophthalmoscope (Fig. 1.23): coaxial light and lenses to neutralize patient and examiner refractive errors, so retinas become conjugate; examiner uses optics of patient's eye as simple magnifier ($M_A = 60/4 = 15 \times$); field of view $\sim 7°$

Indirect ophthalmoscope (Fig. 1.24): enlarged field of view (25°) with stereopsis by adding condensing lens between patient and examiner; binocular eyepiece reduces interpupillary distance to 15 mm ($\sim 4 \times$); $M_A = D_{eye}/D_{lens} = 60/20 = 3 \times$; $M_{Ax} = 3^2 = 9$, but eyepiece reduces depth $4 \times$; therefore $M_{Ax} = 9/4 = 2.25 \times$

Retinoscope: instrument to objectively measure refractive state of eye

The blurred image of the filament on the patient's retina is considered a new light source returning to examiner's eye; by observing the characteristics of the reflex, examiner can determine patient's refractive error

If examiner is at far point of patient's eye, all light rays emanating from patient's pupil pass through retinoscope and examiner's pupil, and patient's pupil will appear uniformly illuminated (neutralization)

If far point is between examiner and patient (myopic), reflex moves in direction opposite to retinoscope sweep ("against" motion)

If far point is behind examiner (hyperopia), reflex has "with" motion

Use correcting lens to determine point of neutralization

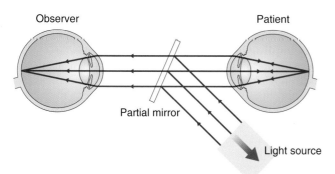

Figure 1.23 Optics of the direct ophthalmoscope. By using a mirror (either half-silvered or with a central aperture), the directions of the light of observation and the light incident to the patient are made concentric (coaxial). (With permission from Miller D, Thall EH, Atebara NH. Ophthalmic instrumentation. In: Yanoff M, Duker JS, eds. *Ophthalmology*, 2nd ed. St Louis: Mosby; 2004.)

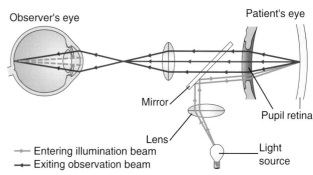

Figure 1.24 Theoretical optics of the indirect ophthalmoscope. The illumination beam enters a small part of the pupil and does not overlap with the observation beam; this minimizes bothersome reflection and backscatter. (With permission from Miller D, Thall EH, Atebara NH: Ophthalmic instrumentation. In: Yanoff M, Duker JS, eds. *Ophthalmology*, 2nd ed. St Louis: Mosby; 2004.)

Correct for working distance to obtain patient's final refraction (add reciprocal of working distance to final finding)

If poor, irregular retinoscopic reflex, try contact lens overrefraction or stenopeic slit refraction

Slit-lamp biomicroscope (Fig. 1.25): illumination and magnification allow stereo viewing of ocular structures; illumination and viewing arms have common pivot point

Applanation tonometry: direct measure of IOP as force/area with split-field prism; at applanated diameter of 3.06 mm,

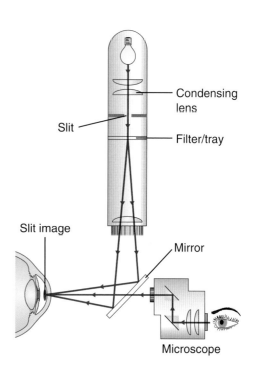

Figure 1.25 The slit lamp. Some slit lamps bring the light to a sharp focus within the slit aperture, and the light within the slit is focused by the condensing lens onto the patient's eyes. The observation system of a modern slit lamp has many potential reflecting surfaces; antireflection coatings on these surfaces help loss of light. (Modified from Spalton DJ, Hitchings RA, Hunter PA. *Atlas of Clinical Ophthalmology*. New York: Grower Medical; 1985.)

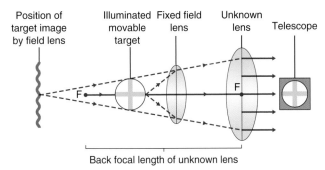

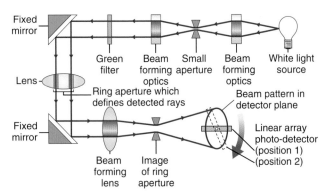

Figure 1.26 The lensometer resembles an optical bench. The movable illuminated target sends light to the field lens, with the target in the endpoint position. Because the focal point of the field coincides with the position of the unknown lens, all final images are of the same size. (With permission from Miller D, Thall EH, Atebara NH: Ophthalmic instrumentation. In: Yanoff M, Duker JS, eds. *Ophthalmology*, 2nd ed. St Louis: Mosby; 2004.)

Figure 1.27 Optics of a typical automated lensometer. Parallel light strikes unknown lens. The refracted light rays (which are confined to a pencil beam within an annulus) ultimately strike an array of electronic photoreceptors. (With permission from Miller D, Thall EH, Atebara NH. Ophthalmic instrumentation. In: Yanoff M, Duker JS, eds. *Ophthalmology*, 2nd ed. St Louis: Mosby; 2004.)

corneal resistance to deformation and attractive force of tear surface tension cancel each other

Lensometer: measures power of spectacle or CL using telescope to detect neutralization point; distance measurement is determined from back vertex power; add measurement is taken from front vertex power; prism measurement is derived from displacement of target pattern (Figs. 1.26 and 1.27)

Keratometer: measures curvature of anterior corneal surface based on power of reflecting surface; measures only 2 paracentral points separated by 90° at the 3- to 4-mm zone; doubling of image prevents interference from eye movements.

　Limitations: only measures small area, measures different regions for corneas of different powers, assumes cornea is spherocylindrical and symmetric with a major and minor axis separated by 90°, ignores spherical aberration, susceptible to focusing and misalignment errors, mire distortion prevents accurate measurement of irregular corneas (Fig. 1.28)

Corneal topographer: measures and images corneal surface; more data than keratometer, quantitates shape and patterns of astigmatism.

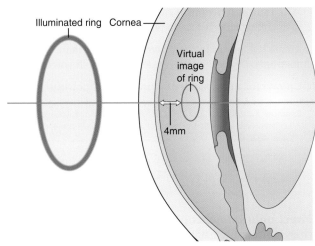

Figure 1.28 Keratometer principle. An illuminated ring is placed in front of the cornea, which acts as a convex mirror and produces a virtual image of the ring approximately 4 mm behind the cornea. (With permission from Miller D, Thall EH, Atebara NH: Ophthalmic instrumentation. In: Yanoff M, Duker JS, eds. *Ophthalmology*, 2nd ed. St Louis. Mosby, 2004.)

　Various technologies: placido based (videokeratoscopy), elevation based (raster photogrammetry, scanning slit), and interferometry based (laser holography, Moiré fringes). Computerized videokeratography (CVK) is most widely used; measures central and peripheral corneal zones and especially useful for evaluating irregular astigmatism; displays data as curvature (axial, instantaneous), power (refractive), elevation, difference, or relative maps; qualitative classification systems and quantitative indices and algorithms for data interpretation (simulated keratometry values, keratoconus screening, surface regularity index, surface asymmetry index, potential corneal acuity, contact lens fitting, etc.).

　Applications: diagnosis of corneal irregularities, screening refractive surgical candidates, evaluating unexplained visual loss, management of refractive, corneal, and cataract surgical patients, and contact lens fitting.

　Limitations: no standardization; depends on reference axis, alignment, and focus; susceptible to artifact (distortion, tear film effect); based on simplified optics (only applies to central cornea); smoothing effect (sampling occurs around the circumference of the mires, no measurement between mires)

Scheimpflug imaging: measures cornea and anterior segment structures with special cameras for greater depth of focus and sharper images. In normal camera, 3 planes (object, lens, and image) are parallel; in Scheimpflug camera, these planes are rotated to intersect at single point or plane resulting in greater depth of field. Data include corneal maps (pachymetry, topography and elevation of anterior and posterior surfaces), tomography, anterior chamber analysis, cataract densitometry

Wavefront aberrometer: measures and maps aberrations of eye, specifically higher-order aberrations (irregular astigmatism); most common is Hartmann-Shack; laser focused on retina acts as point source, reflected light travels back through eye, detected and analyzed to produce wavefront image

Optical biometer: measures ocular dimensions with laser interferometry for IOL calculations, including corneal curvature, anterior chamber depth, lens thickness, axial length, white to white, and others

Ultrasonography: measure acoustic reflectivity of interfaces to provide axial measurements and 2-dimensional images of ocular structures; various devices (A-scan, B-scan, ultrasound biomicroscope [UBM], pachymeter) (see Chapter 11, Posterior Segment)

Ocular coherence tomography: measures optical reflectivity to provide cross-sectional image of ocular structures; principle similar to B-scan ultrasonography but light (no sound), noncontact, higher-resolution pictures. Wavelength dependent: 1310 nm for anterior segment imaging; 820 nm for retinal imaging (see Chapter 11, Posterior Segment)

EQUATIONS

Vergence equation:

$n_1/u + P = n_2/v$

n = refractive index, u = object distance, P = lens power, v = image distance

$U + P = V$ (simple form)

U = object vergence, P = lens power, V = image vergence, n = refractive index

Lens power (diopters):

$P = 1/f$

f = focal length (meters)

Snell's law:

$n_1 \sin(i) = n_2 \sin(r)$

n = refractive index, i = angle of incidence, r = angle of refraction

Prismatic power:

$$\Delta = \frac{\text{image deflection (cm)}}{\text{meters}} = 100 \tan(\beta)$$

β = angle of deviation

Prentice rule:

$\Delta = h\text{D}$

h = distance from optical axis (cm), D = lens power

Reduced schematic eye (calculations of retinal image size):

$$\frac{I}{17\,\text{mm}} = \frac{O}{X}$$

I = retinal image size, O = object size, X = distance to object

Spherical equivalent:

spherical equivalent = sphere + (cylinder/2)

Refracting power of a spherical surface:

$$P = \frac{n_2 - n_1}{r}$$

n_2 = refractive index to right, n_1 = refractive index to left, r = radius of curvature of surface (m), (+ = convex; − = concave)

Lensmaker's equation (reflecting power of a spherical mirror):

$$P = \frac{-1}{f} = \frac{-2}{r}$$

f = focal length of mirror, r = radius of curvature of mirror (− = convex; + = concave)

Power of a thin lens immersed in fluid:

$$\frac{P_{\text{air}}}{P_{\text{aqueous}}} = \frac{n_{\text{IOL}} - n_{\text{air}}}{n_{\text{IOL}} - n_{\text{aqueous}}}$$

Power of lens at new vertex distance:

$$P_2 = P = S(P_1)^2$$

P_1 = original dioptric power of lens, P_2 = new dioptric power, S = difference in location (m)

Transverse (lateral or linear) magnification:

$M_T = I/O$

I = image distance or height, O = object distance or height

Longitudinal (axial) magnification:

$$M_L = (M_T)^2$$

Angular magnification:

$M_A = xP$

x = distance, P = dioptric power of lens

Simple magnifier:

$M_A = P/4$

(divide by 4 because distance set as reading distance of 0.25 m)

Example: 1 × magnifier = +4 lens; 2 × magnifier = +8 lens

Telescope (Galilean and astronomical):

$$M_A = -P_e / P_o$$

P_e = power of eyepiece, P_o = power of objective

Total accommodation through telescope:

$$A_T = A_N (M_A)^2$$

A_N = normal accommodation required, M_A = telescope magnification

IOL power (SRK):

$$P = A - 2.5\,L - 0.9\,K$$

A = A constant for type of IOL, L = axial length, K = average keratometry value

AC/A ratio (accommodative converge/ accommodation): (see Chapter 5, Pediatrics/Strabismus)

normal = 3 : 1 to 5 : 1 (expressed as PD of deviation per D of accommodation)

Calculations:

HETEROPHORIA METHOD: measure deviation with fixation target at 6 m and at 1/3 m

$$AC/A = \frac{\text{deviation at near} - \text{deviation at distance}}{\text{accommodative demand}} + PD$$

PD = interpupillary distance (cm)

LENS GRADIENT METHOD: stimulate accommodation by measuring deviation with target at 6 m, then remeasuring with −1 D sphere in front of both eyes; or, relax accommodation by measuring deviation with target at 1/3 m, then remeasuring with +3 D sphere in front of both eyes

$$AC/A = \frac{\text{deviation with lens} - \text{deviation without lens}}{\text{lens power}}$$

REVIEW QUESTIONS *(Answers start on page 407)*

1. A Prince rule is helpful in determining all of the following, *except*
   a. amplitude of accommodation
   b. near point of accommodation
   c. far point of accommodation
   d. accommodative convergence
2. A myope who pushes his spectacles closer to his face and tilts them is
   a. decreasing effectivity, increasing cylinder
   b. decreasing effectivity, decreasing cylinder
   c. increasing effectivity, decreasing cylinder
   d. increasing effectivity, increasing cylinder
3. The Prentice position refers to
   a. glass prism perpendicular to visual axis
   b. glass prism in frontal plane
   c. plastic prism perpendicular to visual axis
   d. plastic prism in frontal plane
4. The purpose of Q-switching a laser is to
   a. increase energy, increase power
   b. decrease energy, increase power
   c. decrease energy, decrease power
   d. increase energy, decrease power
5. A 50-year-old woman with aphakic glasses wants a new pair of spectacles to use when applying makeup. How much power should be added to her distance correction so that she can focus while sitting 50 cm in front of her mirror?
   a. −2.00 D
   b. −1.00 D
   c. +1.00 D
   d. +2.00 D
6. How far from a plano mirror must a 6-ft-tall man stand to see his whole body?
   a. 2 feet
   b. 3 feet
   c. 6 feet
   d. 12 feet
7. A 33-year-old woman with a refraction of −9.00 + 3.00 × 90 OD at vertex distance 10 mm and keratometry readings of 46.00 @ 90/43.00 @ 180 is fit for a rigid gas-permeable (RGP) contact lens 1 D steeper than flattest K. What power lens is required?
   a. −5.00 D
   b. −6.00 D
   c. −7.00 D
   d. −8.00 D
8. What is the size of a 20/60 letter on a standard 20-ft Snellen chart (tangent of 1 minute of arc = 0.0003)?
   a. 9 mm
   b. 15 mm
   c. 18 mm
   d. 27 mm
9. A Galilean telescope with a +5 D objective and a −20 D eyepiece produces an image with what magnification and direction?
   a. 4×, erect
   b. 4×, inverted
   c. 100×, erect
   d. 100×, inverted
10. An object is placed 33 cm in front of an eye. The image formed by reflection from the front surface of the cornea (radius of curvature equals 8 mm) is located
    a. 4 mm in front of cornea
    b. 4 mm behind cornea
    c. 8 mm in front of cornea
    d. 8 mm behind cornea
11. A convex mirror produces what type of image?
    a. virtual, inverted, magnified
    b. real, inverted, minified
    c. real, erect, magnified
    d. virtual, erect, minified

12. In general, the most bothersome problem associated with bifocals is
    a. image jump
    b. image displacement
    c. induced prism
    d. anisophoria

13. A refraction with a stenopeic slit gives the following measurements: +1.00 at 90° and −2.00 at 180°. The corresponding spectacle prescription is
    a. −2.00 + 1.00 × 90
    b. −2.00 + 1.00 × 180
    c. −2.00 + 3.00 × 180
    d. +1.00 + 3.00 × 90

14. A point source of light is placed 1/3 of a meter to the left of a +7 D lens. Where will its image come to focus?
    a. 25 cm to the right of the lens
    b. 25 cm to the left of the lens
    c. 10 cm to the right of the lens
    d. 10 cm to the left of the lens

15. What is the equivalent sphere of the following cross cylinder: −3.00 × 180 combined with +0.50 × 90?
    a. −1.00
    b. −1.25
    c. −1.50
    d. −1.75

16. What is the size of a letter on a standard 20-ft Snellen chart if it forms an image of 0.5 mm on a patient's retina?
    a. 59 cm
    b. 30 cm
    c. 25 cm
    d. 18 cm

17. The image of a distant object is largest in which patient?
    a. aphake with contact lens
    b. hyperope with spectacles
    c. emmetrope
    d. myope with spectacles

18. What type of image is produced if an object is placed in front of a convex lens within its focal length?
    a. erect and real
    b. erect and virtual
    c. inverted and real
    d. inverted and virtual

19. What is the correct glasses prescription if retinoscopy performed at 50 cm shows neutralization with a plano lens?
    a. −2.00
    b. −1.50
    c. plano
    d. +2.00

20. An anisometropic patient experiences difficulty while reading with bifocals. Which of the following is *not* helpful for reducing the induced phoria?
    a. dissimilar segments
    b. slab-off lens
    c. progressive lenses
    d. Fresnel "press-on" prisms

21. A Geneva lens clock is used to measure what?
    a. thickness
    b. power
    c. index of refraction
    d. base curve

22. What is the induced prism when a 67-year-old woman reads 10 mm below the upper segment optical center of her bifocals, which measure +2.50 + 1.00 × 90 OD and −1.50 + 1.50 × 180 OS add +2.50 OU
    a. 4.0 Δ
    b. 3.5 Δ
    c. 2.5 Δ
    d. 2.0 Δ

23. The optimal size of a pinhole for measuring pinhole visual acuity is approximately
    a. 2.50 mm
    b. 2.00 mm
    c. 1.25 mm
    d. 0.75 mm

24. A person looking at an object 5 m away through a 10 Δ prism placed base-in over the right eye would see the image displaced
    a. 20 cm to the right
    b. 50 cm to the right
    c. 20 cm to the left
    d. 50 cm to the left

25. Calculate the soft CL power for a 40-year-old hyperope who wears +14.00 D glasses at a vertex distance of 11 mm.
    a. +15.00 D
    b. +16.00 D
    c. +17.00 D
    d. +18.00 D

26. After cataract surgery, a patient's refraction is −0.75 + 1.75 × 10. In what meridian should a suture be cut to reduce the astigmatism?
    a. 180°
    b. 100°
    c. 90°
    d. 10°

27. What is the appropriate correction in the IOL power if the A constant for the lens to be implanted is changed from 117 to 118?
    a. decrease IOL power by 1.0 D
    b. increase IOL power by 1.0 D
    c. decrease IOL power by 0.5 D
    d. increase IOL power by 0.5 D

28. An IOL labeled with a power of +20 D has a refractive index of 1.5. If this lens were removed from the package and measured with a lensometer, what power would be found?
    a. +10 D
    b. +13 D
    c. +30 D
    d. +59 D

29. The total cylindrical power of a 0.50 D cross cylinder is
    a. plano
    b. 0.25 D
    c. 0.50 D
    d. 1.00 D

30. To minimize image displacement in a hyperope, the best type of bifocal segment style is
    a. flat top
    b. progressive
    c. round top
    d. executive

31. The logMAR equivalent to 20/40 Snellen acuity is
    a. 0.4
    b. 0.3
    c. 0.2
    d. 0.1

32. A patient who is pseudophakic in one eye and phakic in the other eye will have what amount of aniseikonia?
    a. 1%
    b. 2.5%
    c. 5%
    d. 7%

33. A patient with 20/80 vision is seen for a low-vision evaluation. What add power should be prescribed so that the patient does not have to use accommodation to read the newspaper?
    a. +3
    b. +4
    c. +8
    d. +16

34. The spherical equivalent of a −2.00 + 1.50 × 90 lens is
    a. +0.50
    b. −0.50
    c. −1.25
    d. −3.50

35. After extracapsular cataract extraction, a patient is found to have 2 D of with-the-rule astigmatism and a tight suture across the wound at 12 o'clock. Corneal topography is obtained, and the placido disc image shows an oval pattern with the mires closest together at
    a. 12 o'clock, with the short axis at 90°
    b. 12 o'clock, with the short axis at 180°
    c. 6 o'clock, with the short axis at 90°
    d. 6 o'clock, with the short axis at 180°

36. A 57-year-old woman has a 0.25 mm macular hole in her left eye. The size of the corresponding scotoma on a tangent screen at 1 m is approximately
    a. 1.0 cm
    b. 1.5 cm
    c. 2.5 cm
    d. 3.0 cm

37. During retinoscopy, when neutralization is reached, the light reflex is
    a. narrowest and slowest
    b. narrowest and brightest
    c. widest and slowest
    d. widest and fastest

38. A patient undergoing fogged refraction with an astigmatic dial sees the 9 to 3 o'clock line clearer than all the others. At what axis should this patient's minus cylinder correcting lens be placed?
    a. 30°
    b. 45°
    c. 90°
    d. 180°

39. Myopia is associated with all of the following conditions, *except*
    a. nanophthalmos
    b. pigment dispersion syndrome
    c. spherophakia
    d. nuclear sclerotic cataract

40. What is the ratio of the magnification from a direct ophthalmoscope to the magnification from an indirect ophthalmoscope with a 20D lens at a distance of 25 cm if the patient and examiner are both emmetropic?
    a. 15 : 2
    b. 10 : 3
    c. 5 : 1
    d. 4 : 1

41. A patient with anisometropia wears glasses with a prescription of +5.00 OD and +1.25 OS. Which of the following actions will *not* reduce the amount of aniseikonia?
    a. decrease base curve of right lens
    b. decrease center thickness of left lens
    c. decrease vertex distance of the glasses
    d. fit the patient with CL

42. The principal measurement determined by a Prince rule and +3 D lens in front of the patient's eye is the
    a. range of accommodation
    b. amplitude of accommodation
    c. near point of accommodation
    d. accommodative convergence

43. The 10× eyepiece of the slit-lamp biomicroscope is essentially a simple magnifier. Using the standard reference distance of 25 cm, what is the dioptric power of the 10× eyepiece?
    a. +2.5 D
    b. +10 D
    c. +25 D
    d. +40 D

44. When refracting an astigmatic patient with a Lancaster dial, the examiner should place the
    a. circle of least confusion on the retina
    b. posterior focal line on the retina
    c. anterior focal line behind the retina
    d. entire conoid of Sturm in front of the retina

45. To increase the magnification of the image during indirect ophthalmoscopy, the examiner should
    a. move closer to the condensing lens
    b. move the eyepiece prisms farther apart
    c. use a higher-dioptric-power condensing lens
    d. remove the plus lens in the eyepiece

46. A patient with which of the following refractive errors is most likely to develop amblyopia?
    a. −4.00 OD, −1.50 OS
    b. +1.00 + 0.50 × 180 OD, −1.00 + 0.50 × 180 OS
    c. +5.00 OD, +5.00 OS
    d. −3.00 + 2.00 × 90 OD, −2.00 + 1.00 × 90 OS

47. A 23-year-old man reports blurry vision at near and wears +1.25 reading glasses to see clearly. Which of the following is most likely to be found on examination?
    a. latent hyperopia
    b. nuclear sclerosis
    c. premature presbyopia
    d. exophoria

48. In 1 year, a diabetic 60-year-old woman has a change in refraction from −5.00 to −6.50 OU, which improves her

vision to 20/20 OU. What is the most likely cause of her refractive change?
a. steepening anterior corneal curvature
b. increasing axial length
c. increasing nuclear sclerosis
d. cystoid macular edema

49. The most common cause of monocular diplopia is
a. uncorrected astigmatism
b. anterior basement membrane dystrophy
c. posterior capsular opacity
d. epiretinal membrane

50. A patient with a prescription of –5.50 sphere OD and –1.00 sphere OS is 20/20 in each eye, but glasses cause headache and double vision. The most likely reason is
a. esophoria
b. spherical aberration
c. image jump
d. aniseikonia

51. A hyperopic refraction is most likely caused by
a. a steep cornea and a short axial length
b. a steep cornea and a long axial length
c. a flat cornea and a short axial length
d. a flat cornea and a long axial length

52. How much accommodation is needed for a patient with a distance correction of +1.50 to read without correction at 40 cm?
a. +1.50
b. +2.50
c. +4.00
d. +5.50

53. The limbal relaxing incision for a patient with a refraction of +0.75 – 1.50 × 180 and no lenticular astigmatism should be placed at
a. 45°
b. 90°
c. 150°
d. 180°

54. The denominator in the Snellen visual acuity notation 20/60 represents
a. the lowest line where the patient was able to read at least three letters
b. the distance in feet from the patient to the chart
c. the angle between the patient and the chart
d. the distance at which the letter subtends the standard visual angle

55. A 26-year-old-woman with a history of myopic LASIK complains of blurriness OD. Her uncorrected visual acuity is 20/20, but corneal topography shows a decentered ablation. Which aberration is most likely to be found on wavefront analysis?
a. 1st order
b. 2nd order
c. 3rd order
d. 4th order

56. If a Snellen chart is not present, then which of the following tests is best for evaluating visual acuity?
a. contrast sensitivity
b. wavefront aberrometry
c. Scheimpflug imaging
d. optical coherence tomography

57. A cycloplegic refraction would be most helpful for a
a. 10-year-old who has headaches
b. 19-year-old who cannot see road signs clearly
c. 44-year-old who notices more trouble reading
d. 65-year-old who has trouble seeing a golf ball

58. The most likely cause of a refractive surprise after uncomplicated cataract surgery is
a. incorrect preoperative refraction
b. failure to obtain cycloplegic refraction
c. lack of corneal pachymetry measurement
d. wrong keratometry readings

59. Decreased color discrimination is most likely to be caused by which type of cataract?
a. nuclear sclerotic
b. cortical
c. anterior subcapsular
d. posterior subcapsular

60. A three-piece acrylic IOL intended for the capsular bag is placed in the sulcus without optic capture through the capsulotomy. This patient is most likely to experience what type of refractive error?
a. astigmatism
b. emmetropia
c. hyperopia
d. myopia

61. Six weeks following manual extracapsular cataract surgery with a superior limbal incision, the patient's refraction is found to be –2.00 + 4.00 × 95. The best initial treatment for this residual refractive error is
a. suture removal
b. limbal relaxing incision
c. photorefractive keratectomy
d. IOL exchange

62. Which test is most useful for following a patient with Fuchs dystrophy?
a. ultrasound biomicroscopy
b. corneal pachymetry
c. keratometry
d. gonioscopy

63. A 28-year-old man with anisometropia and amblyopia has a best-corrected visual acuity of 20/15 OD and 20/40 OS. His refraction is +0.25 + 0.25 × 75 OD and +3.75 + 0.25 × 90 OS. Which of the following is the best treatment option?
a. full spectacle prescription
b. +3.75 contact lens in the left eye
c. cycloplegia of the right eye
d. patching of the right eye

64. A patient with cataracts and best-corrected visual acuity of 20/50 complains that glasses do not work well enough. Which is the best nonsurgical option to help this patient?
a. increase pantoscopic tilt
b. use dissimilar curves
c. increase add power
d. increase refractive index

65. Which higher-order aberration has the least effect on visual quality?
a. coma
b. spherical aberration
c. secondary astigmatism
d. trefoil

SUGGESTED READINGS

Basic and Clinical Sciences Course. (2021). *Section 3: Clinical optics*. San Francisco: AAO.

Benjamin, W. J. (2006). *Borish's clinical refraction* (2nd ed.). Philadelphia: Elsevier.

Milder, B., Rubin, M. L., & Weinstein, G. W. (1991). *The fine art of prescribing glasses without making a spectacle of yourself*. Gainesville: Triad Scientific Publications.

Rubin, M. L. (1993). *Optics for clinicians*. Gainesville: Triad Scientific Publications.

2

Pharmacology

OCULAR PHARMACOLOGY

Pharmacodynamics: the study of the biochemical and physiologic effects of drugs and their mechanisms of action

Pharmacokinetics: the study of the factors that determine the relationship between drug dosage and the change in concentration over time in a biological system; the movement of drug through the body, including absorption, distribution, metabolism, and excretion

Bioavailability: the amount of drug absorbed (penetration into ocular tissues)
  Depends on concentration, rate of absorption, tissue binding, transport, metabolism, and excretion
  Methods of improving bioavailability:
    INCREASE CONCENTRATION: limited by solubility and tonicity (hypertonicity causes reflex tearing, which dilutes and washes drug from the eye); drug with poor solubility can be formulated as suspension or emulsion
    SURFACTANTS: surface-active agents alter cell membranes, increasing permeability of the corneal epithelium
    OSMOTICS: alter tonicity to make more isotonic
    LIPID SOLUBILITY: increasing improves corneal penetration
    INCREASE PH: increases nonionized (lipid-soluble) form of drug, increasing corneal penetration (pH of tears = 7.4)
    INCREASE VISCOSITY: viscous additives (methylcellulose, polyvinyl alcohol) increase contact time and therefore penetration

    INCREASE CONTACT TIME: gels and oil-based ointment formulations (mineral oil, petrolatum), polymer matrix (DuraSite); must be able to release drug

Toxicity: adverse effects of drug and other components of medications (preservatives); affected by pharmacodynamics and pharmacokinetics
  Topical ocular medications absorbed through mucous membranes (conjunctiva, nasopharynx), iris, and ciliary body, which avoids first-pass metabolism of liver, increasing risk of systemic effects, particularly in children; 50%–99% of dose can be absorbed systemically, but amount limited by tear dilution and washout
  Preservatives: can enhance corneal permeability and have corneal toxicity
    QUATERNARY AMMONIUMS (CATIONIC SURFACTANTS, DETERGENTS): benzalkonium chloride (BAK), benzododecinium bromide, cetrimide, polyquaterniu apraclonidine m-1
    ORGANOMERCURIALS: thimerosal
    BIGUANIDES: chlorhexidine
    ALCOHOLS: chlorobutanol, phenylethanol
    PARABENS: methylparaben, propylparaben
    OXIDANTS: sodium perborate, stabilized oxychloro complex, stabilized chlorite peroxide (less toxicity, dissipate to inert substances with light exposure)
  Ethylenediaminetetraacetic acid (EDTA) is common buffering agent; ionic buffers with borate, sorbitol, propylene glycol, and zinc become inert when they react with tear film cations
  Toxicity: thimerosal > BAK > chlorobutanol > methyl paraben > sodium perborate
  Preservative-free drops are least toxic

25

Therapeutic index: a method of comparing potency of different antibiotics; a measure of relative effective (therapeutic) concentration of antibiotic at target site against a target organism

Inhibitory quotient (IQ): The most potent antibiotic has the lowest minimum inhibitory concentration (MIC) (or highest inhibitory quotient)

ROUTES OF ADMINISTRATION

Topical: absorption related to corneal penetration

1 drop = 50 μL (20–40 drops in most bottles)

Conjunctival cul-de-sac holds only 10 μL (20% of drop)

Drop diluted by reflex tearing and normal tear turnover: only ~50% of drug that reaches the cul-de-sac is present 4 minutes later (10% of drop), and only 17% (3.4% of drug) is present after 10 minutes

Corneal barriers to penetration:

    TIGHT JUNCTIONS (epithelium and endothelium): limit passage of hydrophilic drugs

    STROMA (water rich): limits passage of lipophilic drugs

Methods of increasing absorption:

1. Add surfactants (disrupts epithelial integrity; e.g., benzalkonium chloride, topical anesthetic).
2. Promote punctal occlusion (decreases drainage).
3. Close eyelid (no blinking) after drops are placed for 5 minutes.
4. Increase lipid solubility of drug (increases pH); more important than water solubility.
5. Increase frequency of drops.

Topical medications have systemic adverse effects because the drugs bypass hepatic "first-pass" metabolism (cul-de-sac → nasolacrimal duct → mucosa → bloodstream).

Examples of other delivery systems:

    PRODRUG: inactive drug derivatives (usually ester or amide) with better ocular penetration that are activated by enzymes in eye; dipivalyl epinephrine (Propine; prodrug of epinephrine, less toxicity), nepafenac (Nevanac; prodrug of amfenac), prostaglandin analogues (latanoprost, travoprost, bimatoprost, tafluprost), valacyclovir (Valtrex; prodrug of acyclovir)

    OINTMENT: drugs that have better uptake in ointment form, including tetracycline, chloramphenicol, and fluorometholone

    SUSTAINED RELEASE GEL: pilocarpine (Pilopine HS; decreased dosing)

    INSERT: may be soluble or insoluble (more constant rate of release but requires removal); pilocarpine (Ocusert; membrane-controlled system; slow release over 1 week); hydroxypropyl cellulose (Lacrisert; artificial tear slow-release pellet)

    IMPLANTS: sustained drug delivery (alternative to repeated injections); ganciclovir, fluocinolone acetonide, and dexamethasone intravitreal implants; bimatoprost (Durysta) intracameral implant

    COLLAGEN CORNEAL SHIELDS: drug-impregnated contact lens–like devices; dissolve within 1–3 days, releasing high drug concentrations (usually antibiotics) on ocular surface

    CONTACT LENS: hydrogel lens presoaked in drug solution

    PUNCTAL PLUG: drug-filled core releases into tear film; plug may cause irritation or may extrude

    GEL FORMING DROP: nonviscous drop that transforms to gel at body temperature

    ENCAPSULATED CELL TECHNOLOGY: cells within semipermeable capsule secrete over time after inserted into vitreous

    LIPOSOMES: synthetic lipid microspheres containing water-soluble drug or hydrophobic drug incorporated into lipid membrane; topical administration but short shelf life, limited drug capacity, and stability issues

    NANOTECHNOLOGY: biodegradable nanoparticles to transport drugs and genes

    IONTOPHORESIS: electrical current to move charged molecules, can achieve high drug concentration (i.e., antibiotic in cornea and anterior chamber); limitations include discomfort and tissue damage

    MICROELECTROMECHANICAL SYSTEMS: implantable device with reservoir, refill port, battery, electronics, electrolysis chamber, and pars plana cannula to deliver microdoses of drug into vitreous (antiangiogenics for age-related macular degeneration [AMD], steroids for uveitis)

Subconjunctival/sub-Tenon: increases duration and concentration, bypasses conjunctival and corneal barriers, avoids systemic toxicity; useful if poor compliance

Retrobulbar/peribulbar: used for anesthesia; alcohol or chlorpromazine (to kill pain fibers and optic nerve [ON] in blind, painful eye)

Intraocular: direct ocular effects; beware toxicity (particularly from preservatives [corneal endothelial damage/failure, toxic anterior segment syndrome (TASS), retinal ischemia, vasculitis]), retinal tear, retinal detachment (RD), endophthalmitis; used intraoperatively (intracameral, intravitreal) and in retinal diseases (intravitreal), including macular edema (cystoid macular edema [CME], diabetic macular edema [DME], retinal vein occlusion [RVO], uveitis), choroidal neovascularization (CNV), endophthalmitis, cytomegalovirus (CMV) retinitis

Systemic: must cross blood–ocular barrier (blood–aqueous for anterior segment, blood–retinal for posterior segment); penetrance is improved with decreased molecular size, decreased protein binding, and increased lipid solubility

Concentration

1% solution = 1 g/100 mL = 10 mg/mL

    Example: How much atropine is contained in 5 mL of a 2% solution?

    2% = 2 g/100 mL = 20 mg/mL = 100 mg in 5 mL

Conversion shortcut: multiply drug percentage by 10 to obtain concentration in mg/mL

Example: 2% = 2 × 10 = 20 mg/mL = 100 mg in 5 mL

FDA approval process: 3 steps for new drug application (NDA)

Phase 1: human testing for toxicology and pharmacokinetic data

Phase 2: randomized controlled trials to determine safety and efficacy

Phase 3: controlled and uncontrolled trials to evaluate risk–benefit and physician labeling

ANESTHETICS

Mechanism: reversible blockade of nerve fiber conduction (block sodium channels); pH dependent (less effective at low pH [inflamed tissue])

Structure: two classes; do not necessarily have allergic cross-reactivity

Ester: hydrolyzed by plasma cholinesterase and metabolized in liver; cocaine, tetracaine, proparacaine, procaine, benoxinate

Amide: longer duration and less systemic toxicity; metabolized in liver; lidocaine, mepivacaine, bupivacaine

Topical: disturb intercellular junction of corneal epithelium (increase permeability)

Proparacaine (Alcaine, Ophthetic, Ophthaine): duration 10–30 minutes, corneal toxicity; may cause allergic dermatitis (also common with atropine and neomycin); does not necessarily have allergic cross-reactivity with tetracaine

Tetracaine (Altacaine, TetraVisc, Pontocaine): similar to proparacaine but longer onset and duration and more toxic to corneal epithelium

Benoxinate (oxybuprocaine): similar to proparacaine

Cocaine: greatest epithelial toxicity; excellent anesthesia, sympathomimetic effect (test for Horner syndrome)

Fluorescein is available in combination with proparacaine (Fluoracaine, Flucaine) or benoxinate (Fluress, Flurox) for tonometry

Parenteral: may be used with epinephrine (1:100,000) to cause vasoconstriction, increasing duration by reducing systemic absorption; also decreases bleeding; hyaluronidase (Wydase) 150 IU breaks down hyaluronic acid in the extracellular matrix, increasing tissue penetration and reducing anesthetic volume needed, but decreases duration; side effect of retrobulbar anesthesia = respiratory depression, bradycardia

Toxicity: hypotension, convulsions, nausea, vomiting

Procaine (Novocain): duration 30–45 minutes (1 hour with epinephrine)

Lidocaine (Xylocaine): duration 1 hour (2 hours with epinephrine); used for local anesthesia, akinesia

Mepivacaine (Carbocaine): duration 2 hours

Bupivacaine (Marcaine): duration 8 hours (8–12 hours with epinephrine); often combined with lidocaine (for rapid onset and long duration) and hyaluronidase (for better diffusion in orbit) for retrobulbar and peribulbar blocks

General: all agents decrease intraocular pressure (IOP) except ketamine, chloral hydrate, N_2O, and ether

Malignant hyperthermia: rare, autosomal-dominant condition that occurs after exposure to inhalation agents (most commonly halothane, also succinylcholine, haloperidol); more common in children and males; thought to be a result of calcium-binding disorder in sarcoplasmic reticulum that causes increased intracellular calcium, which stimulates muscle contraction

Interference with oxidative phosphorylation causes hypermetabolic crisis

Most have defect in ryanodine receptor (*RYR-1* gene on chromosome 19q13.1)

FINDINGS: tachycardia (first sign), elevated CO_2 levels, tachypnea, unstable blood pressure (BP), arrhythmias, cyanosis, sweating, muscle rigidity (trismus from masseter rigidity), increased temperature (later sign); later, heart failure and disseminated intravascular coagulation develop; laboratory tests show respiratory and metabolic acidosis and increased K, Mg, myoglobin, and creatine phosphokinase, as well as hypoxemia, hypercarbia, and myoglobinuria

SCREENING: elevated creatine phosphokinase, muscle biopsy/contracture test, platelet bioassay (decreased adenosine triphosphate in platelet exposed to halothane)

TREATMENT: stop anesthesia, hyperventilate with 100% oxygen, give sodium bicarbonate, cool patient (iced saline intravenous [IV] and lavage; surface cooling), mannitol and furosemide (Lasix), IV dantrolene (prevents release of calcium from sarcoplasmic reticulum), procainamide, insulin (do not use lactated Ringer solution, which increases potassium)

PROGNOSIS: <5% mortality

AUTONOMIC SYSTEM

Sympathetic

Extensive system for mass response ("fight or flight") (Table 2.1)

Synapses near cord (superior cervical ganglion)

Long postganglionic nerves

Adrenergic receptors:

α_1: smooth muscle contraction (arteries [decrease aqueous production by reducing ciliary body blood flow], iris dilator, Müller muscle)

α₂: feedback inhibition, ciliary body (decreases production and/or increases outflow)

β₁: cardiac stimulation

β₂: pulmonary and gastrointestinal (GI) smooth muscle relaxation, ciliary body/trabecular meshwork (increase aqueous production, increase outflow facility)

Neurotransmitter: acetylcholine (ACh) at preganglionic terminal, epinephrine and norepinephrine (NE) at postganglionic terminal

Monoamine oxidase (MAO) breaks down NE in nerve terminal; blocked by MAO inhibitors (avoid with phenylephrine, epinephrine, and pseudoephedrine-based cold remedies)

Catechol-*O*-methyltransferase breaks down NE in effector cell

Reserpine prevents storage of NE in nerve terminal

Cocaine, tricyclics block reuptake of NE by nerve terminal (thus potentiate its action)

Hydroxyamphetamine increases release of NE from nerve terminal

Table 2.1	Autonomic system responses	
Organ/Function	**Sympathetic (fight/flight)**	**Parasympathetic (homeostasis)**
HR	Increase	Decrease
BP	Increase	Decrease
GI motility	Decrease	Increase
Bronchioles	Dilate	Constrict
Bladder	Constrict	Dilate
Vessels	Constrict	Dilate
Sweat	Decrease	Increase
Pupils	Dilate	Constrict
Eyelids	Elevate	Normal

BP, *Blood pressure;* GI, *gastrointestinal;* HR, *heart rate.*

Parasympathetic

More limited system for discrete response (homeostatic)
Synapses near end organ (ciliary ganglion)
Short postganglionic nerves

Cholinergic receptors:

Nicotinic: somatic motor and preganglionic autonomic nerves (extraocular muscles, levator, orbicularis [outside eye])

Muscarinic: postganglionic parasympathetic nerves (iris sphincter, ciliary muscle [inside eye])

Neurotransmitter: ACh

Acetylcholinesterase (AChE) breaks down ACh

Cholinergic Drugs

Direct-acting agonists: act on end organ; therefore, do not need intact innervation; cause shallowing of anterior chamber (AC); disruption of blood–aqueous barrier, miosis, brow ache, and decrease in IOP

Acetylcholine (Miochol: very short acting, unstable, used intracamerally), methacholine, carbocholine (carbamylcholine, carbachol; direct and indirect acting), pilocarpine (less potent than ACh, but resistant to AChE; no miosis if IOP > 40 mm Hg)

Varenicline (Tyrvaya nasal spray; causes lacrimation to treat dry eye disease)

Indirect-acting agonists: anticholinesterases (AChE inhibitor); strongest agents; cause miosis and decrease in IOP (contract longitudinal fibers of ciliary muscle = increased outflow of trabecular meshwork)

Reversible: carbocholine, physostigmine (eserine; treat lid lice), edrophonium (Tensilon; for diagnosis of myasthenia gravis), neostigmine (treat myasthenia gravis and urinary retention); can cause bradycardia, treat with atropine

Irreversible: echothiophate (phospholine iodide; treat glaucoma and accommodative esotropia; may cause iris cysts and subcapsular cataracts), isoflurophate (very long-acting, not used clinically), demecarium

Adverse effects: cataract, RD, pupillary block, blocks metabolism of succinylcholine (prolonged respiratory paralysis) and ester anesthetics, can mimic acute abdomen (GI effects); antidote is pralidoxime (PAM) or atropine

Muscarinic antagonists: anticholinergics; cause deepening of AC, stabilization of blood–aqueous barrier, mydriasis, and cycloplegia

Atropine (1- to 2-week duration; most allergenic, supersensitivity seen in Down syndrome), scopolamine (hyoscine; 1-week duration; greater central nervous system [CNS] toxicity than atropine), homatropine (1- to 3-day duration), cyclopentolate (Cyclogyl; 24-hour duration; beware CNS side effects with 2% solution, especially in children), tropicamide (Mydriacyl; 4- to 6-hour duration)

Toxicity: mental status changes, hallucinations, tachycardia, urinary retention, dry mouth/skin, fever

Antidote: physostigmine (1–4 mg IV)

Nicotinic antagonists:

Nondepolarizing agents: gallamine, pancuronium, vecuronium, rocuronium; do not cause muscle contraction

Depolarizing agents: succinylcholine, decamethonium; cause muscle contraction and elevated IOP; contraindicated for ruptured globe (extraocular muscle contraction can cause extrusion of intraocular contents)

Adrenergic Drugs

Sympathomimetics: may cause mydriasis, vasoconstriction, decreased IOP

Direct-acting α-agonists: epinephrine, phenylephrine, dipivefrin, clonidine, apraclonidine (Iopidine), brimonidine (Alphagan, Lumify), methyldopa, naphazoline (Naphcon, Vasocon, Opcon), oxymetazoline (Afrin, OcuClear, Visine LR, Upneeq), tetrahydrozoline (Visine)

Direct-acting β-agonists: epinephrine, isoproterenol, terbutaline, dopamine, albuterol (salbutamol)

Indirect-acting agonists: cocaine, hydroxyamphetamine (Paredrine), ephedrine

Sympatholytics: may cause decreased IOP

General blockers: guanethidine, bethanidine, protriptyline, 6-hydroxydopamine

α-blockers: thymoxamine, dibenamine, phentolamine, prazosin, labetalol, dapiprazole (Rev-Eyes; miosis)

β-blockers: timolol, levobunolol, betaxolol, metipranolol, carteolol, propranolol, metoprolol, atenolol, nadolol, pindolol

OCULAR HYPOTENSIVE (GLAUCOMA) MEDICATIONS

β-Blockers

Mechanism: reduce aqueous production (inhibit Na^+/K^+ pump) by decreasing cyclic adenosine monophosphate production in ciliary epithelium; ~20% IOP reduction

Loss of effectiveness over time as a result of downregulation of β-receptors (long-term drift)

Adverse effects: dry eye syndrome (decreased corneal sensitivity), bradycardia, heart block, bronchospasm, impotence, lethargy, depression, headache, rarely diarrhea and hallucinations, alopecia, dermatitis; may mask hypoglycemia

Nonselective ($β_1$ and $β_2$): *timolol* (Timoptic), *levobunolol* (Betagan), *metipranolol* (Optipranolol), *carteolol* (Ocupress)

10% do not show a therapeutic effect; inhibit lipoprotein lipase (break down chylomicrons and very-low-density lipoprotein [VLDL]) and cholesterol acyltransferase (incorporate cholesterol into high-density lipoprotein [HDL]); may cause decreased serum HDL levels (except carteolol)

Carteolol has intrinsic sympathomimetic activity

Cardioselective ($β_1 \gg β_2$): *betaxolol* (Betoptic)

Fewer pulmonary adverse effects

Indications: patients with pulmonary problems who cannot tolerate nonselective β-blockers; often used for normal-tension glaucoma; may not cause as much vasoconstriction of vessels supplying ON

α₂-Agonists

Apraclonidine (Iopidine), **brimonidine** (Alphagan P):

Mechanism: reduce aqueous production by decreasing episcleral venous pressure, increase uveoscleral outflow. Brimonidine may have neuroprotective properties by upregulating neurotrophin, basic fibroblast growth factor, and cellular regulatory genes.

Adverse effects: allergy, superior lid retraction, dry mouth, blanching of conjunctival vessels (vasoconstrictive effect, apraclonidine > brimonidine; can prolong iris sphincter ischemia in angle closure), miosis,

lethargy, headache, stomach cramps; avoid in children, especially <3 years of age: increased risk of somnolence, seizures, apnea as a result of CNS penetration; contraindicated in infants because of systemic toxicity with hypotension, hypothermia, and bradycardia

Dipivefrin (Propine): prodrug of epinephrine (converted into epinephrine in cornea by esterases), lower concentration and increased solubility versus epinephrine (penetrates cornea 17 × better); thus, less toxicity and fewer adverse effects

Mechanism: improves aqueous outflow, slightly reduces aqueous production

Adverse effects: allergy, CME in aphakia, hypertension, tachycardia (fewer systemic adverse effects than epinephrine)

Epinephrine: 1%–2% is equivalent to Propine 0.1%; 3 salt forms: hydrochloride, borate, bitartrate (first 2 are equivalent, 2% bitartrate is equivalent to 1% hydrochloride or borate)

Mechanism: improves aqueous outflow, slightly reduces aqueous production

Adverse effects: allergy, CME in aphakia (reversible), hypertension, tachycardia, arrhythmias, adrenochrome (black) deposits in conjunctiva

Miotics

Mechanism: increase aqueous outflow (contraction of ciliary muscle opens trabecular meshwork), decrease uveoscleral outflow

Pilocarpine: only direct cholinergic agonist; peak action at 2 hours, 8-hour duration

Beware for treatment of angle closure: causes shallowing of AC and narrowing of angle, but miosis pulls peripheral iris away from angle, balancing out the other effects

Adverse effects: headache, brow ache, accommodative spasm, miosis (dimming, reduction of vision), induced myopia (forward shift of lens–iris diaphragm), pupillary block, follicular conjunctivitis, dermatitis, nyctalopia, rarely retinal tear or even RD

Other effects: breakdown of blood–aqueous barrier, reduction of uveoscleral outflow, increased depth of field (result of miosis; to treat presbyopia [Vuity])

Carbachol: direct and indirect cholinergic agonist; stronger effect and longer duration of action; poor corneal penetration; needs corneal surface disrupter (benzalkonium chloride); intraocular formulation (Miostat 0.01%) used intracamerally during surgery for pupillary miosis (more effective, longer duration, and decreased IOP compared with acetylcholine [Miochol 1%], which is faster acting)

Echothiophate (phospholine iodide): indirect cholinergic agonist (cholinesterase inhibitor); 3-week duration; also used in accommodative esotropia

Adverse effects: greater orbicularis, ciliary, and iris muscle spasm; cataracts in adults (therefore, use only in aphakic or pseudophakic patients); iris cysts in children (proliferation of iris pigment epithelium; phenylephrine prevents cyst formation); decreased serum pseudocholinesterase activity (can accentuate succinylcholine effects during general anesthesia)

Carbonic Anhydrase Inhibitors (CAIs)

Mechanism: decrease bicarbonate formation in ciliary body epithelium; bicarbonate formation is linked to Na+ and fluid transport, so CAIs reduce aqueous production
Carbonic anhydrase catalyzes the reaction:
$$CO_2 + H_2O \leftrightarrow H_2CO_3$$
Amount of carbonic anhydrase is 100 × that needed for aqueous production; so >99% must be inhibited to achieve IOP decrease
Sulfonamide derivative (do not administer to patients with sulfa allergy)

Oral: *acetazolamide* (Diamox; per os [PO]/IV), *methazolamide* (Neptazane, PO; more lipid soluble, less toxicity); also for treatment of idiopathic intracranial hypertension, may be effective for cystoid macular edema
Adverse effects: dry eye syndrome (decreased tear production), metabolic acidosis (IV administration causes greater metabolic acidosis), kidney stones (reduced excretion of urinary citrate or magnesium; less risk with methazolamide which is metabolized in liver), hypokalemia (especially when used with other diuretics; very dangerous with digoxin), paresthesias (hands/feet /lips), GI upset, diarrhea, lethargy, loss of libido, weight loss, metallic taste, aplastic anemia, Stevens-Johnson syndrome; transient myopia

Topical: *dorzolamide* (Trusopt), *brinzolamide* (Azopt); ~15% IOP reduction
Adverse effects: metallic taste, paresthesias, malaise, weight loss, depression, skin rash, corneal endothelial decompensation/toxicity (consider stopping before cataract surgery)

Prostaglandin Analogues/Prostanoids

Mechanism: increase uveoscleral outflow, ~30% IOP reduction

Latanoprost (Xalatan), **bimatoprost** (Lumigan, Durysta implant), **travoprost** (Travatan), **tafluprost** (Zioptan), **latanoprostene bunod** (Vyzulta), **unoprostone isopropyl** (Rescula): prostaglandin $F_{2\alpha}$ analogues (Vyzulta is a nitric oxide–donating prostaglandin analogue that also increases trabecular outflow; Rescula is a related docosanoid compound)
Adverse effects: flu-like symptoms, hyperemia, eyelash growth, periocular skin and iris pigmentation (increases number of melanosomes but not melanocytes), prostaglandin-associated periorbitopathy (upper lid ptosis, deepening of upper lid sulcus, involution of dermatochalasis, periorbital fat atrophy,

mild enophthalmos, inferior scleral show, increased prominence of lid vessels, tight eyelids), CME, reactivation of herpes simplex virus (HSV) keratitis

Rho Kinase (ROCK) Inhibitors

Mechanism: increase trabecular outflow, reduce aqueous production, reduce episcleral venous pressure (regulates smooth muscle tone, relaxation of vascular endothelial smooth muscle)

Netarsudil (Rhopressa):
Adverse effects: conjunctival hyperemia, conjunctival hemorrhage, cornea verticillata

Hyperosmotic Agents

Mechanism: low-molecular-weight substances that increase serum osmolality to draw fluid out of eye (reduces vitreous volume)
Adverse effects: headache, thirst, nausea, vomiting, diarrhea, diuresis, dizziness, and rebound IOP elevation; IV agents can cause subarachnoid hemorrhage

Urea (IV; 30% solution): not commonly used; extravasation causes tissue necrosis

Mannitol (Osmitrol; IV; 20% solution): most potent; may exacerbate congestive heart failure

Glycerin (Osmoglyn; PO; 50% solution): may cause hyperglycemia in diabetics (metabolized by liver into glucose; discontinued in 2004, can compound by diluting 100% solution)

Isosorbide (Ismotic; PO): not metabolized (can be used in diabetics); secreted 95% unchanged in urine

Other hyperosmotic agents: used topically for corneal edema
Glycerin (Ophthalgan; topical; 100% solution): used to clear corneal edema for examination or laser procedure
Muro 128 (hypertonic saline; topical; drops or ointment; 2.5% or 5% strength): used to reduce epithelial edema of cornea, especially in treatment of recurrent erosions

Combinations

Brimonidine-timolol (Combigan)

Brinzolamide-brimonidine (Simbrinza)

Dorzolamide-timolol (Cosopt)

Netarsudil-latanoprost (Rocklatan)

Allergenicity

apraclonidine > epinephrine > dipivefrin brimonidine > β-blocker > pilocarpine

ANTI-INFLAMMATORY DRUGS

Inflammatory Pathway

Arachidonic acid, released from cell membrane phospholipids, produces mediators of inflammation. Arachidonic acid is converted into hydroperoxides (by lipoxygenase) or endoperoxides (by cyclooxygenase); hydroperoxides form a chemotactic agent and leukotrienes (slow-reacting substance of anaphylaxis); endoperoxides form prostaglandins (mediate inflammation), prostacyclin (vasodilator and platelet antiaggregant), and thromboxane (vasoconstrictor and platelet aggregator) (Fig. 2.1).

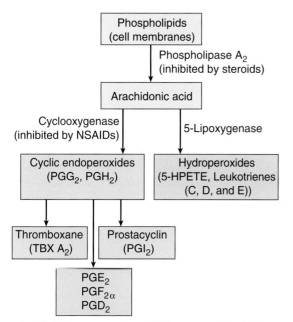

Figure 2.1 The inflammatory pathway. *NSAIDs,* nonsteroidal anti-inflammatory drugs; *PG,* prostaglandin; *5-HPETE,* 5-hydroperoxyeicosatetraenoic acid.

Nonsteroidal Anti-Inflammatory Drugs (NSAIDs)

Mechanism: block inflammatory mediators by inhibiting cyclooxygenase pathway

Classes:

Salicylates: acetylsalicylic acid (ASA; aspirin), diflunisal, salicylamide

Acetic acids: indomethacin (indometacin), diclofenac (Voltaren), sulindac, etodolac, ketorolac (Acular, Toradol), nepafenac (Nevanac, Ilevro), bromfenac (Xibrom, Bromday, BromSite, Prolensa)

Phenylalkanoic acids: ibuprofen, suprofen (Profenal), flurbiprofen (Ocufen), naproxen, fenoprofen, ketoprofen

Cyclooxygenase-2 (COX-2) inhibitors: celecoxib (Celebrex); rofecoxib (Vioxx; discontinued) and valdecoxib (Bextra; discontinued)

Indications:

Prevent miosis during intraocular surgery: Profenal, Ocufen

Allergic conjunctivitis, corneal pain, postsurgical inflammation, CME: Voltaren, Acular, Nevanac, Ilevro, Xibrom, Bromday, BromSite, Prolensa (topical NSAIDs without concomitant steroid have been associated with corneal melting)

Scleritis, uveitis: oral agents

Adverse effects:

Oral: GI (peptic ulcers), cardiovascular (heart attack, stroke), nephrotoxicity, hepatotoxicity; Reye syndrome (associated with aspirin use in children with febrile viral infections); hypersensitivity reactions (mediated by leukotrienes), cornea verticillata (i.e., indomethacin, ibuprofen, naproxen)

Topical: corneal melting

Glucocorticoids (Corticosteroids, Steroids)
(Table 2.2)

Table 2.2 Common ophthalmic steroids	
Generic name	**Trade name**
Topical	
Prednisolone acetate 1%	Pred Forte, Omni Pred
Fluorometholone acetate 0.1%	Flarex
Dexamethasone alcohol 0.1%	Maxidex
Fluorometholone alcohol 0.1%	FML
Prednisolone phosphate 1%	Inflamase
Dexamethasone phosphate 1%	Decadron
Difluprednate 0.05%	Durezol
Loteprednol etabonate 1%	Inveltys
Loteprednol etabonate 0.5%/0.38%	Lotemax, Lotemax SM
Loteprednol etabonate 0.25%	Eysuvis
Loteprednol etabonate 0.2%	Alrex
Subconjunctival	
Dexamethasone phosphate	Decadron
Methylprednisolone acetate	Solu Modrol, Depo Modrol
Prednisolone acetate	Durapred, Omnipred
Triamcinolone acetonide	Kenalog
Betamethasone	Celestone
Intravitreal	
Triamcinolone acetonide	Kenalog, Triesence

Mechanism: block release of arachidonic acid from phospholipids by inhibiting phospholipase A₂; anti-inflammatory and immunosuppressive effects, including inhibiting release of lysosomal enzymes, preventing macrophage migration, interfering with lymphocyte function, decreasing fibroblast activity, inhibiting neovascularization, and reducing capillary permeability

Classes:

Ester: loteprednol

Ketone: all others

Preparations (ketones):

Phosphate: hydrophilic; poor penetration of intact corneal epithelium (improved penetration with epithelial defect)

Alcohol: biphasic; penetrate intact cornea

Acetate: more biphasic; best corneal penetration

Potency: increased by 1 or 2 double bond(s), 9 fluorination, 6 methylation, O at C11; IOP elevation from deoxygenation at C21 (Table 2.3)

Derivatives of progesterone (weaker): fluorometholone (FML), medrysone

Table 2.3	Relative anti-inflammatory activity of steroids
Steroid	**Relative anti-inflammatory activity**
Hydrocortisone	1 (the standard)
Cortisone	0.8
Medrysone	4
Prednisone	4
Prednisolone	5
Triamcinolone	5
Dexamethasone	25
Betamethasone	25
Rimexolone	25
Loteprednol	25
Fluorometholone	40
Difluprednate	60
Fluocinolone	240

Subconjunctival/sub-Tenon injection: produces higher ocular concentration and longer duration; beware in IOP responder

Other routes of administration: oral, IV, intraocular

Oral dose of 7.5 mg dexamethasone results in intravitreal concentration of therapeutic levels

Indications: conjunctivitis, keratitis, scleritis, uveitis, hyphema, CME, macular edema, CNV, endophthalmitis

Adverse effects:

Systemic: adrenal insufficiency, hyperglycemia, hypertension, hypokalemia, peptic ulcers, delayed wound healing, superinfection, emotional lability, psychosis, insomnia, growth retardation, muscle atrophy, osteoporosis (most common cause of osteoporosis before age 50; 30%–50% of patients have fracture, and up to 40% develop osteonecrosis on long-term steroids), aseptic necrosis of the hip, hirsutism, weight gain, Cushingoid appearance, pseudotumor cerebri

Check purified protein derivative (PPD) and controls, complete blood count (CBC), blood glucose, lipid profile, and chest radiographs before starting systemic steroids, and follow height, bone mineral density, and spinal x-ray during long-term treatment. Peptic ulcer prophylaxis with H_2-blocker (ranitidine [Zantac], famotidine [Pepcid]) or proton pump inhibitor (omeprazole [Prilosec], lansoprazole [Prevacid]), and preventive treat-

ment of steroid-induced osteoporosis with calcium (1000–1500 mg qd), vitamin D (800 IU qd), and possibly a bisphosphonate (alendronate, risedronate, or zoledronate) or teriparatide during long-term treatment.

Ocular: posterior subcapsular cataract (PSC), elevated IOP/glaucoma, delayed wound healing/corneal reepithelialization, scleral melting, secondary infections (e.g., HSV, fungal), mydriasis, ptosis, eyelid skin atrophy

IOP-elevating potential: difluprednate > dexamethasone > prednisolone > fluorometholone > hydrocortisone > tetrahydrotriamcinolone > medrysone (after 6 weeks of dexamethasone therapy, 42% have IOP > 20 mm Hg; 6% have IOP > 31 mm Hg); depends on potency, formulation, and delivery method

Steroids with less IOP-elevating potential: rimexolone (Vexol), loteprednol (Inveltys, Lotemax, Alrex, Eysuvis)

OCULAR DECONGESTANTS

Sympathomimetic α-agonists, reduce conjunctival hyperemia by vasoconstriction; available over the counter (OTC)

Naphazoline (Naphcon, Opcon, Vasocon), **oxymetazoline** (0.025%; Afrin, OcuClear, Visine LR), **tetrahydrozoline** (Visine)

Indications: eye redness

Adverse effects: rebound vasodilation and conjunctival injection with chronic use

Oxymetazoline hydrochloride (0.1%; Upneeq): elevates upper eyelid by stimulating Müller muscle; prescription only (4 × concentration of OTC product)

Indications: acquired blepharoptosis

Adverse effects: punctate keratitis, dry eye, blurred vision, headache

Brimonidine (0.025%; Lumify): less risk of rebound vasodilation (OTC, ≤ 1/4 concentration of Alphagan)

Phenylephrine hydrochloride (Mydfrin): used diagnostically, dilates pupil, elevates eyelid, reduces conjunctival injection

ANTIALLERGIC MEDICATIONS

Antihistamines/Vasoconstrictors (OTC)

Naphazoline hydrochloride/pheniramine maleate (OcuHist, Opcon-A, Naphcon-A), **naphazoline hydrochloride/antazoline phosphate** (Vasocon-A): vasoconstrictor naphazoline temporarily relieves redness, but can cause rebound redness with chronic use

Mast Cell Stabilizers

Cromolyn (cromoglicate; Crolom; Opticrom), **nedocromil** (Alocril), **pemirolast** (Alamast), **lodoxamide** (Alomide, 2500 times more effective than cromolyn): reduce permeability of mast cell plasma membrane, preventing release of histamine; reduce phosphodiesterase activity (facilitator of mast cell degranulation); inhibit activation of neutrophils, monocytes, and eosinophils; do not interfere with binding of antigen to previously sensitized cells; no antihistamine activity and therefore useful for chronic allergies, not for acute symptomatic relief

H₁-Blockers (Antihistamines)

Levocabastine (Livostin; discontinued), **emedastine** (Emadine), **cetirizine** (Zerviate): pure H_1-specific receptor antagonists; bind to histamine receptors (inhibit itching and hyperemia)

H₁-Blockers + Mast Cell Stabilizers

Ketotifen (Zaditor, Alaway), **olopatadine** (Patanol, Pataday, Pazeo), **azelastine** (Optivar), **epinastine** (Elestat), **bepotastine** (Bepreve), **alcaftadine** (Lastacaft): stabilize mast cells and bind to H_1 receptors (inhibit itching); bind to H_2 receptors at low level (inhibit hyperemia)

IMMUNOMODULATORY THERAPY

Immunomodulatory therapy (IMT) agents (immunosuppressives or disease-modifying antirheumatic drugs [DMARDS]) modify or regulate immune functions; used in uveitis when vision-threatening or steroid inadequate, contraindicated, or dependent; classified as nonbiologic (antimetabolites, alkylating agents, and T-cell inhibitors; response may take months) and biologic (tumor necrosis factor [TNF] inhibitors, other immune mediators; faster response); maintain steroids, then taper after IMT response
> *Indications:* ocular cicatricial pemphigoid, necrotizing scleritis, Behçet disease, sympathetic ophthalmia, Vogt-Koyanagi-Harada (VKH) syndrome, serpiginous choroidopathy, and other severe, chronic noninfectious uveitis
> *Contraindications:* infection, recent live vaccination, liver/kidney/blood disorder, pregnant or breastfeeding
> *Adverse effects:* serious complications, including nephrotoxicity, hepatotoxicity, bone marrow suppression, malignancy, infection (opportunistic and secondary), sterility; therefore must monitor CBC with differential, liver and renal function tests

Nonbiologic Agents (Conventional Immunosuppressives)

Antimetabolites

Inhibit purine-ring biosynthesis

Azathioprine (Imuran): purine analogue, interferes with DNA replication and ribonucleic acid (RNA) transcription, alters purine metabolism; efficacy depends on thiopurine S-methyltransferase (TPMT) enzyme activity level in patient (should be normal to high); inflammation control in ~50%
> *Adverse effects:* GI upset, nausea, emesis, cytopenias, hepatitis

Methotrexate (Rheumatrex, Trexall): folate analogue; inhibits enzyme dihydrofolate reductase and folate metabolism; inhibits synthesis of deoxythymidine monophosphate nucleotide and DNA replication; anti-inflammatory effect from adenosine release; given with folate to reduce risk of side effects; effective in sarcoidosis, panuveitis, scleritis, juvenile idiopathic arthritis (JIA)–associated anterior uveitis, and primary intraocular lymphoma; steroid sparing in 67%
> *Adverse effects:* cytopenias, liver, lung or renal toxicity, GI upset, anorexia; teratogenic; periorbital edema, hyperemia

Mycophenolate mofetil (CellCept): purine analogue; inhibits inosine monophosphate dehydrogenase, purine synthesis, and DNA replication; steroid sparing in 85%
> *Adverse effects:* GI upset, diarrhea, hepatitis, cytopenias

Alkylating Agents

Create cross-linkage between DNA strands, resulting in inhibition of transcription of messenger RNA (mRNA) and prevention of DNA synthesis; increased risk of malignancy; therefore used for recalcitrant vision-threatening or life-threatening disease (necrotizing scleritis associated with systemic vasculitis, sympathetic ophthalmia, Behçet disease, VKH syndrome, intermediate uveitis)

Chlorambucil (Leukeran): interacts with 7-guanine of DNA, resulting in strand breakage or cross-linkage; drug-free remission in up to 75%
> *Adverse effects:* cytopenias, hematologic malignancy, sterility; must monitor CBC

Cyclophosphamide (Cytoxan): alkylates purines, interferes with DNA replication; inflammation control in 85%
> *Adverse effects:* hemorrhagic cystitis (oral > IV; prevent with high water intake), bladder cancer, renal transitional cell cancer, cytopenias, alopecia, opportunistic infections (prophylaxis with trimethoprim-sulfamethoxazole), sterility; must monitor CBC and urinalysis

T-Cell Inhibitors

Cyclosporine (Neoral, Sandimmune): calcineurin inhibitor, blocks production of interleukin-2 (IL-2) and IL-2 receptors, inhibits proliferation of lymphocytes, inhibits T-cell activation and recruitment; macrolide product of fungus *Beauveria nivea*; inflammation control in ~50%
> *Indications:*
> > TOPICAL: dry eye disease, ligneous conjunctivitis, atopic keratoconjunctivitis, vernal keratoconjunctivitis

SYSTEMIC: Mooren ulcer, uveitis in Behçet disease or sympathetic ophthalmia, prevention of corneal transplant rejection; also used in ocular cicatricial pemphigoid (OCP) and thyroid eye disease

Adverse effects: systemic administration is associated with renal toxicity (renal tubular atrophy, interstitial fibrosis), hypertension, anemia, fatigue, paresthesia, peripheral neuropathy, elevated erythrocyte sedimentation rate (ESR), hypertrichosis, hepatotoxicity, hyperuricemia; must monitor blood pressure, CBC, creatinine

Tacrolimus (Prograf, Envarsus, Astagraf, Protopic): calcineurin inhibitor, blocks production of IL-2 and IL-2 receptors, and T-cell receptor expression, inhibits T-cell activation; product of *Streptomyces tsukubaensis*; steroid sparing in 85%

Indications: chronic posterior and intermediate uveitis

Adverse effects: renal toxicity and hypertension (less than cyclosporine), neurotoxicity

Sirolimus (Rapamune): inhibits T-cell activation, reduces T- and B-cell responses to lymphokines

Adverse effects: pulmonary toxicity, malignancy, impaired wound healing, diabetes-like symptoms

Lifitegrast (Xiidra): small-molecule integrin antagonist, inhibits T-cell–mediated inflammation (blocks binding of lymphocyte function-associated antigen-1 (LFA-1; T-cell surface receptor) to intercellular adhesion molecule-1 (ICAM-1; expressed in cornea and conjunctiva)

Indications: topical for dry eye disease

Biologic Agents

Genetically engineered proteins made from living organism or its products that inhibit targeted cytokine and cell interactions (e.g., antibodies, interleukins, vaccines, cells, genes); specific indications or when nonbiologics are ineffective

Tumor Necrosis Factor-α (TNF-α) Inhibitors

TNF-α may be important in JIA, ankylosing spondylitis, spondyloarthropathies

Adalimumab (Humira; human monoclonal IgG1 antibody against TNF-α), **infliximab** (mouse/human chimeric antibody; less tolerated); others include **certolizumab, golimumab:** inflammation control in up to 100%

Indications: noninfectious intermediate, posterior, and panuveitis in adults, Behçet disease, HLA-B27-associated uveitis, JIA-associated uveitis, sarcoidosis, VKH syndrome

Adverse effects: increased risk tuberculosis and opportunistic infections, lymphoma, anaphylaxis, hepatitis B reactivation, demyelinating disease, cytopenia, heart failure, stroke, psoriasis, and lupus-like syndrome

Lymphocyte Inhibitors

Rituximab (Rituxan; chimeric antibody against CD20 cells (B lymphocytes); also **abatacept, daclizumab:** Behçet disease, necrotizing scleritis, pemphigoid

Specific Receptor Antagonists

Tocilizumab (Actemra): interleukin-6 antagonist

Indications: with steroid taper for giant cell arteritis in adults

Adverse effects: runny nose, sinus pain, sore throat, headache, dizziness, itching, abdominal pain, urinary tract infection, hypertension, increase blood cholesterol, increase risk of cancer and infection

Others

Interferon alfa-2a (IFN-α2a, Roferon, Pegasys): antiviral, immunomodulatory, and antiangiogenic properties; inflammation control in 90% with Behçet uveitis and 60% in non-Behçet uveitis.

Adverse effects: flu-like symptoms, cytopenias, depression

Interferon alfa-2b: subconjunctival, intralesional, or topical for conjunctival intraepithelial neoplasia, squamous cell carcinoma, and Kaposi sarcoma; systemic for melanoma, lymphoma, hairy cell leukemia, genital warts, hepatitis B and C

Adverse effects: headache, GI upset, nausea, diarrhea, fatigue, back pain, dizziness

Teprotumumab (Tepezza): monoclonal antibody inhibitor of insulin-like growth factor-1 receptor

Indications: thyroid eye disease

Adverse effects: muscle spasm, nausea, alopecia, diarrhea, fatigue, hyperglycemia, hearing loss, dysgeusia, headache, dry skin

Repository corticotropin (Acthar gel): adrenocorticotropic hormone (ACTH)

Indications: severe acute and chronic allergic and inflammatory processes of eye and adnexa

Adverse effects: infection, stomach ulcers, mood changes, depression, insomnia, acne, dry skin, bruising, skin thinning, delayed wound healing, sweating, headache, dizziness, vertigo, blurred vision, swelling, weight gain, shortness of breath, seizures, bloody stool, pancreatitis, low potassium, hypertension

Cenegermin (Oxervate): recombinant human nerve growth factor (rhNGF; first topical biologic)

Indications: neurotrophic keratitis

ANTINEOPLASTIC DRUGS

Various mechanisms of action to cause cell death; biologic therapy also used for cancer to regulate immune system

Alkylating agents: act directly on DNA, prevent cell division; busulfan, carboplatin, chlorambucil, cyclophosphamide, melphalan, thiotepa (topically in pterygium surgery to prevent recurrence)

Angiogenesis inhibitors: inhibit angiogenesis, endothelial proliferation, and other signaling pathways.

Vascular endothelial growth factor (VEGF) inhibitors

Antibodies: bevacizumab (Avastin; monoclonal antibody), ranibizumab (Lucentis; a fragment antibody), brolucizumab (Beovu; an antibody fragment), aflibercept (Eylea; a fusion protein that acts like antibody), pegaptanib (Macugen; an aptamer) intravitreal for neovascular age-related macular degeneration (wet AMD), diabetic retinopathy, retinal vein occlusions, retinopathy of prematurity; systemic aflibercept and bevacizumab for colorectal cancer and other solid tumors

Tyrosine kinase inhibitors (TKIs): pazopanib, sunitinib, sorafenib; for soft tissue sarcomas

Antimetabolites: interfere with metabolic pathways, cell-cycle specific; methotrexate (folate antagonist), 6-mercaptopurine (purine antagonist), 5-fluorouracil (5-FU, pyrimidine antagonist; topically in glaucoma surgery)

Antitumor antibiotics: bind DNA, stopping RNA and protein synthesis, not cell-cycle specific; bleomycin, dactinomycin, mitomycin-C (topically in glaucoma, corneal, and pterygium surgery to prevent scarring), daunorubicin (daunomycin), doxorubicin (hydroxydaunorubicin, Adriamycin), mitoxantrone

Hormones: block androgen or estrogen receptors; tamoxifen (may cause corneal opacities, retinopathy), leuprorelin, flutamide

Inorganic ions: interfere with DNA uncoiling; cisplatin

Mitotic inhibitors/plant alkaloids: bind to tubulin, blocking microtubule formation and preventing cell division; vincristine, vinblastine, vinorelbine, estramustine, paclitaxel

Nitrosoureas: alkylate DNA, preventing uncoiling and replication; carmustine, lomustine

Topoisomerase inhibitors: block enzymes necessary for DNA replication; etoposide, teniposide, topotecan

ANTI-INFECTIVE DRUGS

Antibiotics

Inhibitors of Cell-Wall Synthesis

β-Lactams: cidal; contain β-lactam ring

Penicillins (PCNs): least toxic; variable protein binding; 5 classes based on spectrum and resistance to bacteria-produced β-lactamases (penicillinases)

1. *Penicillin G* (intravenous), *penicillin V* (oral): renal excretion inhibited by probenecid

    SPECTRUM: gram-positive and gram-negative cocci, anaerobes, *Listeria, Actinomyces, Leptospira, Treponema;* but most *Staphylococcus aureus,* *Staphylococcus epidermidis,* anaerobes, and *Neisseria gonorrhoeae* now resistant

    INDICATIONS: syphilis

2. *Isoxazolyl PCNs:* penicillinase-resistant; methicillin, nafcillin, oxacillin, cloxacillin, dicloxacillin, floxacillin

    SPECTRUM: extended to penicillinase-producing *S. aureus* (non–methicillin resistant)

3. *Amino PCNs:* broader spectrum; ampicillin, amoxicillin, bacampicillin

    SPECTRUM: gram-positives (except *Staphylococcus*), extended to gram-negatives, not resistant to penicillinase or broad-spectrum β-lactamases; *Neisseria, Haemophilus, Proteus, Shigella, Salmonella, Listeria, Escherichia coli; Haemophilus influenzae* becoming more resistant

    INDICATIONS: preseptal cellulitis

4. *Carboxy PCNs:* antipseudomonal; carbenicillin, ticarcillin

    SPECTRUM: extended to gram-negative rods (*Pseudomonas, Enterobacter, Proteus*) and anaerobes (*Bacteroides*) not resistant to penicillinase, less active against gram-positives and *Listeria*

5. *Acyl ureido PCNs:* increased potency to gram-negatives; piperacillin, mezlocillin, azlocillin

    SPECTRUM: increased activity to gram-negatives (*Pseudomonas, Klebsiella, Enterobacter*), anaerobes (*Bacteroides*), and *Listeria;* retain activity to gram-positives not resistant to penicillinase

β-lactamase inhibitors: combined with PCNs to increase spectrum of activity; clavulanate (amoxicillin/clavulanate = Augmentin), sulbactam (ampicillin/sulbactam = Unasyn), tazobactam (piperacillin/tazobactam = Zosyn)

Cephalosporins: more resistant to β-lactamases, not effective against enterococci, *Listeria, Legionella,* and methicillin-resistant *S. aureus* (MRSA); ~10% cross-reactivity in PCN-allergic patients

First generation: cefazolin (Ancef, Kefzol), cefalexin (cephalexin, Keflex), cephalothin (Keflin; most resistant to β-lactamases), cefadroxil (Duricef), cephradine (Velosef)

    SPECTRUM: gram-positives (*Staphylococcus, Streptococcus*) and some gram-negatives (*Klebsiella, E. coli;* especially cefazolin)

    INDICATIONS: cefazolin for keratitis, endophthalmitis

Second generation: cefamandole (Mandol), cefonicid (Monocid), cefaclor (Ceclor), cefotetan (Cefotan), cefoxitin (Mefoxin), cefuroxime (Zinacef)

    SPECTRUM: better gram-negative but less gram-positive; anaerobes (*Proteus, Serratia, Bacteroides fragilis;* cefoxitin, cefotetan, cefamandole), *H. influenzae, Enterobacter,* and *Neisseria* (cefuroxime)

Third generation: cefoperazone (Cefobid), cefotaxime (Claforan), ceftazidime (Tazidime), ceftizoxime (Cefizox), ceftriaxone (Rocephin; most effective), moxalactam (Moxam)

    SPECTRUM: better gram-negative bacilli, weaker gram-positive cocci; *Enterobacter, Pseudomonas* (ceftazidime, cefoperazone), *Neisseria, Serratia, Proteus;* Lyme disease and gonorrhea (ceftriaxone)

Fourth generation: cefepime (Maxipime), cefpirome (Cefrom, Cefir)
    SPECTRUM: most gram-negatives and gram-positives, more resistant to β-lactamases
Fifth generation: ceftaroline (Teflaro), ceftobiprole (Zevtera), ceftolozane/tazobactam (Zerbaxa)
    SPECTRUM: extended to *Pseudomonas* (ceftobiprole); serious abdominal and urinary tract infections (ceftolozane)

Carbacephems (loracarbef [Lorabid]): similar structure to cephalosporins; more β-lactamase resistant, broader spectrum (most gram-positives and gram-negatives)

Monobactams (aztreonam): monocyclic; similar coverage as aminoglycosides but safer (no ototoxicity or nephrotoxicity)
    Spectrum: aerobic gram-negative, including *Pseudomonas aeruginosa*; poor activity to gram positives and anaerobes

Carbapenems: different ring structure, β-lactamase resistant, very broad activity; imipenem rapidly inactivated by renal dehydropeptidase (combined with cilastatin, which inhibits this enzyme), newer carbapenems are more resistant to the enzyme
    Imipenem/cilastatin (Primaxin), *ertapenem, meropenem, biapenem, panipenem, faropenem, tomopenem, ritipenem, doripenem* (Doribax, most effective)
    SPECTRUM: almost all gram-positives (not MRSA), gram-negatives, and anaerobes, including Enterobacter and P. aeruginosa
    INDICATIONS: serious systemic and mixed infections, septicemia; doripenem for carbapenem-resistant gram-negative bacilli and penicillin-resistant streptococci
    ADVERSE EFFECTS: GI upset

Non–β-Lactams: cidal

Polymyxin B: basic peptide; acts as detergent, disrupts cell membrane
    Spectrum: gram-negatives (*Haemophilus, Enterobacter, E. coli, Klebsiella, Pseudomonas*)
    Indications: conjunctivitis (combined with trimethoprim [Polytrim])
    Adverse effects: systemic administration is associated with severe nephrotoxicity

Bacitracin: polypeptides; often used in combination with neomycin or polymyxin to broaden activity
    Spectrum: gram-positives, *Neisseria, Haemophilus, Actinomyces,* most MRSA
    Indications: blepharitis, conjunctivitis

Glycopeptides: interfere with polymerization of cell wall
    Vancomycin: produced by *Streptococcus orientalis*
    SPECTRUM: very good for gram-positives; *Staphylococcus,* including MRSA; *Streptococcus,* including penicillin-resistant strains; *Bacillus, Propionibacterium acnes, Clostridium difficile,*

Corynebacterium, diphtheroids; *Enterococcus* becoming resistant
    INDICATIONS: keratitis, endophthalmitis; endocarditis, pseudomembranous colitis
    ADVERSE EFFECTS: systemic administration is associated with ototoxicity and nephrotoxicity, red man syndrome (flushing with rapid IV infusion); intracameral associated with hemorrhagic occlusive retinal vasculitis (HORV)
    Teicoplanin (Targocid), *oritavancin* (Orbactiv), *dalbavancin* (Dalvance): extended activity to *Streptococcus, Enterococcus,* and vancomycin-resistant bacteria; longer half-life, less toxicity; used for staph infections, endocarditis, osteomyelitis, septic arthritis, bacteremia

Inhibitors of Folate Metabolism

Sulfonamides: static; derivatives of para-aminobenzenesulfonamide, analogues of para-aminobenzoic acid (PABA), inhibit folic acid synthesis;
    Sulfacetamide, sulfadiazine, sulfisoxazole, sulfamethoxazole: resistance is problem; increased efficacy in combination with trimethoprim or pyrimethamine (dihydrofolate reductase inhibitors, block next step in folate metabolism)
    SPECTRUM: gram-positives and gram-negatives; toxoplasmosis, *Chlamydia, Actinomyces, Pneumocystis*
    INDICATIONS: blepharitis, conjunctivitis, toxoplasmosis
    ADVERSE EFFECTS: allergy (mild to severe including toxic epidermal necrolysis and Stevens-Johnson syndrome), transient myopia
    Sulfonamide (sulfa) antibiotic hypersensitivity is to the N1 heterocyclic ring; not present in nonantibiotic sulfonamide drugs, so cross-reactivity is unlikely, and no cross-reactivity to drugs with sulfate group (structurally different)

Trimethoprim: not a sulfonamide; inhibits dihydrofolate reductase; often combined with sulfamethoxazole (TMP/SMX, Bactrim, Septra) for broad-spectrum activity and concomitant administration with metronidazole (Flagyl) for coverage; better than 3rd-generation cephalosporins
    Spectrum: gram-positives and gram-negatives (*Staphylococcus, Streptococcus, Listeria monocytogenes, Serratia, Proteus, Haemophilus, Enterobacter, E. coli, Klebsiella*)
    Indications: toxoplasmosis; pneumocystis prophylaxis; urinary tract, respiratory, gastrointestinal, skin, and ear infections (TMP-SMX)

Dapsone: diaminodiphenyl sulfone (DDS); effective against bacteria and protozoa
    Indications: OCP, dermatitis, leprosy (in combination with rifampicin and clofazimine)

Pyrimethamine (Daraprim): in combination with sulfonamide; antiprotozoal
    Indications: malaria, toxoplasmosis
    Adverse Effects: bone marrow depression (anemia, thrombocytopenia; prevent with use of folinic acid [Leucovorin])

Inhibitors of Protein Synthesis

Tetracyclines: static; inhibit 30S ribosomal subunit; take on empty stomach (chelates with milk, calcium, antacids, and iron causing decreased absorption); use with caution in women of childbearing age; also decreases efficacy of oral contraceptive medications and bactericidal medications (penicillins)

Produced by *Streptomyces: chlortetracycline, oxytetracycline, demeclocycline*

Semisynthetic: *tetracycline, doxycycline, minocycline*

  SPECTRUM: gram-positive and gram-negative, *Chlamydia, Rickettsia, Mycoplasma, Nocardia, Actinomyces;* most *S. aureus* and gram-negative bacilli (*Klebsiella, H. influenzae, Proteus vulgaris,* and *P. aeruginosa*) are resistant

  INDICATIONS: prophylaxis and treatment of ophthalmia neonatorum, *Chlamydia;* also rosacea, meibomian gland dysfunction, scleral melting (excreted into oil glands and have anti-inflammatory properties (i.e., inhibit leukocyte migration, inhibit phospholipase A$_2$, anticollagenolytic, decrease free radicals); bronchitis, Rocky Mountain spotted fever, syphilis

  ADVERSE EFFECTS: GI upset, candidiasis (oral, vaginal), phototoxic dermatitis, damages developing bone and teeth (discoloration) and thus contraindicated in pregnancy and children younger than 10 years of age, nephrotoxicity (Fanconi syndrome), hepatotoxicity, decreased prothrombin activity (potentiates warfarin [Coumadin]), photosensitivity (UV light, beware extended sun exposure), idiopathic intracranial hypertension

Aminoglycosides: cidal; inhibit 30S and 50S ribosomal subunits; poor GI absorption

Gentamycin (better for *Serratia*), *tobramycin* (better for *Pseudomonas*), *amikacin* (best for *Pseudomonas* and *Mycobacterium;* resistant to enzymatic inactivation, less nephrotoxic than gentamycin), *streptomycin* (*Streptococcus viridans* endocarditis, tularemia, brucellosis, plague), *neomycin* (*Acanthamoeba*), *paromomycin* (*Acanthamoeba*), *kanamycin* (less effective for gram-negative bacilli)

  SPECTRUM: gram-negative bacilli and some *Staphylococcus* (gentamycin and tobramycin are active against *S. aureus* and *S. epidermidis*); increased efficacy when combined with antibiotics that disrupt cell-wall synthesis (penicillins) except gentamycin, which is inactivated

  INDICATIONS: conjunctivitis, keratitis, endophthalmitis

  ADVERSE EFFECTS: systemic administration is associated with ototoxicity and nephrotoxicity; topical neomycin causes allergy (~8%) and corneal toxicity

Spectinomycin: cidal; inhibits 30S ribosomal subunit; aminocyclitol (not an aminoglycoside)

Spectrum: gram-positives, some gram-negatives, *Mycoplasma, Neisseria*

Indications: gonorrhea

Macrolides: static; inhibit 50S ribosomal subunit

Erythromycin, azithromycin (Zithromax; an azalide, better for *H. influenzae, N. gonorrhoeae, Chlamydia*), *clarithromycin* (Crixan, Biaxin; better for staphylococci, streptococci, *Mycobacterium leprae*)

  SPECTRUM: gram-positives (*Streptococcus pyogenes, S. pneumoniae, Corynebacterium diphtheriae, L. monocytogenes*) and a few gram-negatives (*N. gonorrhoeae*), *Chlamydia, Mycoplasma, Legionella;* atypical mycobacteria, *Mycobacterium avium-intracellulare,* and *Toxoplasma gondii* (azithromycin and clarithromycin)

  INDICATIONS: blepharitis, conjunctivitis, chlamydia, gonorrhea, community-acquired pneumonia, *M. avium-intracellulare*

  ADVERSE EFFECTS: GI upset, increased risk of cardiac arrhythmias (especially azithromycin)

Lincosamide: static; inhibits 50S ribosomal subunit

Clindamycin (Cleocin), *lincomycin* (Lincocin)

  SPECTRUM: gram-positives and anaerobes, including *B. fragilis,* toxoplasmosis

  INDICATIONS: toxoplasmosis

  ADVERSE EFFECTS: GI upset, may cause pseudomembranous colitis (from overgrowth of *C. difficile;* treat with oral vancomycin or metronidazole [Flagyl])

Chloramphenicol (Chloromycetin): static; inhibits 50S ribosomal subunit; semisynthetic, originally from *Streptomyces venezuelae;* no longer used because of serious adverse effects

Spectrum: gram-positives and gram-negatives, *Neisseria, H. influenzae,* anaerobes, *Chlamydia, Rickettsia, Mycoplasma;* some activity to *S. aureus, S. pneumoniae, Klebsiella pneumoniae, Enterobacter, Serratia, Proteus mirabilis; P. aeruginosa* resistant

Indications: meningitis, plague, cholera, typhoid fever; conjunctivitis, blepharitis

Adverse effects: aplastic anemia (even topically), reversible bone marrow suppression, lymphoma, hemolysis, neurotoxicity

Inhibitors of Nucleic Acid Synthesis

Fluoroquinolones: cidal; analogues of nalidixic acid; inhibitors of genetic replication; inhibit DNA gyrase (topoisomerase II) and topoisomerase IV; high penetration into ocular tissue

Ciprofloxacin (Ciloxan), *ofloxacin* (Ocuflox), *norfloxacin* (Chibroxin), *levofloxacin* (Quixin, Iquix), *gatifloxacin* (Zymar, Zymaxid), *moxifloxacin* (Vigamox), *besifloxacin* (Besivance); *temafloxacin, lomefloxacin, gemifloxacin*

  SPECTRUM: aerobic gram-negatives and gram-positives, increased activity with newer generations; *H. influenzae, Pseudomonas* (ciprofloxacin), *Enterobacter, S. aureus;* also, *Chlamydia, Rickettsia, Mycoplasma,* and *Mycobacterium.* Gati-, moxi-, and besi- have extended spectrum with enhanced activity against gram-positives, fluoroquinolone-resistant organisms, and atypical mycobacteria

  INDICATIONS: conjunctivitis, keratitis, surgical prophylaxis; prophylaxis in penetrating trauma (oral Cipro achieves high levels in vitreous); genitourinary, GI, pulmonary, skin and bone infections

  ADVERSE EFFECTS: systemic administration is associated with GI upset, tendon rupture, peripheral neuropathy, cartilage damage in children, increased risk aortic dissection; topical ciprofloxacin and norfloxacin may cause crystalline deposits in cornea

Rifampicin (Rifampin): inhibits RNA polymerase, developed as anti-TB drug
  Indications: Mycobacterium, Legionella, N. meningitidis prophylaxis, *H. influenzae* carriers
  Adverse effects: hepatotoxicity, turns body fluids orange-red

Anti-TB Agents

Isoniazid: cidal; inhibits cell-wall synthesis of mycobacteria
  Adverse effects: hepatotoxicity, vitamin B_6 deficiency

Rifampin (see above)

Pyrazinamide: unknown mechanism; analogue of nicotinamide
  Adverse effects: hepatotoxicity, gout

Ethambutol: chelates metals
  Adverse effects: optic neuropathy

Fumagillin: treatment of microsporidia keratoconjunctivitis

Antivirals

Mechanism: static; inhibit genetic replication; most are nucleoside analogues

Topical: treatment of HSV keratitis
  Idoxuridine (IDU, Stoxil): can cause follicular conjunctivitis, corneal epitheliopathy, punctal stenosis
  Vidarabine (Vira-A): adverse effects less severe than IDU
  Trifluorothymidine (Viroptic): inhibits thymidylate synthetase (virus-specific enzyme)
  Ganciclovir (Zirgan): guanosine analogue; activated only by thymidine kinase (virus-specific enzyme) and selectively interferes with viral DNA replication. Similar efficacy as topical acyclovir (not available in United States); more effective than Viroptic and less toxic to cornea; best tolerated

Systemic:
  Acyclovir (Zovirax; acycloguanosine, guanosine analogue; activated only by thymidine kinase (virus-specific enzyme), *valacyclovir* (Valtrex; prodrug of acyclovir, better bioavailability), *penciclovir* (Denavir, activated by thymidine kinase), *famciclovir* (Famvir; prodrug of penciclovir): treatment of HSV and varicella-zoster virus (VZV)
    ADVERSE EFFECTS: may cause GI upset; high doses can cause nephrotoxicity and neurotoxicity
  Ganciclovir (Cytovene), *valganciclovir* (Valcyte, oral prodrug of ganciclovir, better bioavailability): treatment of CMV
    ADVERSE EFFECTS: bone marrow suppression (cannot use with azidothymidine [AZT])
  Foscarnet (Foscavir, blocks pyrophosphate receptor on CMV DNA polymerase): treatment of CMV
    ADVERSE EFFECTS: nephrotoxicity, less myelosuppression, electrolyte abnormalities, neurotoxicity
  Cidofovir (Vistide, cytidine analogue): treatment of CMV, longer duration
    ADVERSE EFFECTS: nephrotoxicity (reduced when given with probenecid and IV fluid), GI upset, neutropenia, uveitis, hypotony (irreversible)

Antifungals

Mechanism: disrupt cell membranes

Classification:
  Yeasts: form pseudohyphae; *Candida, Cryptococcus*
  Molds: filamentous; form hyphae
    SEPTATE: *Fusarium, Aspergillus, Penicillium, Curvularia, Paecilomyces, Phialophora*
    NONSEPTATE: *Phycomycetes, Rhizopus, Mucor, Absidia*
  Dimorphic fungi: grow as yeast or mold; *Histoplasma, Blastomyces, Coccidioides*

Polyenes: bind to ergosterol
  Amphotericin B (Fungizone): topical, IV, subconjunctival, intravitreal
    SPECTRUM: broad (especially *Candida*; also, *Cryptococcus, Blastomyces, Histoplasma, Coccidioides,* mucormycosis; not as good for *Aspergillus, Fusarium*)
    INDICATIONS: keratitis, endophthalmitis (intravenous drug abuse [IVDA], immunosuppression, hyperalimentation)
    ADVERSE EFFECTS: fever, hypotension, headache, phlebitis, GI upset, nephrotoxicity, anemia, retinal toxicity (with IV use)
  Natamycin (pimaricin, Natacyn): topical only; too toxic for IV use, toxic to retina intravitreally
    SPECTRUM: filamentous fungi (especially *Aspergillus, Fusarium*), not as good for *Candida*; not effective against *Mucor* (nonseptate, branching hyphae)
    INDICATIONS: keratitis (removal of epithelium improves penetration)

Azoles: inhibit ergosterol synthesis; second-line agents to amphotericin; also used for *Acanthamoeba*
  Spectrum: Aspergillus, Blastomyces, Histoplasma, Coccidioides, Cryptococcus, Candida
  Adverse effects: GI upset, headache, rash
  Imidazoles:
    KETOCONAZOLE (Nizoral; topical, oral): limited spectrum *(Candida, Cryptococcus)*
    ADVERSE EFFECTS: reversible hepatotoxicity
    MICONAZOLE (topical, IV, intravitreal): broad spectrum (filamentous fungi and yeast)
    ADVERSE EFFECTS: may cause corneal erosions, anemia
    CLOTRIMAZOLE (oral): good for *Aspergillus*
    ADVERSE EFFECTS: hepatotoxicity
  Triazoles: safer (less effect on human sterol synthesis) and more effective, but increase plasma concentrations of other drugs

FLUCONAZOLE (Diflucan; oral, IV, subconjunctival): limited spectrum (*Candida*, *Cryptococcus*)

ITRACONAZOLE (Sporanox; oral, IV): broader spectrum than ketoconazole

VORICONAZOLE (topical, oral, IV, intravitreal): broadest spectrum, better for *Aspergillus*, high intraocular concentration

Echinocandins: inhibit glucan, component of fungal cell wall; IV only

Caspofungin, micafungin, anidulafungin

SPECTRUM: broad coverage, especially *Candida*, *Aspergillus*

Fluorinated pyrimidine (antimetabolite): most fungi are resistant, except *Cryptococcus* and some *Candida*

Flucytosine: converted to 5-FU, disrupts DNA synthesis

ADVERSE EFFECTS: myelosuppression, nausea, vomiting, diarrhea

Antiamebics

Mechanism: cidal (amoebae and cysts); cationic surface-active properties; interfere with cell membranes and inhibit enzymes

Indications: topical for *Acanthamoeba* keratitis

Biguanides: *polyhexamethylene biguanide* (PHMB), *chlorhexidine*; first-line agents, less corneal toxicity

Diamidines: *propamidine* (Brolene), *hexamidine*; synergistic effect with biguanides, corneal toxicity

Antihelmintics

Mebendazole, thiabendazole, albendazole: inhibit glucose uptake and microtubule synthesis

Adverse effects: GI upset

Pyrantel pamoate: neuromuscular junction blocker

Adverse effects: nausea, vomiting, headache, rash

Diethylcarbamazine: enables phagocytosis of microfilaria

Ivermectin: increases gamma-aminobutyric acid (GABA) release, paralyzing microfilaria

Adverse effects: fever, headache, rash

Praziquantel: causes calcium loss, paralyzing worm

Adverse effects: GI upset, fever

MISCELLANEOUS

Antifibrinolytic agents: synthetic lysine analogues; safety concerns with oral administration, efficacy concerns with topical administration

Aminocaproic acid (Amicar), *tranexamic acid*

MECHANISM: antifibrinolytic; stabilizes blood clot, delays lysis, decreases secondary hemorrhages

INDICATIONS: hyphema (to prevent rebleed; larger and delayed presentation have higher risk; usually 2–6 days later)

CONTRAINDICATIONS: hypercoagulable states, pregnancy, renal disease, liver disease, patients at risk for myocardial infarction (MI), pulmonary embolism, cerebrovascular accident (CVA)

ADVERSE EFFECTS: nausea, vomiting, diarrhea, muscle cramps, hypotension, arrhythmias, headache, rash (aminocaproic acid); nausea, vomiting, hypotension (tranexamic acid)

Botulinum toxin type A (Botox, Dysport, Xeomin, Jeuveau): neurotoxin from *C. botulinum* that blocks release of acetylcholine from nerve terminal; paralyzes muscle (1–3 months)

Indications: blepharospasm, hemifacial spasm, strabismus, cosmetic to reduce wrinkles; also to treat overactive bladder, chronic migraine, axillary hyperhidrosis

Adverse effects: ptosis, diplopia, exposure keratopathy

Fluorescein dye: IV for fluorescein angiography

Adverse effects: nausea, vomiting, dizziness, headache, dyspnea, hypotension, skin necrosis, phototoxic reactions, anaphylaxis

Indocyanine green (ICG) dye: IV for ICG angiography; contraindicated in patients allergic to iodine

Adverse effects: GI upset, hypotension, urticaria, anaphylaxis

Povidone-iodine solution (5%; Betadine): broad-spectrum antimicrobial activity; topical sterile prep for surgical procedures, reduces risk of postsurgical endophthalmitis; *not* contraindicated in patients allergic to IV contrast agents or shellfish (allergy is to tropomyosin, not iodine)

OCULAR TOXICOLOGY (TABLE 2.4)

Anticholinergics (atropine, scopolamine, hyoscyamine): toxicity causes flushing, agitation, tachycardia, somnolence, dry mouth, dry eye, mydriasis, cycloplegia, blurry vision, angle closure; increased sensitivity in albinism, Down syndrome, and neonates

Antihistamines (diphenhydramine): dry eye, mydriasis, cycloplegia, blurry vision, angle closure

Antibiotics:

Aminoglycosides: intraocular administration may cause macular infarction (intravenous fluorescein angiography [IVFA]: pruned-tree appearance of retinal vasculature)

Chloramphenicol: aplastic anemia, optic neuropathy; peripheral neuritis can precede visual complaints by 1–2 weeks

Penicillin and *tetracycline:* idiopathic intracranial hypertension

Sulfonamides: conjunctivitis, transient myopia, angle closure, optic neuropathy

Isoniazid, rifampin, ethambutol: optic neuropathy

Table 2.4 Ocular toxicology

Ocular structure	Effect	Drug
Extraocular muscles	Nystagmus, diplopia	Anesthetics, sedatives, anticonvulsants, propranolol, antibiotics, phenothiazines, pentobarbital, carbamazepine, monoamine oxidase inhibitors
Lid	Edema	Chloral hydrate
	Discoloration	Phenothiazines
	Ptosis	Guanethidine, propranolol, barbiturates
Conjunctiva	Hyperemia	Reserpine, methyldopa, dupilumab
	Allergy	Antibiotics, sulfonamides, atropine, antivirals, glaucoma medications
	Discoloration	Phenothiazines, chlorambucil, phenylbutazone
Cornea	Keratitis	Antibiotics, phenylbutazone, barbiturates, chlorambucil, steroids, dupilumab
	Edema	Amantadine
	Deposits	Chloroquine, amiodarone, tamoxifen, indomethacin, ibuprofen, naproxen, clofazimine, suramin, phenothiazines, gold
	Pigmentation	Vitamin D
Increased IOP	Open angle	Anticholinergics, caffeine, steroids, anti-VEGF agents (ranibizumab, bevacizumab, aflibercept)
	Narrow angle	Anticholinergics, antihistamines, phenothiazines, tricyclic antidepressants, haloperidol, sulfonamides (Topamax)
Anterior chamber	Uveitis	Rifabutin, bisphosphonates, sulfonamides, diethylcarbamazine, metipranolol, cidofovir, oral contraceptives, immune checkpoint inhibitors
Lens	Opacities / cataract	Steroids, phenothiazines, ibuprofen, allopurinol, long-acting miotics, busulfan, tamoxifen
	Myopia	Sulfonamides, tetracycline, prochlorperazine, autonomic antagonists, duloxetine (Cymbalta)
Retina	Edema	Chloramphenicol, indomethacin, tamoxifen, carmustine
	Hemorrhage	Anticoagulants, ethambutol
	Vascular damage	Oral contraceptives, oxygen, aminoglycosides, vancomycin, talc, carmustine, interferon
	Pigmentary degeneration	Phenothiazines, indomethacin, nalidixic acid, ethambutol, isotretinoin, chloroquine, hydroxychloroquine, pentosan
	Exudative retinal detachment	MEK inhibitors, immune checkpoint inhibitors
Optic nerve	Neuropathy	Ethambutol, isoniazid, rifampin, sulfonamides, streptomycin, chloramphenicol, chloroquine, quinine, digitalis, imipramine, busulfan, cisplatin, vincristine, disulfiram, linezolid, cyclosporine
	Papilledema	Steroids, vitamin A, tetracycline, phenylbutazone, amiodarone, nalidixic acid, isotretinoin, lithium

VEGF, *vascular endothelial growth factor.*

Antimalarials (chloroquine/hydroxychloroquine): cornea verticillata, fine pigmentary macular changes (bull's-eye maculopathy); patients may complain of halos around lights; visual acuity usually unchanged; dose related, both total daily (more important) and cumulative

Quinine: overdose can result in acute visual loss (to no light perception [NLP]), tinnitus, weakness, confusion

Barbiturates (phenobarbital): nystagmus, diplopia, ptosis, conjunctivitis

Phenothiazines (chlorpromazine, thioridazine): pigmentary retinopathy, corneal deposits, cataracts, angle closure

Tricyclic antidepressants: mydriasis, cycloplegia, dry eye, angle closure

Dilantin: diplopia, nystagmus, papilledema

Gold: deposits in inferior corneal stroma and anterior lens capsule (chrysiasis)

Talc: multiple tiny yellow-white glistening particles scattered through posterior pole with macular edema, venous engorgement, hemorrhages, arterial occlusion, retinal nonperfusion, and peripheral neovascularization (NV)

Amiodarone (Cordarone): cornea verticillata, occasionally anterior subcapsular opacities

Digoxin: changes in color vision (xanthopsia [yellow vision]), optic neuropathy

Diuretics (hydrochlorothiazide): xanthopsia, transient myopia, angle closure

Phosphodiesterase 5 inhibitors (Viagra, Cialis, Levitra): decreased retinal blood flow by up to ~30%; altered color and light perception; possibly ischemic optic neuropathy

Carmustine: retinal infarction, retinal pigment epithelium (RPE) changes, arterial occlusions, hemorrhages, macular edema, glaucoma, optic neuritis, internuclear ophthalmoplegia (INO)

Narcotics (opiates): miosis

NSAIDs (indomethacin): corneal deposits, diplopia, optic neuritis, pigmentary macular changes; may have changes in vision, dark adaptation, and visual fields

Corticosteroids: posterior subcapsular cataracts, increased IOP, delayed wound healing, secondary infections, pseudotumor cerebri

Dupilumab (Dupixent): blepharitis, conjunctivitis, dry eye, keratitis

Pentosan polysulfate (Elmiron): pigmentary maculopathy

Oral contraceptives: dry eye, vascular occlusions, perivasculitis, optic neuritis, pseudotumor cerebri

Tamoxifen: deposits in cornea and macula, posterior subcapsular cataracts, may have macular edema

MEK inhibitors: exudative retinal detachments

Immune checkpoint inhibitors (ICIs; cemiplimab, pembrolizumab, nivolumab, atezolizumab, avelumab, durvalumab, ipilimumab): uveitis, subretinal fluid, may have corneal erosions, subconjunctival hemorrhage, hypotony maculopathy, cystoid macular edema, choroiditis, optic neuritis

Isotretinoin: impairment of dark adaptation

Interferon: reversible vasoocclusive disease

REVIEW QUESTIONS (Answers start on page 410)

1. Which antibiotic results in the highest intravitreal concentration when administered orally?
   a. ciprofloxacin
   b. penicillin
   c. bactrim
   d. clindamycin

2. Which anesthetic agent would most interfere with an intraocular gas bubble?
   a. isoflurane
   b. propofol
   c. sodium thiopental
   d. nitrous oxide

3. Which of the following is *not* an adverse effect of CAIs?
   a. death
   b. paresthesias
   c. iris cysts
   d. stevens-Johnson syndrome

4. Which β-blocker has the *least* effect on β_2 receptors?
   a. levobunolol
   b. betaxolol
   c. carteolol
   d. timolol

5. Which drug has the *least* effect on uveoscleral outflow?
   a. atropine
   b. latanoprost
   c. pilocarpine
   d. dorzolamide

6. Which enzyme is inhibited by steroids?
   a. cyclooxygenase
   b. phospholipase A_2
   c. lipoxygenase
   d. endoperoxide

7. Which of the following steroid formulations has the best corneal penetrability?
   a. prednisolone acetate
   b. dexamethasone phosphate
   c. prednisolone phosphate
   d. dexamethasone alcohol

8. Adverse effects of foscarnet include all of the following, *except*
   a. seizures
   b. infertility
   c. electrolyte abnormalities
   d. myelosuppression

9. Which glaucoma medication is *not* effective when IOP is > 60 mm Hg?
   a. acetazolamide
   b. timolol
   c. pilocarpine
   d. apraclonidine

10. Which medicine is *not* associated with OCP-like conjunctival shrinkage?
    a. phospholine iodide
    b. pilocarpine
    c. epinephrine
    d. timolol

11. Which β-blocker is β_1-selective?
    a. carteolol
    b. timolol
    c. betaxolol
    d. levobunolol

12. The most appropriate treatment for neurosyphilis is
    a. penicillin G
    b. erythromycin
    c. penicillin V
    d. tetracycline

13. Which is the correct mechanism of action of botulinum toxin?
    a. it prevents the release of acetylcholine
    b. it blocks acetylcholine receptors
    c. it inhibits the reuptake of acetylcholine
    d. it is an acetylcholinesterase inhibitor

14. Fluoroquinolones are *least* effective against
    a. *klebsiella*
    b. *h. influenzae*
    c. anaerobic cocci
    d. *serratia*

15. Hydroxychloroquine toxicity depends most on
    a. patient age
    b. daily dose
    c. patient race
    d. cumulative dose

16. Calculate the amount of cocaine in 2 mL of a 4% solution.
    a. 2 mg
    b. 8 mg
    c. 20 mg
    d. 80 mg

17. NSAIDs block the formation of all of the following substances, *except*
    a. thromboxane
    b. leukotrienes
    c. prostaglandins
    d. prostacyclin

18. Systemic effects of steroids may include all of the following, *except*
    a. papilledema
    b. hirsutism
    c. potassium depletion
    d. renal tubular acidosis

19. Which drug does *not* produce decreased tear production?
    a. pilocarpine
    b. diphenhydramine (Benadryl)
    c. timolol
    d. atropine

20. Natamycin is a
    a. diamine
    b. imidazole
    c. polyene
    d. aminoglycoside

21. Which glaucoma medicine does *not* decrease aqueous production?
    a. apraclonidine
    b. pilocarpine
    c. acetazolamide
    d. timolol

22. β-blockers may cause all of the following, *except*
    a. constipation
    b. impotence
    c. alopecia
    d. depression

23. Idoxuridine may cause all of the following, *except*
    a. filamentary keratitis
    b. punctal stenosis
    c. corneal hypesthesia
    d. nonhealing epithelial erosion

24. Which of the following antifungal agents has the broadest spectrum against yeast-like fungi?
    a. miconazole
    b. natamycin
    c. ketoconazole
    d. amphotericin

25. All of the following medications are combination antihistamine and mast cell stabilizers, *except*
    a. alomide
    b. zaditor
    c. optivar
    d. patanol

26. The antidote for atropine toxicity is
    a. edrophonium
    b. physostigmine
    c. carbachol
    d. pilocarpine

27. Which of the following agents is contraindicated for ruptured globe repair?
    a. gallamine
    b. halothane
    c. pancuronium
    d. succinylcholine

28. The duration of action of 1 drop of proparacaine is
    a. 5 minutes
    b. 20 minutes
    c. 45 minutes
    d. 60 minutes

29. Which of the following medications is *not* commercially available as a topical formulation?
    a. ganciclovir
    b. azithromycin
    c. cyclosporine
    d. vancomycin

30. All of the following are complications of CAIs, *except*
    a. hypokalemia
    b. aplastic anemia
    c. metabolic alkalosis
    d. kidney stones

31. Topiramate is associated with
    a. open-angle glaucoma
    b. normal-tension glaucoma
    c. angle-closure glaucoma with pupillary block
    d. angle-closure glaucoma without pupillary block

32. A patient with ocular hypertension and an allergy to sulfonamides should *not* be treated with
    a. bimatoprost
    b. dorzolamide
    c. timolol
    d. brimonidine

33. Infectious keratitis caused by *Candida albicans* is best treated with topical
    a. amphotericin B
    b. natamycin
    c. fluconazole
    d. clotrimazole

34. Which of the following oral agents should be used to treat a patient with ocular cicatricial pemphigoid?
    a. pyrazinamide
    b. 5-fluorouracil
    c. cyclophosphamide
    d. flucytosine

35. The glaucoma medication contraindicated in infants is
    a. timolol
    b. brimonidine
    c. latanoprost
    d. dorzolamide

36. Which systemic antibiotic is used to treat *Chlamydia* during pregnancy?
    a. doxycycline
    b. ceftriaxone
    c. penicillin
    d. erythromycin

37. The local anesthetic with the longest duration of action is
    a. mepivacaine
    b. procaine
    c. bupivacaine
    d. lidocaine

38. A 33-year-old man has had follicular conjunctivitis with a watery discharge for 5 weeks. Elementary bodies are present on a conjunctival smear; therefore, the most appropriate treatment is
    a. oral azithromycin
    b. oral acyclovir
    c. topical cromolyn
    d. topical prednisolone

39. The most appropriate treatment for *Fusarium* keratitis is topical
    a. tobramycin
    b. pimaricin
    c. chloramphenicol
    d. ciprofloxacin

40. All of the following are associated with vitamin A toxicity, *except*
    a. cranial nerve (CN) 6 palsy
    b. retinal hemorrhages
    c. papilledema
    d. band keratopathy

41. Which of the following is a serious adverse effect of a long-acting cycloplegic agent?
    a. somnolence
    b. bradycardia
    c. urinary retention
    d. hypothermia

42. An oral NSAID should *not* be used in a patient with
    a. renal insufficiency
    b. diabetes mellitus
    c. sulfa allergy
    d. hyperthyroidism

43. Ocular rosacea is best treated with which of the following oral medications?
    a. acyclovir
    b. cyclosporine
    c. doxycycline
    d. tacrolimus

44. A patient taking which of the following medications is at increased risk for complications at the time of cataract surgery?
    a. β-adrenergic antagonist
    b. muscarinic antagonist
    c. α$_1$-adrenergic antagonist
    d. carbonic anhydrase inhibitor

45. A patient suddenly stops breathing after administration of a peribulbar injection of anesthetic. The most likely reason is
    a. retrobulbar hemorrhage
    b. globe perforation
    c. injection into the medial rectus
    d. injection into the optic nerve sheath

46. Which of the following anesthetic agents is most likely to increase IOP?
    a. halothane
    b. chloral hydrate
    c. thiopental
    d. ketamine

47. Which of the following medications is most likely to cause hallucinations?
    a. prednisolone acetate
    b. cyclopentolate
    c. ketorolac
    d. neomycin

48. A 10-year-old African American boy with a hyphema develops increased intraocular pressure. Which of the following drugs should be avoided?
    a. carbonic anhydrase inhibitors
    b. prostaglandin analogs
    c. β-adrenergic antagonists
    d. α-adrenergic agonists

49. General anesthesia for cataract surgery is most likely the best option in a patient with
    a. previous pars plana vitrectomy
    b. nanophthalmos
    c. dementia
    d. sleep apnea

50. All of the following medications are causes of cornea verticillata, *except*
    a. hydroxychloroquine
    b. indomethacin
    c. netarsudil
    d. tobramycin

51. Which eye drop preservative is *least* toxic?
    a. chlorobutanol
    b. methylparaben
    c. sodium perborate
    d. thimerosal

52. Bladder cancer is most commonly associated with which drug?
    a. methotrexate
    b. cyclophosphamide
    c. tacrolimus
    d. adalimumab

53. For topical eye medications, the volume of 1 drop is approximately
    a. 10 µL
    b. 50 µL
    c. 100 µL
    d. 150 µL

54. Which of the following statements regarding Miostat and Miochol is true?
    a. Miochol reduces IOP
    b. Miostat has a shorter duration
    c. Miochol is faster acting
    d. Miochol is more effective

55. Methazolamide can be used to treat all of the following, *except*
    a. fungal keratitis
    b. increased IOP
    c. cystoid macular edema
    d. idiopathic intracranial hypertension

Please visit the eBook for an interactive version of the review questions. See front cover for activation details.

SUGGESTED READINGS

Doughty, M. (2001). *Ocular pharmacology and therapeutics: A primary care guide*. Philadelphia: Butterworth-Heinemann.

Fraunfelder, F. T., Fraunfelder, F. W., & Chambers, W. A. (2014). *Drug-induced ocular side effects* (7th ed.). Philadelphia: Butterworth-Heinemann.

Grant, W. M., & Schuman, J. S. (1993). *Toxicology of the eye* (4th ed.). Springfield, IL: Charles C. Thomas.

Greenbaum, S. (1997). *Ocular anesthesia*. Philadelphia: WB Saunders.

Medical Economics. (2002). *Physicians' desk reference for ophthalmic medicines*. Montvale, NJ: Author.

Roy, F. H., & Fraunfelder, F. T. (2007). *Roy and Fraunfelder's current ocular therapy* (6th ed.). Philadelphia: WB Saunders.

Zimmerman, T. J. (1997). *Textbook of ocular pharmacology* (3rd ed.). Philadelphia: Lippincott-Raven.

3

Embryology/Pathology

EMBRYOLOGY

Embryogenesis controlled by series of genetic programs, gene expression from external cues, process regulated by homeobox genes *(HOX)*

Eye development genes: paired box 6 *(PAX6, most* important), also paired box 2 *(PAX2)*, retinal and anterior neural fold homeobox *(RAX)*, and paired like homeodomain 2 *(PITX2)*

Formation of eye: embryonic plate → neural plate → neural tube → optic pits → optic vesicles → optic cups

Embryonic plate (Fig. 3.1): 3 germ layers
1. Ectoderm (outer layer; forms eye and brain): neuroectoderm, surface ectoderm, and neural crest (migrating stem cells from crest of neural folds, form tissue with characteristics of ectoderm and mesoderm)
2. Mesoderm (middle layer)
3. Endoderm (inner layer; does not contribute to ocular tissue)

Optic pits: evaginations of the forebrain; form at day 23 of gestation

Optic vesicle: anterolateral outpouching of primitive brainstem; evaginates on day 25 and becomes the globe
Optic vesicle induces the lens placode at day 28

Abnormalities of evagination: may result in anophthalmia, cyclopia (synophthalmia), congenital cystic eye, congenital nonattachment of the retina; apical forebrain lesions such as synophthalmia are associated with arrhinencephaly, proboscis, ethmocephaly, trisomy 13

Optic cup (Fig. 3.2): forms on day 27 as optic vesicle invagination upon itself
Inner layer becomes the retina
Outer layer becomes the retinal pigment epithelium (RPE)
Potential space between the two becomes the subretinal space (which was the cavity of the neural tube and optic vesicle)
Cells at anterior margin of optic cup form the posterior pigment epithelium of the iris
Cells between the future iris and the future retina form the ciliary body

Embryonic fissure: on undersurface of optic cups; closes on day 33, allowing pressurization of globe
Closure occurs first in midzone/equator, then extends posteriorly and anteriorly
Serves as portal for mesoderm to enter eye (i.e., hyaloid artery)
Coloboma: failure of closure of embryonic fissure; sporadic or autosomal dominant (AD); typical (located in inferonasal quadrant) or atypical (located elsewhere)
May involve retina and choroid (associated with basal encephalocele, cleft palate, and CHARGE syndrome), iris, and/or optic nerve
An eyelid coloboma is not related to closure of embryonic fissure

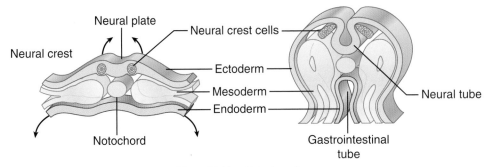

Figure 3.1 Neural tube formation.

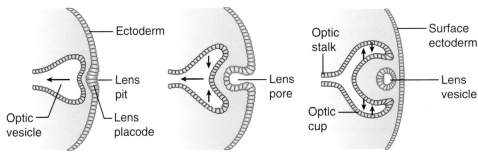

Figure 3.2 Optic cup formation.

Microphthalmos with cyst: small, abnormal eye with cystic expansion extending posteriorly into orbit

Arises in area of and external to a choroidal coloboma; cyst usually contains dysplastic neuroectodermal tissue and may not directly connect with the eye

Optic pit: considered an atypical coloboma; associated with basal encephalocele

Hyaloid artery (Fig. 3.3): enters through embryonic fissure and forms vasa hyaloidea propria (blood supply to primary vitreous)

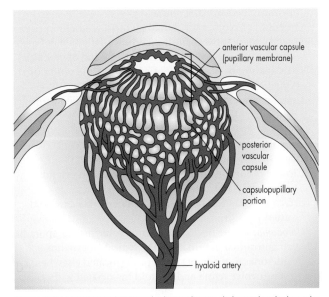

Figure 3.3 Hyaloid vasculature and primary vitreous during embryologic ocular development. (With permission from Dass AB, Trese MT: Persistent hyperplastic primary vitreous. In: Yanoff M, Duker JS, eds. *Ophthalmology*. London: Mosby; 1999.)

Intravitreal portion regresses by 8½ months; intraneural portion becomes central retinal artery

Posterior tunica vasculosa lentis supplies the posterior lens

Retinal vascular development begins during 16th week: mesenchymal cells next to hyaloid artery form capillary network, then form arteries and veins; vessels grow centrifugally from optic disc, reach nasal ora serrata during eighth month and temporal ora 1–2 months later

3% of normal neonates have a patent hyaloid artery

Remnants of hyaloid vasculature system:

BERGMEISTER PAPILLAE: at optic nerve head; glial sheath of Bergmeister envelops posterior third of hyaloid artery and begins to atrophy during seventh month; epipapillary veil results if it does not fully regress

PERIPAPILLARY LOOP: vascular loop extending from optic nerve head; risk of artery obstruction or vitreous hemorrhage

MITTENDORF DOT: small opacity on posterior lens capsule at which hyaloid artery is attached to posterior tunica vasculosa lentis, usually inferonasal

PERSISTENT PUPILLARY MEMBRANE: thin iris strands bridging pupil; may attach to anterior lens capsule; remnants of anterior tunica vasculosa lentis

Optic nerve: neuroectoderm surrounded by neural crest cells; develops from optic stalk (connects optic vesicle to forebrain)

At 6 weeks, neural crest cells degenerate creating space for retinal ganglion cell axons

Primitive epithelial papillae: cells from inner layer of optic cup at superior end of embryonic fissure, which becomes the optic disc; hyaloid artery in and ganglion cell axons out during 7th week

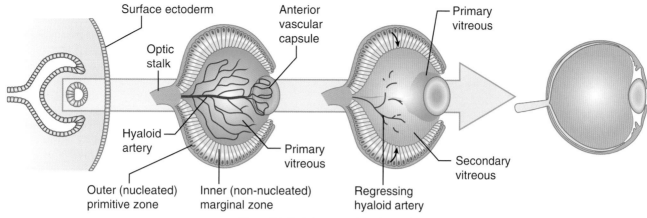

Surface ectoderm

Optic stalk

Anterior vascular capsule

Primary vitreous

Hyaloid artery

Outer (nucleated) primitive zone

Inner (non-nucleated) marginal zone

Primary vitreous

Secondary vitreous

Regressing hyaloid artery

Figure 3.4 Posterior segment development.

Meninges from neural crest cells

Oligodendrocytes from neuroectoderm form myelin sheath (compared with peripheral nerves, in which Schwann cells produce myelin sheath; reason why the optic nerve more prone to neuritis)

Myelination starts centrally, reaches chiasm at 7½ months and lamina cribrosa at birth; complete approximately 1 month after birth

Inner limiting membrane (ILM) of Elschnig: covers ON contiguous with ILM

ON may show deceptively exaggerated cupping because nerve fibers posterior to lamina cribrosa are incompletely myelinated at birth

ON hypoplasia is associated with DeMorsier syndrome; 13% have pituitary abnormalities

Vitreous: produced by lens (surface ectoderm), retina (neuroectoderm), and vascular endothelium of hyaloid artery (mesoderm); contains mesenchymal cells

Primary vitreous: formed by hyaloid vascular system (vasa hyaloidea propria, which includes hyaloid canal, hyaloid vessels, and posterior portions of tunica vasculosa lentis); eventually replaced by secondary vitreous; failure to regress causes persistent hyperplastic primary vitreous (PHPV) (Fig. 3.4)

Secondary vitreous: formed by retina

Area of Martegiani: extends from disc into vitreous to become Cloquet's canal

Cloquet's canal: junction of primary and secondary vitreous

Tertiary vitreous: zonule fibers formed from ciliary processes and lens capsule

Berger's space: retrolental space

Retina: neuroectoderm; starts to form during 4th–6th week, cells of 2 neuroblastic layers form during 3rd month

Inner neuroblastic layer: forms ganglion, amacrine, and Müller cells

Outer neuroblastic layer: forms bipolar, horizontal, and photoreceptor cells

In 5th week, RPE melanization

Vascularization begins at 4 months; temporal periphery is last portion to become vascularized

Development of fovea is not complete until ≥4 weeks after birth

Retinal dysplasia: abnormal proliferation of developing retina produces tubular structures with a rosette-like appearance; represents nonspecific response to disorganizing influence during development; associated with maternal LSD ingestion, Patau syndrome (trisomy 13), microphthalmos, congenital glaucoma, Peter anomaly, uveal and optic nerve colobomas, cyclopia, and synophthalmia

Choroid: requires RPE for development; stroma from neural crest cells, vascular endothelium from mesoderm, vessel walls from neural crest cells

At 3 months, choriocapillaris forms posterior to anterior

At 6–7 months, uveal melanization starts at disc, continues after birth

Sclera: neural crest cells and mesoderm (temporal aspect); forms anterior to posterior

Scleral spur and Tenon capsule develop during extraocular muscle insertion

Blue hue at birth as a result of thinness (see underlying uveal pigment)

Cornea: neural crest cells; 3 waves of limbal migration to center

1st wave: grows between epithelium and lens, forming double layer of corneal endothelium

2nd wave: grows between epithelium and endothelium, forming stroma, rich in hyaluronic acid and collagen fibrils

3rd wave: iris stroma

At 4 months, Descemet membrane develops

At 5 months, Bowman layer develops

Angle: neural crest cells from peripheral cornea differentiate into chamber angle during 7th week

In 4th month, Schlemm canal forms

In 7th month, angle moves posteriorly

In 8th month, formation is complete; trabecular meshwork appears just before birth

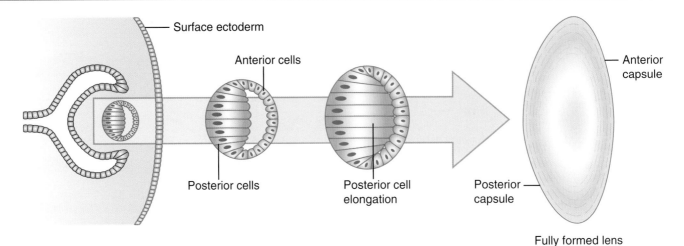

Figure 3.5 Lens development.

Lens: at 27 days, surface ectoderm adjacent to optic vesicle enlarges to form lens placode (lens plate)

Circular indentation then occurs on lens plate, forming lens pit, which invaginates the wall of the optic vesicle until it closes to form a sphere

Basement membrane of the surface ectoderm forms the surface of the sphere (the lens vesicle) and subsequently becomes the lens capsule

Lens epithelial cells on posterior aspect of this sphere elongate and migrate first (primary lens fibers); these cells fill the core of the lens vesicle at approximately 40 days (embryonal nucleus)

At 7 weeks, anterior cells migrate toward equator and proliferate to form secondary lens fibers that encase the embryonal nucleus and form the Y sutures; Y sutures represent the meeting of embryonal and fetal nuclei (upright anteriorly, inverted posteriorly)

After 3 months, zonules of Zinn (zonular fibers) develop (Fig. 3.5)

Lens development:

3 weeks	Lens placode from surface ectoderm
6 weeks	Lens vesicle; further development requires normal neuroretina
12 weeks	Tunica vasculosa lentis
28–38 weeks	Degeneration of tunica vasculosa lentis

Lens of a newborn is more spherical than that of an adult; therefore, anterior chamber appears shallow

Iris: rim of optic cup grows around lens and forms iris

Epithelial layers (iris pigment epithelium [IPE]; anterior nonpigmented and posterior pigmented) are from inner and outer layers of the optic cup (neuroectoderm); forms part of the blood–aqueous barrier

In 7th week, stroma forms from neural crest cells, and tunica vasculosa lentis forms

In 6th month, sphincter and dilator muscles form from neuroectoderm

In 7th month, blood vessels enter iris

In 9th month, tunica vasculosa lentis disappears

Newborn iris is usually gray-blue; development of iris color takes weeks to months, as stromal chromatophores (dendritic melanocytes from neural crest) complete their migration into uvea shortly after birth

Iris dilator muscle is immature, causing relative miosis in infancy

RPE and posterior pigment epithelium of the iris form from the outer layer of the optic cup (have mature coloration because pigment granules develop very early in gestation)

Ciliary body (CB): formation begins in third month; fold in optic cup becomes epithelial layers of ciliary processes

In 4th month, filaments from surface cells form zonules; the major arterial circle of the iris (located in CB), the longitudinal ciliary muscle, and the ciliary processes develop

In 5th month, pars plana develops, and CB stroma and ciliary muscle develop from neural crest cells adjacent to cornea

In 7th month, circular fibers of ciliary muscle differentiate

Patient's age can be determined by analysis of CB cellularity

Nasolacrimal system: at 6 weeks, surface ectoderm is buried in mesoderm, between maxillary and lateral nasal processes

In 3rd month, the cord canalizes

Defects: may result in imperforate valve of Hasner; rarely, absent puncta or canaliculi

At 6–7 weeks, lacrimal gland begins to develop from conjunctiva in temporal fornix and mesenchyme

Reflex tearing occurs 20 days after birth

Eyelids: at 8 weeks, upper lids form by fusion of medial and lateral frontonasal processes; lower lids by fusion of maxillary processes and medial nasal processes

At 8–10 weeks, lid folds fuse, glands and cilia begin to develop

At 12 weeks, orbicularis muscle present in folds

At 24 weeks, separation begins from nasal side

Orbit: ectoderm, mesoderm, and neural crest components

At 4 weeks, frontonasal and maxillary processes of neural crest cells surround optic cups, develop into bone, cartilage, fat, and connective tissue

At 3 months, ossification begins

At 6–7 months, bones fuse

Orbital bones are membranous except sphenoid (initially cartilaginous)

Embryologic tissues and their components:

Neuroectoderm: sensory retina, nonpigmented ciliary body epithelium, RPE, pigmented CB epithelium (extension of RPE), IPE, iris sphincter and dilator muscle, optic nerve (neural and glial elements), lateral geniculate body, peripheral nerves related to eye function, erector pili muscle associated with hair follicles of the skin

Mnemonic: **MORE** (**M**uscles of pupil, **O**ptic nerve, **R**etina (and RPE), **E**pithelium of iris and ciliary body)

Surface ectoderm: crystalline lens, corneal and conjunctival epithelium, eyelid skin, glands, and cilia, caruncle, lacrimal gland, nasolacrimal system

Mnemonic: **S1L2E3** (**S**kin of eyelids/appendages, **L**ens, **L**acrimal gland, **E**pithelium of cornea, **E**pithelium of conjunctiva, **E**pithelium of nasolacrimal system)

Surface and neuroectoderm: vitreous, zonules

Neural crest cells: corneal stroma and endothelium, iris stroma, trabecular meshwork (TM), chamber angle, Schlemm canal, sclera (except temporal portion), extraocular muscle sheaths and tendons, ciliary muscle (nonpigmented layer of ciliary body), choroidal stroma, melanocytes, meningeal sheaths, orbital bones, orbital fat and connective tissue, muscular and connective tissue layers of blood vessels, ciliary ganglion

S-100 STAIN: specific for neural crest–derived structures

3 WAVES OF NEURAL CREST CELL MIGRATION (DURING 7TH WEEK): corneal and TM endothelium, keratocytes (corneal stroma), iris stroma

ANTERIOR SEGMENT DISORDERS RESULTING FROM NEURAL CREST ABNORMALITIES:

ABNORMAL MIGRATION: congenital glaucoma, posterior embryotoxin, Axenfeld-Rieger syndrome, Peter anomaly, sclerocornea

ABNORMAL PROLIFERATION: iridocorneal endothelial (ICE) syndromes

ABNORMAL TERMINAL INDUCTION: corneal endothelial dystrophies

Mesoderm: blood vessel endothelium, anterior chamber angle outflow apparatus, sclera (temporal portion), extraocular muscles, Schlemm canal, iris stroma, ciliary body, choroid, portion of vitreous, fat

Mesenchyme: primitive connective tissue; originates from neural crest cells and mesoderm (Fig. 3.6)

PATHOLOGY

MICROBIAL STUDIES

Stains

Gram: bacteria, fungi

Giemsa: *Acanthamoeba*, fungi, and cytology; best for intranuclear inclusion bodies

Acid fast (Ziehl-Neelsen): *Mycobacterium*, *Nocardia*

Acridine orange: bacteria, fungi, *Acanthamoeba*

Periodic acid-Schiff (PAS): fungi

Gomori methenamine silver: fungi

Calcofluor white: fungi and *Acanthamoeba* (binds to cell wall, visible with fluorescent microscopy)

KOH: fungi

Culture Media

Blood agar: most bacteria (except *Haemophilus*, *Neisseria*, and *Moraxella*) and fungi; very good for atypical *Mycobacterium*

Blood agar in 5% to 10% carbon dioxide: *Moraxella*

Chocolate (contains hemin and nicotinamide adenine dinucleotide [NAD]): *Haemophilus*, *Neisseria*, and *Moraxella*

Thioglycolate broth: aerobic and anaerobic bacteria

Cooked meat broth: anaerobic bacteria

Sabouraud agar: fungi

Brain-heart infusion agar: fungi

Löwenstein-Jensen agar: *Mycobacteria*, *Nocardia*

Loeffler: *Corynebacteria*

Non-nutrient agar with *Escherichia coli* overgrowth: *Acanthamoeba*

Period after conception	Event	Period after conception	Event
22nd day	Optic groove appears	3rd month	Differentiation of precursors of rods and cones
25th day	Optic vesicle forms from optic pit		Ciliary body develops
26th day	Primordia of superior rectus, inferior rectus, medial rectus, and inferior oblique appear		Appearance of limbus
			Anterior chamber appears as a potential space
27th day	Formation of lens plate from surface ectoderm		Sclera condenses
	Primordium of lateral rectus appears		Eyelid folds lengthen and fuse
28th day	Embryonic fissure forms	4th month	Formation of retinal vasculature begins
	Cells destined to become retinal pigment epithelium acquire pigmentation		Beginning of regression of hyaloid vessels
			Formation of physiologic cup of optic disc
29th day	Primordium of superior oblique appears		Formation of lamina cribrosa
5th week	Lens pit forms and deepens into lens vesicle		Major arterial circle of iris forms
	Hyaloid vessels develop		Development of iris sphincter muscle
	Primary vitreous develops		Development of longitudinal ciliary muscle and processes of ciliary body
	Osseous structures of the orbit begin to develop		Formation of tertiary vitreous
6th week	Closure of embryonic fissure		Bowman's membrane forms
	Corneal epithelial cells develop interconnections		Canal of Schlemm appears
	Differentiation of retinal pigment epithelium		Eyelid glands and cilia form
	Proliferation of neural retinal cells	5th month	Photoreceptors differentiate
	Formation of secondary vitreous		Eyelid separation begins
	Formation of primary lens fibers	6th month	Cones differentiate
	Development of periocular vasculature		Ganglion cells thicken in macula
	Appearance of eyelid folds and nasolacrimal duct		Differentiation of dilator pupillae muscle
	Ciliary ganglion appears		Nasolacrimal system becomes patent
7th week	Migration of ganglion cells toward optic disc	7th month	Rods differentiate
	Formation of embryonic lens nucleus		Ora serrata forms
	Development of choroidal vessels from periocular mesenchyme		Migration of ganglion cells to form nerve fiber layer of Henle
	Three waves of neural crest migration: first wave: formation of corneal and trabecular endothelium second wave: formation of corneal stroma third wave: formation of iris stroma		Choroid becomes pigmented
			Circular ciliary muscle fibers develop
			Myelination of optic nerve
			Posterior movement of anterior chamber angle
	Formation of tunica vasculosa lentis		Orbicularis muscle differentiation
	Sclera begins to form	8th month	Completion of anterior chamber angle formation
			Hyaloid vessels disappear
		9th month	Retinal vessels reach the temporal periphery
			Pupillary membrane disappears
		After birth	Development of macula

Figure 3.6 Timeline of ocular embryogenesis. (With permission from Azar NJ, Davis EA: Embryology in the eye. In: Yanoff M, Duker JS, eds. *Ophthalmology*. 2nd ed. St Louis: Mosby; 2004.)

Cytology

Intracytoplasmic basophilic inclusions (Giemsa stain): *Chlamydia*

Intranuclear eosinophilic inclusions (Papanicolaou stain): herpes (Tzanck smear)

TISSUE STAINS

Hematoxylin and eosin (H&E): hematoxylin is specific for nucleic acids within nuclei and stains blue (basophilic);

eosin is specific for most cytoplasmic organelles (such as mitochondria) and stains pink (eosinophilic)

Periodic acid-Schiff (PAS): stains basement membrane material magenta (Descemet, lens capsule, Bruch membrane, ILM, guttae, drusen); also stains glycogen, fungi, conjunctival goblet cells (useful for differentiation of corneal from conjunctival epithelium)

Masson trichrome: stains collagen blue or green, and hyaline red; used for granular dystrophy

Congo red: stains amyloid orange; used for lattice dystrophy

Crystal violet: stains amyloid red-purple; used for lattice dystrophy

Alcian blue: stains acid mucopolysaccharide (glycosaminoglycan) blue; used for macular dystrophy

Colloidal iron: stains acid mucopolysaccharide (glycosaminoglycan) blue; used for macular dystrophy

Oil red O: stains neutral lipids red-orange in frozen section; must be used on fresh tissue because formalin leaches out lipid

Sudan black: stains phospholipids; myelin in optic nerve

Luxol fast blue: stains myelin blue; demyelinated plaques lose affinity for stain

Bodian: stains nerve fibers black

Mucicarmine: stains mucus pink/red; mucus-secreting adenocarcinomas (i.e., mucoepithelioid variant of squamous cell carcinoma, gastrointestinal, breast)

Verhoeff Van Gieson: stains elastic tissue black; used for elastotic degeneration

Movat pentachrome: stains elastic tissue black

Wilder: stains reticulin fibers black

Alizarin red: stains calcium red-orange

von Kossa: stains calcium black; used for band keratopathy

Prussian blue: stains iron (hemosiderin, ferric ions) blue

Fontana-Masson: stains melanin black; used for amelanotic melanoma

S-100 protein: stains nevi, melanomas, schwannomas, neurofibromas, and other heterologous cell lines

Polarizing filters: for evaluating structures or deposits that have a regular molecular structure (amyloid, calcium oxalate crystals), as well as suture granulomas and vegetable foreign bodies

TISSUE FIXATION

Orientation of globe: identify superior oblique (SO) (tendinous insertion) and inferior oblique (IO) (muscular insertion) muscles

Paraffin: embedding process for histologic examination: water is removed, and organic solvents leach out lipids; polymethylmethacrylate (PMMA) is dissolved completely; to preserve lipids, fresh or frozen tissue specimens are used; paraffin must be removed before different stains are applied

Glutaraldehyde: for electron microscopy

Formalin and Bouin fixative: for light microscopy; 10% buffered formalin (formalin = 40% solution of formaldehyde in water); formalin stabilizes protein, lipid, and carbohydrates, and prevents postmortem enzymatic destruction of tissue

Ethyl alcohol: cytology

Fixation artifacts:

Lange's fold: retinal fold at ora serrata in newborn eyes probably caused by unequal shrinkage of retinociliary tissues during fixation

Artifactual RD: common histologic finding, differentiated from true retinal detachment by lack of subretinal fluid, preservation of photoreceptors, and pigment attached to outer surface of rods and cones (Fig. 3.7)

Clefts in corneal stroma: clear spaces within stroma; obliterated in corneal edema

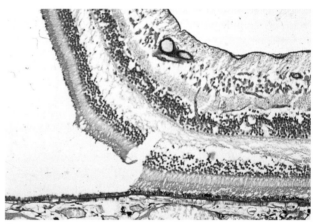

A

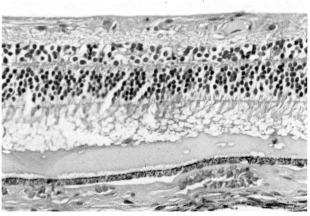

B

Figure 3.7 (A) Artifact retinal detachment (RD) with no fluid, pigment adherent to photoreceptors, and normal retinal architecture. (B) True RD with material in subretinal space and degeneration of outer retinal layers. (With permission from Yanoff M, Fine BS: *Ocular pathology*. 5th ed. St Louis: Mosby; 2002.)

ADAPTIVE IMMUNE-TRIGGERED INFLAMMATORY RESPONSES

Immune response arc: 3 phases (afferent, processing, effector)

Coombs and Gell Classification (Hypersensitivity Reactions): Prior to discovery of T lymphocytes

Type I: anaphylactic/immediate hypersensitivity (immunoglobulin E [IgE])

Example: hay fever, vernal, atopic, giant papillary conjunctivitis (GPC)

Type II: cytotoxic/antibody-dependent hypersensitivity (complement mediated, immunoglobulin M [IgM], immunoglobulin G [IgG])

Example: ocular cicatricial pemphigoid (OCP), Mooren ulcer

Type III: immune complex reactions (Ag–Ab complex, IgG)

Example: Stevens-Johnson, marginal infiltrates, disciform keratitis, subepithelial infiltrates, Wessely ring, scleritis, Behçet disease, phacoanaphylaxis, rheumatoid arthritis, systemic lupus erythematosus

Type IV: cell-mediated reaction/delayed hypersensitivity (CD4 lymphocytes)

Example: phlyctenule, graft reaction, contact dermatitis, interstitial keratitis, granulomatous disease (tuberculosis [TB], syphilis, leprosy, sarcoidosis), sympathetic ophthalmia, Vogt-Koyanagi-Harada (VKH) syndrome

Type V: autoimmune/stimulatory hypersensitivity (IgM or IgG, complement)

Example: Graves' disease, myasthenia gravis

Type of effector responses to adaptive immunity: More accurate classification

Antibody mediated: B-cell tissue infiltration and Ab secretion

Lymphocyte mediated: T-cell delayed hypersensitivity and cytotoxic T cell

Combined antibody and cellular mechanisms: antibody-dependent cellular cytotoxicity (ADCC) and acute IgE-mediated mast cell degranulation

Immune privilege: protects vital structures (i.e., central nervous system, eyes, testicles)

Ocular immune privilege (immunoregulatory mechanisms to modulate intraocular response) discovered when no inflammatory reaction from foreign antigen in anterior chamber

Iris, ciliary body, and RPE important in immune homeostasis; RPE regulation includes limiting T-cell activation and converting effector cells to regulatory cells

Anterior chamber–associated immune deviation (ACAID): attenuated effector phase of immune response

Effector blockade: T-cell and complement activation less effective in anterior uvea; various mechanisms, including Fas ligand (FasL, CD95 ligand; on iris and cornea (endothelium), downregulates inflammation by causing T-cell apoptosis)

IMMUNOGLOBULINS

IgG: most abundant; crosses the placenta; binds complement

IgA: second most abundant; monomeric or joined by J chain; important against viral infection; found in secretions

IgM: largest; binds complement; important in primary immune response

IgD: present in newborns; not in tear film; major receptor on B-cell surface

IgE: sensitizes mast cells and tissue leukocytes; role in atopy

Table 3.1	Human leukocyte antigen associations
Uveitis	
A2, DR5, DR8, DR11, DP2	Juvenile idiopathic arthritis (JIA)
A11, DR4	Sympathetic ophthalmia
A29	Birdshot chorioretinopathy (90%)
B7, DR2	Presumed ocular histoplasmosis syndrome (80%), acute posterior multifocal placoid pigment epitheliopathy (APMPPE)
B8, B13	Sarcoidosis
B8, B51, DR2, DR15	Intermediate uveitis
B27 (8% of population)	Adult iridocyclitis (usually unilateral): reactive arthritis syndrome (50%–75%), ankylosing spondylitis (90%), inflammatory bowel disease (60%), psoriatic arthritis (also B17)
	Whipple disease (also DRB1, DQB1)
Bw54	Posner-Schlossman syndrome
B5 (subtypes Bw51, Bw52), B12	Behçet disease (70%)
DR1, DR4, Dw53	Vogt-Koyanagi-Harada syndrome
DR15	Multiple sclerosis intermediate uveitis
DQw7, Bw62, DR4, Aw33, B44, DRw6	Acute retinal necrosis (50%)
DQA1, DQB1, DRB1	Tubulointerstitial nephritis and uveitis syndrome
External Disease	
B5, DR3, DR4	Herpes simplex virus keratitis
B8, DR3	Sjögren syndrome
B12	Ocular cicatricial pemphigoid
B15	Scleritis
DR3	Thygeson superficial punctate keratitis (SPK)
Neuro-Ophthalmology	
A1, B8, DR3	Myasthenia gravis (MG)
B7, DR2	Multiple sclerosis (MS)
DR3	Graves' disease

HLA (HUMAN LEUKOCYTE ANTIGEN) SYSTEM

Major histocompatibility complex (MHC) proteins found on surfaces of all nucleated cells

In humans, MHC proteins are the human leukocyte antigen (HLA) molecules

Gene loci are located on chromosome 6; 3 classes:
Class I: antigen presentation to cytotoxic T cells (CD8+); loci A, B, C
Class II: antigen presentation to helper T cells (CD4+); loci DR, DP, DQ
Class III: complement system; 3 pathways: classical (triggers bacterial cell wall attack), alternative (triggers phagocytosis), lectin (triggers inflammation)

INFLAMMATION

Inflammatory pathway (see Chapter 2, Pharmacology)

Tissue infiltration by inflammatory cells

Types of Inflammatory Cells

Leukocytes (white blood cells) divided into 2 categories: myeloid (neutrophils, eosinophils, basophils, mast cells, monocytes, macrophages, dendritic cells, and Langerhans cells) and lymphoid (T lymphocytes, B lymphocytes, natural killer cells)

Neutrophils: polymorphonuclear leukocytes (PMNs)
Primary cell in acute inflammation; migrate from bloodstream to site of inflammation by chemotaxis; primary functions are phagocytosis (mediated by antibody Fc receptors and complement receptors) and effector cells (release granule products and cytokines)
Multilobed nucleus
Abscess: focal collection of PMNs
Pus: PMNs and tissue necrosis

Eosinophils:
Allergic and parasite-related reactions (mnemonic: "worms, wheezes, weird diseases"); activated by many mediators (especially interleukin-5 [IL-5]), modulation of mast cell reactions, phagocytosis of Ag–Ab complexes
Bilobed nucleus, abundant lysosomes, cytoplasmic granules (i.e., major basic protein and ribonucleases effective for destroying parasites)

Mast cells: tissue basophils, 2 subtypes (connective tissue and mucosal)
IgE bound to surface, Ag causes degranulation; also involved in induction of cell-mediated immunity and wound healing
Connective tissue mast cells: release histamine and heparin, synthesize prostaglandin D_2
Mucosal mast cells: stimulated by cytokines from T cells to produce leukotrienes (C4), have low levels of histamine
Example: anaphylaxis, allergic conjunctivitis
Looks like plasma cell

Macrophages: derived from monocytes (Fig. 3.8)
Primary phagocytic cell; second line of cellular defense; regulation of lymphocytes via Ag presentation and monokine production
Kidney-shaped nucleus
Transformation into epithelioid histiocytes and fuse into multinucleated giant cells

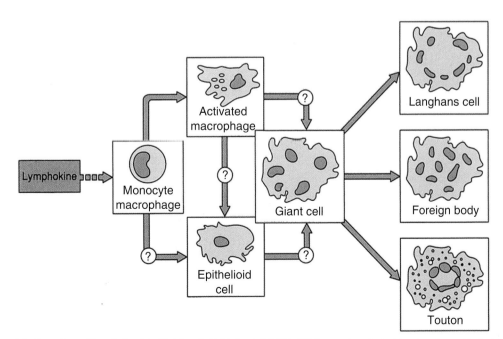

Figure 3.8 Macrophage differentiation. (Modified from Roitt IM, Brostoff J, Male DK: *Immunology*. 2nd ed. London: Gower Medical; 1989.)

Epithelioid histiocyte: activated macrophage with vesicular nucleus and eosinophilic cytoplasm; cells resemble epithelium; hallmark of granulomatous inflammation; fuse to form giant cells

Giant cells: 3 types

LANGHANS: nuclei arranged around periphery in ring/ horseshoe pattern
Example: TB, sarcoidosis

TOUTON: midperipheral ring of nuclei; central eosino-philic cytoplasm; nuclei are surrounded by clear zone of foamy lipid
Example: juvenile xanthogranuloma (JXG)

FOREIGN BODY: nuclei randomly distributed; surrounds or contains foreign body

Dendritic cells:

Bone marrow–derived mononuclear cells, located in blood and migrate to epithelial and lymphoid tissue

Upregulate costimulatory molecules, produce cytokines, activate immune cells

Langerhans cells:

Present in mucosal epithelium

When activated, degranulate and transform into dendritic-like cells; functions include antigen presentation, lymphoid cell regulation, differentiation of T lymphocytes, induction of delayed hypersensitivity

Lymphocytes:

Main cell in humoral and cell-mediated immune reactions; mature in peripheral lymphoid organs; 3 types:

B lymphocytes: activated by antigen receptor stimulation and helper T-cell interaction to differentiate and eventually become **plasma cells** (synthesis and secretion of antibodies, initially IgM, then switch to other classes); eccentric "cartwheel" nucleus, basophilic cytoplasm; **plasmacytoid cell** (granular eosinophilic cytoplasm), **Russell body** (immunoglobulin crystals)

T lymphocytes: helper (CD4+; differentiate into subsets producing different cytokines [Treg, Th1, Th2, Th17]; promote Ab secretion from B cells, eliminate pathogens, involved in hypersensitivity reactions), cytotoxic (CD8+; release cytokines and other cytotoxic molecules to destroy tumor cells and virus-infected cells, antigen specific)

Non-T, non-B lymphocytes: natural killer cells (similar to cytotoxic T cells, destroy tumor cells and virus-infected cells, but not antigen specific), lymphokine-activated cells, killer cells (mediate ADCC)

Scant cytoplasm

Types of Inflammation

Acute:

Suppurative: neutrophils
Nonsuppurative: lymphocytes

Chronic:

Nongranulomatous: lymphocytes and plasma cells
Granulation tissue in reparative phase; exuberant response causes pyogenic granuloma

Granulomatous: epithelioid histiocytes; 3 patterns

DIFFUSE: epithelioid cells distributed randomly against background of lymphocytes and plasma cells
Example: sympathetic ophthalmia, fungal infection, JXG, lepromatous leprosy

DISCRETE: epithelioid cells form nodules with giant cells, surrounded by rim of lymphocytes and plasma cells
Example: sarcoidosis, miliary TB, tuberculoid leprosy

ZONAL: palisaded giant cells surround central nidus
Example: phacoantigenic endophthalmitis (phacotoxic uveitis is nongranulomatous); rheumatoid scleritis (nidus = scleral collagen); chalazion

Endophthalmitis: inflammation involving at least one ocular coat and adjacent cavity; sclera is not involved

Panophthalmitis: suppurative endophthalmitis also involving sclera and orbit

Sequelae of Inflammation

Cornea: scarring

Calcific band keratopathy: basophilic granules in Bowman membrane

Inflammatory pannus: subepithelial fibrovascular and inflammatory ingrowth with destruction of Bowman membrane
Example: trachoma

Degenerative pannus: fibrous tissue between epithelium and intact Bowman membrane
Example: chronic corneal edema

Anterior chamber: organization of hypopyon; retrocorneal fibrous membranes

Peripheral anterior synechiae: seclusio pupillae (if 360°)
Pupillary membrane: occlusion pupillae

Lens:

Anterior subcapsular cataract: fibrous plaque beneath folded anterior capsule, secreted by irritated metaplastic anterior epithelial cells

Posterior subcapsular cataract: bladder cells adjacent to capsule

Ciliary body:

Cyclitic membrane: retrolental collagenous membrane attached to ciliary body; contraction leads to detachment of pars plana, ciliary muscle remains adherent to scleral spur attachment; attributable to organization and scarring of vitreous, metaplastic ciliary epithelium, organized inflammatory residua

Retina:

CME: retinal vascular leakage or Müller cell edema

RPE changes: hypertrophy, hyperplasia, and migration (pseudoretinitis pigmentosa); fibrous metaplasia (collagen and basement membrane material deposited on Bruch membrane, contain lacunae of RPE cells [pseudoadenomatous proliferation]); intraocular bone from osseous metaplasia

Reactive gliosis

Phthisis: rectus muscle traction on hypotonus globe causes squared-off appearance; thickened sclera, high incidence of retinal detachment and disorganization, calcareous degeneration of lens

EYELID EPITHELIAL CHANGES

Hyperkeratosis: thickening of the keratin layer; clinically appears as white, flaky lesion (leukoplakia)

Parakeratosis: thickening of the keratin layer with retention of nuclei; indicates shortened epidermal regeneration time; granular layer is thin or absent

Dyskeratosis: keratin formation within the basal cell layer or deeper

Acanthosis: thickening of the squamous cell layer resulting from proliferation of prickle cells

Acantholysis: loss of cohesion between epidermal cells with breakdown of intercellular junctions, creating spaces within the epidermis; occurs in pemphigus and produces intraepithelial bullae

Dysplasia: disorderly maturation of epithelium with loss of polarity, cytologic atypia, and mitotic figures found above the basal layer
  Mild: <50% epidermal thickness involved
  Severe: >50% involved

Carcinoma in situ: full-thickness replacement of epithelium by malignant cells without invasion through the basement membrane

Squamous cell carcinoma: malignant epithelial cells invade below basement membrane

Anaplasia: cytologic malignancy with pleomorphism, anisocytosis, abnormal nuclei, and mitotic figures

Papillomatosis: proliferation of dermal papillae, causing surface undulation

Pseudoepitheliomatous hyperplasia: inflammatory response with hyperplasia of epithelium, which mimics carcinoma; acanthosis with protrusion of broad tongues of benign epidermis into the dermis

Elastosis: actinic damage; seen as blue staining (normally pink) of superficial dermal collagen with H&E stain; damaged collagen stains with elastic tissue stains but is not susceptible to digestion with elastase (Fig. 3.9)

AGING CHANGES

Cornea: Hassal-Henle warts (excrescences and thickenings of Descemet membrane in corneal periphery)

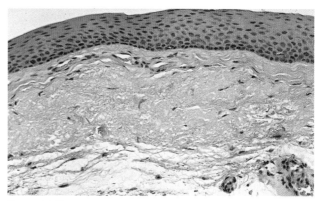

Figure 3.9 Elastosis demonstrating basophilic degeneration of conjunctival substantia propria in a pinguecula. (With permission from Yanoff M, Fine BS: *Ocular pathology.* 5th ed. St Louis: Mosby; 2002.)

Ciliary epithelium: hyperplasia and proliferation

Pars plana and pars plicata: clear (teardrop) cysts

Retina: wounds loss of retinal cells and replacement with glial tissue; chorioretinal adhesions and pigmentary lesions in periphery; peripheral microcystoid degeneration (Blessig-Iwanoff cysts): located in outer plexiform layer; bubbly appearance just behind ora serrata; lined by Müller cells; contain mucopolysaccharides

WOUNDS

Wound Healing

Cornea: stromal healing is avascular; fibrosis; neutrophils arrive via tears in 2–6 hours; wound edges swell and glycosaminoglycans (keratan sulfate, chondroitin sulfate) disintegrate at edge of wound; activated fibroblasts migrate across wound and produce; takes 4–6 weeks to return to full corneal thickness collagen and fibronectin, anterior surface reepithelializes; endothelium migrates and regenerates Descemet membrane (Box 3.1)

Sclera: does not heal itself; it is avascular and acellular; ingrowth of granulation tissue from episclera and choroid

Iris: no healing

Retina: scars are produced by glial cells rather than fibroblasts

Box 3.1 Collagen
Type 1: normal corneal stroma; Bowman membrane (highly disorganized type 1, basal lamina has type 4)
Type 2: vitreous
Type 3: stromal wound healing
Type 4: basement membranes

Wound Complications

Epithelial ingrowth: sheet of multilayered nonkeratinized squamous epithelium over any intraocular surface; may form cyst (free-floating or attached to iris); implanted cells tend to be 2–4 cell layers thick and have conjunctival characteristics (more than corneal)

Fibrous downgrowth: proliferating fibroblasts originate from episcleral or corneal stroma; contraction can occur; can occur with a puncture wound if there is a break in Descemet membrane

Hemorrhage:

Corneal blood staining: hemoglobin (Hgb) breakdown products are forced through endothelial cells by increased intraocular pressure (IOP); Hgb molecules are removed by phagocytic and biochemical processes

Hemosiderosis bulbi: hemosiderin contains iron; can damage essential intracellular enzyme systems

Ochre membrane: hemorrhage that accumulates on posterior surface of detached vitreous

Synchysis scintillans: accumulation of cholesterol within vitreous following breakdown of red blood cell membranes; angular, birefringent, flat crystalline particles with golden hue located in dependent portions of globe; cholesterol dissolves during preparation of tissues in paraffin; cholesterol clefts are negative image of cholesterol crystals, surrounded by serous fluid

OCULAR INJURIES

Blunt Trauma

Scleral rupture (weak spots):
1. Limbus (superonasal or on opposite side from trauma as circumferential arc parallel to limbus)
2. Posterior to rectus muscle insertions
3. Equator
4. Lamina cribrosa (ON)

Uveal tract is connected to sclera in 3 places:
1. Scleral spur
2. Internal ostia of vortex veins
3. Peripapillary tissue

Cyclodialysis: disinsertion of longitudinal fibers of ciliary muscle from scleral spur

Angle recession: rupture of face of ciliary body; plane of relative weakness at ciliary body face extending posteriorly between longitudinal fibers and more central oblique and circular fibers; oblique and circular muscles atrophy, changing cross-sectional shape of ciliary body from triangular to fusiform

Iridodialysis: disinsertion of iris root from ciliary body

Vossius ring: compression and rupture of IPE cells against anterior surface of lens deposit ring of melanin concentric to pupil

Lens capsule rupture: capsule is thinnest at posterior pole; cataract can form immediately; epithelium may be stimulated by trauma to form anterior lenticular fibrous plaque

Descemet rupture: causes acute edema (hydrops); results from minor trauma (keratoconus) or major trauma (forceps injury)

Choroidal rupture: often concentric to optic disc; risk of choroidal neovascularization (CNV)

Sclopetaria: high-speed projectiles (e.g., bullet injury); choroidal rupture with overlying rupture/necrosis of retina

Retinal dialysis: retina anchored anteriorly to nonpigmented epithelium of pars plana and reinforced by vitreous base, which straddles the ora serrata; circumferential tear of retina at point of attachment of ora or immediately posterior to vitreous base attachment

Commotio retinae: temporary loss of retinal transparency; results from disruption of photoreceptor elements, not true retinal edema

Penetrating Trauma

Penetration: partial-thickness wound (into)

Perforation: full-thickness wound (through) (globe penetration results from perforation of the cornea or sclera; globe perforation is a double-penetrating injury)

Sequelae of Trauma

Phthisis bulbi:

Atrophia bulbi without shrinkage: initially, size and shape of eye are maintained; with loss of nutrition: cataract develops, retina atrophies and separates from RPE by serous fluid accumulation, synechiae cause increased IOP

Atrophia bulbi with shrinkage: eye becomes soft as a result of ciliary body dysfunction; internal structures are atrophic but histologically recognizable; globe becomes smaller, with squared-off shape (because of tension of rectus muscles); anterior chamber collapses; corneal endothelial cell damage leads to corneal edema and opacification

Atrophia bulbi with disorganization (phthisis bulbi): globe shrinks to average diameter of 16–19 mm; most ocular contents are disorganized; calcification of Bowman layer, lens, retina, and drusen; bone formation in uveal tract

Intraocular Foreign Body

Copper:

≥85%: noninfectious suppurative endophthalmitis

<85% *(chalcosis):* copper deposits in basement membranes (Kayser-Fleischer ring, sunflower cataract, retinal degeneration)

Steel (contains iron): siderosis bulbi; follow with electroretinogram (early increased a wave, normal b wave; later decreased b wave leading to extinguished)

Organic (vegetable matter): severe granulomatous foreign body response

Chemical Injury

Acid: precipitates proteins; zone of coagulative necrosis acts as barrier to deeper penetration

Alkali: denatures proteins and lyses cell membranes; no effective barrier is created—therefore deeper penetration; vascular occlusion, ischemia, corneal damage during healing phase owing to collagenase released by regenerating tissue; limbal bleaching in severe cases (if limbal stem cells are depleted the corneal surface is repopulated with conjunctival cells)

Radiation

Nonionizing: depends on wavelength
Microwave: cataract
Infrared: true exfoliation of lens capsule (glassblower's cataract)
Ultraviolet: keratitis (welder's flash, snow blindness)

Ionizing: tissue damage is direct (actively reproducing cells) or indirect (blood vessels); epithelial atrophy and ulceration, dermatitis of eyelids, dysfunction of adnexa, destructive ocular surface disease with keratinization, cataract; retinal necrosis, ischemia, neovascularization, optic atrophy (retina is relatively radioresistant, but retinal blood vessels are vulnerable)

INFECTION (TABLE 3.2)

Table 3.2 Most common cause of infections

Endophthalmitis:	
Acute postoperative (<6 weeks)	Coagulase-negative *Staphylococcus*, *Staphylococcus aureus*
Delayed postoperative	*Propionibacterium acnes*, coagulase-negative *Staphylococcus*
From filtering bleb	*Streptococcus pneumoniae*, *Staphylococcus*, *Haemophilus influenzae*
Posttraumatic	*Staphylococcus* species, *Bacillus cereus*, gram-negative organisms
Endogenous (intravenous drug abuse [IVDA])	*Candida*
Dacryocystitis	*S. pneumoniae*, *Staphylococcus*
Dacryadenitis	*Staphylococcus*
Canaliculitis	*Actinomyces*
Orbital cellulitis (children)	*S. aureus*
Preseptal cellulitis	*S. aureus*
Angular blepharitis	*Staphylococcus*, *Moraxella*

TUMORS (BOX 3.2, 3.3, 3.4)

Box 3.2 Tumors

Congenital:
    Hamartoma: composed of tissues normally found in that area
    Example: hemangioma
    Choristoma: composed of tissues not normally found in that area
    Example: choroidal osteoma

Most common primary malignant intraocular tumor in adults: uveal melanoma

Second most common primary malignant intraocular tumor in adults: lymphoma

Most common primary malignant intraocular tumor in children: retinoblastoma

Second most common primary malignant intraocular tumor in children: medulloepithelioma

Most common malignant lacrimal gland tumor: adenocystic carcinoma

Most common benign orbital tumor in adults: cavernous hemangioma

Most common benign orbital tumor in children: capillary hemangioma

Most common primary malignant orbital tumor in children: rhabdomyosarcoma

Most common metastasis to orbit in children: neuroblastoma

Box 3.3 Differential diagnostics of intraocular calcification

Retinoblastoma
Choroidal osteoma
Choroidal hemangioma
Phthisis
Osseous choristoma

Box 3.4 Differential diagnostics of intraocular cartilage

Persistent hyperplastic primary vitreous (retrolental plaque)
Medulloepithelioma
Teratoma
Trisomy 13 (Fig. 3.10)
Complex choristoma of conjunctiva

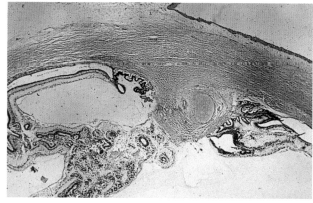

Figure 3.10 Trisomy 13 demonstrating intraocular cartilage and retinal dysplasia. (Reported in Hoepner J, Yanoff M: Ocular anomalies in trisomy 13–15: an analysis of 13 eyes with two new findings. *Am J Ophthalmol.* 1972;74:729–737.)

REVIEW QUESTIONS *(Answers start on page 412)*

1. Which stain is the most helpful in the diagnosis of sebaceous gland carcinoma?
   a. giemsa
   b. hematoxylin and eosin
   c. oil-red-O
   d. methenamine silver

2. Pagetoid spread is most commonly associated with
   a. malignant melanoma
   b. squamous cell carcinoma
   c. sebaceous gland carcinoma
   d. Merkel cell tumor

3. A melanoma occurring in which of the following locations has the best prognosis?
   a. iris
   b. ciliary body
   c. choroid, anteriorly
   d. choroid, posterior pole

4. Calcification in retinoblastoma is caused by
   a. RPE metaplasia
   b. necrosis
   c. hemorrhage
   d. metastasis

5. The type of organism that causes Lyme disease is a
   a. bacillus
   b. spirochete
   c. protozoan
   d. tick

6. Characteristics of ghost cells include all of the following, *except*
   a. khaki-colored
   b. rigid
   c. Heinz bodies
   d. biconcave

7. A gland of Moll is best categorized as
   a. mucinw
   b. apocrine
   c. sebaceous
   d. holocrine

8. Which of the following is *not* a gram-positive rod?
   a. *Corynebacterium*
   b. *Bacillus*
   c. *Serratia*
   d. *Listeria*

9. Trantas dots are composed of what cell type?
   a. macrophage
   b. neutrophil
   c. eosinophil
   d. mast cell

10. Types of collagen that can be found in the cornea include all of the following, *except*
    a. I
    b. II
    c. III
    d. IV

11. Lens nuclei are retained in all of the following conditions, *except*
    a. Leigh syndrome
    b. Lowe syndrome
    c. Rubella
    d. Alport syndrome

12. VKH syndrome is best described by which type of hypersensitivity reaction?
    a. I
    b. II
    c. III
    d. IV

13. Lacy vacuolization of the iris pigment epithelium occurs in which disease?
    a. central retinal vein occlusion
    b. diabetes
    c. central retinal artery occlusion
    d. hypercholesterolemia

14. Antoni A and B cells occur in which tumor?
    a. neurilemmoma
    b. meningioma
    c. glioma
    d. neurofibroma

15. Which tumor is classically described as having a "Swiss cheese" appearance?
    a. rhabdomyosarcoma
    b. adenoid cystic carcinoma
    c. benign mixed tumor
    d. meningioma

16. Which iris nodule is correctly paired with its histopathology?
    a. JXG, inflammatory cells
    b. Lisch nodule, neural crest hamartoma
    c. Koeppe nodule, stromal hyperplasia
    d. Brushfield spot, histiocytes and Touton giant cells

17. Which of the following statements is true concerning immunoglobulin?
    a. IgG crosses the placenta
    b. IgA binds complement
    c. IgM is present in newborns
    d. IgD is the second most abundant

18. A retinal detachment caused by fixation artifact can be differentiated from a true retinal detachment by all of the following, *except*
    a. a fold at the ora serrata
    b. no subretinal fluid
    c. normal retinal architecture
    d. pigment adherent to photoreceptors

19. Which of the following epithelial changes in the eyelid refers to thickening of the squamous cell layer?
    a. parakeratosis
    b. acanthosis
    c. dysplasia
    d. papillomatosis

20. Intraocular hemorrhage may cause all of the following sequelae, *except*
    a. synchysis scintillans
    b. ochre membrane
    c. asteroid hyalosis
    d. hemosiderosis bulbi

21. Intraocular calcification may occur in all of the following, *except*
    a. retinoblastoma
    b. medulloepithelioma
    c. choroidal hemangioma
    d. phthisis

22. The histopathology of which tumor is classically described as a storiform pattern of tumor cells?
    a. rhabdomyosarcoma
    b. plasmacytoma
    c. neurilemmoma
    d. fibrous histiocytoma

23. Which of the following findings is a histologic fixation artifact?
    a. Lange's fold
    b. Mittendorf dot
    c. Berger's space
    d. Cloquet's canal

24. The corneal stroma is composed of
    a. surface ectoderm
    b. neural crest cells
    c. mesoderm
    d. neural ectoderm

25. *Neisseria* is best cultured with which media?
    a. Loeffler
    b. Sabouraud
    c. thioglycolate
    d. chocolate agar

26. Which of the following stains is used to detect amyloid?
    a. colloidal iron
    b. alcian blue
    c. crystal violet
    d. Masson trichrome

27. HLA-B7 is associated with
    a. Behçet disease
    b. presumed ocular histoplasmosis syndrome
    c. iridocyclitis
    d. sympathetic ophthalmia

28. Which of the following conjunctival lesions should be sent to the pathology lab as a fresh unfixed tissue specimen?
    a. lymphoma
    b. squamous cell carcinoma
    c. Kaposi sarcoma
    d. melanoma

29. Subepithelial infiltrates in the cornea from epidemic keratoconjunctivitis are thought to be
    a. lymphocytes and dead adenovirus
    b. polymorphonuclear leukocytes surrounding live adenovirus
    c. macrophages containing adenoviral particles
    d. lymphocytes and polymorphonuclear leukocytes

30. Which is the correct order of solutions for performing a Gram stain?
    a. iodine solution, crystal violet stain, ethanol, safranin
    b. crystal violet stain, safranin, ethanol, iodine solution
    c. iodine solution, safranin, ethanol, crystal violet stain
    d. crystal violet stain, iodine solution, ethanol, safranin

31. The iris sphincter is derived from what embryologic tissue?
    a. neural crest cells
    b. surface ectoderm
    c. neural ectoderm
    d. mesoderm

32. Blepharitis is most commonly associated with
    a. *Streptococcus pneumoniae*
    b. *Staphylococcus aureus*
    c. *Haemophilus pneumoniae*
    d. *Propionibacterium acnes*

33. Which type of radiation causes lens capsule scrolling?
    a. infrared
    b. ionizing
    c. microwave
    d. ultraviolet

34. Which of the following measures is most likely to reduce the risk of postoperative endophthalmitis following cataract surgery?
    a. preoperative povidone-iodine drops
    b. eyelid draping
    c. intracameral injection of gentamicin
    d. subconjunctival injection of gentamicin

35. The most common causative organism of canaliculitis is
    a. *Candida albicans*
    b. Herpes simplex virus
    c. *Actinomyces israelii*
    d. *Nocardia asteroides*

36. The crystalline lens is formed from which embryologic tissue?
    a. neural crest
    b. ectoderm
    c. mesoderm
    d. endoderm

37. Which of the following bacteria can penetrate an intact corneal epithelium?
    a. *Staphylococcus aureus*
    b. *Staphylococcus epidermidis*
    c. *Neisseria gonorrhoeae*
    d. *Proprionibacterium acnes*

38. Which immunoglobulin is *not* found in the tear film?
    a. IgA
    b. IgD
    c. IgE
    d. IgG

39. Where is the major arterial circle of the iris located?
    a. iris stroma
    b. iris dilator muscle
    c. iris pigment epithelium
    d. ciliary body

40. The zonules are formed from
    a. primary vitreous
    b. secondary vitreous
    c. tertiary vitreous
    d. quaternary vitreous

Please visit the eBook for an interactive version of the review questions. See front cover for activation details.

SUGGESTED READINGS

Embryology

Mann, I. (1964). *The development of the human eye.* New York: Grune & Stratton.

Pathology

Apple, D. J. (1998). *Ocular pathology: Clinical applications and self-assessment* (5th ed.). St. Louis: Mosby.

Basic and Clinical Science Course. (2021). *Section 2: Fundamentals and principles of ophthalmology.* San Francisco: AAO.

Basic and Clinical Science Course. (2021). *Section 4: Ophthalmic pathology and intraocular tumors.* San Francisco: AAO.

Char, P. H. (2001). *Tumors of the eye and ocular adnexa.* Ontario, Canada: BC Decker.

Eagle, R. C. (2011). *Eye pathology: An atlas and basic text* (2nd ed.). Philadelphia: Lippincott Williams & Wilkins.

Spencer, W. H. (1996). *Ophthalmic pathology: An atlas and textbook* (4th ed.). Philadelphia: W. B. Saunders.

Yanoff, M., & Sassani, J. W. (2019). *Ocular pathology* (8th ed.). Philadelphia: Saunders.

4

Neuro-Ophthalmology

ANATOMY OF THE VISUAL PATHWAY

Optic nerve → chiasm → optic tract → lateral geniculate body → optic radiation → occipital lobe (Fig. 4.1)

Optic nerve (ON): composed of 1.2 million nerve fibers; ON head diameter ~1.8 mm, enlarges to 3.5 mm posterior to lamina cribrosa as a result of myelin sheath; located 3–4 mm from fovea; causes absolute scotoma (blind spot) 15° temporal to fixation and slightly below horizontal meridian; ~45–50 mm in length (1 mm intraocular, 25–30 mm intraorbital, 4–10 mm intracanalicular, 3–16 mm [usually ~10 mm] intracranial) (Fig. 4.2); acquires myelin posterior to lamina cribrosa

Surrounded by 3 layers of meninges: dura mater (outer layer; merges with sclera), arachnoid layer, pia mater (inner layer, fused to surface of nerve); space between arachnoid and pia contains cerebrospinal fluid (CSF)

ON runs through annulus of Zinn (ring of tendinous origins of the rectus muscles) and enters the optic canal

Optic canal: 9 mm long and 5–7 mm wide; thinnest medially, adjacent to ethmoid and sphenoid sinuses; dura of ON fuses with periosteum of canal

Intracranial ON: above are found the frontal lobe, olfactory tract, and anterior cerebral and anterior communicating arteries; laterally, the internal carotid artery (ICA) emerges from the cavernous sinus

Blood supply (Fig. 4.3)

    INTRAORBITAL PORTION: pial vessels, branches of central retinal and ophthalmic arteries

    INTRACANALICULAR PORTION: branches of ophthalmic artery

    INTRACRANIAL PORTION: branches of ophthalmic, anterior cerebral, and superior hypophysial arteries

Chiasm: 10 mm above pituitary gland, ~12 mm wide, 8 mm long, 4 mm thick

53% of ON fibers cross in chiasm: nasal retinal fibers cross in chiasm to contralateral optic tract (decussating nasal fibers); inferior fibers (subserving the superior visual field) are the first to cross; temporal fibers remain uncrossed; macular fibers run posteriorly (posterior compression leads to bitemporal defect)

"Knee of von Willebrand": inferonasal retinal fibers cross in chiasm and course anteriorly ~4 mm into contralateral ON before running posteriorly; produces junctional scotoma

Carotid arteries course on either side of chiasm (Fig. 4.4)

Blood supply: ICA; occasionally by anterior cerebral and anterior communicating arteries

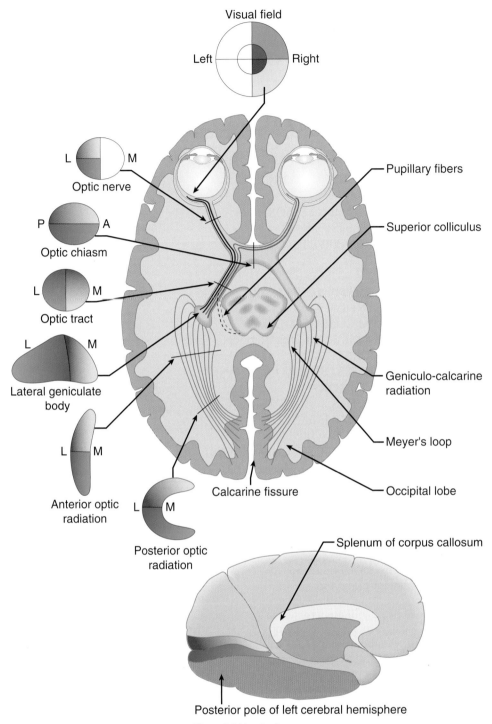

Figure 4.1 Visual pathway.

Optic tract: lower fibers lie laterally (90° rotation of fibers); tract courses laterally around cerebral peduncle; 70% fibers travel to lateral geniculate body (LGB) and 30% to superior colliculus

    Damage to optic tract results in contralateral relative afferent pupillary defect (RAPD) because 53% of fibers cross (greater quantity of nasal fibers [nasal to foveal]), including the large monocular crescent (which corresponds with the extreme nasal retina)

Special fibers run to the hypothalamus, contributing to neuroendocrine systems that control diurnal rhythms

A major projection leaves the optic tract just before the LGB to form the brachium of the superior colliculus (also called optic tectum)

Superior colliculus: involved in foveation reflexes (receives input from pupillary fibers); injury disrupts eye movements but does not cause visual field (VF) defect

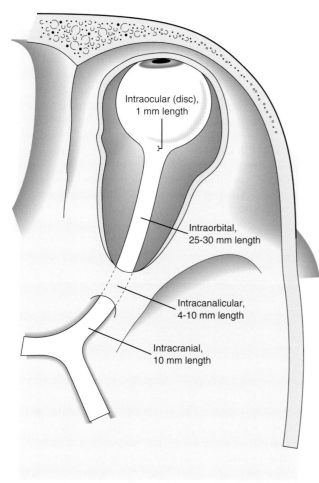

Figure 4.2 The four portions of the optic nerve. The lengths are given. (With permission from Sadun AA: Anatomy and physiology. In: Yanoff M, Duker JS, eds. *Ophthalmology*. 2nd ed. St Louis: Mosby; 2004.)

Pupillary fibers pass through brachium of superior colliculus to pretectal area, which innervates both Edinger-Westphal subnuclei of CN 3

Optic tract provides retinal input to visual nucleus (pulvinar) in the thalamus

Blood supply: anterior choroidal artery; branches from posterior communicating artery

Lateral geniculate body (LGB): part of the thalamus (Fig. 4.5)

Lower fibers lie laterally in optic tract and LGB (90° rotation of fibers)

Crossed fibers (contralateral eye): project to layers 1, 4, and 6

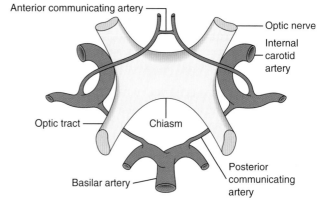

Figure 4.4 Relationship of the optic chiasm, optic nerves, and optic tracts to the arterial circle of Willis. The chiasm passes through the circle of Willis and receives its arterial supply from the anterior cerebral and communicating arteries from above and the posterior communicating, posterior cerebral, and basilar arteries from below. (Adapted from Reed H, Drance SM. *The essentials of perimetry: static and kinetic*. 2nd ed. London: Oxford University Press; 1972.)

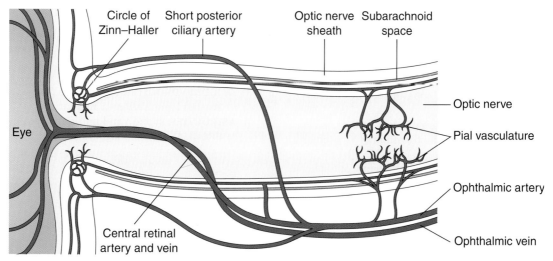

Figure 4.3 Anterior optic nerve. The sheath and the vascular supply to the intraocular and intraorbital portions are shown. (With permission from Sadun AA: Anatomy and physiology. In: Yanoff M, Duker JS, eds. *Ophthalmology*. 2nd ed. St Louis: Mosby; 2004.)

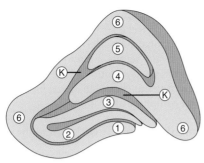

Figure 4.5 Lateral geniculate body section. The layers are numbered from ventral to dorsal in this posterior view. K fibers travel between the lamellae. (With permission from Lawton AW: Retrochiasmal pathways, higher cortical function, and nonorganic visual loss. In: Yanoff M, Duker JS, eds. *Ophthalmology*. 2nd ed. St Louis: Mosby; 2004.)

Uncrossed fibers (ipsilateral eye): project to layers 2, 3, and 5

Layers of LGB can also be categorized by neuronal size:
MAGNOCELLULAR NEURONS (M cells): layers 1 and 2; subserve motion detection, stereoacuity, and contrast sensitivity; project to layer 4C alpha of visual cortex
PARVOCELLULAR NEURONS (P cells): layers 3–6; subserve fine spatial resolution and color vision; project to layer 4C beta of visual cortex
KONIOCELLULAR NEURONS (K cells): sit in interlaminar zones and superficial layers; receive input from both retinas and the superior colliculus; may modulate information among other pathways

Blood supply: anterior communicating artery and choroidal arteries

Optic radiation: myelinated nerve fibers; connect LGB to occipital cortex
Superior retinal fibers (inferior VF): travel in white matter underneath parietal cortex to occipital lobe
Inferior retinal fibers (superior VF): travel around ventricular system into temporal lobe (Meyer's loop); Meyer's loop is ~5 cm from tip of temporal lobe; temporal lobe injury causes incongruous homonymous superior quadrantanopia, or a "pie-in-the-sky" VF defect
Macular fibers: travel more centrally than do inferior retinal fibers
Blood supply: middle cerebral arteries

Primary visual cortex (striate cortex, V1, Brodmann's area 17): medial face of occipital lobe, divided horizontally by calcarine fissure
Visual cortex contains a topographic map of the contralateral hemifield; central portion of VF is highly magnified
Macular region is posterior, extending slightly onto lateral aspect of occipital lobe
Peripheral VF is located anteriorly along calcarine fissure
Temporal crescent in each VF (from 55°–100°) is seen only by nasal retina of ipsilateral eye; located most anteriorly; only site posterior to chiasm that, if injured, would cause a monocular VF defect; temporal crescent may also be the only portion of VF spared after occipital lobe damage

Blood supply: middle and posterior cerebral arteries

Visual association areas: areas 18 and 19

Other areas:
Ganglia:
CILIOSPINAL CENTER OF BUDGE: sympathetic fibers from hypothalamus synapse; located at level C8 to T2
SUPERIOR CERVICAL: second-order sympathetic fibers synapse
CILIARY: small parasympathetic ganglion; 1 cm from optic foramen between ON and lateral rectus muscle
RECEIVES 3 ROOTS:
Long sensory: sensory from cornea, iris, and ciliary body
Short parasympathetic (synapse): motor to ciliary body and iris sphincter
Sympathetic (do not synapse): conjunctival vasoconstrictor fibers and iris dilator
GENICULATE: traversed by CN 7; contains cell bodies that provide taste from anterior 2/3 of tongue
SPHENOPALATINE: parasympathetic fibers to lacrimal gland
Horizontal gaze center: controls gaze to ipsilateral side; located in paramedian pontine reticular formation (PPRF) at level of CN 6 nucleus; projects to ipsilateral CN 6 nucleus and (via medial longitudinal fasciculus [MLF]) to contralateral CN 3 nucleus (Fig. 4.6)
Medial longitudinal fasciculus: extends from anterior horn cells of the spinal cord to the thalamus; connects CN 3 nuclei and gaze centers (ipsilateral CN 3 and contralateral CN 6)
Vertical gaze center: originates in frontal eye fields or in superior colliculus; requires bilateral cortical input; projections travel to rostral interstitial nucleus of the MLF (riMLF) located behind red nucleus in midbrain; fibers travel to nuclei of CN 3 and 4 (Fig. 4.7)
UPGAZE (lateral portion of riMLF): stimulates CN 3 nucleus (superior rectus [SR] and inferior oblique [IO])
DOWNGAZE (medial portion of riMLF): stimulates CN 3 nucleus (inferior rectus [IR]) and CN 4 nucleus
TORSIONAL MOVEMENTS: via interstitial nucleus of Cajal
Glial cells:
OLIGODENDROCYTES: myelination (begins at LGB and reaches lamina cribrosa after birth)
ASTROCYTES: support and nutrition
MICROGLIAL CELLS: phagocytosis

PHYSIOLOGY

Testing

Color vision tests: Ishihara pseudoisochromatic or Hardy-Rand-Ritter plates; Farnsworth tests
Congenital defects: usually red/green

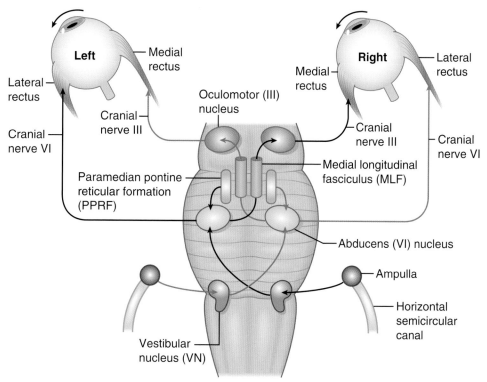

Figure 4.6 Horizontal eye movement pathways. (With permission from Bajandas FJ, Kline LB: *Neuro-ophthalmology review manual*. Thorofare, NJ: Slack; 1998.)

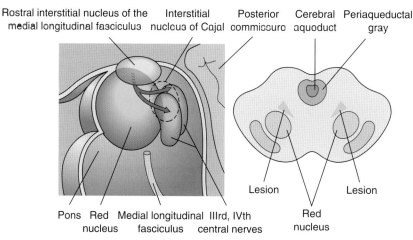

Upgaze

Rostral interstitial nucleus of the medial longitudinal fasciculus

Posterior commissure

Lesion B Lesion A Lesion B Lesion C

Pons Red nucleus IIIrd, IVth central nerves

Red nucleus

Downgaze

Rostral interstitial nucleus of the medial longitudinal fasciculus

Interstitial nucleus of Cajal

Posterior commissure

Cerebral aquoduct

Periaqueductal gray

Lesion Lesion

Pons Red nucleus Medial longitudinal fasciculus IIIrd, IVth central nerves

Red nucleus

Figure 4.7 Pathways for vertical gaze. Upgaze pathways originate in the rostral interstitial nucleus of the medial longitudinal fasciculus and project dorsally to innervate the oculomotor and trochlear nerves, traveling through the posterior commissure. Lesions to both axon bundles are necessary to produce upgaze paralysis *(lesions B or C)*. Upgaze paralysis is a feature of the dorsal midbrain syndrome as a result of the lesion's effect on the posterior commissure *(lesion A)*. Downgaze pathways also originate in the rostral interstitial nucleus of the medial longitudinal fasciculus but probably travel more ventrally. Bilateral lesions also are needed to affect downgaze and usually are located dorsomedial to the red nucleus. (With permission from Donahue SP, Lavin PJM: Disorders of supranuclear control of ocular motility. In: Yanoff M, Duker JS, eds. *Ophthalmology*. London: Mosby; 1999.)

Acquired macular disease: may diminish blue/yellow in early stages (blue cones concentrated in perifoveal ring)

Fovea has mostly red/green cones, so red/green defects are detected in ON diseases. Perception of red object indicates gross macular function

Photostress recovery test: determine best-corrected vision, shine bright light into eye for 10 seconds, record time for vision to recover within 1 line of best-corrected vision; test each eye separately; invalid for eyes with vision worse than 20/80

Optic nerve disease: normal recovery time (<60 seconds)

Macular disease: prolonged time (>90 seconds)

Contrast sensitivity: Pelli-Robson chart; Regan contrast sensitivity chart; VectorVision chart

Visually evoked potential/response (VEP, VER): measures macular visual function, integrity of primary and secondary visual cortex, and continuity of ON and tract radiations; fovea has large area in occipital cortex, close to recording electrodes; smaller area representing more peripheral retina lies deep within calcarine fissure (Fig. 4.8)

Can measure vision in preverbal infants

Flash VER: strobe light

Pattern VER: checkerboard pattern or bar grating (amacrine and ganglion cell layer of retina)

P100 wave: positive deflection at 100 ms; amplitude is height from peak to trough, latency is time from onset of flash to peak of wave

Toxic or compressive optic neuropathies: reduction of amplitude more pronounced than prolongation of latency

Demyelination: latency is prolonged; amplitude may be only mildly reduced

Amsler grid: tests central 10° of the visual field (held at 35 cm); 10 cm × 10 cm grid composed of 5-mm squares; primarily used to evaluate foveal pathology

Optokinetic nystagmus (OKN): presence suggests visual input is present; slow phase is noted in direction of moving stimulus

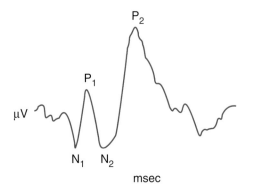

Figure 4.8 Normal visual evoked cortical response. (Reprinted with permission from Slamovits TL: *Basic and clinical science course. Section 12: Retina and Vitreous.* San Francisco: American Academy of Ophthalmology; 1993.)

Parieto-occipital area controls slow pursuit, frontal lobe controls saccades

Pathway in visual association area terminates in ipsilateral pontine gaze center, resulting in pursuit movements to the same side (i.e., right visual association area controls pursuit to the right)

Can use to diagnose functional visual loss

Normal (symmetric) OKN response: occipital lobe, temporal lobe, LGB, or optic tract lesions do not interfere with pursuit

Deficient pursuit movements to side of lesion (asymmetric OKN): parietal lobe lesion

Cogan's dictum (for homonomous hemianopia): asymmetric OKN indicates parietal lobe lesion; symmetric OKN indicates occipital lobe lesion

Reversal of OKN response: 60% of patients with congenital motor nystagmus

Dorsal midbrain syndrome: downward-moving OKN drum causes convergence–retraction nystagmus

Congenital ocular motor apraxia: loss of voluntary horizontal gaze (vertical gaze intact); abnormal OKN (fast phase absent); maintained tonic deviation; requires neuroimaging

Red glass test: evaluation of diplopia

Potential acuity meter (PAM): projects image of letter chart onto retina to test macular potential in patients with media opacities

Purkinje vascular phenomena and blue field entopic test: visualization of retinal vasculature; indicates gross retinal function

Visual Field Defects (Fig. 4.9)

Types:

Blind spot: physiologic as a result of ON; 15° temporal to fixation and slightly below horizontal midline

Baring of blind spot: glaucoma, normal patients

Cecocentral scotoma: involves blind spot and macula (within 25° of fixation); can occur in any condition that produces a central scotoma, dominant optic atrophy, Leber hereditary optic neuropathy (LHON), toxic/nutritional optic neuropathy, optic pit with serous retinal detachment, optic neuritis

Central scotoma: unilateral (optic neuritis, compressive lesion of ON, retinal lesion [macular edema, disciform scar]); bilateral (toxic optic neuropathy, nutritional deficiency, macular lesions)

Arcuate scotoma: glaucoma, optic neuritis, anterior ischemic optic neuropathy (AION), branch retinal artery occlusion (BRAO), branch vein occlusion (BVO), ON drusen

Altitudinal defect: damage to upper or lower pole of optic disc; optic neuritis, AION, hemiretinal artery or vein occlusion

Spiraling of VF: suggests malingering/functional visual loss

Pseudo-bitemporal hemianopia (slope and cross-vertical meridian): uncorrected refractive error, tilted optic disc, enlarged blind spot (papilledema), large central or

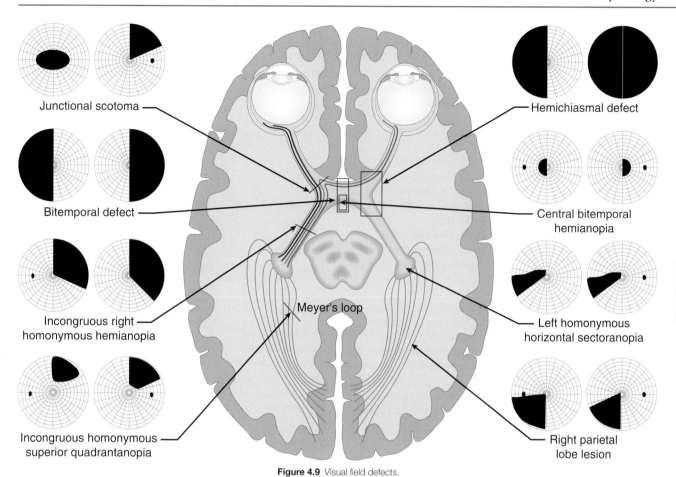

Figure 4.9 Visual field defects.

cecocentral scotoma, sector retinitis pigmentosa (nasal quadrant), overhanging lid, coloboma

Binasal defect: most nasal defects result from arcuate scotomas (glaucoma); also, pressure on temporal aspect of ON and anterior angle of chiasm, aneurysm, pituitary adenoma, infarct

Constricted field (ring scotoma): retinitis pigmentosa, advanced glaucoma, thyroid eye disease, ON drusen, vitamin A deficiency, occipital stroke, panretinal photocoagulation, functional visual loss

Neurologic defect: bilateral and respects vertical midline

Localizing VF defects:

Nerve fiber layer: arcuate, papillomacular, temporal wedge

Chiasm: bitemporal hemianopia (junctional scotoma if involving Willebrand's knee)

Optic tract: incongruous homonymous hemianopia

Temporal lobe (Meyer's loop): "pie-in-the-sky" (denser superiorly, spares central)

Parietal lobe: denser inferiorly

Occipital lobe: congruous; ± macular sparing

Neurologic VF defects:

Congruity of VF defect (retrochiasmal lesions): the more congruous the defect, the more posterior the lesion

Superior field: anterior retinal ganglion cells → lateral portion of optic tract → temporal lobe (Meyer's loop) → inferior bank of calcarine fissure

Vision not reduced by unilateral lesion posterior to the chiasm (20/20 acuity with macula-splitting hemianopia)

Chiasm: pituitary tumor, pituitary apoplexy, craniopharyngioma, meningioma, ON glioma, aneurysm, trauma, infection, metastatic tumor, multiple sclerosis (MS), sarcoid

ANTERIOR CHIASMAL SYNDROME: lesion at junction of ON and chiasm; involves fibers in Willebrand's knee (contralateral nasal retinal loop); causes **junctional scotoma** (central scotoma in one eye and superotemporal defect in the other)

BODY OF CHIASM: bitemporal hemianopia; vision may be preserved

POSTERIOR CHIASM: bitemporal hemianopia; primarily involves crossing macular fibers

LATERAL COMPRESSION: very rare; binasal hemianopia (more commonly caused by bilateral ON or retinal lesions)

Optic tract: posterior sellar or suprasellar lesions; homonymous hemianopia, contralateral RAPD

Retro-LGB lesions: 90% of isolated homonymous hemianopias result from stroke

Optic radiations:

TEMPORAL LOBE (MEYER'S LOOP): "pie-in-the-sky" (superior homonymous hemianopia), formed visual hallucinations, seizures

PARIETAL LOBE: inferior homonymous hemianopia, hemiparesis, visual perception difficulty, agnosia, apraxia, OKN asymmetry

GERSTMANN SYNDROME: lesion of dominant parietal lobe; acalculia, agraphia, finger agnosia, left–right confusion, associated with inferior homonymous hemianopia if optic radiation involved

Occipital lobe:

HOMONYMOUS HEMIANOPIA WITH MACULAR SPARING: suggests infarct in area supplied by posterior cerebral artery; macular region receives dual supply from both middle cerebral artery (MCA) and posterior cerebral artery

BILATERAL CONGRUOUS CENTRAL ISLANDS WITH VERTICAL STEP: equivalent to homonymous hemianopia with macular sparing; vertical step does not occur in retinal or ON lesions

CHECKERBOARD FIELD: bilateral incomplete homonymous hemianopias, superior on one side and inferior on opposite side (left upper and right lower homonymous quadrant defects)

BILATERAL HOMONYMOUS ALTITUDINAL DEFECTS: infarction or trauma to both occipital lobes, above or below calcarine fissure

MONOCULAR TEMPORAL CRESCENT DEFECT: anterior occipital infarct; far temporal field is seen by only one eye

Cortical blindness: bilateral occipital lobe destruction; pupillary response intact, blindsight (rudimentary visual capacity), unformed visual hallucinations, Riddoch phenomenon (perceive moving targets but not stationary ones); may deny blindness (**Anton syndrome**)

Eye Movements Under Supranuclear Control

Horizontal gaze center (Figs. 4.10 and 4.11):

Saccades: contralateral frontal eye fields (frontal lobe) → superior colliculus → PPRF → horizontal gaze center (CN 6 nucleus) → ipsilateral lateral rectus (LR) and contralateral medial rectus (MR) (via MLF)

Smooth pursuit: ipsilateral parieto-occipital lobe → superior colliculus (SC) → PPRF → horizontal gaze center → ipsilateral LR and contralateral MR (via MLF)

Saccadic system: generates fast eye movements (FEMs) (refixation); 300°–700°/s

Tests: refixation, rotation, calorics, and optokinetic nystagmus (fast saccadic return phase)

Abnormalities: progressive external ophthalmoplegia, myasthenia gravis, Wilson disease, Huntington disease, ataxia-telangiectasia, spinocerebellar degeneration, progressive supranuclear palsy, olivopontocerebellar atrophy, Whipple disease, Gaucher disease, MS, Pelizaeus-Merzbacher disease

Ocular motor apraxia: failure to initiate a saccade

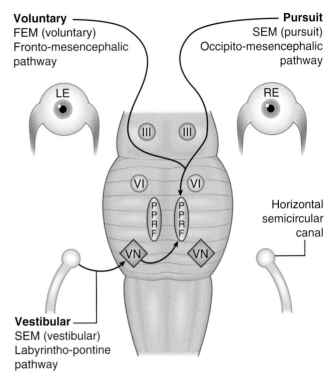

Figure 4.10 Fast eye movement (voluntary), slow eye movement (SEM; pursuit), and SEM (vestibular). Pathways all converge on paramedian pontine reticular formation for horizontal eye movements. *VN,* Vestibular nuclei. (With permission from Bajandas FJ, Kline LB: *Neuro-ophthalmology review manual.* Thorofare, NJ: Slack; 1998.)

Smooth pursuit system: slow eye movements (SEMs); following movements; ipsilateral parieto-occipital junction (horizontal); interstitial nucleus of Cajal (vertical)

Tests: Doll's head, rotation, OKN (pursuit movement)

Abnormalities: demyelination (young patients), microvascular disease (older patients)

Vergence system: maintains foveal fixation on approaching object; controlled by frontal and occipital lobes, and possibly midbrain

Types: voluntary, accommodative, fusional

Test: look from distance to near

Position maintenance system (vestibulo-ocular reflex [VOR]): maintains specific gaze position during head movements

Teleologically oldest eye movement system; also fastest (shortest latency)

Semicircular canals → CN 8 → vestibular nucleus → contralateral horizontal gaze center → extraocular muscles (EOMs)

Test: calorics, rotation

Abnormalities cause oscillopsia

Nonoptic reflex systems: integrate eye movements with body movements

Normal caloric and Doll's head responses when nuclear and internuclear connections are intact

Calorics: irrigate water into ears and observe induced eye movements; mnemonic: **COWS (Cold Opposite,**

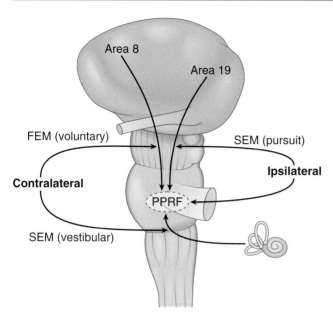

Figure 4.11 Composite reminder of the course and lateralization of the three conjugate horizontal eye movement pathways. (With permission from Bajandas FJ, Kline LB: *Neuro-ophthalmology review manual*. Thorofare, NJ: Slack. 1988, p 55.)

Warm **S**ame) refers to direction of fast phase of nystagmus in awake patient (jerk nystagmus); in comatose patient, get tonic deviation in opposite direction of mnemonic (sustained slow phase movement only [Fig. 4.12])

Bilateral cold-water irrigation produces nystagmus with fast phase upward in awake patient and downward tonic deviation in comatose patient; opposite effects with warm water

PATHWAY: vestibular nuclei → contralateral CN 6 nuclei → ipsilateral LR and contralateral MR (via MLF); no connection to the PPRF

Doll's head (oculocephalic reflex): turn head and observe direction of eye movements; vestibular system moves eyes; use when patient cannot voluntarily move eyes

Eyes should have tonic movement in direction opposite head rotation

INTACT DOLL'S HEAD: supranuclear lesion (cranial nerve pathways to muscles are intact) (i.e., progressive supranuclear palsy)

ABNORMAL DOLL'S HEAD: lesion is infranuclear paresis or restrictive disease (perform forced ductions)

Bell's phenomenon: upward turning of eyes with forced closure of eyelids

INTACT BELL'S PHENOMENON: supranuclear lesion

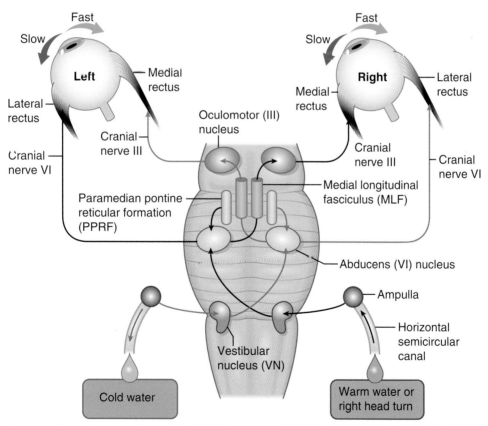

Figure 4.12 Vestibulo-ocular reflex demonstrating right beating nystagmus. Right COWS (cold opposite, warm same). (Calorics should be performed with head back 60°.) (With permission from Bajandas FJ, Kline LB: *Neuro-ophthalmology review manual*. Thorofare, NJ: Slack; 1988.)

DIPLOPIA

Types:

Comitant: amount of deviation same in all fields of gaze

Incomitant: amount of deviation varies in different fields of gaze

Etiology:

Monocular: high astigmatism, chalazion or lid mass, corneal abnormality, iris atrophy, polycoria, cataract, subluxed crystalline lens, decentered intraocular lens (IOL), posterior capsular opacity, retinal pathology, functional

Binocular: neuropathic (cranial nerve palsies, MS), myopathic (thyroid eye disease, orbital pseudotumor), neuromuscular junction (myasthenia gravis [MG])

DDx:

Supranuclear (resulting from inadequate convergence): skew deviation, progressive supranuclear palsy, Parkinson disease, Huntington disease, dorsal midbrain syndrome

Intermittent: MG, MS, migraine, thyroid eye disease, convergence spasm, decompensated phoria, convergence–retraction nystagmus, ocular myotonia

Vertical: MG, MS, thyroid eye disease, orbital disease (tumor, trauma, inflammation), CN 3 or CN 4 palsy, Brown syndrome, skew deviation

Aberrant regeneration: Duane syndrome, Marcus-Gunn jaw-winking syndrome

Restrictive syndromes: intraocular pressure (IOP) elevation >4 mm Hg when eyes directed into restricted field (thyroid, trauma, inflammatory orbital disease, neoplastic process)

EYE MOVEMENT DISORDERS

Central Disorders (Supranuclear) (Fig. 4.13)

Often no symptoms or complaints

Horizontal Gaze Palsies

Congenital

Must distinguish between supranuclear and infranuclear causes; often abnormality of CN 6 or interneurons; vertical movements usually unaffected

Möbius Syndrome

Horizontal gaze palsy with CN 6, 7, 8, and 9 palsies (facial diplegia, deafness, abnormal digits)

Ocular Motor Apraxia

Saccadic palsy; impairment of voluntary horizontal eye movements with preservation of reflex movements; male > female; congenital or acquired **(Balint syndrome)**; extensive bilateral cerebral disease involving supranuclear pathways (usually bilateral frontoparietal); usually benign and resolves in congenital disease

Associations: Gaucher disease, spinocerebellar degeneration, MR, ataxia-telangiectasia, Wilson disease, hypoplasia of corpus callosum, hydrocephalus; rarely cerebellar mass lesion (perform magnetic resonance imaging [MRI])

Findings:

Head thrusting: patient must move head to look at objects; head thrust toward desired direction of gaze results in contralateral slow eye movement, so patient must overshoot target; lessens with age; may resolve by age 20; patient may also blink to break fixation

Abnormal OKN: fast phase absent

Abnormal vestibular nystagmus: fast phase absent

Normal pursuits

Normal vertical saccades

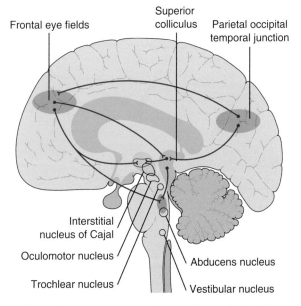

Frontal eye fields
Superior colliculus
Parietal occipital temporal junction
Interstitial nucleus of Cajal
Oculomotor nucleus
Trochlear nucleus
Abducens nucleus
Vestibular nucleus

Rostral interstitial nucleus of the medial longitudinal fasciculus
Paramedian pontine reticular formation

Fig. 4.13 Supranuclear control of eye movements. The pontine horizontal gaze center *(blue)* and the vertical gaze center in the midbrain *(yellow)* receive input from the frontal eye fields to initiate saccades and from the parietal occipital temporal junction to control pursuit. These gaze centers control ocular motility by synapsing upon the ocular motor nerve nuclei (III, IV, and VI). (With permission from Lavin PJM, Donahue SP: Disorders of supranuclear control of ocular motility. In: Yanoff M, Duker JS, eds. *Ophthalmology.* 2nd ed. St Louis: Mosby; 2004.)

Acquired

Frontoparietal lesion (stroke, trauma, or infection): tonic deviation of eyes to side of lesion (contralateral area 8 unopposed); seizure will move eyes *away* from lesion

> *Doll's head testing and calorics:* can turn eyes contralateral to lesion (intact vestibular pathway)

Parieto-occipital lesion: ipsilateral pursuit palsy (cogwheel pursuit)

Tegmental lesion: ipsilateral pursuit and saccadic palsy

Pontine lesion (PPRF)**:** ipsilateral horizontal gaze palsy

Parkinson disease: reduced blinking, reduced saccades, reduced glabellar reflex suppression, blepharospasm, oculogyric crisis

Huntington disease: abnormal vertical and horizontal saccades, fixation, and pursuit

Metabolic disorders: hyperglycemia, Wernicke encephalopathy, Wilson disease

Drug-induced: tricyclic antidepressants, phenytoin, phenothiazines

Pseudo-gaze palsies: MG, chronic progressive external ophthalmoplegia (CPEO), Duane syndrome

Internuclear ophthalmoplegia (INO) (Fig. 4.14): lesion of MLF; inability to adduct ipsilateral eye with nystagmus of fellow eye; may have skew deviation, vertical diplopia, and gaze-evoked upbeat nystagmus; rule out myasthenia gravis

> *Unilateral:* ischemia (young), demyelination (older patients), tumor, infection (meningitis, encephalitis), trauma, compression

> *Bilateral* (involves both MLF near junction with the 3rd nerve nucleus in midbrain): demyelination/MS (most common), trauma, ischemia, infection, Chiari malformation, toxicity (amitriptyline, ethanol, benzodiazepine)

> *Types:*

> **ANTERIOR (MIDBRAIN):** preserved convergence

> **POSTERIOR (PONS):** impaired convergence
> (WEBINO = wall-eyed bilateral INO)

One-and-a-half syndrome (Fisher syndrome)

(Fig. 4.15): lesion of CN 6 nucleus and ipsilateral MLF; causes ipsilateral gaze palsy and INO; only movement is abduction of contralateral eye (with nystagmus); supranuclear lesion and thus convergence is intact; called *paralytic pontine exotropia* when patient appears exotropic; myoclonus patients with recovery from one-and-a-half syndrome may develop oculopalatal myoclonus

> *Etiology:* stroke (most common), MS, basilar artery occlusion, pontine metastases

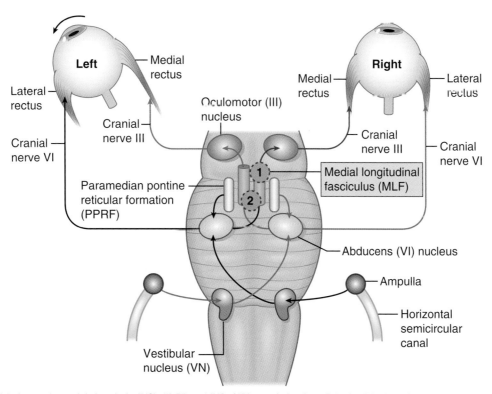

Figure 4.14 (1) Right internuclear ophthalmoplegia (INO). (2) Bilateral INO. (With permission from Bajandas FJ, Kline LB: *Neuro-ophthalmology review manual.* Thorofare, NJ: Slack; 1988.)

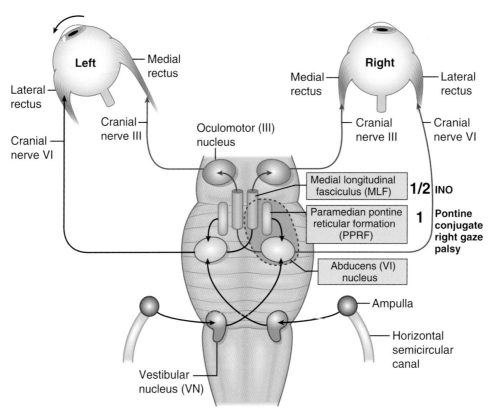

Figure 4.15 Right acute one-and-a-half syndrome (paralytic pontine exotropia). (With permission from Bajandas FJ, Kline LB: *Neuro-ophthalmology review manual*. Thorofare, NJ: Slack; 1988.)

Vertical Gaze Abnormalities

Parinaud Syndrome (Dorsal Midbrain Syndrome)

Supranuclear gaze palsy with nuclear CN 3 palsy

Etiology: 90% caused by pineal tumor; also, demyelination, infarction, trauma

Findings: supranuclear paresis of upgaze (Doll's head intact), bilateral mid-dilated pupils, convergence–retraction nystagmus on attempted upgaze (synchronous backward jerking movements of both eyes resulting from cocontraction of horizontal recti), light-near dissociation, vertical OKN, skew deviation, eyelid retraction (Collier's sign); mnemonic: **CLUES** (**C**onvergence-retractions nystagmus, **L**ight-near dissociation, **U**pgaze paralysis, **E**yelid retraction, **S**kew deviation)

Diagnosis: MRI; human chorionic gonadotropin (hCG) level

Treatment: radiation therapy (XRT)

Progressive Supranuclear Palsy (Steele-Richardson-Olszewski Syndrome)

Progressive vertical (early) and horizontal (late) gaze palsy (downward gaze usually affected first); no Bell's phenomenon; doll's head maneuver gives full range of

movement (ROM), indicating supranuclear nature of disorder; eventually frozen globe to all stimuli, spasm of fixation, decreased blink rate, blepharitis, blepharospasm; occasionally, apraxia of eye opening; also, axial rigidity, dysarthria, and dementia

Skew Deviation

Vertical misalignment of visual axes resulting from imbalance of prenuclear inputs; comitant or incomitant, nonlocalizing

Vertical tropia, hyperdeviation usually increases on ipsilateral downgaze, no cyclodeviation; hypodeviated eye usually ipsilateral to lesion, except when associated with INO, in which hyperdeviated eye is ipsilateral; does not obey the Parks–Bielschowsky 3-step test and misalignment is resolved or different when lying down (altered peripheral vestibular input); may occur with other brainstem symptoms or cerebellar disease; MRI of posterior fossa recommended

Etiology: lesion of the central vestibular pathway or cerebellum including brainstem infarct, MS, increased intracranial pressure (ICP), pseudotumor cerebri, vestibulo-ocular imbalance, cerebellar disease; vertebral–basilar insufficiency may cause transient skew deviation

Treatment: often transient and requires observation only; chronic deviations may be treated with prism spectacles or surgery

Whipple Disease

Oculomasticatory myorhythmia (vertical eye movements and facial activity similar to myoclonus)

Olivopontocerebellar atrophy

Hereditary or sporadic; onset early adulthood; unsteady gait, slurred speech, dementia, optic atrophy, retinal degeneration

Eye movements progressively slow in all directions, finally complete external ophthalmoplegia

Pathology: cerebellar and pontine atrophy

Kernicterus

Progressive loss of eye movements

Also, metabolic diseases (maple syrup disease, Wernicke encephalopathy), drug induced

NYSTAGMUS

Rhythmic involuntary oscillations of the eyes resulting from disorder of SEM system. Direction named after fast phase (horizontal, vertical, torsional, or combination; brain's attempt to correct problem), even though abnormality is noted with slow phase

Etiology: abnormal slow eye movement, high gain instability (SEM is working at high gain), vestibular tone imbalance, integrator leak (gaze-evoked nystagmus), OKN abnormality

Characteristics: may be fast or slow, pendular (equal speed) or jerk (designated by direction of fast phase), unidirectional or multidirectional, conjugate (same direction and amplitude in both eyes) or dissociated (different amplitude in each eye) or disconjugate (different directions in each eye), congenital or acquired
   Gain: eye moves 15° (output) in response to a retinal image position error of 15° (gain = 1)
   Foveation: bring an image onto, or maintain an image on, the fovea
   Frequency: oscillations per second (Hz)
   Amplitude: excursion of oscillation
   Intensity: product of amplitude and frequency
   Null point: position in which intensity of nystagmus is least
   Neutral point: position in which a reversal of the direction of jerk nystagmus occurs

Childhood Nystagmus

Most commonly, congenital, latent, sensory, and spasmus nutans (see Chapter 5, Pediatrics/Strabismus)

Physiologic Nystagmus

Several forms of nystagmus, including end-gaze, optokinetic, caloric, rotational (VOR), head shaking, pneumatic, compression, flash induced, flicker induced

Acquired Nystagmus

Pattern helps localize pathology, may have oscillopsia

Bruns

Combination of gaze-paretic nystagmus when looking toward lesion (fast phase toward the lesion) and vestibular imbalance nystagmus when looking away from lesion (fast phase away from lesion) (i.e., with right-sided lesion: high-amplitude, low-frequency, right-beating nystagmus on right gaze; low-amplitude, high-frequency, left-beating nystagmus on left gaze)

Gaze-paretic component is of high amplitude and low frequency (because of impairment of horizontal gaze mechanism on side of lesion)

Vestibular component is of low amplitude and high frequency, with fast phase away from damaged vestibular nuclei on side of lesion

Caused by cerebellopontine angle mass (usually acoustic neuroma or meningioma)

Convergence–Retraction

Cocontraction of lateral recti produces rhythmic convergence movement (abnormal saccades) and retraction of both eyes on attempted upgaze; not a true nystagmus (not initiated by a slow phase)

Caused by periaqueductal gray matter or dorsal midbrain lesion (Parinaud syndrome, pinealoma, trauma, brainstem arteriovenous malformation [AVM], obstructive hydrocephalus, stroke, MS)/compression of vertical gaze center at riMLF

Dissociated

Asymmetric between the two eyes (different direction, amplitude, frequency, etc.); always pathologic

Caused by posterior fossa disease, MS

Downbeat

Jerk nystagmus with fast phase down (eyes drift upward with corrective saccade downward); worsens in downgaze, improves in upgaze; oscillopsia

Caused by lesion that affects pathways responsible for downgaze; cervicomedullary junction lesion (Arnold-Chiari malformation, tumor, syrinx: 33%), spinocerebellar degeneration, intoxication, lithium, paraneoplastic cerebellar degeneration, 50% with no identifiable cause

Mnemonic: **DoWNBEAT** (**D**egeneration demyelination or drugs, **W**ernicke encephalopathy, **N**eoplasm, **B**rainstem disease, **E**ncephalitis, **A**rnold-Chiari malformation, **T**rauma or toxin)

Treatment: may respond to potassium channel blocker, gabapentin, clonazepam, baclofen

Drug Induced

Usually jerk nystagmus, often gaze-evoked nystagmus (left-beating on left gaze, right-beating on right gaze); may be absent in downgaze

Associated with anticonvulsants (phenytoin, carbamazepine), barbiturates, tranquilizers, and phenothiazines

Gaze Evoked

Nystagmus in direction of gaze, absent in primary position, fast phase toward lesion (cerebellar)

Results from impaired neural integrator function:

Physiologic: fatiguable with prolonged eccentric gaze, symmetric

Pathologic: prolonged, asymmetric; from brainstem or posterior fossa lesions (acoustic neuroma, cerebellar hemisphere tumor) or intoxication (alcohol, sedatives, anticonvulsants)

If asymmetric, must obtain neuroimaging

Waveform: exponentially decreasing

Periodic Alternating Nystagmus (PAN)

Changes horizontal direction; jerks right 90 seconds, 5- to 10-second pause, jerks left 90 seconds, repeats; remains horizontal in vertical gaze; very rare, usually acquired

Results from disease of vestibulocerebellar system or cervicomedullary junction (albinism, craniovertebral junction lesion [Arnold-Chiari malformation], MS, syphilis, tumor, vascular, Dilantin, spinocerebellar degeneration)

Treatment: baclofen; surgery (large recession of all four recti muscles)

See-Saw

Combination of conjugate torsional nystagmus and disconjugate vertical nystagmus with one eye rising and intorting while fellow eye falls and excyclotorts, then reverses; may have INO

Caused by large suprasellar or diencephalon lesions (can be associated with a visual field defect, often bitemporal hemianopsia resulting from a craniopharyngioma), cerebrovascular accident (CVA), trauma, or congenital achiasma

MRI: rule out large parasellar tumors expanding into third ventricle

Treatment: baclofen

Upbeat

Jerk nystagmus with fast phase up (eyes drift downward with corrective saccade upward); non-localizing

Caused by medullary lesions, midline cerebellar (vermis) lesions, medulloblastoma, cerebellar degeneration, MS, Wernicke syndrome or intoxication

Vestibular

Horizontal, rotary, jerk nystagmus in primary gaze; same in all fields of gaze; slow component is linear; remains horizontal in vertical gaze

Caused by vestibular disease, infection (labyrinthitis), Ménière disease, vascular, trauma, toxicity

Peripheral vestibular disease: fast phase toward good side; slow phase toward lesion; associated with tinnitus, vertigo, deafness; fixation inhibits vertigo and nystagmus; direction of Romberg fall changes with head turning

Central vestibular disease: nonlocalizing; no tinnitus or deafness; fixation does not inhibit nystagmus

Voluntary

Unsustainable for >30 seconds; associated with hysteria and malingering

Other Eye Movement Disorders

Ocular Bobbing

Intermittent conjugate rapid downward eye movements. followed by slow return to primary position

Often secondary to hemorrhage; patient usually comatose

Ocular Dipping

Opposite of ocular bobbing; intermittent rapid upward eye movements followed by slow return to primary position

Ocular Myoclonus

Vertical pendular nystagmus associated with synchronous palatal (uvula) beating

Caused by bilateral pseudohypertrophy of inferior olives in medulla, lesion in myoclonic triangle (red nucleus, ipsilateral inferior olive, contralateral dentate nucleus)

Opsoclonus (Saccadomania)

Rapid, chaotic eye movements in all directions; persists in sleep

Associated with dancing hands and feet

Abnormality of pause cells (normally suppress burst cells of PPRF)

Caused by remote paraneoplastic effect on cerebellum from metastatic neuroblastoma (check urine vanillylmandelic acid [VMA]), occasionally with encephalitis

Waveform: no slow phase; repetitive, random; no intersaccadic interval

Oscillopsia

Illusion of movement in the seen world

Usually occurs in SO myokymia and acquired nystagmus; rarely in congenital nystagmus

Caused by vestibulo-ocular reflex abnormality

CRANIAL NERVE PALSIES (FIG. 4.16)

Oculomotor Nerve (CN 3) Palsy

Anatomy: nucleus in rostral midbrain; fascicle travels ventrally through midbrain, traversing red nucleus, and corticospinal tract in cerebral peduncle; nerve enters subarachnoid space, passes between posterior cerebral and superior cerebellar arteries, then courses lateral to posterior communicating artery and enters lateral wall of cavernous sinus; receives sympathetics from internal carotid plexus; passes through superior orbital fissure and divides into superior (supplies SR and levator) and inferior (supplies IR, MR, IO, iris sphincter, and ciliary muscle) divisions.

Only one subnucleus (midline location) supplies both levator palpebrae superioris; fibers from SR subnucleus supply contralateral SR; Edinger-Westphal nucleus supplies both pupils (Fig. 4.17)

Types: complete, partial, pupil sparing

Findings: ptosis, hypotropia, exotropia; may involve pupil (fixed and dilated); may cause pain

7 syndromes (Fig. 4.18):
   Nuclear CN 3 palsy (see Fig. 4.18, ①): extremely rare; contralateral SR paresis and bilateral ptosis; pupil involvement is both or neither
   Fascicle syndromes (see Fig. 4.18, ②): ischemic, infiltrative (tumor), or inflammatory (rare)
      NOTHNAGEL SYNDROME: lesion of fascicle and superior cerebellar peduncle that causes ipsilateral CN 3 paresis and cerebellar ataxia
      BENEDIKT SYNDROME: lesion of fascicle and red nucleus that causes ipsilateral CN 3 paresis,

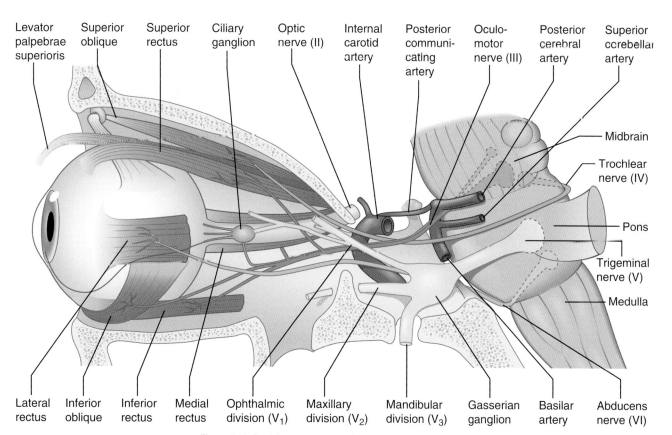

Figure 4.16 Cranial nerve pathways. (Copyright Peter K. Kaiser, MD.)

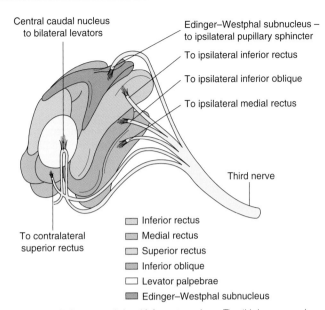

Figure 4.17 Anatomy of the third nerve nucleus. The third nerve nucleus consists of a single, central, caudally located nucleus for the levator palpebrae; paired bilateral subnuclei with crossed projections that innervate the superior recti; and paired bilateral subnuclei with uncrossed projections that innervate the medial recti, inferior recti, and inferior oblique muscles. Parasympathetic input to the ciliary body and iris sphincter arises from the Edinger-Westphal nucleus. (Redrawn from Warwick R: Representation of the extraocular muscles in the oculomotor nuclei of the monkey. *J Comp Neurol.* 1953;98:449–503.)

contralateral hemitremor (resting and intentional), and contralateral decreased sensation

WEBER SYNDROME: lesion of fascicle and pyramidal tract that causes ipsilateral CN 3 paresis and contralateral hemiparesis

CLAUDE SYNDROME: combination of Nothnagel and Benedikt syndromes

Uncal herniation (see Fig. 4.18, ③): supratentorial mass may cause uncal herniation compressing CN 3

Posterior communicating artery (PCom or PCA) aneurysm (see Fig. 4.18, ④): most common nontraumatic isolated pupil involving CN 3 palsy; aneurysm at junction of PCom and carotid artery compresses nerve, particularly external parasympathetic pupillomotor fibers; usually painful

Cavernous sinus syndrome (see Fig. 4.18, ⑤): associated with multiple CN palsies (3, 4, V_1, 6) and Horner; CN 3 palsy often partial and pupil sparing; may lead to aberrant regeneration

Orbital syndrome (see Fig. 4.18, ⑥): tumor, trauma, pseudotumor, or cellulitis; associated with multiple CN palsies (3, 4, V_1, 6), proptosis, chemosis, injection; ON can appear normal, swollen, or atrophic

After passing through the superior orbital fissure, CN 3 splits into superior and inferior divisions; therefore, CN 3 palsies distal to this point may be complete or partial

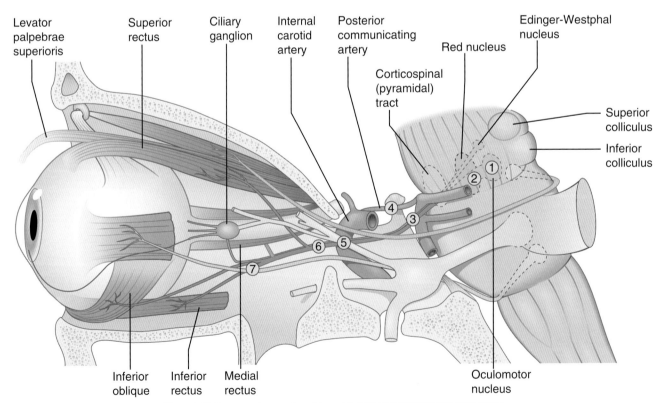

Figure 4.18 Seven syndromes of cranial nerve 3 palsy. (Copyright Peter K. Kaiser, MD.)

Pupil-sparing isolated CN 3 palsy (see Fig. 4.18, ⑦): small-caliber parasympathetic pupillomotor fibers travel in outer layers of nerve closer to blood supply (but more susceptible to damage by compression); fibers at core of nerve are compromised by ischemia; may explain pupil sparing in 80% of ischemic CN 3 palsies and pupil involved in 95% of compressive CN 3 palsies (trauma, tumor, aneurysm)

ETIOLOGY:
  ADULTS: vasculopathic/ischemic (diabetes mellitus [DM], hypertension [HTN]), trauma, giant cell arteritis (GCA), occasionally tumor, aneurysm (very rare)
  CHILDREN: congenital, trauma, tumor, aneurysm, migraine
  14% of Pcom aneurysms initially spare pupil
  20% of diabetic CN 3 palsies involve pupil
  Microvascular CN 3 palsies usually resolve in 3–4 months
  MG may mimic CN 3 palsy

Aberrant regeneration:
IR and/or MR fibers may innervate levator and/or iris sphincter; sign of previous CN 3 palsy caused by aneurysm or tumor (occasionally trauma); never occurs after vasculopathic injury

Findings:
  LID-GAZE DYSKINESIS: lid retracts on downgaze (pseudo–von Graefe's sign) and/or adduction
  PUPIL-GAZE DYSKINESIS: more pupillary constriction with convergence than to light (pseudo–Argyll-Robertson pupil) and/or pupillary constriction on downgaze

2 forms:
  PRIMARY: no preceding acute CN 3 palsy; insidious development of CN 3 palsy with accompanying signs of misdirection, caused by intracavernous lesion (meningioma, aneurysm, neuroma)
  SECONDARY: occurs months after CN 3 palsy from trauma, aneurysm (carotid-cavernous [C-C]), or tumor compression, but never after vasculopathic/ischemic lesion

Other causes of CN 3 palsy:
Congenital: variable degrees of aberrant regeneration; 75% have smaller pupil on involved side (caused by aberrant regeneration); ptosis and anisocoria
  TREATMENT: muscle surgery to straighten eye in primary gaze
Ophthalmoplegic migraine: onset in childhood; positive family history of migraine; paresis of CN 3 occurs as headache abates; usually resolves in 1 month (can be permanent)
Cyclic oculomotor palsy: usually at birth or early childhood; very rare; occurs after complete CN 3 palsy, can be a result of diabetic ischemia
  FINDINGS: spastic movements of muscles innervated by CN 3 occur at regular intervals for 10 to 30 seconds (spasms of lid elevation, adduction, miosis)
  MRI: rule out aneurysm

Workup:
If age <11: MRI/magnetic resonance angiography (MRA)
If age 11–50 years: MRI/MRA and medical workup
If age >50 years:
  WITH PUPIL INVOLVEMENT: MRI/MRA; if normal, cerebral angiography (catheter)
  WITH PUPIL SPARING: usually microvascular; no invasive investigation needed initially; check blood pressure (BP) (HTN), blood glucose (DM), erythrocyte sedimentation rate (ESR), C-reactive protein (CRP; GCA), complete blood count (CBC), antinuclear antibody (ANA), Venereal Disease Research Laboratory (VDRL), fluorescent treponemal antibody absorption (FTA-ABS); if it persists >3 months, MRI/MRA with cerebral angiography (aneurysm) if negative

Trochlear Nerve (CN 4) Palsy

Anatomy: nucleus in caudal mesencephalon at level of inferior colliculus; decussates in anterior medullary velum next to aqueduct of Sylvius; fascicle passes between posterior cerebral artery and superior cerebellar artery; nerve travels in lateral wall of cavernous sinus, enters orbit via superior orbital fissure outside annulus of Zinn; innervates superior oblique muscle

Longest intracranial course (75 mm); only CN that exits dorsally from brainstem; only CN that decussates (except for CN 3 subnucleus that innervates SR); most commonly injured CN following closed head injury (owing to long course)

Etiology: congenital (most common in kids); in adults: 40% trauma, 30% ischemia, 20% miscellaneous or undetermined, 10% aneurysm

Findings: ipsilateral hypertropia (caused by superior rectus overaction)

5 syndromes:
Nuclear/fascicular syndrome (see Fig. 4.19, ①): hemorrhage, infarction, demyelination, trauma; may have contralateral Horner or INO
Subarachnoid space syndrome (see Fig. 4.19, ②): injury as nerve emerges from dorsal surface of brainstem; trauma (contrecoup forces transmitted to brainstem by free tentorial edge), tumor (pinealoma, tentorial meningioma), meningitis, neurosurgical trauma
Cavernous sinus syndrome (see Fig. 4.19, ③): multiple CN palsies (3, 4, V₁, 6) and Horner
Orbital syndrome (see Fig. 4.19, ④): multiple CN palsies (3, 4, V₁, 6) and Horner; proptosis, chemosis, injection
Isolated CN 4 palsy (see Fig. 4.19, ⑤):
  CONGENITAL: most common; may occur in elderly due to decompensation; large, vertical fusion amplitudes (10–15Δ); check old photos for head tilt
  ACQUIRED: acute onset of vertical diplopia; head position (chin down, face turn to opposite side, head tilt to opposite shoulder)

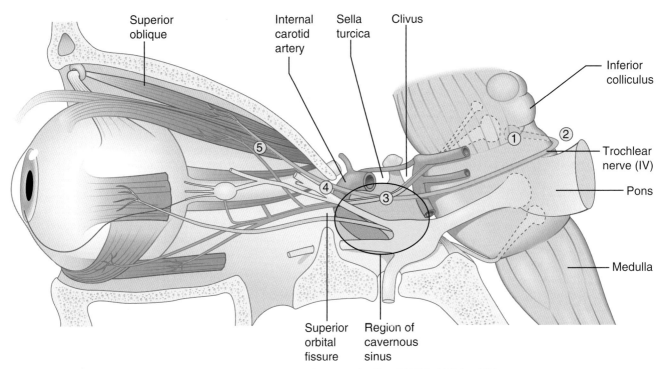

Figure 4.19 Five syndromes of cranial nerve 4 palsy. (Copyright Peter K. Kaiser, MD.)

DDx of vertical diplopia: myasthenia gravis, thyroid eye disease, orbital disease (tumor, trauma, inflammation), CN 3 palsy, CN 4 palsy, Brown syndrome, skew deviation, MS

Diagnosis: Parks–Bielschowsky 3-step test (used for hypertropia resulting from weakness of a single muscle)
  Step 1: Which eye has hypertropia?
    LEFT HYPER: paresis of OD (*oculus dextrus,* right eye) elevators (right superior rectus [RSR] or right inferior oblique [RIO]) or OS (*oculus sinister,* left eye) depressors (left inferior rectus [LIR] or left superior oblique [LSO])
  Step 2: Worse on right or left gaze?
    If hyper is worse in left gaze:
      Problem with OS muscles that have greatest vertical action during abduction (SR and IR)
      Problem with OD muscles that have greatest vertical action during adduction (SO and IO)
    SR and IR work best when eye is ABducted
      So if left hyper is worse on gaze left: LIR
    SO and IO work best when eye is ADducted
      So if left hyper is worse on gaze left: RIO
    If left hyper is worse on gaze right: RSR or LSO
  Step 3: Worse on right or left head tilt?
    With head tilt, eyes undergo corrective torsion (with right head tilt, OD intorts and OS extorts)
    If one of the intorters is the cause of the hyper, then tilting head will worsen hyper on side of head tilt
    If worse hyper on left head tilt, problem with left intorters (LSR, LSO) or right extorters (RIR, RIO)

Bilateral CN 4 palsies: usually result from severe head trauma (contusion of anterior medullary velum)

Vertical deviation in primary gaze may or may not be present
Right head tilt (RHT) in left gaze; left head tilt (LHT) in right gaze
Either eye can be hyper on step 3 of 3-step test
V-pattern esotropia (ET > 25Δ)
>10° of torsion with double Maddox rod test

Workup: check BP, blood glucose, CBC, ESR, VDRL, FTA-ABS, ANA; neuroimaging if history of head trauma or cancer, signs of meningitis, young age, other neurologic findings, or isolated palsy that does not improve after 3–4 months

Treatment:
  Glasses: occlude lens or prisms for diplopia
  Muscle surgery:
    KNAPP'S PRINCIPLES FOR CN 4 PALSY: strengthen (tuck) the palsied SO, weaken the antagonist (ipsilateral IO), or weaken the yoke (contralateral IR) to correct hyperdeviation
    HARADA-ITO PROCEDURE: anterior and lateral displacement of palsied muscle to correct excyclotorsion

Abducens Nerve (CN 6) Palsy

Anatomy: nucleus in dorsal pons medial to CN 7; travels anterior and lateral to PPRF, then through pyramidal tract, and exits lower pons in pontomedullary groove in subarachnoid space; climbs over clivus (vulnerable to elevated ICP) over petrous ridge, along base of skull, through Dorello's canal, under Gruber's ligament; enters cavernous sinus and then orbit through superior orbital fissure; passes laterally to supply lateral rectus

2nd most common CN to be injured following closed head injury

CN 6 lesions occur in conditions that cause increased ICP

6 syndromes (Fig. 4.20):

Brainstem syndromes (see Fig. 4.20, ①):

MILLARD-GUBLER SYNDROME: lesion of CN 6 and 7 fascicles and pyramidal tract causing CN 6 and 7 palsies with contralateral hemiparesis

RAYMOND SYNDROME: lesion of CN 6 and pyramidal tract causing CN 6 palsy and contralateral hemiparesis

FOVILLE SYNDROME: lesion of CN 6 nucleus, CN 5 and 7 fascicles, and sympathetics causing ipsilateral 5, 6, and 7 palsies, horizontal conjugate gaze palsy, and ipsilateral Horner

MÖBIUS SYNDROME: associated with CN 7 lesion, supernumerary digits, skeletal abnormalities, mental retardation

Subarachnoid space syndrome (see Fig. 4.20, ②): increased ICP can cause downward displacement of brainstem with stretching of CN 6 (tethered at exit from pons and Dorello's canal); occurs in 30% of patients with pseudotumor cerebri; also hemorrhage, meningitis, inflammation (sarcoidosis), infiltration (lymphoma, leukemia, carcinoma)

Petrous apex syndrome (see Fig. 4.20, ③): portion of CN 6 within Dorello's canal is in contact with tip of petrous pyramid and is susceptible to processes affecting the petrous bone

GRADENIGO SYNDROME: localized inflammation or extradural abscess of petrous apex (mastoiditis) following otitis media; CN 6 palsy with ipsilateral decreased hearing, facial pain, and facial paralysis

PSEUDO-GRADENIGO SYNDROME: various etiologies

NASOPHARYNGEAL CANCER: obstruction of eustachian tube can cause serous otitis media, can invade cavernous sinus, causing CN 6 palsy

CEREBELLOPONTINE ANGLE TUMOR: CN 5, 6, and 7 palsies; decreased hearing, papilledema

PETROUS BONE FRACTURE: may have CN 5, 6, 7, or 8 lesions, hemotympanum, Battle's sign (bruising over mastoid bone), CSF otorrhea

BASILAR ANEURYSM

CLIVUS CHORDOMA

Cavernous sinus syndrome (see Fig. 4.20, ④):

ETIOLOGY: trauma, vascular (diabetes, migraine, aneurysms, arteriovenous [AV] fistula), tumor, inflammation, granuloma

FINDINGS: CN 3, 4, V₁, Horner, ON, chiasm, and pituitary involvement

Orbital syndrome (see Fig. 4.20, ⑤):

ETIOLOGY: trauma, tumor, orbital pseudotumor, cellulitis

FINDINGS: proptosis, chemosis, conjunctival injection; may have ON edema or atrophy; CN V₁ may be involved

Isolated CN 6 palsy (see Fig. 4.20, ⑥):

CHILDREN: often postviral (resolves over weeks), associated with otitis media; consider tumor (pontine glioma), trauma

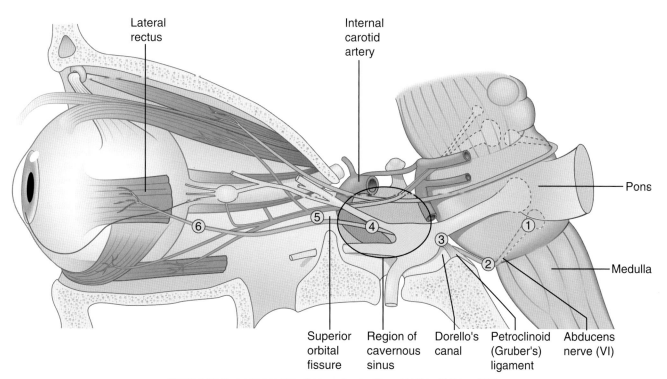

Figure 4.20 Six syndromes of cranial nerve 6 palsy. (Copyright Peter K. Kaiser, MD.)

ADULTS: vasculopathic, undetermined, MS, tumor (nasopharyngeal CA, cavernous sinus meningioma, chordoma), trauma, GCA, syphilis

Pseudo–CN 6 palsy: thyroid eye disease, convergence spasm, strabismus, medial wall fracture, myasthenia gravis, orbital myositis, Miller Fisher syndrome

Workup:

Congenital: usually resolves by 6 weeks

Acquired: same as for CN 4 palsy; consider lumbar puncture (LP) and Tensilon test

Trigeminal Nerve (CN 5) Palsy

Anatomy: nerve emerges from ventral pons; passes below tentorium to ganglion; divides into 3 divisions (Fig. 4.21)

Ophthalmic (V_1): passes through lateral wall of cavernous sinus; divides into lacrimal, frontal, and nasociliary nerves

Maxillary (V_2): passes through lateral wall of cavernous sinus; exits cranium through foramen rotundum

Mandibular (V_3): exits cranium through foramen ovale
Supplies sensory to face and eye, motor to muscles of mastication (Fig. 4.22)

Trigeminal neuralgia (tic douloureux): caused by compression of CN 5 at root (superior cerebellar artery aneurysm or tumor); facial pain involves entire CN 5 division; lasts seconds; 95% unilateral; usually involves maxillary or mandibular distribution, ophthalmic distribution alone is rare

Diagnosis: neuroimaging

Treatment: medical (carbamazepine) or surgical (radiofrequency destruction of trigeminal ganglion through foramen ovale)

Facial Nerve (CN 7) Palsy

Anatomy: passes around CN 6 nucleus; exits brainstem ventrally at cerebellopontine angle; enters internal auditory canal (of petrous portion of temporal bone) with nervus intermedius and cochlear and vestibular nerves; enters facial nerve canal; exits temporal bone via stylomastoid foramen; branches in parotid gland. Supplies facial muscles and lacrimal and salivary glands; posterior two-thirds of tongue; external ear sensation; dampens stapedius

Lacrimal gland innervation (parasympathetic): originates in superior salivatory nucleus, fibers leave brain with nervus intermedius (glossopalatine) and travel with CN 7 through geniculate ganglion, emerges from petrous portion of sphenoid bone as greater superficial petrosal nerve; enters pterygoid canal and enters sphenopalatine ganglion, where primary parasympathetic fibers synapse and second-order fibers join zygomatic nerve, which sends a branch to lacrimal gland.

Frontal lobe (precentral motor cortex) provides input to CN 7 nuclei in pons (control voluntary facial movements); upper face innervation is bilateral (from both supranuclear motor areas), lower-face innervation is mainly from contralateral supranuclear motor area (Fig. 4.23)

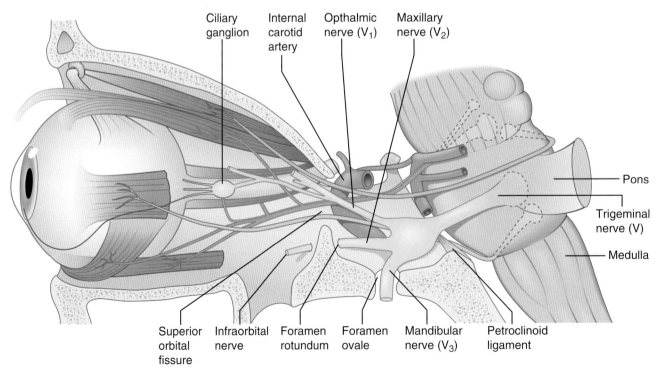

Figure 4.21 Cranial nerve 5 pathway. (Copyright Peter K. Kaiser, MD.)

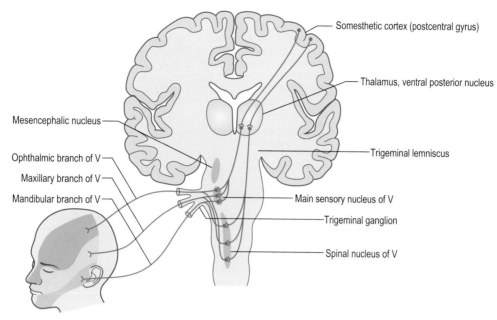

Figure 4.22 Cranial nerve 5 innervation.

Supranuclear palsy: lesion in precentral gyrus of cerebral cortex results in contralateral paralysis of volitional facial movement involving lower face more severely than upper

Emotional and reflex movements (smiling, spontaneous blinking) are preserved (extrapyramidal)

Brainstem lesion (pons): ipsilateral facial weakness involving both upper and lower face; results from tumor, vascular causes
  Associated with CN 5 and 6 palsies, lateral gaze palsy, cerebellar ataxia, and contralateral hemiparesis
  With CN 5 palsy: cerebellopontine angle tumors, infratemporal fossa tumors
  With CN 6 palsy: brainstem injury or injury near anteromedial portion of temporal bone (Gradenigo syndrome)

Peripheral CN 7 lesion: acute unilateral facial nerve palsy is most common cranial neuropathy
  Bell palsy: idiopathic facial nerve palsy; may be preceded by preauricular or mastoid pain
  Facial weakness progressing to paralysis over months
  Associated with progressive twitching or facial spasm; suggests neoplasm; most common between ages 15–45 years; 10% have positive family history
  TREATMENT: consider oral steroids
  PROGNOSIS: 70% have complete recovery in 6 weeks; 85% will fully recover; 10% recurrence (ipsilateral or contralateral)
    POOR PROGNOSTIC SIGNS: complete facial paralysis at presentation, impairment of lacrimation, advanced age; if incomplete recovery, aberrant regeneration is common

Trauma: fracture of temporal bone
  FINDINGS: hearing loss, vertigo, hemotympanum, perforated tympanic membrane, Battle's sign (bruising over mastoid bone)
  Delayed onset or incomplete paralysis usually caused by nerve contusion or swelling
  Complete facial paralysis immediately after head trauma suggests nerve transection
  BIRTH TRAUMA WITH FORCEPS: congenital CN 7 lesion; tends to resolve
Infection:
  RAMSAY-HUNT SYNDROME: herpes zoster virus (HZV) oticus (infection of outer ear and nerves of inner auditory canal); 20% have sensorineural hearing loss and dizziness
    Preauricular or mastoid pain precedes facial paralysis by 1–3 days; associated with a vesicular rash of outer ear or on tympanic membrane
  TREATMENT: acyclovir and prednisone
  PROGNOSIS: poor; only 10% recovery in patients with complete paralysis; 66% recovery with partial paralysis
  May develop postherpetic neuralgia
  Also HIV, Lyme disease, otitis media, malignant otitis externa (usually elderly individuals with diabetes; can progress to cellulitis of inner ear canal and osteomyelitis of temporal bone; usually caused by *Pseudomonas*)
Sarcoidosis: most frequent cause of bilateral seventh resulting from infiltration of CN 7, usually at parotid gland
Erosive cholesteatoma: pressure on segment of CN 7 that travels through middle ear
Tumor: most intracranial and bone tumors that cause

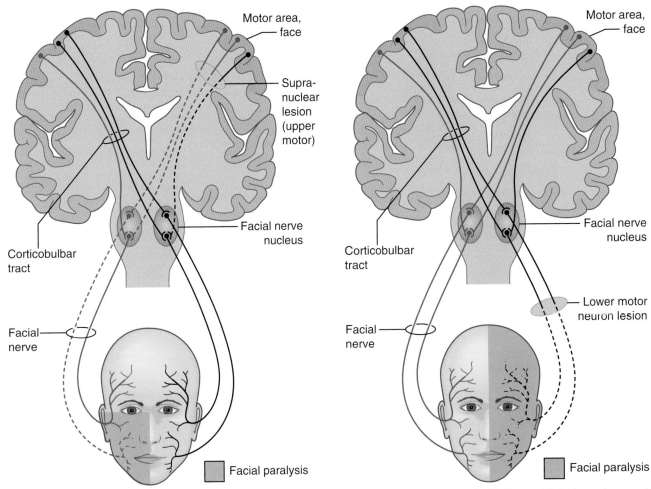

Figure 4.23 Facial weakness resulting from upper and lower motor neuron lesions. (With permission from Bajandas FJ, Kline LB: *Neuro-ophthalmology review manual.* Thorofare, NJ: Slack; 1988.)

facial paralysis are benign (including acoustic neuroma, meningioma, glomus tumors [triad of facial paralysis, pulsatile tinnitus, and hearing loss]); tumors of parotid gland are usually malignant (adenoid cystic carcinoma)

Guillain-Barré syndrome (Miller Fisher variant): facial diplegia can occur with ophthalmoplegia and ataxia; absent deep tendon reflexes; CSF protein elevated with normal cell count; often bilateral

Melkersson-Rosenthal syndrome: recurrent facial paralysis with chronic facial swelling and lingua plicata (furrowing of tongue); unilateral or bilateral; occurs in childhood or adolescence

Aberrant facial innervation:

  MARCUS-GUNN JAW WINKING: activation of muscles of mastication induces orbicularis oculi contraction

  CROCODILE TEARS: lacrimation evoked by chewing

Other findings: lacrimation (damage to greater superficial petrosal nerve), impaired stapedius muscle reflex (damage to stapedial nerve), impaired taste (damage to chorda tympani nerve), swelling of parotid gland or cervical lymphatics

(suggests malignant tumor or inflammatory condition of parotid [sarcoidosis, tuberculosis (TB)])

Disorders of CN 7 overactivity:

Benign essential blepharospasm: frequent bilateral blinking proceeds to involuntary spasms and forceful contractures of orbicularis; may cause functional blindness; unknown etiology; usually affects women age >50; absent during sleep

  TREATMENT: botulinum toxin (Botox) injections, rarely surgery (orbicularis myomectomy)

Hemifacial spasm: unilateral contractions of facial muscles; usually caused by vascular compression of CN 7 at brainstem; rarely caused by tumor; present during sleep; obtain MRI

Facial myokymia: fasciculations of facial muscles; if multifocal and progressive, consider MS

Eyelid myokymia: benign fasciculations of eyelid

Multiple CN Palsies

CN 3, 4, 5, and 6: caused by lesion of brainstem, cavernous sinus (Fig. 4.24), and/or superior orbital fissure; may have CN 2 dysfunction (orbital apex syndrome)

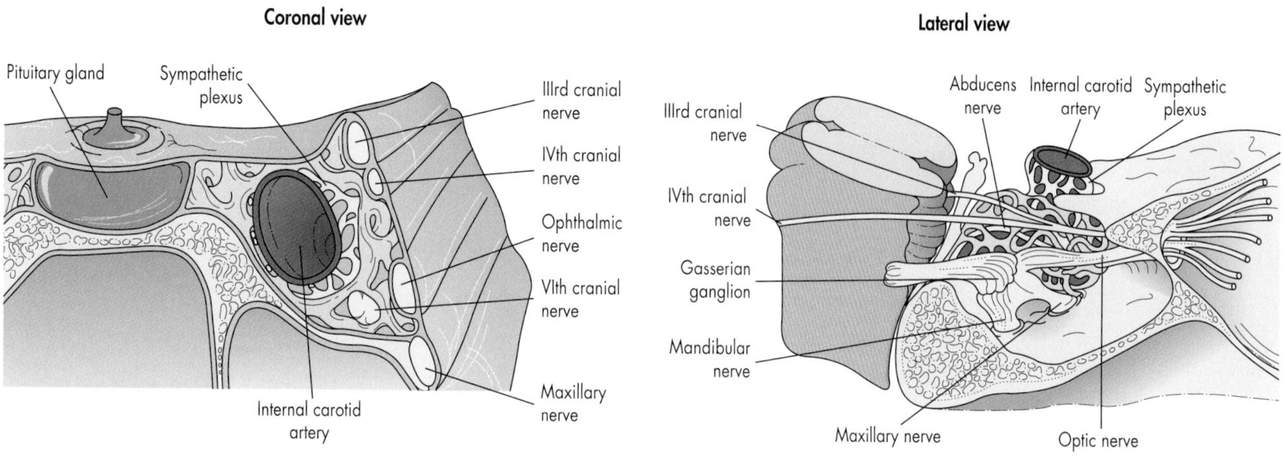

Figure 4.24 Anatomy of the cavernous sinus. (With permission from Moster M: Paresis of isolated and multiple cranial nerves and painful ophthalmoplegia. In: Yanoff M, Duker JS, eds. *Ophthalmology*. London: Mosby; 1999.)

Etiology: AV fistula, cavernous sinus thrombosis, metastases to cavernous sinus, skin malignancy with perineural spread to cavernous sinus, meningioma, mucormycosis, HZV, Tolosa-Hunt syndrome, mucocele, nasopharyngeal cancer, carcinomatous meningitis, pituitary apoplexy (headache with bilateral signs and decreased vision)

DDx: thyroid eye disease, orbital disease, MG, GCA, Miller Fisher variant of Guillain-Barré syndrome, chronic progressive external ophthalmoplegia

Herpes zoster ophthalmicus (HZO): CN 3, 4, and 6 palsies occur in ~15%; pain and skin eruption in trigeminal distribution, decreased corneal sensation, pupil may be involved (tonic pupil)

Hutchinson's rule: if tip of nose involved (nasociliary nerve), eye will probably (but not always) be involved

Mimics of multiple cranial nerve palsies: MG, CPEO, orbital lesions (thyroid, pseudotumor, tumor), progressive supranuclear palsy, Guillain-Barré syndrome

PUPILS

Innervation (Fig. 4.25)

Iris Sphincter

Parasympathetic innervation from Edinger-Westphal nucleus

Pathway of pupillary light reflex: ON → chiasm (fibers split) → optic tract → pretectal nucleus (synapse) → cross to both Edinger-Westphal nuclei (synapse) → travel via CN 3 though subarachnoid space and cavernous sinus, then travel in inferior division of CN 3 to ciliary ganglion → postganglionic fibers travel via short ciliary nerves to ciliary body and iris sphincter

Iris Dilator

Sympathetic innervation

Pathway: posterior hypothalamus → down spinal cord → synapse in ciliospinal center of Budge (C8–T2 level) → second-order neuron ascends sympathetic chain → over apex of lung → synapse at superior cervical ganglion → third-order neuron ascends with ICA) and joins CN 6 in cavernous sinus → enters orbit via long ciliary nerve (through superior orbital fissure next to CN V_1) to iris dilator and Müller muscle

Disorders

Relative Afferent Pupillary Defect (RAPD; Marcus-Gunn Pupil)

Large retinal lesion, asymmetric ON disease, chiasm lesion, optic tract lesion (contralateral RAPD)

No RAPD: cataract, acute papilledema, amblyopia, refractive error, functional visual loss, lesions posterior to lateral geniculate body

Light-Near Dissociation

Pupil does not react to light but near response intact

Etiology: syphilis (Argyll-Robertson), Adie pupil, familial dysautonomia (Riley-Day syndrome), Parinaud syndrome, RAPD, physiologic, severe retinal disease, aberrant regeneration of CN 3, diabetes, myotonic dystrophy, encephalitis, alcoholism, HZO

Abnormal Light and Near Response

Pharmacologic, trauma, CN 3 palsy

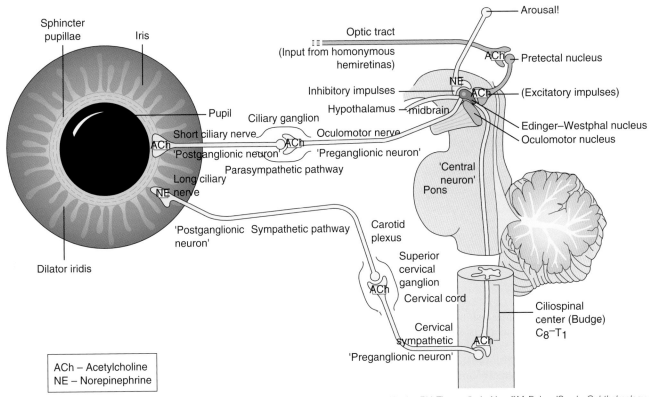

Figure 4.25 Parasympathetic and sympathetic innervation of the iris muscles. (With permission from Kardon RH: The pupils. In: Yanoff M, Duker JS, eds. *Ophthalmology.* 2nd ed. St Louis: Mosby; 2004.)

Anisocoria

Pupils of unequal size

Miosis: small pupil
   DDx: Horner syndrome, pharmacologic (pilocarpine, brimonidine, narcotics, insecticides), Argyll-Robertson pupil, iritis, diabetes, spasm of near reflex, senescence

Mydriasis: large pupil
   DDx: CN 3 palsy, Adie tonic pupil, pharmacologic (mydriatics, cycloplegics, cocaine), iris damage (trauma, ischemia, surgery [Urrets-Zavalia syndrome]), Hutchinson pupil
   Both Horner and Adie are examples of denervation hypersensitivity (sympathetic tone loss in Horner, parasympathetic tone loss in Adie)

Horner Syndrome

Sympathetic lesion causing ptosis, miosis, and anhidrosis; anhidrosis often present in both first- and second-order lesions; may also have facial numbness, diplopia, and vertigo; may have mild inverse ptosis of lower lid, dilation lag; anisocoria most pronounced in dim light; congenital (forceps injury, shoulder dystocia); can cause iris heterochromia (ipsilateral lighter iris)

Preganglionic: from hypothalamus to superior cervical ganglion

1st-order neuron (central Horner): hypothalamus to spinal cord level C8 to T2 (ciliospinal center of Budge)
   ETIOLOGY:
      MIDBRAIN: neuron located near CN 4 nucleus in dorsolateral tegmentum; lesion at this level (usually ischemia) causes Horner and SO palsy
      PONS: near CN 6 nucleus; ischemia, tumor, demyelination, polio, syringomyelia, and inflammation, Foville syndrome (lesion of CN 5, 6, and 7 and Horner)
      MEDULLA: lateral medullary syndrome of Wallenberg (stroke of vertebral artery or posterior inferior cerebellar artery [PICA] causing lateral medullary infarction); ipsilateral lesion of CN 9, 10, and 11; Horner, vertigo, cerebellar signs, skew deviation, ipsilateral decreased pain/temperature sensation of face, contralateral decreased pain/temperature sensation of trunk and limbs); no extremity weakness
      VERTEBROBASILAR STROKES AND VERTEBRAL ARTERY DISSECTION
      CERVICAL DISC DISEASE: arthritis, demyelination, inflammation, tumors
      SYRINGOMYELIA: spinal cord cavities surrounded by gliosis involving spinothalamic tracts; causes ipsilateral loss of pain/temperature sensation but preservation of touch; muscle wasting and weakness (especially small hand muscles); Charcot arthropathy (35%)

2nd-order neuron: majority of preganglionic Horner's; ciliospinal center of Budge to superior cervical ganglion

ETIOLOGY: mediastinal or apical tumor (neuroblastoma [most common], Pancoast), thyroid disease, neurofibroma, pneumothorax, cervical infections, upper respiratory tract tumors, brachial plexus syndromes, carotid artery dissection, aneurysm, trauma

Postganglionic: superior cervical ganglion to iris dilator

3rd-order neuron: anhidrosis limited to ipsilateral forehead

ETIOLOGY:

INTERNAL CAROTID ARTERY DISSECTION: transient ischemic attack (TIA), stroke, neck pain, amaurosis, dysacousia, bad taste in mouth

LESIONS INVOLVING MECKEL'S CAVE OR CAVERNOUS SINUS: associated with CN 3, 4, V_1, V_2, and 6 palsies

TRIGEMINAL HERPES ZOSTER

HEADACHE SYNDROMES: migraine, cluster headaches, Raeder syndrome (middle-aged men with Horner and daily unilateral headaches)

TUMOR OF PAROTID GLAND, NASOPHARYNX, SINUSES

TRAUMA

Diagnosis: pharmacologic testing

Cocaine test: topical cocaine (4%, 10%) blocks reuptake of norepinephrine (NE), causing pupil dilation

Determines presence of Horner syndrome

Functioning neuron will release NE, and pupil will dilate

ABNORMAL RESULT: no pupil dilation

Hydroxyamphetamine 1% (Paredrine) test: releases NE from nerve terminal

Distinguishes between preganglionic and postganglionic lesions

POSITIVE IN PREGANGLIONIC LESIONS: pupil dilates because postganglionic neuron is intact

NEGATIVE IN POSTGANGLIONIC LESIONS: pupil does not dilate because neuron does not have NE

Treatment: ptosis surgery to shorten Müller muscle (Putterman procedure [conjunctival–Müller muscle resection], Fasanella-Servat procedure [tarsoconjunctival resection])

Adie Tonic Pupil

Dilated, tonic pupil due to postganglionic parasympathetic pupillomotor damage; 90% women; 20–40 years of age; 80% unilateral

Findings: initially, pupil is dilated and poorly reactive; later becomes miotic; segmental contraction of pupil (vermiform movements); light-near dissociation with slow (tonic) redilation after near stimulus

Adie syndrome: Adie pupil and decreased deep tendon reflexes; orthostatic hypotension

Pathology: loss of ganglion cells in ciliary ganglion, degenerated axons in short ciliary nerves

DDx: HZV, GCA, syphilis, orbital trauma, diabetes, alcoholism, and dysautonomia associated with cancer and amyloidosis

Diagnosis: dilute pilocarpine (0.125%) or Mecholyl 2.5% will constrict the tonic pupil but not the normal pupil; false-positive test can occur in CN 3 palsy

Argyll-Robertson Pupil

Bilateral small, irregular pupils with light-near dissociation caused by tertiary syphilis

Hutchinson Pupil

Unilateral dilated, poorly reactive pupil in comatose patient caused by ipsilateral supratentorial mass causing displacement of hippocampal gyrus (uncal herniation) entrapping CN 3; pupillomotor fibers travel in peripheral portion of nerve and are susceptible to early damage from compression

Simple Anisocoria

Most common cause of relative difference (<1 mm) between pupils; occurs in up to 20% of general population

OCULAR MUSCLE DISORDERS

Ophthalmoplegia

Static

Agenesis of extraocular muscles, congenital fibrosis syndrome, congenital myopathies

Progressive

Chronic Progressive External Ophthalmoplegia (CPEO)

(See Chapter 5, Pediatrics/Strabismus)

Mitochondrial disease, isolated or hereditary; bilateral; affects all directions of gaze; several types

Kearns-Sayre Syndrome (mitochondrial DNA): Onset before age 20; gene deletion impairs oxidative phosphorylation

Findings: triad of ophthalmoplegia with ptosis, pigmentary retinopathy, cardiac conduction defects (arrhythmias, heart block, cardiomyopathy; workup includes electrocardiogram [EKG])

Other findings: mental retardation, short stature, deafness, ataxia, elevated CSF protein

Pathology: ragged red fibers

Oculopharyngeal Muscular Dystrophy (AD)

Onset in 5th-6th decade; increased frequency in French-Canadian and Bukharan Jewish populations; progressive dysphagia followed by ptosis; CPEO develops in most

Mutations in *PABPN1* gene on chromosome 14q11

Pathology: vacuolar myopathy

Myotonic Dystrophy (AD)

Most common form of adult muscular dystrophy; myotonia of peripheral muscles; worse in morning and with cold, excitement, fatigue

2 types: type 1 caused by mutations in *DMPK* gene on chromosome 19q13; type 2 caused by mutations in *CNBP* gene on chromosome 3q21; signs and symptoms overlap (type 1 more severe)

Findings: Christmas tree cataract (presenile cataract with polychromatic subcapsular cortical crystals), mild pigmentary retinopathy, ptosis, lid lag, light-near dissociation, miotic pupils, may develop ocular hypotony

Other findings: myotonia, testicular atrophy, frontal baldness, cardiac abnormalities, bilateral facial weakness, insulin resistance, mental retardation

Diagnosis: electroretinogram (ERG; low voltage), electromyogram (EMG; myotonic discharge)

Inflammatory Disorders

Thyroid eye disease, orbital pseudotumor, amyloidosis

Others

Vitamin E deficiency, muscle tumors

Episodic

Familial periodic paralysis, trauma, ischemia, vasculitis, disorders of neuromuscular junction (myasthenia gravis, Eaton-Lambert syndrome, organophosphate poisoning, botulism)

Myasthenia Gravis (MG)

Weakness of voluntary muscles resulting from autoimmunity to motor endplates (antibodies to postsynaptic acetylcholine [ACh] receptors or other proteins of striated muscle), hallmark is fatigability; 90% have eye symptoms, 50% present with eye symptoms; females > males; onset age,

15–50 years old; 80% with ocular presentation will develop generalized disease; 15% spontaneously resolve; does not affect pupillary fibers

Neonatal form: transplacental transfer of ACh receptor antibody

Congenital form: genetic defect in ACh receptor

Types:
 Ocular: consists of ptosis and extraocular weakness only
 Systemic: other skeletal muscles involved; Graves' disease develops in 5% of patients

Associations: thymic hyperplasia (70%), thymoma (occurs in 10% of MG patients; 30% of people with thymoma have MG), other autoimmune diseases (rheumatoid arthritis, lupus, thyroid disease)

Drugs that exacerbate MG: steroids, antibiotics (aminoglycosides, clindamycin, erythromycin), β-blockers, D-penicillamine, phenytoin, curare, methoxyflurane, lidocaine

Findings: asymmetric variable ptosis (worse with fatigue, sustained upgaze, and at end of day), see-saw ptosis ("curtaining"; when more ptotic lid is lifted, other lid falls owing to Hering's law), Cogan's lid twitch (when patient looks from downgaze to primary position, lid will overshoot), ipsilateral hypotropia, negative forced ductions, ophthalmoplegia, pseudo-INO, nystagmus (on extreme gaze); great masquerader: can look like any neuropathy or myopathy affecting eye movement

Other findings: facial muscle weakness, dysphagia, dysarthria, dyspnea, weakness of neck, extremities, and trunk; muscle bulk usually preserved until late

DDx: Myotonic dystrophy, CPEO, involutional ptosis, toxins (snake, arthropod, bacteria [botulism]), thyroid eye disease, IOI, MS, INO
 Eaton-Lambert syndrome: paraneoplastic syndrome consisting of profound proximal muscle pain and weakness, dysarthria, dysphagia; associated with small cell lung cancer
  MECHANISM: impaired presynaptic release of ACh; 50% demonstrate specific antibodies against presynaptic voltage-gated calcium channels
  DIAGNOSIS: muscle strength and reflexes are enhanced with exercise; no improvement with edrophonium
   EMG: increased muscle action potentials with repeated nerve stimulation

Diagnosis:
 Tensilon test (edrophonium [IV]; [AChE]) inhibitor that prolongs action of ACh, resulting in stronger muscle contraction): not commonly done anymore

because drug is unavailable; consider short-acting pyridostigmine 60 mg po trial in clinic or at home instead; historically, Tensilon test positive 80%–90% but high false-negative rate; may cause bradycardia therefore, test dose of 1–2 mg first; other adverse effects include sweating, nausea, vomiting, salivation, fever, elevated IOP; antidote is atropine sulfate (0.5 mg)

ACh receptor antibody (Ab): 3 types (binding Ab, blocking Ab, modulating Ab); 50% sensitive in ocular MG, 80% sensitive in general MG, 90% positive in MG with thymoma, 99% specific; seronegative MG caused by antigen excess, ocular-specific Ab; Ab against other components of ACh receptor

EMG: fatigue with repetitive nerve stimulation; single-fiber EMG of peripheral orbicularis muscle most sensitive

Photos: check old photos; morning versus evening for variability in lid position

Rest test: rest with eyes closed × 30 minutes; positive if improvement in ptosis occurs

Ice test: neuromuscular transmission improves in cold; therefore, apply ice pack × 2 minutes; positive if improvement occurs

Others: chest CT/MRI, thyroid function and lupus tests

Treatment: pyridostigmine (Mestinon [AChE inhibitor]), steroids, plasmapheresis, IV gamma globulin, immunomodulatory therapy (mycophenolate, methotrexate, rituximab), thymectomy (33% resolve, 33% improve, 33% no benefit); prism spectacles and consider surgery for stable strabismus (>6–12 months)

Primary Overaction Syndromes

Convergence Spasm

Miosis with increasing esodeviation

Superior oblique myokymia

Episodic repetitive firing of SO causes intermittent oscillopsia, shimmering vision, and vertical and/or torsional diplopia; chronic; unknown etiology; treat with carbamazepine (Tegretol) or propranolol; consider simultaneous weakening of ipsilateral SO and IO

Ocular Neuromyotonia

Failure of muscle to relax; occurs after radiation therapy to parasellar lesions; may affect CN 3 or 6; diagnose by having patient look in direction of action of muscle (up and in for CN 3, laterally for CN 6); treat with carbamazepine (Tegretol)

Oculogyric Crisis

Bilateral tonic supraduction of eyes and neck hyperextension resulting from acute effect of phenothiazine overdose; also described with postinfectious Parkinson disease

EYE MOVEMENTS IN COMA

Normal Eye Movements and Pupils

Bilateral cerebral depression

Limited Eye Movements and Normal Pupils

Metabolic, drugs

Horizontal Limitation

Eyes straight: pontine damage

Eyes deviated to side: cerebral damage

Bilateral horizontal limitations (gaze palsy, INO, CN 6 palsy): pontine damage

Ipsilateral horizontal deviation with contralateral limb weakness: basal ganglia damage

Contralateral horizontal deviation without limb weakness: cerebellar lesions

Vertical Limitation

Eyes straight: midbrain or pretectal damage

Upward deviation: hypoxic encephalopathy (severe cerebellar damage), lithium toxicity, phenothiazine overdose, heatstroke

Downward deviation (more common and more ambiguous than upward deviation): pretectal, metabolic, thalamic hemorrhage; tentorial herniation; pineal tumors; meningitis; hepatic encephalopathy

Vertical-gaze paresis and bilateral CN 3 palsy: midbrain damage

Total Ophthalmoplegia

Midbrain stroke, pituitary apoplexy, meningitis

Skew Deviation

Posterior fossa dysfunction

Bilateral Lid Retraction

Pretectal dysfunction

Nystagmus

Upbeat (structural), downbeat (hypoxic, Arnold-Chiari malformation, toxic [lithium], paraneoplastic), convergence–retraction (dorsal midbrain)

Calorics

Water irrigated into ear produces nystagmus; mnemonic for direction of nystagmus (fast phase): **COWS** (**C**old **O**pposite, **W**arm **S**ame); jerk nystagmus in awake patient; tonic deviation in comatose patient in opposite direction of mnemonic; bilateral cold-water irrigation produces upbeat nystagmus in awake patient; downward tonic deviation in comatose patient

OPTIC NERVE

Developmental Anomalies

(See Chapter 5, Pediatrics/Strabismus)

Optic Disc Swelling

Nerve fibers anterior to lamina cribrosa swell as a result of obstruction of axoplasmic flow at level of lamina choroidalis or lamina scleralis

Orthograde transport (ganglion cells to LGB): slow component = 2 mm/day; fast component = 500 mm/day

Retrograde transport (LGB to ganglion cells)

Mechanism: ischemia, inflammation, increased ICP, compression

Findings: elevated hyperemic nerve head (3 diopters = 1 mm), blurred disc margins, loss of physiologic cup, peripapillary nerve fiber layer (NFL) edema, chorioretinal folds, dilated / tortuous veins, peripapillary flame-shaped hemorrhages, exudates, cotton-wool spots (NFL infarcts)

Chronic swelling may cause Paton's lines (radial or concentric folds of peripapillary retina), gliosis, high water marks, pale disc, disc pseudodrusen, attenuated vessels, vision loss

DDx of optic disc edema/pseudoedema:
papilledema, ischemic optic neuropathy, optic neuritis, central retinal vein occlusion (CRVO), diabetic papillitis, malignant hypertension, neuroretinitis (cat-scratch disease), infiltration of the optic disc (sarcoidosis, tuberculosis,

leukemia, metastases), optic disc drusen, ON head tumors (astrocytic hamartoma, gliomas, capillary hemangioma), orbital disease/compressive optic neuropathy (thyroid eye disease, orbital pseudotumor, orbital mass), inflammatory diseases (syphilis, acute posterior multifocal placoid pigment epitheliopathy [APMPPE], Vogt-Koyanagi-Harada [VKH] syndrome), LHON

Papilledema

Disc edema resulting from increased intracranial pressure

Etiology: congenital caused by hydrocephalus or perinatal hemorrhage; acquired caused by intracranial neoplasm or other masses, infection (meningitis, encephalitis), subdural or subarachnoid hemorrhage, pseudotumor cerebri ([IIH]; see below)

Findings: disc edema (may be asymmetric), disc hyperemia, reduced physiologic cup, thickened nerve fiber layer obscuring retinal vessels, peripapillary nerve fiber layer hemorrhages, cotton-wool spots, exudates, choroidal folds, Paton's lines (circumferential peripapillary retinal folds caused by optic nerve edema), loss of spontaneous venous pulsations (absent in 20% of normal individuals with congenitally small cup:disc ratios); transient visual obscurations (visual blackouts lasting <10 seconds associated with postural changes); diplopia (caused by unilateral or bilateral CN 6 palsies); normal color vision, acuity, and pupils; enlarged blind spot on VF; headache, pulsatile tinnitus, dizziness, nausea, vomiting, neck or back pain, meningismus and radiating pain, altered mental status, other cranial nerve paresis or neurologic deficits
  Chronic cases: pale atrophic nerve, arteriolar attenuation, poor vision, VF loss, refractile small hyaline bodies on the disc

DDx: optic disc edema without elevated ICP, which includes malignant hypertension, diabetic papillitis, optic neuritis, uveitis, infections, anterior ischemic optic neuropathy, anemia, LHON, hypotony, ON infiltration (lymphoma, leukemia) or masses, optic disc drusen, and pseudopapilledema; central retinal vein occlusion and neuroretinitis are more commonly unilateral but can sometimes occur bilaterally

Diagnosis: check BP; emergent neuroimaging (orbit and brain MRI/CT), if no mass, perform lumbar puncture (measure opening pressure)

Idiopathic Intracranial Hypertension (IIH; Pseudotumor Cerebri)

Papilledema with normal neuroimaging and CSF; diagnosis of exclusion

90% female; usually childbearing age (mean 33 years old), obese (body mass index [BMI] >30 kg/m²)

IIH is sometimes known as pseudotumor cerebri (PTC) because it causes signs and symptoms similar to a tumor. However, PTC refers to papilledema with a known cause, and IIH refers to cases that are truly idiopathic:

IIH: associated with recent weight gain, polycystic ovari syndrome, obstructive sleep apnea

PTC: associated with endocrine disorder (Addison; steroid withdrawal), chronic obstructive lung disease, radical neck surgery, thrombosis of dural sinus (trauma, childbirth, middle ear infection, hypercoagulable state); use of steroids, birth control pills, vitamin A, tetracyclines (doxycycline), fluoroquinolones, levothyroxine, nalidixic acid, isotretinoin, lithium, amiodarone; may be exacerbated with pregnancy

Findings: headache, nausea, vomiting, optic disc edema (may be asymmetric), transient visual obscurations, photopsias, VF defect (enlarged blind spot, constriction, or arcuate scotoma), retrobulbar pain, pulsatile intracranial noises; may have visual loss, positive RAPD, diplopia (CN 6 palsy)

In children: irritability; no disc swelling if fontanelles open

DDx: (see Optic Disc Swelling, above)

Diagnosis: normal brain MRI, elevated CSF pressure (≥250 mm H$_2$O) with normal composition (diagnosis of exclusion)

Treatment:

No vision loss: headache treatment and weight loss; for PTC, treat underlying cause (discontinue associated medication)

Mild vision loss: acetazolamide (Diamox), furosemide, weight loss

Advanced VF loss: consider high dose steroids, ON sheath decompression, serial lumbar punctures (temporary relief), lumbar–peritoneal shunt

Optic Neuritis

Inflammation of ON (any part); idiopathic or associated with systemic disease; most common optic neuropathy in people <45 years old; female preponderance

Papillitis: inflammation is anterior, optic disc swelling is present

Retrobulbar: inflammation is behind the globe, no optic disc swelling; more common

Etiology: most commonly isolated or associated with demyelination (MS), also vasculitis (sarcoidosis, granulomatosis with polyangiitis), infectious (syphilis, tuberculosis, Lyme disease), autoimmune (systemic lupus erythematosus [SLE], neuromyelitis optica [NMO, Devic

disease; bilateral optic neuritis and transverse myelitis], anti–myelin-associated oligodendrocytes glycoprotein [anti-MOG] syndrome)

Isolated form: usually females (77%), mean onset = 32 years of age; 65% retrobulbar

Findings: subacute unilateral visual loss (can evolve over 1st week, then spontaneous improvement over weeks [70% regain 20/20]), ocular pain exacerbated by eye movements, decreased color vision (especially red-green) and contrast sensitivity, positive RAPD (unless bilateral and symmetric optic neuritis), VF defect (50% diffuse, 20% central scotoma, rarely altitudinal), ON appears normal or swollen (35%), disc pallor late

Other findings:

Pulfrich phenomenon: motion of pendulum appears elliptical owing to altered depth perception from delayed conduction in the demyelinated nerve

Uhthoff symptom/sign/phenomenon: worsening of symptoms with heat or exercise; present in 50% after recovery

Phosphenes: flashes of light induced by eye movements or sound

Auditory clicks: CN 7 innervates stapedius, and patient hears click with effective transmission

DDx: intraocular inflammation, malignant hypertension, DM, cat-scratch disease, optic perineuritis, LHON, ON glioma, orbital tumor, anterior ischemic optic neuropathy, central serous retinopathy, multiple evanescent white-dot syndrome, acute idiopathic blind spot enlargement syndrome

Lab test: for atypical findings (i.e., older age, no pain, acute severe or persistent [>1 month] visual loss, bilateral involvement, papillitis with peripapillary hemorrhages, exudates, intraocular inflammation, other cranial nerve involvement), include serum or CSF aquaporin-4 autoantibodies (AQP4-IgG) (for NMO), RPR and FTA-ABS (for syphilis); serum ESR, ANA (for SLE), C-ANCA (for granulomatosis with polyangiitis); Lyme and *Bartonella* titers; ACE, CXR or CT, gallium or PET scan (for sarcoidosis); and consider genetic testing (for LHON)

MRI: to rule out MS (periventricular white matter lesions), NMO (spinal lesions), and compressive or infiltrative lesions

Treatment: consider systemic steroids for patients who require rapid return of vision (ONTT; see accompanying box); if evidence of MS, then immunomodulatory therapy with injectables (interferon), oral agents, and/or infusions; if evidence of NMO, then high-dose IV steroids and other treatment if not responsive (see below)

Optic Neuritis Treatment Trial (ONTT)

Objective: to evaluate the role of corticosteroids in the treatment of unilateral optic neuritis

Methods: patients with unilateral optic neuritis were randomly assigned to three treatment groups:

IV steroids: 250 mg IV methylprednisolone qid × 3 days, followed by oral prednisone (1 mg/kg/day) × 11 days
Oral steroids: prednisone (1 mg/kg/day) × 14 days
Oral placebo: 14 days

Results:

IV steroids: more rapid recovery of visual acuity at 2 weeks; did not reduce risk of subsequent attacks; decreased incidence of MS at 2 years versus placebo, but no difference at 3 years
Oral prednisone: associated with higher rate of new attacks in either eye at 1 year; highest relapse rate of optic neuritis at 5 years (41% vs. 25% for IV and placebo groups)
Brain MRI: periventricular white-matter lesions were associated with MS
Lesions in 50% of patients with first attack of optic neuritis
5-YEAR RESULTS: 30% risk for MS, regardless of treatment group
   WITH NO LESIONS: 16% developed MS
   ≥ 3 LESIONS: 51% developed MS
Increased risk of developing MS if previous neurologic symptoms (regardless of MRI status)
10-YEAR RESULTS:
   WITH NO LESIONS: 22% developed MS
   ≥ 1 LESIONS: 56% developed MS
   Optic neuritis recurred in 35% overall and 48% who developed MS
15-YEAR RESULTS:
   WITH NO LESIONS: 25% developed MS
   ≥ 1 LESIONS: 72% developed MS
   92% had ≥20/40 vision, 3% had ≤20/200 vision
   Up to 90% have abnormality in visual function (i.e., color, contrast, visual field, stereopsis, visual field)
If normal MRI and no previous neurologic findings or fellow eye involvement: decreased risk of MS if optic neuritis was painless, if disc swelling was present, and vision loss was only mild
No patients developed MS who had normal MRI with peripapillary hemorrhage or macular exudates
Abnormal MRI: 43% progress to MS by 3 years; progression to MS at 1 year was 7.5% with IV steroids, 14.7% with oral steroids, and 16.7% with placebo

Conclusions:

In general, ~ 30% develop MS within 4 years, and 38% develop MS by 10 years (risk is higher in women than men)

Consider treating optic neuritis with IV steroids; do not initiate treatment with oral steroids

Steroid treatment speeds visual recovery by 1–2 weeks but has no long-term visual advantage and after 3 years has no protective effect against MS

Regardless of MRI status, there is a higher risk for MS if the patient has previous neurologic symptoms or a history of optic neuritis in the fellow eye.

Neuromyelitis Optica Spectrum Disorder (NMOSD, NMO, Devic Disease)

Rare autoimmune demyelinating disease causing severe optic neuritis and transverse myelitis (usually within weeks to months but may be separated by years)

Onset ~40 years old; more common in females, increased risk in Asians and African Americans (2–3 ×)

2 forms: monophasic or relapsing

Findings: acute severe decreased vision (usually <20/200 and bilateral), eye pain; may have VF defects (bitemporal or homonymous hemianopia), motility abnormalities (nystagmus, internuclear ophthalmoplegia, opsoclonus); may develop central retinal artery occlusion

Other findings: weakness/numbness of extremities, exaggerated deep tendon reflexes, genitourinary (sphincter dysfunction) and gastrointestinal (hiccups, vomiting, weight loss) involvement; may develop paralysis

DDx: optic neuritis (see above), multiple sclerosis, anti-MOG syndrome

Lab tests: AQP4-IgG (negative in 25%), lumbar puncture (pleocytosis, increased polymorphonuclear cells, eosinophils)

MRI: ON inflammation (more extensive than MS and may involve optic chiasm and tracts), spinal cord lesions (length ≥3 vertebral segments, often cervical and upper thoracic lesions), brain lesions (up to 70%; usually around 3rd ventricle and cerebral aqueduct, dorsal brainstem, area postrema)

Treatment: acute cases require hospitalization for workup and step-wise therapy with immediate high-dose IV methylprednisolone (1000 mg qd × 3–5 days; to prevent strokes to ON and retina), then plasmapheresis (in patients who do not respond to steroids), and then eculizumab (Soliris; for complement inhibition), inebilizumab-cdon

(Uplizna; for B-cell depletion), or satralizumab (Enspryng; for anti–interleukin-6 [IL-6- activity). These medications are also used in AQP4-positive patients with relapsing form. Immunosuppressive agents, including azathioprine, mycophenolate, or rituximab, can reduce recurrence

Prognosis: worse than optic neuritis with MS; poor in 83% with spinal cord lesions and 67% with optic neuritis; >50% develop <20/200 vision within 5 years; respiratory failure causes death

Optic Neuropathies

Anterior Ischemic Optic Neuropathy (AION)

Ischemia of ON head just posterior to lamina cribrosa resulting from inadequate perfusion by posterior ciliary arteries; results in acute visual loss

2 forms: arteritic (GCA; 5% of AION); nonarteritic (ischemic; 95% of AION)

Findings: decreased color vision and acuity, positive RAPD, VF loss (altitudinal or arcuate defects most common, central scotomas also occur), unilateral optic disc edema (often involving one sector), contralateral disc appears crowded (small C/D ratio)

Arteritic: caused by giant cell (temporal) arteritis (inflammatory vasculopathy affecting medium-sized to large vessels), stroke affecting the posterior ciliary arteries; female > male (2:1); aged > 55 years; most common in Caucasians; may have amaurosis fugax or diplopia

Other findings: scalp tenderness, jaw or tongue claudication, polymyalgia rheumatica (PMR), fever, malaise, anorexia, weight loss, anemia, headache, tender temporal artery, neck pain, brainstem stroke (resulting from involvement of vertebral artery); cotton-wool spots, choroidal ischemia (seen as patchy choroidal filling on fluorescein angiography [FA])

Pathology: granulomatous inflammation with epithelioid cells, lymphocytes, giant cells; disruption of internal elastic lamina and proliferation of intima with aneurysm formation (Fig. 4.26)

Diagnosis: elevated ESR (for men > [age/2]; for women > [(age + 10)/2]; may be normal in 10%), CRP (above 2.45 mg/dL), low hematocrit (anemia of chronic illness), FA (patchy choroidal filling, nonperfusion), temporal artery biopsy (inflammation in artery wall with disruption of internal elastica lamina, skip lesions [specimen at least 3 cm], perform within 2 weeks of steroid treatment)

Treatment (emergent): steroids (prednisone 60–120 mg orally; consider IV initially [1 g × 3 days]) to prevent fellow eye involvement (65% risk of involvement of fellow eye without treatment; usually affected within 10 days); some patients lose vision despite treatment

Nonarteritic (NAION): ischemic; no associated symptoms; usually aged 50–75 years; often occurs upon

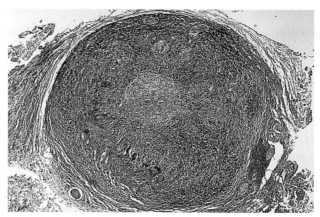

Figure 4.26 Arteritic anterior ischemic optic neuropathy demonstrating vasculitis of all coats of temporal artery with giant cells. (Courtesy MM Rodrigues. From Yanoff M, Fine BS: *Ocular pathology*. 5th ed. St Louis: Mosby; 2002.)

awakening; etiology unclear but not a stroke, associated with anatomic (disc-at-risk or small cup:disc ratio, small optic disc size, recent posterior vitreous detachment) and systemic (diabetes [30%], hypertension [40%], ischemic heart disease [20%], hypercholesterolemia [70%], smoking [50%], obstructive sleep apnea, hypercoagulable states) risk factors; recurrence in same eye is rare; 25%–40% risk of fellow eye involvement; normal ESR; NAION may be mimicked by amiodarone, phosphodiesterase-5 inhibitors, linezolid, ethambutol, isoniazid, and others; may be associated with optic disc drusen in young-onset cases

Treatment: none, consider daily aspirin if significant vascular risk factors

ISCHEMIC OPTIC NEUROPATHY DECOMPRESSION TRIAL (IONDT): ON sheath fenestration is not effective

Smokers had earlier mean onset (age 64) than nonsmokers (age 70)

43% of control patients regained ≥3 lines of vision at 6 months (vs. 34% of those having surgery)

Surgery conferred higher risk of loss of 3 lines of vision (24% vs. 12% with observation)

Pseudo-Foster-Kennedy syndrome: AION is the most frequent cause of unilateral disc edema and contralateral optic atrophy; disc not hyperemic as in true Foster-Kennedy syndrome

DDx of AION: malignant HTN, DM, retinal vascular occlusion, compressive lesion, collagen vascular disease, syphilis, herpes zoster (multifocal varicella zoster virus [VZV] vasculopathy): with temporal artery involvement causes arteritic or atypical nonarteritic AION (confirmed by viral antigen in temporal artery biopsy (both GCA-positive and GCA-negative); features overlap with GCA (headache, polymyalgia rheumatica, temporal artery tenderness, central retinal artery occlusion, retinal necrosis, posterior ischemic optic neuropathy) or may have atypical NAION findings (pain, larger cup:disc ratios, retinal involvement, slow progression); also migraine, postoperative, massive blood loss, normal-tension glaucoma

Retrobulbar Optic Neuropathy (Posterior Ischemic Optic Neuropathy)

Rare; usually bilateral; occurs with severe anemia and hypotension (i.e., major blood loss from surgery, trauma, gastrointestinal [GI] bleed, dialysis); associated with medications (antibiotics [ethambutol, isoniazid, sulfonamides, chloramphenicol], anticancer drugs [cisplatin, vincristine, busulfan])

Findings: disc swelling may occur if ischemic process extends anteriorly

Treatment: treat acute cause (prompt reversal of hypotension, blood transfusion)

Compressive Optic Neuropathy

Intraorbital, intracanalicular, or intracranial (prechiasmal)

Etiology: ON tumor, pituitary tumor or apoplexy, thyroid eye disease, hematoma

Findings: slow progressive vision loss, decreased color vision, positive RAPD, VF defect (central scotoma that extends to periphery), proptosis; disc may be normal, pale, or swollen; may have endocrine abnormalities (parachiasmal lesions), chemosis and restricted motility (thyroid)

Diagnosis: orbit CT/MRI

Infiltrative Optic Neuropathy

Etiology: leukemia, lymphoma, multiple myeloma, plasmacytoma, metastatic carcinoma (breast and lung most common), sarcoidosis, TB, cryptococcus, toxoplasmosis, toxocariasis, CMV, coccidiomycosis

Findings: disc may appear grayish-white with associated hemorrhages; mass may be visible

Toxic/Nutritional Optic Neuropathy

Painless symmetric progressive vision loss

Etiology: ethambutol (most common; toxicity is dose and duration dependent: after 2 months, incidence is 1% for 15 mg/kg/day, 6% for 25 mg/kg/day, 18% for >35 mg/kg/day), rarer causes include isoniazid (less severe and reversible), rifampin, chloramphenicol, sulfonamides, streptomycin, chloroquine, quinine, linezolid, digitalis, amiodarone, isotretinoin, cyclosporine, vincristine, methotrexate, chlorambucil, tamoxifen, penicillamine, disulfiram, cisplatin, arsenic, lead, mercury, thallium, carbon monoxide, and tobacco-related or alcohol-related (ethyl alcohol, ethylene glycol, methanol) amblyopia

Findings: decreased vision ($\leq$ 20/200), VF loss (cecocentral scotomas), disc hyperemia, then pallor; alcohol-related has nonreactive pupils, nystagmus, optic disc swelling, retinal edema

Traumatic Optic Neuropathy

ON contusion or compression due to trauma

Occurs in 3% of patients with severe head trauma and 2.5% of patients with midfacial fractures

Findings: decreased vision, VF defects, positive RAPD

CT scan/MRI: rule out canal fracture, orbital hematoma, ON hematoma

Treatment: lateral canthotomy for tense orbit, drain subperiosteal hematoma
> *IV steroids* (methylprednisolone): 30 mg/kg loading dose, then 5.4 mg/kg/h × 48 hours
> If vision improves, switch to 80 mg oral and taper by 20 mg every 2–3 days; if vision worsens on oral steroids, restart high-dose IV and consider surgical decompression of canal
> Consider surgical decompression of optic canal if no response to steroids after 48 hours
> If no improvement in vision after 3 days, stop steroids

Hereditary Optic Neuropathy

(See Chapter 5, Pediatrics/Strabismus)

Mnemonic (causes of optic neuropathy): NIGHT TIC (**N**euritis, **I**schemic, **G**ranulomatous infiltration, **H**ereditary, **T**raumatic, **T**oxic, **I**rradiation, **C**ompressive)

Optic Atrophy

Pale, white appearance of ON head caused by injury to any part of pathway from retinal ganglion cells to LGB

Etiology: optic neuropathy, optic neuritis, glaucoma, central retinal artery occlusion (CRAO), tumors, aneurysms

Pathology: increased number of astrocytes (gliosis) within nerve; normal parallel architecture of glial columns seen in sagittal sections is lost; widened space between nerve and meninges; loss of myelin; thickened pial septa

ON Tumors

ON Glioma (Fig. 4.27)

Low-grade astrocytoma: usually in children aged <10

"Benign" but 14% mortality rate (highest with hypothalamus involvement)

10%–15% have neurofibromatosis (15% of patients with neurofibromatosis have ON gliomas)

50% intraorbital, 50% intracranial
> *Findings:* vision loss, strabismus, nystagmus, disc edema or atrophy; may have proptosis (intraorbital ON glioma); can spread to chiasm and contralateral ON
> *MRI:* fusiform thickening and kinking of ON

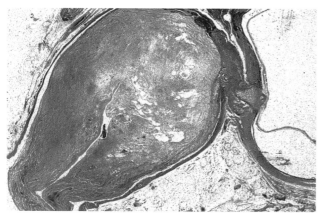

Figure 4.27 Glioma demonstrating central necrosis. (With permission from Yanoff M, Fine BS: *Ocular pathology*. 5th ed. St Louis: Mosby; 2002.)

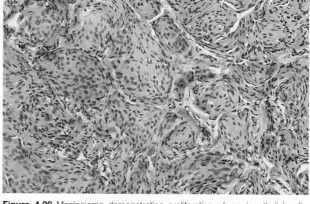

Figure 4.28 Meningioma demonstrating proliferation of meningothelial cells. (With permission from Yanoff M, Fine BS: *Ocular pathology*. 5th ed. St Louis: Mosby; 2002.)

Malignant ON glioma (glioblastoma multiforme): occurs in adults

Painful vision loss; becomes bilateral; death in 3–9 months

ON Meningioma

Derived from outer arachnoid; may arise from ectopic nests of meningeal cells; female > male (3:1)

Findings: triad of decreased vision, optic atrophy, optociliary shunt vessels; also, proptosis, ON edema, retinal vascular occlusions

Sphenoid wing meningioma: fullness of temporal orbital fossa and orbit

Pathology: psammoma bodies and whorls of concentrically packed spindle cells (Fig. 4.28)

CT/MRI: railroad track sign (caused by calcification)

CHIASM COMPRESSION

Chiasm anatomy: location with respect to pituitary gland
  Prefixed: chiasm is forward; pituitary tumor will compress the optic tracts
  Normal: chiasm is aligned with pituitary; pituitary tumor will compress chiasm
  Postfixed: chiasm is behind; pituitary tumor will compress ONs

Etiology: pituitary tumor (most common), pituitary apoplexy, craniopharyngioma, meningioma, glioma, aneurysm, trauma, infection, metastasis, MS, sarcoidosis

VF defects: central scotoma, bitemporal hemianopia, incongruous homonymous hemianopia, junctional scotoma (ipsilateral central scotoma with contralateral superotemporal defect caused by lesion at junction of ON and chiasm)

DDx of bitemporal VF defect: sector retinitis pigmentosa, coloboma, tilted disc

Pituitary Tumor

Most commonly chromophobe (often prolactinoma); can also secrete adrenocorticotropin (ACTH) (Cushing disease); basophil can secrete ACTH; eosinophil can secrete growth hormone (GH) (acromegaly); secreting tumors usually present with endocrine dysfunction, except prolactin-secreting tumor in males (presents with signs of chiasmal compression); 30% nonsecreting (present with vision loss)

Findings: VF defect (bitemporal hemianopia), hormone imbalance, optic atrophy

Diagnosis: x-ray shows large pituitary fossa, double floor sign, bony erosion

Treatment: dopamine antagonist (bromocriptine) for prolactinoma, hormone replacement, transsphenoidal surgery for nonsecreting tumor, XRT

Meningioma

Derived from meningothelial cells of arachnoid; often at sphenoid ridge; occurs in adults, especially middle-aged women

Tuberculum sellae meningioma: compression of ON just before chiasm, may cause unilateral VF defect
  Findings: optic atrophy, hyperostosis

Pathology: whorled cellular pattern; may see psammoma bodies

Pituitary Apoplexy

Acute hemorrhage and expansion of a pituitary tumor, usually secondary to ischemic necrosis

Findings: headache, decreased vision, ocular motility disturbance; progresses to no light perception (NLP) and complete ophthalmoplegia

Sheehan Syndrome

Panhypopituitarism in pregnancy resulting from hemorrhage

Craniopharyngioma

Usually causes compression of chiasm from above and behind; occurs in children and young adults

Findings: initial damage to upper nasal fibers (inferior bitemporal field defect); later, upper temporal defect papilledema, optic atrophy

MRI: calcification

DDx of calcification of sella turcica: craniopharyngioma, supraclinoid aneurysm, meningioma, atrioventricular (AV) malformation, glioma of chiasm (very rare), chordoma (extremely rare)

Glioma

Occurs in children and adults; may extend into both ONs, causing bilateral vision loss with complicated bilateral VF defects

Aneurysm

ICA and anterior cerebral artery; middle-aged adults; present with vision loss, ophthalmoplegia

Subfrontal Mass Lesion

Slow progressive asymmetric bilateral visual loss, late ON pallor

Other Chiasmal Lesions

MS, trauma, basal meningitis, sphenoid sinus mucocele or carcinoma

RETROCHIASMAL DISORDERS

Cause homonymous VF defects (see Fig. 4.9)

Cogan's dictum: causes homonymous hemianopia
With asymmetric OKN = parietal lobe lesion (usually mass)
With symmetric OKN = occipital lobe lesion (usually infarction)

Optic Tract

Vascular, craniopharyngioma extending posteriorly

Findings: incongruous homonymous hemianopia, bilateral optic atrophy (bow-tie appearance), contralateral RAPD

Lateral Geniculate Body

Very rare

Findings: incongruous homonymous hemianopia or congruous homonymous sectoranopia (sectoral optic atrophy), normal pupils

Temporal Lobe

Glioma, vascular

Findings: "Pie-in-the-sky" VF defect (inferior macular fibers do not travel as far anteriorly into Meyer's loop)

Other findings: déjà vu symptoms, foul odors; may have formed visual hallucinations

Parietal Lobe

Glioma, meningioma, metastases, MCA thrombosis

Findings: affect fibers from superior retina first (contralateral inferior homonymous quadrantanopia) or contralateral inferior homonymous hemianopia denser inferiorly; spasticity of conjugate gaze (tonic deviation of eyes to opposite side of parietal lesion); OKN asymmetry (nystagmus dampened when stimuli moved in direction of damaged parietal lobe); may have contralateral motor paresis

Gerstmann syndrome: lesion of dominant parietal lobe (inferior homonymous hemianopia, acalculia, agraphia, finger agnosia, left–right confusion)

Occipital Lobe

Vascular (90%), tumors, trauma

Findings:
Central homonymous hemianopia (periphery spared): fibers from macula terminate at tip of occipital lobes
Macula sparing: fibers from retinal periphery terminate on mesial surface of occipital lobe (supplied by PCA)
Temporal crescent: homonymous hemianopia with sparing of far temporal periphery (supplied by nasal retina and travels to most anterior portion of mesial surface of contralateral occipital lobe)

Other findings: unformed visual hallucinations, paliopia (perseveration in homonymous field), prosopagnosia (inability to recognize faces; bilateral medial occipitotemporal lesion), Riddoch phenomenon (ability to perceive moving objects but not stationary ones)

Disconnection syndrome: dominant occipital lobe and splenium of corpus callosum; usually caused by posterior artery stroke (right homonymous hemianopia with alexia [cannot read] but not agraphia [can write])

CORTICAL LESIONS

Cause disorders of visual integration

Visual information from LGB goes to primary visual cortex (V1) of both occipital lobes; further processing occurs in areas V2-V5

To read, information travels from visual cortex to angular gyrus in parietal lobe of dominant hemisphere (usually on left side); visual information from right hemifield is transmitted directly from left occipital lobe to ipsilateral angular gyrus, and information from left hemifield is transmitted through splenium of corpus callosum to contralateral angular gyrus

Disorders

Alexia

Inability to read despite normal vision

Pseudo-Alexia

Can be caused by inability to read, hemianopias with split fixation, and expressive (Broca) or conduction aphasias

Alexia With Agraphia (Inability to Write)

Parietal lesions involving angular gyrus

Alexia Without Agraphia

Large left occipital lesions that also disrupt fibers crossing in splenium of corpus callosum from right occipital cortex to left angular gyrus; information from left VF cannot travel to left parietal lobe (angular gyrus); patient is blind in right visual field, can see and write but not read, even what they have just written

Dyslexia

Central nervous system problem in which letters appear reversed; male > female (3:1); visual training does not improve academic abilities of children with dyslexia or learning disabilities

Visual Neglect

Patient ignores one side of visual space

Visual Extinction

Patient ignores one side of visual space when presented with simultaneous stimuli to both visual fields; occurs more often with right parietal lesions

Visual Agnosia

Bilateral lesions of occipitotemporal area; inability to recognize objects by sight, although can recognize by touch, language, and intellect

Anomia

Inability to name objects

Prosopagnosia

Bilateral infero-occipital lesions; inability to recognize faces

Cerebral Achromatopsia

Unilateral or bilateral lesion in infero-occipital area; loss of color vision in opposite hemifield

DISORDERS DURING PREGNANCY

Occur more commonly with eclampsia and preeclampsia

Conditions: central serous retinopathy (CSR), hypertensive retinopathy, Purtscher-like retinopathy, RD, cerebral venous thrombosis, CRAO, carotid cavernous fistula, Sheehan syndrome (postpartum pituitary infarct causing panhypopituitarism; secondary hemorrhage can cause CN 2–6 palsies)

Conditions that worsen during pregnancy: uveal melanoma, pituitary adenoma, meningioma, DM, Graves' disease, orbital and choroidal hemangiomas

Conditions that improve during pregnancy: MS, optic neuritis, sarcoidosis, lupus

Migraines: may improve or worsen

Preeclampsia: transient visual loss in 50%, cerebral blindness in 15%; ischemic cerebrovascular complication risk increases 13 × during pregnancy and postpartum due to hypercoagulable state
> *Arterial abnormalities:* occur in 60%–90%; most common during second and third trimesters and first week postpartum
> *Venous abnormalities:* during first 6 weeks postpartum (venous sinus thrombosis presents with headache and papilledema).

BRAIN TUMORS (TABLE 4.1)

Foster-Kennedy Syndrome

Frontal lobe mass (usually olfactory or sphenoid ridge meningioma) causing anosmia (loss of smell), ipsilateral optic atrophy (tumor compression), and contralateral ON edema (elevated ICP)

Pseudo–Foster-Kennedy syndrome: bilateral AION (pale nerve from old AION and fellow nerve edema from new AION)

Table 4.1 Classification of brain tumors

By origin:	
Glial (gliomas)	Astrocytoma
Neuronal	Neuroblastoma, medulloblastoma
Connective tissue	Sarcoma
Lymphoreticular	Primary (non-Hodgkin) central nervous system (CNS) lymphoma
Blood vessels	Hemangioma, angioma
Bone	Osteoma
Neural crest	Meningioma (arachnoid cells), primary CNS
Congenital rests:	melanoma
Notochord	Chordoma
Adipose cells	Lipoma
Ectodermal derivatives	Craniopharyngioma, teratoma, dermoid
Glands:	Adenoma
Pituitary gland	Pineocytoma, pineoblastoma,
Pineal gland	germ cell tumors
By age:	
<20 years old	CNS tumors are second-most-common type of malignancy (leukemia is first); approximately 66% located in posterior fossa; gliomas of cerebellum, brainstem, optic nerve; pinealomas; primitive neuroectodermal tumors; craniopharyngiomas
20–60 years old	Meningiomas, gliomas of cerebral hemispheres, pituitary tumors
>60 years old	Malignant gliomas, metastases

Cerebellopontine Angle Tumors

Usually acoustic neuroma; associated with neurofibromatosis; peripheral CN 7 lesion (orbicularis weakness, inability to wrinkle forehead), CN 6 lesion, CN 5 lesion (decreased corneal sensation), nystagmus (vestibular to contralateral side, gaze paretic to ipsilateral side)

Posterior Fossa Tumors

Cause most severe papilledema because encroach on cerebral aqueduct and fourth ventricle with rapid rise in ICP

Metastases

In order of frequency at autopsy: melanoma, lung, breast, renal, colorectal, ovarian

HEADACHES

(Fig. 4.29)

Migraines

Etiology: cerebral vasospasm; slow-moving concentric wave of suppressed electrical activity

Types:

Common (without aura) (80%): male = female; any age; little or no prodrome; throbbing headache, photophobia, nausea

Classic (with aura) (15%–20%): male = female; any age; trigger factors; visual prodrome followed by hemicranial pain, nausea, vomiting, dizziness, photophobia

Scintillating scotoma (5–30 minutes, half visual field; may have macropsia, micropsia, hallucinations, achromatopsia); may have tingling on one side of face and/or ipsilateral hand; rarely, hemiparesis, vertigo, mood changes, distortion of hearing and smell

Acephalgic (migraine equivalent) (5%): aura without headache

Most common after age 40 years; history of migraines with or without aura; rule out TIA

Hemiplegic: familial or sporadic; rare; unilateral motor weakness or partial paralysis

Basilar-type (Bickerstaff syndrome): rare; usually in teenage girls and young women; aura mimics vertebrobasilar artery insufficiency with brain-stem or bilateral occipital lobe symptoms (blindness, diplopia, vertigo, difficulty with speech or coordination)

Childhood periodic syndromes: migraine features, usually precursors to migraine; brief attacks of cyclical vomiting, abdominal migraine, benign paroxysmal vertigo; usually no headache

Retinal (ocular): temporary scotoma or monocular blindness; headache may precede or occur within an hour Examination during attack reveals venous constriction

Complications of migraine:

OPHTHALMOPLEGIC: headache and recurrent paresis of one or more ocular motor nerves (usually CN 3); may last > 1 week; rarely, permanent ophthalmoplegia

MIGRAINE INFARCTION: stroke during migraine or neurologic deficit for >1 week; corresponding lesion on neuroimaging

STATUS MIGRAINOSUS: attack lasting >72 hours (with or without treatment); continuous headache or intermittent with interruptions at <4 hours

MIGRALEPSY: seizures during or immediately after a migraine

Precipitating factors:

Diet: tyramine (bananas, avocado, yogurt, aged cheese), phenylethylamine (chocolate, cheese, wine), sodium nitrite (preservatives, food coloring, processed meats and fish), monosodium glutamate (Chinese food, processed meats, frozen dinners, canned soup), caffeine, alcohol, artificial sweeteners

Lifestyle: excessive sleep, fasting or dieting, exertion, fatigue, stressful events, depression

Hormonal: supplemental estrogen, menses, oral contraceptives, ovulation

Environmental: sun exposure, loud noise, bright lights, glare, flickering lights, strong odors

Treatment:

General: alter diet, lifestyle, hormonal and environmental factors

Abortive: ice pack, cold shower, exercise, massage, local scalp pressure; analgesics; oral ergotamine or dihydroergotamine (DHE); antiemetics; sumatriptan (Imitrex; serotonin agonist; works on peripheral trigeminal nerve terminals that supply pain-sensitive vascular and meningeal structures; also causes constriction of certain intracranial blood vessels; oral and injectable forms; 83% obtain relief within 4 hours,

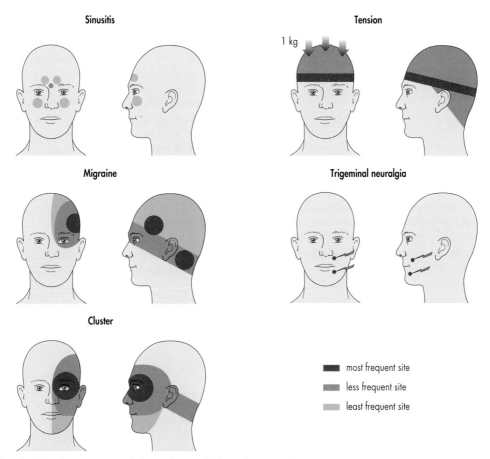

Figure 4.29 Location of pain for the common headache syndromes. (With permission from Weinstein JM: Headache and facial pain. In: Yanoff M, Duker JS, eds. *Ophthalmology*. London: Mosby; 1999.)

45% have recurrence 24 hours later; adverse effects include flushing or tingling, chest pain)

Prophylactic: consider if attacks occur once every 2 months or more often, if severity limits normal activity, or if acute therapies have failed or are contraindicated

β-BLOCKERS: reduce frequency of attacks by half (in 70% of patients)

TRICYCLIC ANTIDEPRESSANTS: amitriptyline, nortriptyline, imipramine, and doxepin

SEROTONIN REUPTAKE INHIBITORS: fluoxetine

CALCIUM CHANNEL BLOCKERS: decrease frequency of attacks, do not affect severity

Tension Headaches

Dull, persistent pain like tight band around head

Cluster Headaches

Severe, unilateral, orbital, supraorbital, and/or temporal pain lasting from 15 minutes to 3 hours; may awaken patient from sleep; usually occur in men 30–40 years of age; more common in smokers; attacks occur in groups and last weeks or months

Findings (ipsilateral): conjunctival injection, lacrimation, nasal congestion, rhinorrhea, forehead/facial sweating,

miosis, ptosis, and/or eyelid edema; *may develop* postganglionic Horner syndrome

Glossopharyngeal Neuralgia

Unilateral pain in region of larynx, tongue, tonsil, and ear; may have hoarseness and coughing; can be stimulated by swallowing or pungent tastes

Treatment: carbamazepine, baclofen, phenytoin

Carotidynia

Pain arising from cervical carotid artery, radiates to ipsilateral face and ear; rule out carotid dissection

Temporomandibular Joint (TMJ) Syndrome

Unilateral ear or preauricular pain, radiates to temple, jaw, or neck; worse with chewing

Findings: limitation of normal jaw movement, audible click on jaw opening

Other Causes of Headache/Facial Pain

Acute: subarachnoid hemorrhage, meningitis, encephalitis, focal scalp inflammation, sinusitis, dental disease, acute uveitis, acute glaucoma, scleritis, HZV, cervical spondylitis, GCA

Recurrent: asthenopia, cerebral aneurysm or angioma, severe hypertension

Chronic: muscle tension, depression, cerebral tumor, pituitary or nasopharyngeal tumor, metastatic carcinoma, Paget disease, increased intracranial pressure, chronic subdural hemorrhage, postherpetic neuralgia, trigeminal neuralgia (tic douloureux), Costen syndrome (temporomandibular osteoarthritis)

VISUAL DISTURBANCES

Functional Visual Loss

Diagnosis of exclusion; trick patient with visual tests

Bottom-up acuity: start with 20/20 line and slowly progress up chart

Deception of eye tested: fogging with phoropter; trial frame with two high-power cylinders of opposite sign in same axis (so net power is zero), then spin one of the cylinders, thus fogging good eye; red-green glasses used with duochrome filter of projection chart (red letters are seen with eye behind red lens), prism test (10 PD lens base out in front of a seeing eye causes gaze shift)

Stereoacuity: minimum amount of acuity is needed to distinguish different stereo images

Binocular integrated multicolored vision assessment test (BIMVAT): red and blue filters placed over near correction in trial frame; blue filter over "bad" eye, then show letters made up of orange, brown, and blue components (orange components seen through blue filter but not red filter); some letters designed so that they can be read as 2 different letters (e.g., P or R) depending on what components are seen, so any letter with all-orange components read correctly was read by the "bad" eye

Visual field testing: spiral field

With complete blindness: OKN, signature (truly blind patients can do this without difficulty), touch nose or other finger (patient may mistake this for a visual task and be unable to perform), mirror test, shock value tests (startle or menace), ERG

Transient Visual Loss

Visual Obscurations

Last seconds; occur in papilledema (change in posture or eye movement) or optic disc drusen

Amaurosis Fugax

Monocular loss or dimming of vision lasting from 2 to >30 minutes; commonly caused by carotid or cardiac disease,

also occurs in GCA, vertebrobasilar insufficiency (bilateral), hypotension, hyperviscosity (anticardiolipin), migraine, eclampsia; brief episodes may indicate impending CRAO

Uhthoff's Phenomena

Blurring of vision with activity or heat; caused by optic neuritis

Scintillating Scotoma

Ocular migraine

Whiteout of Vision or "Chicken-Wire" Pattern

Occipital ischemia

Gradual Peripheral Constriction of Vision With Visual Phenomena

Cerebrovascular disease or occipital migraine

Other Visual Phenomena

Visual Hallucinations

Release hallucinations (Charles Bonnet syndrome): formed (faces, objects) or unformed (flashes of light); occur in areas of absent vision; usually continuous and variable; common in age-related macular degeneration (AMD) and patients with large VF defects; associated with lesions anywhere in visual pathway; stop with eye movement

Ictal hallucinations: stereotyped, paroxysmal visual hallucinations; unformed (occipital lobe lesion) or formed (associated with strange odor; temporal lobe lesion)

Palinopsia: abnormal perseveration of visual images; can be hallucinatory (creation of image that does not exist; either simple/unformed or complex/formed; caused by dysfunction of visual memory from seizures or cortical lesions) or illusory (altered perception of real image; caused by migraine, head trauma, drug/medication)

Phosphenes

Unstructured flashes of light

Photopsias

Structured geometric figures

VASCULAR DISORDERS

Cerebral Aneurysm

Occurs in 5% of population; rarely symptomatic before age 20; associated with hypertension

Risk factors: HTN, AV malformation, coarctation of the aorta, polycystic kidney disease, fibromuscular dysplasia, Marfan syndrome, Ehlers-Danlos syndrome

Types: fusiform or saccular ("berry"; most common at arterial bifurcations; 90% supratentorial; >10 mm have highest risk of rupture)

Location:

Internal carotid artery (85%): main trunk (PCA, ophthalmic artery, cavernous sinus), anterior communicating artery, MCA trifurcation, anterior cerebral artery; most common site is at origin of posterior communicating artery, leading to CN 3 palsy with pupil involvement

Basilar artery (5%)

Vertebral artery (5%)

Findings:

Anterior communicating artery: ON compression, chiasm compression, paraplegia

Origin of PCA: sudden-onset severe headache, complete CN 3 palsy

Bifurcation of MCA: hemiparesis, aphasia

Bifurcation of ICA: ON compression, chiasm compression, hemiparesis

Subarachnoid hemorrhage: neurosurgical emergency; severe headache ("worst headache of life"), nausea, vomiting, stiff neck; **Terson syndrome** (vitreous and subarachnoid hemorrhages [when ICP in ON sheath exceeds ocular venous pressure])

Sentinel bleed: headache with transient neurologic symptoms before major rupture

Diagnosis:

Cerebral arteriogram: 4-vessel study of both carotid and vertebral arteries

MRI: detects aneurysms >5 mm in size

Magnetic resonance angiography (MRA): can detect 3-mm aneurysm

CT scan: acutely to screen for subarachnoid and intraparenchymal bleed; unacceptable screen for unruptured aneurysms (if negative, perform lumbar puncture to determine presence of subarachnoid blood)

Treatment:

Medical (symptomatic, unruptured): stabilize, lower ICP with hyperventilation and mannitol; prevent vasospasm with calcium channel blockers and blood volume expansion; control blood pressure

Surgery: clip aneurysm; if unable, may need to ligate feeding artery

Prognosis: risk of bleed is 1%/year

30% mortality at time of rupture; if untreated, 33% mortality at 6 months; survivors have neurologic deficits

Rebleed risk is highest in first 24 hours; untreated patients have 25% risk of rebleed during first 2 weeks

Vasospasm is major cause of morbidity and death; 30% within first 2 weeks, highest risk between days 4–10

Arteriovenous Malformation (AVM)

Congenital, may be familial; symptoms usually before age 20; 90% supratentorial, 70% cortical, 20% deep, 10% in posterior fossa or dura mater; 6% have intracranial aneurysm

Findings: intracranial bleed (50%), sometimes with subarachnoid hemorrhage; neurologic symptoms before bleed (50%) (seizures, headaches, other neurologic deficits); may hear bruit

Cortical AVM in occipital lobe: visual symptoms and migraines

Hemispheric AVM: can get homonymous hemianopia

Brainstem AVM: diplopia, nystagmus, gaze palsy, pupil abnormality

Diagnosis:

CT scan: hemorrhage; calcified AVMs visible on plain x-ray

MRI: better for small AVMs

Cerebral angiogram: demonstrate anatomy

Treatment: resection, ligation of feeding vessel, embolization, stereotactic radiosurgery

Prognosis: 20% mortality when bleeding begins; rebleed rate is 2.5%/year

Carotid Artery Dissection

Intracranial or extracranial

Etiology:

Trauma: blunt (head, neck), carotid artery compression, hanging, manipulative neck therapy, surgery, carotid artery cannulation during angiography

Spontaneous: fibromuscular dysplasia, Marfan syndrome, Ehlers-Danlos, polycystic kidney disease, syphilis, atherosclerosis, moyamoya, idiopathic

Findings:

Traumatic: ipsilateral headache and ophthalmic signs, contralateral neurologic deficits; may hear bruit

Symptoms can be delayed (weeks to months); severe cases can present with cerebral ischemia and coma

Spontaneous: transient or permanent neurologic defects; amaurosis fugax, monocular visual loss, or ipsilateral Horner syndrome; intracranial extension may cause CN palsies, diplopia, tongue paralysis, facial numbness

Visual loss from embolic occlusion of ophthalmic artery, central retinal artery, or short posterior ciliary arteries

Rarely, ocular ischemia from reduced blood flow

Diagnosis: MRI

Treatment: controversial

Vertebrobasilar Dissection

40% of all dissecting aneurysms; basilar more common than vertebral

General findings: headache, neck pain, signs of brainstem and cerebellar dysfunction

Basilar artery dissection: ocular motor palsies, progresses to coma and death

Vertebral artery dissection (various presentations): fatal brainstem infarction (usually young adults); subarachnoid hemorrhage; aneurysmal dilation with brainstem and lower cranial nerve signs from mass effect; chronic dissection with recurrent TIAs, strokes, and subarachnoid hemorrhages

Vertebrobasilar Insufficiency (VBI)

Posterior circulation ischemia; vertebrobasilar system (vertebral, basilar, posterior cerebral arteries) supplies occipital cortex and areas involved with ocular motility in brainstem and cerebellum

Etiology: thrombus, emboli, hypertension, arrhythmias, arterial dissection, hypercoagulable state, subclavian steal syndrome

Findings: ataxia, vertigo (may also have tinnitus, deafness, or vomiting), dysarthria, dysphagia, hemiparesis, hemiplegia, drop attack (patient suddenly drops to ground without warning, no loss of consciousness), bilateral dimming of vision lasting seconds to minutes, photopsias, homonymous VF loss without other neurologic findings

Cerebral Blindness/Cortical Blindness

Bilateral occipital lobe lesions; pupils react normally; may deny blindness (Anton syndrome)

Cerebral Venous and Dural Sinus Thrombosis

Occlusion of cortical and subcortical veins produces neurologic symptoms; most commonly, cavernous sinus, lateral sinus, and superior sagittal sinus

Etiology: inflammation (Behçet, SLE), infection, trauma, invasion of vessel wall by tumor (leukemia, lymphoma, meningioma), altered blood flow (hypoperfusion, hematologic disorders, venous emboli, hypercoagulability, oral contraceptives, pregnancy, sickle cell disease, protein C or S deficiency, antithrombin III deficiency, lupus anticoagulant)

Cavernous sinus thrombosis: aseptic or septic (infection of sinus or face; rarely otitis or orbital cellulitis)
   Findings: usually unilateral; orbital congestion, lacrimation, chemosis, eyelid swelling, ptosis, proptosis, ophthalmoplegia (CN 6 most common); may have corneal anesthesia, facial numbness, Horner syndrome
   Other findings: headache, nausea, vomiting, somnolence, fever, chills, evidence of meningitis or sepsis
   Treatment: antibiotics, anticoagulants, corticosteroids, surgery

Lateral sinus thrombosis: usually septic from chronic otitis media
   Findings: CN 6 palsy most common (severe facial pain [Gradenigo syndrome] if compressed against petroclinoid ligament), papilledema
   Other findings: symptoms of infection, neck pain, tenderness of ipsilateral jugular vein, retroauricular edema; may have facial weakness

Superior sagittal sinus (SSS) thrombosis: usually aseptic
   Aseptic: occurs during pregnancy, immediately postpartum, or with oral contraceptives; risk factors include vasculitis and systemic inflammatory disorders
   Septic: most commonly from meningitis; also paranasal sinus infection, pulmonary infection, tonsillitis, dental infection, pelvic inflammatory disease, and otitis media
   Findings:
      THROMBOSIS OF ANTERIOR 1/3 OF SINUS: mild symptoms
      THROMBOSIS OF POSTERIOR SINUS: may cause pseudotumor cerebri (headaches and papilledema; consider in pseudotumor that occurs in thin patients), seizures, altered mental status, focal neurologic signs; may be fatal from brain hemorrhage and herniation
   Treatment: anticoagulation, fibrinolytic agents, ICP-lowering agents

Diagnosis: CT, MRI, MRA (venous phase)

INTRACRANIAL ARACHNOID CYST

Congenital malformation; CSF-filled cyst, most commonly in middle cranial fossa (Sylvian fissure)

Findings: seizures, headaches, CN palsy, exophthalmos, hydrocephalus (compression of foramen of Munroe, aqueduct, or fourth ventricle), increased intracranial pressure, papilledema

Cyst rupture may cause subdural hematoma

Treatment: fenestration, shunt

NEURO-OPHTHALMIC MANIFESTATIONS OF AIDS

CNS Lymphoma

High-grade B-cell non-Hodgkin lymphoma; second-most-common malignancy in AIDS

Findings: diplopia (from CN 3, 4, 6 involvement; may have disc swelling from infiltration of orbit and ON)

Progressive Multifocal Leukoencephalopathy (PML)

Papovavirus destroys oligodendrocytes; gray matter relatively spared; can affect central visual pathway and ocular motor fibers

Findings: ataxia, altered mental status, dementia, hemiparesis, focal neurologic defects

Diagnosis: MRI (demyelination; usually parieto-occipital areas, typically involves subcortical white matter with focal or confluent lesions; may see focal enhancement with contrast)

Treatment: none; death common within 6 months

REVIEW QUESTIONS *(Answers start on page 413)*

1. The VF defect most characteristic of optic neuritis is
   a. altitudinal
   b. central
   c. centrocecal
   d. arcuate

2. Which cranial nerve is most prone to injury in the cavernous sinus?
   a. 3
   b. 4
   c. 5
   d. 6

3. Which of the following agents is *least* toxic to the ON?
   a. isoniazid
   b. dapsone
   c. methanol
   d. ethambutol

4. See-saw nystagmus is produced by a lesion located in which area?
   a. chiasm
   b. posterior fossa
   c. suprasellar
   d. cervicomedullary junction

5. What is the location of a lesion that causes an ipsilateral Horner syndrome and a contralateral CN 4 palsy?
   a. midbrain
   b. pons
   c. cavernous sinus
   d. orbit

6. The *least* useful test for functional visual loss is
   a. confrontation VF
   b. OKN
   c. HVF
   d. tangent screen at 1 m and 2 m

7. Optociliary shunt vessels may occur in all of the following conditions, *except*
   a. chronic glaucoma
   b. central retinal vein occlusion
   c. meningioma
   d. ischemic optic neuropathy.

8. Which is *not* a symptom of pseudotumor cerebri?
   a. diplopia
   b. entoptic phenomena
   c. visual obscurations
   d. headache

9. A 63-year-old woman reports sudden onset of jagged lines in the right peripheral vision. She has experienced three episodes, which lasted approximately 10 to 20 minutes, in the past month. She denies headaches and any history or family history of migraines. The most likely diagnosis is
   a. vertebrobasilar insufficiency
   b. occipital AVM
   c. migraine variant
   d. posterior vitreous detachment

10. A 60-year-old man with optic disc swelling in the right eye and left optic atrophy most likely has
    a. ischemic optic neuropathy
    b. left sphenoid ridge meningioma
    c. Leber hereditary optic neuropathy
    d. left ON glioma

11. Which of the following findings may not be present in a patient with an INO?
    a. dissociated horizontal nystagmus
    b. limitation of adduction
    c. absent convergence
    d. abnormal abduction saccades

12. A paradoxical pupillary reaction is *not* found in which condition?
    a. achromatopsia
    b. albinism
    c. Leber congenital amaurosis
    d. ON hypoplasia

13. Inheritance of Leber hereditary optic neuropathy is
    a. sporadic
    b. autosomal dominant
    c. mitochondrial DNA
    d. X-linked recessive

14. An OKN strip moved to the left stimulates what parts of the brain?
    a. right frontal, left occipital
    b. right frontal, right occipital
    c. left frontal, left occipital
    d. left frontal, right occipital

15. The smooth pursuit system does *not* involve the
    a. PPRF.
    b. prestriate cortex
    c. occipital motor area
    d. frontal motor area

16. Dorsal midbrain syndrome is *not* associated with
    a. absent convergence
    b. gaze palsy
    c. light-near dissociation
    d. nystagmus

17. The location of Horner syndrome is best differentiated by which drug?
    a. cocaine
    b. hydroxyamphetamine (Paredrine)
    c. pilocarpine 0.125%
    d. pilocarpine 1%

18. The blood supply to the prelaminar ON is the
    a. meningeal arteries
    b. ophthalmic artery
    c. short posterior ciliary arteries
    d. central retinal artery

19. ON hypoplasia is associated with all of the following, *except*
    a. paradoxic pupillary response
    b. midline abnormalities
    c. maternal ingestion of LSD
    d. spasmus nutans

20. A lesion in the pons causes
    a. anisocoria
    b. miosis
    c. light-near dissociation
    d. mydriasis

21. Which of the following syndromes is characterized by abduction deficit and contralateral hemiplegia?
    a. Foville
    b. Gradenigo
    c. Millard-Gubler
    d. Weber

22. All of the following are features of progressive supranuclear palsy, *except*
    a. hypometric saccades
    b. loss of oculovestibular reflex
    c. full motility with doll's head maneuver
    d. limitation of downgaze

23. Pituitary apoplexy is characterized by all of the following, *except*
    a. nystagmus
    b. facial numbness
    c. headache
    d. diplopia

24. Which of the following is most likely to produce a junctional scotoma?
    a. craniopharyngioma
    b. multiple sclerosis
    c. pituitary adenoma
    d. meningioma

25. All of the following are characteristics of an optic tract lesion, *except*
    a. relative afferent pupillary defect
    b. decreased vision
    c. homonymous hemianopia
    d. ON pallor

26. The saccade system does *not* involve the
    a. occipital motor area
    b. premotor cortex
    c. frontal motor area
    d. PPRF

27. A 22-year-old man sustains trauma resulting in a transected left ON. Which of the following is true regarding the right pupil?
    a. it is larger than the left pupil
    b. it is smaller than the left pupil
    c. it is equal in size to the left pupil
    d. it reacts consensually

28. Characteristics of spasmus nutans include all of the following, *except*
    a. spontaneously disappears within 3 years
    b. may mimic chiasmal glioma
    c. begins before 1 year of age
    d. signs present during sleep

29. A congenital CN 4 palsy can be distinguished from an acquired palsy by
    a. vertical fusional amplitude > 10Δ
    b. incyclotropia of 5°
    c. excyclotropia of 5°
    d. spontaneous head tilt to the opposite side

30. Characteristics of a diabetic CN 3 palsy may include all of the following, *except*
    a. pain
    b. spontaneous recovery within 90 days
    c. sluggish pupillary response
    d. aberrant regeneration

31. A CN 3 lesion may cause all of the following, *except*
    a. contralateral ptosis
    b. ipsilateral ptosis
    c. bilateral ptosis
    d. no ptosis

32. ON drusen is associated with all of the following, *except*
    a. retinitis pigmentosa
    b. CRAO
    c. cystoid macular edema
    d. CNV

33. A lesion causing limited upgaze with an intact Bell's phenomenon is located where?
    a. supranuclear
    b. nuclear
    c. tract
    d. cavernous sinus

34. An acute subarachnoid hemorrhage caused by a ruptured aneurysm may produce all of the following, *except*
    a. ptosis.
    b. orbital hemorrhage
    c. vitreous hemorrhage
    d. efferent pupillary defect

35. The typical length of the intracranial portion of the ON is approximately
    a. 5 mm
    b. 10 mm
    c. 15 mm
    d. 20 mm

36. Findings in ocular motor apraxia include all of the following, *except*
    a. abnormal OKN response
    b. abnormal pursuits
    c. head thrusting
    d. abnormal vestibular nystagmus

37. Which of the following statements is true regarding the optic chiasm?
    a. 53% of temporal retinal fibers remain uncrossed in the ipsilateral optic tract
    b. 47% of temporal retinal fibers cross to the contralateral optic tract
    c. 53% of nasal retinal fibers cross to the contralateral optic tract
    d. 47% of nasal retinal fibers cross to the contralateral optic tract

38. Which of the following statements is false regarding the LGB?
    a. M cells are important for stereoacuity
    b. the LGB is part of the thalamus
    c. there is a 90° rotation of ON fibers in the LGB
    d. P cells are important for motion detection

39. A patient with a homonymous hemianopia is found to have an asymmetric OKN response. The location of the lesion is
    a. parietal lobe
    b. occipital lobe
    c. temporal lobe
    d. LGB

40. The only intact eye movement in one-and-a-half syndrome is
    a. abduction of ipsilateral eye
    b. adduction of ipsilateral eye
    c. abduction of contralateral eye
    d. adduction of contralateral eye

41. A pineal tumor is most likely to cause
    a. Balint syndrome
    b. Fisher syndrome
    c. Nothnagel syndrome
    d. Parinaud syndrome

42. Metastatic neuroblastoma is most likely to be associated with
    a. opsoclonus
    b. ocular bobbing
    c. ocular dipping
    d. ocular myoclonus

43. Which of the following statements regarding pupillary innervation is true?
    a. sympathetic innervation of the iris sphincter involves three neurons from the Edinger-Westphal nucleus
    b. parasympathetic innervation of the iris sphincter involves two neurons and the ciliospinal center of Budge
    c. parasympathetic innervation of the iris dilator involves two neurons from the Edinger-Westphal nucleus
    d. sympathetic innervation of the iris dilator involves three neurons and the ciliospinal center of Budge

44. Which is the most important test to order in a patient with chronic progressive external ophthalmoplegia?
    a. ERG
    b. EKG
    c. EMG
    d. ESR

45. Pseudotumor cerebri is most likely to cause a palsy of which cranial nerve?
    a. 3
    b. 4
    c. 5
    d. 6

46. A CT scan of a patient with visual loss shows a railroad-track sign. The most likely diagnosis is
    a. ON glioma
    b. pituitary adenoma
    c. ON meningioma
    d. craniopharyngioma

47. The most likely etiology of homonymous hemianopia with macular sparing is
    a. vascular
    b. infectious
    c. neoplastic
    d. traumatic

48. All of the following findings are associated with optic neuritis, *except*
    a. abnormal color perception
    b. abnormal depth perception
    c. flashes of light with eye movements
    d. metamorphopsia

49. Which of the following findings is *not* associated with an acoustic neuroma?
    a. lagophthalmos
    b. light-near dissociation
    c. decreased corneal sensation
    d. nystagmus

50. A superior oblique muscle palsy is most commonly caused by
    a. a tumor
    b. multiple sclerosis
    c. an aneurysm
    d. trauma

51. A 29-year-old obese woman with headaches, papilledema, and a normal head CT scan is diagnosed with idiopathic intracranial hypertension. All of the following findings are consistent with her diagnosis, *except*
    a. visual obscurations
    b. homonymous hemianopia
    c. enlarged blind spot
    d. incomitant esotropia

52. Transection of the left ON adjacent to the chiasm results in
    a. a VF defect in the right eye
    b. decreased corneal sensation in the right eye
    c. an afferent pupillary defect in the right eye
    d. pseudoproptosis of the right eye

53. The Amsler grid viewed at 30 cm tests how many degrees of central vision?
    a. 5
    b. 10
    c. 15
    d. 30

54. Aberrant regeneration of CN 3 may cause all of the following, *except*
    a. lid elevation on abduction
    b. pupillary constriction on adduction
    c. monocular dampening of the OKN response
    d. lid elevation on downgaze

55. A 42-year-old woman admitted to the hospital with severe headache and neck stiffness suddenly becomes disoriented and vomits. On examination, her left pupil is dilated and does not react to light. She most likely has
    a. encephalitis
    b. meningitis
    c. brainstem herniation
    d. subarachnoid hemorrhage

56. A healthy 19-year-old woman presents with gradual loss of vision OD and pain when looking side to side. Her past medical history and review of systems are negative. Exam shows visual acuity of 20/50, reduced color vision, a relative afferent pupillary defect, and a normal-appearing optic nerve OD. The most important test to obtain is
    a. VF
    b. lumbar puncture
    c. MRI
    d. blood work (ANA, ACE, VDRL)

57. A 68-year-old patient with diabetes reports double vision. Exam is normal except for a right abducens palsy. Further questioning reveals recent weight loss and scalp and jaw pain. Which of the following tests is most useful?
    a. Fasting blood glucose
    b. CRP
    c. Tensilon test
    d. CT of orbits

58. A patient is found to have anisocoria, which is greater in a dim room. The most likely etiology is
    a. CN 3 palsy
    b. Horner syndrome
    c. pharmacologic
    d. traumatic

59. A middle-aged man relates a history of double vision and hearing loss from his left ear. On exam, he has a left esotropia and facial palsy. The most likely location of his lesion is
    a. cavernous sinus
    b. inferior colliculus
    c. sella turcica
    d. cerebellopontine angle

60. A risk factor for nonarteritic anterior ischemic optic neuropathy is
    a. obesity
    b. hypertension
    c. polymyalgia rheumatica
    d. MS

61. A 73-year-old man complains of reduced vision in his right eye. His visual acuity is found to be 20/400 OD and 20/25 OS. Upon further questioning, he reports recent headaches, scalp tenderness, and pain when eating. The most appropriate initial course of action is to
    a. start treatment with systemic steroids immediately
    b. start treatment with systemic steroids after obtaining routine ESR and CRP results
    c. start treatment with systemic steroids after obtaining stat MRI/MRA results
    d. start treatment with systemic steroids after obtaining temporal artery biopsy

62. A. 23-year-old woman notices transient episodes of blurred vision and sometimes double vision. She also reports frequent headaches. Fundus exam shows blurred optic disc margins in both eyes. The most likely diagnosis is
    a. optic neuritis
    b. migraine
    c. pituitary adenoma
    d. increased ICP

63. The swinging flashlight test would be most helpful in diagnosing a patient with
    a. Adie tonic pupil
    b. Argyll-Robertson pupil
    c. Horner syndrome
    d. prechiasmal afferent lesion

64. Cervicomedullary junction lesions are associated with which types of nystagmus?
    a. downbeat and see-saw
    b. downbeat and periodic alternating
    c. upbeat and see-saw
    d. upbeat and periodic alternating

Please visit the eBook for an interactive version of the review questions. See front cover for activation details.

SUGGESTED READINGS

Basic and Clinical Sciences Course. (2021). *Section 5: Neuro-ophthalmology*. San Francisco: AAO.

Burde, R. M., Savino, P. J., & Trobe, J. D. (2002). *Clinical decisions in neuro-ophthalmology* (3rd ed.). Philadelphia: Mosby.

Foroozan, R., & Vaphiades, M. S. (2017). *Kline's neuro-ophthalmology review manual* (8th ed.). Thorofare, NJ: Slack.

Liu, G. T., Volpe, N. J., & Galetta, S. (2018). *Neuro-ophthalmology diagnosis and management* (3rd ed.). Philadelphia: WB Saunders.

Loewenfeld, I. E., & Lowenstein, O. (1999). *The pupil anatomy: Physiology and clinical applications* (2nd ed.). Philadelphia: Butterworth-Heineman.

Miller, N. R., Newman, N. J., Biousse, V., & Kerrison, J. B. (2007). *Walsh & Hoyt's clinical neuro-ophthalmology: The essentials* (2nd ed.). Philadelphia: Lippincott Williams & Wilkins.

5

Pediatrics/Strabismus

PEDIATRICS

ANATOMY

At birth, diameter of eye is 66% that of the adult eye

Eye enlarges until 2 years of age, then further growth in puberty (Table 5.1)

Infants have variable levels of astigmatism

Majority of children are hyperopic; increases up to 7 years of age, then diminishes

Eye color darkens during first few months of life

Dilator pupillae poorly developed at birth

Fovea matures during first few months of life

Myelinization of optic nerve (ON) completed shortly after birth

PHYSIOLOGY

Visual acuity levels (see *Strabismus* section)
  Documented by visual evoked potentials in infancy and preferential looking tests in first months of life
  Premature infants reach landmarks later
Decreased vision in infants and children

History: family history, complications in pregnancy, perinatal problems
  Examination: visual response (assess each eye independently), pupillary reactions (paradoxical response suggests achromatopsia, congenital stationary night blindness [CSNB], ON hypoplasia), ocular motility (strabismus, nystagmus, torticollis), cycloplegic refraction, fundus examination
  Additional tests: optokinetic nystagmus (OKN) response, forced preferential looking, electroretinogram (ERG), visual evoked response (visually evoked cortical potential [VEP], visually evoked cortical response [VER]), ultrasonography, imaging studies

Table 5.1 Changes in ocular measurements with age

Ocular dimensions	Infant (mm)	Adult (mm)
Axial length	17	24
Corneal diameter	9.5–10.5	12
Corneal radius of curvature	6.6–7.4	7.4–8.4
Scleral thickness	Half of adult	

DDx of infant with poor vision and normal ocular structures: Leber congenital amaurosis, achromatopsia, blue cone monochromatism, CSNB, albinism, ON hypoplasia, optic atrophy, congenital infection (**TORCH syndrome** [**T**oxoplasmosis, **O**ther infections (syphilis; also hepatitis B, varicella-zoster virus, HIV, parvovirus B19), **R**ubella, **C**ytomegalovirus (CMV), **H**erpes simplex virus (HSV)]), cortical visual impairment (resulting from extensive occipital lobe damage), delay in visual maturation

ORBITAL DISORDERS

Congenital Anomalies

Anophthalmos

Bilateral absence of eye resulting from failure of primary optic vesicle to form; extremely rare

Findings: hypoplastic orbits

Buphthalmos

Large eye as a result of increased intraocular pressure (IOP) in congenital glaucoma

Cryptophthalmos

Failure of differentiation of lid and anterior eye structures

Partial or complete absence of the eyebrow, palpebral fissure, eyelashes, and conjunctiva

Attenuation of the levator, orbicularis, tarsus, and conjunctiva

Often associated with severe ocular defects

Microphthalmos

Small, disorganized eye

Disruption of ocular development occurs after budding of optic vesicle

Usually unilateral

Microphthalmos With Cyst

Caused by failure of embryonic fissure to close

Usually blue mass of lower lid

Associated with congenital rubella, congenital toxoplasmosis, maternal vitamin A deficiency, maternal thalidomide ingestion, trisomy 13, trisomy 15, and chromosome 18 deletion

Nanophthalmos

Small eye with normal features

Normal-size lens and thickened sclera

Associated with hyperopia and angle-closure glaucoma

Increased risk of choroidal effusion during intraocular surgery

Infections

Preseptal Cellulitis

Infection anterior to orbital septum; spares globe

Penetrating skin trauma, dacryocystitis, sinusitis (most common pediatric cause)

Most common organism: *Staphylococcus aureus*

Findings: lid edema, erythema, and pain; may have fever; may progress to orbital cellulitis

Treatment: CT scan if questioning orbital involvement, systemic antibiotics (IV in severe cases, children <5 years old, and failed oral treatment)

Orbital Cellulitis

Infection posterior to orbital septum; involves globe

Most common cause of proptosis in children

Usually secondary to sinusitis (ethmoid sinus is most common)

Associated with subperiosteal abscesses

Etiology: extension of infection from periorbital structures, sinusitis, dacryocystitis, dacryoadenitis, endophthalmitis, dental infections, intracranial infections, trauma or previous surgery, endogenous (bacteremia with septic embolization)

Organisms: *S. aureus* (most common organism in children), *Streptococcus pneumoniae*, *Haemophilus influenzae* (nontypeable) in children <5 years old, fungi (*Phycomycetes*, most aggressive; usually immunocompromised patient; causes necrosis, vascular thrombosis, orbital invasion)

Findings: fever, decreased vision, positive relative afferent pupillary defect (RAPD), proptosis, restriction of ocular motility, pain on eye movement, periorbital swelling, chemosis, optic disc swelling

CT scan: diagnosis, localization, and involvement of adjacent structures

Treatment: IV antibiotics, surgical drainage, observation of subperiosteal abscess unless any of the following are present requiring emergent drainage: age >9 years old, frontal sinusitis, nonmedial location, large size, anaerobic infection (gas on CT scan), recurrence after prior drainage, chronic sinusitis (polyps), optic neuropathy, or dental origin

Complications: subperiosteal abscess, cavernous sinus thrombosis, or intracranial extension causing blindness or death

Benign Lesions

Dermoid Cyst (Choristoma)

Arises from dermal elements (neural crest origin)

Lined by keratinizing epithelium with dermal appendages

Most common orbital mass in childhood

Usually located in superotemporal quadrant near brow, often adjacent to bony suture

Often filled with keratin

Generally do not enlarge after 1 year of age

May induce bony erosion

Rupture can cause intense inflammatory reaction

CT scan: well circumscribed with bony molding

Treatment: complete excision, remove en bloc because contents may cause granulomatous inflammation

Epidermoid Cyst (Choristoma)

Arises from epidermal elements

Lined by epidermis only (no dermal appendages)

Usually filled with keratin

Rupture can lead to an acute inflammatory process

Lipodermoid

Solid tumor usually located beneath the conjunctiva over lateral surface of globe

May appear similar to prolapsed orbital fat, prolapsed lacrimal gland, or lymphoma

Usually no treatment is needed

Difficult to excise completely

Teratoma

Rare cystic tumor arising from ≥2 germinal layers

Usually composed of ectoderm along with either endoderm or mesoderm (or both)

Can cause dramatic proptosis at birth

Rarely malignant

Capillary hemangioma

Most common benign tumor of the orbit in children

Often manifests in the first few weeks of life and enlarges over the first 6-12 months, with complete regression by age 5-8 years in 80% of cases

Spontaneous involution over the next few years

Predilection for the superior nasal quadrant of the orbit and medial upper eyelid

Female > male (3:2)

Diffuse irregular mass of plump endothelial cells and small vascular channels

High-flow lesion

Findings:
Strawberry nevus: skin involvement; appears as red, irregularly dimpled, elevated surface; blanches with direct pressure (port wine stain does not blanch)
Orbital location: can present with proptosis; bluish appearance of eyelids and conjunctiva

Pathology: numerous blood-filled channels lined by endothelium; little contribution from larger vessels or stroma; unencapsulated (Fig. 5.1)

CT/MRI scan: well-circumscribed lesion

Treatment: required if tumor causing ptosis or astigmatism with resultant anisometropia, strabismus, or amblyopia; options include observation, intralesional steroid injection, systemic steroids, interferon, topical timolol, propanolol (requires monitoring), laser, radiation, or excision

Complications:
Eyelid involvement may cause: ptosis with occlusion amblyopia, astigmatism and anisometropia with refractive amblyopia, strabismus with strabismic amblyopia
Kasabach-Merritt syndrome: consumptive coagulopathy with platelet trapping, resulting in thrombocytopenia

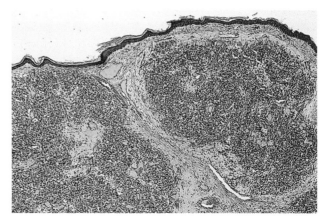

Figure 5.1 Capillary hemangioma demonstrating abnormal proliferation of blood vessels and endothelial cells. (From Yanoff M, Fine BS. *Ocular Pathology*, 5th ed. St Louis: Mosby; 2002.)

and cardiac failure; acute hemorrhage is possible; mortality ~ 30%

High-output congestive heart failure can occur with multiple visceral capillary hemangiomas

Respiratory compromise with subglottic hemangiomas

Lymphangioma (Lymphatic Malformation)

Rare, lymphatic-filled choristoma

Often superonasal

Appears in 1st decade of life

Involves the eyelids, conjunctiva, and deeper orbital tissues

Lesion waxes and wanes, but does not involute

Findings: acute pain, proptosis (often increasing with upper respiratory infection), bluish hue to overlying lid, may hemorrhage into channels (chocolate cyst)

Pathology: lymph-filled vascular channels lined by endothelium; unencapsulated (Fig. 5.2)

CT scan: may show layered blood in a lobular, cystic mass with infiltrative pattern

MRI: infiltrating pattern with indistinct margins; grapelike cystic lesions with fluid-fluid layering of serum and red blood cells

Treatment: observation (spontaneous regression common); rarely surgical evacuation because complete excision difficult and recurrence common

Complications: anisometropia, amblyopia, strabismus

Varix

Most common vascular abnormality

Dilations of preexisting venous channels

Findings: proptosis (increases with crying or straining; can occur when head is in a dependent position), orbital

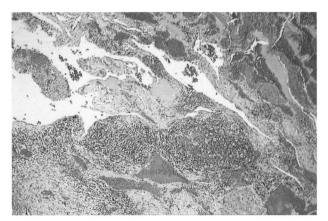

Figure 5.2 Lymphangioma demonstrating lymph-filled spaces, some with blood. (From Yanoff M, Fine BS. *Ocular Pathology*, 5th ed. St Louis: Mosby; 2002.)

hemorrhage (especially after trauma), motility disturbance (usually restricted upgaze), disc swelling, optic atrophy

Radiograph: phlebolith present in 30% of cases

Treatment: surgery
  Indications: cosmetic, severe proptosis, ON compression, pain; surgery is often difficult because of intertwining of normal structures and direct communication with cavernous sinus

Fibrous Dysplasia

Tumor of fibrous connective tissue, cartilage, and bone

Progressive disease of childhood and young adulthood

Monostotic (in young adults) or polyostotic

Orbital involvement: usually monostotic; frontal (most common), sphenoid, and ethmoid bones; causes unilateral proptosis during first 2 decades of life

Polyostotic: multiple bones involved; can cause narrowing of optic canal and lacrimal drainage system

Albright syndrome: polyostotic fibrous dysplasia, short stature, premature closure of epiphysis, precocious puberty, and hyperpigmented macules
  Findings: diplopia, proptosis, headaches, facial asymmetry, decreased visual acuity (compromised optic canal), hearing loss (compromised external ear canal)
  Pathology: normal bone is replaced by immature woven bone and osteoid in a cellular fibrous matrix, stroma of the bone is highly vascularized, no osteoblasts present

Neurofibroma

Hamartoma

18% have neurofibromatosis type 1 (NF-1)

Nearly all adults with NF-1 have neurofibromas

Plexiform neurofibroma: most commonly involves the upper lid (S-shaped deformity); tortuous, fibrous cords infiltrate orbital tissues

Nodular: firm and rubbery consistency

Findings: often involves eyelid or causes proptosis, may cause glaucoma; absence of greater wing of sphenoid bone

Pathology: well-circumscribed, nonencapsulated proliferation of Schwann cells, perineural cells, and axons; stains with S-100 (specific for neural crest–derived structures) (Fig. 5.3)

Treatment: surgical excision

Optic Nerve Glioma (Grade I Astrocytoma)

Considered pilocytic astrocytoma of the juvenile type

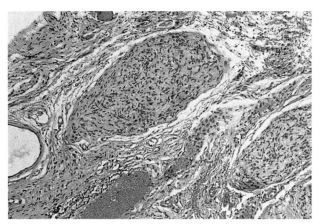

Figure 5.3 Neurofibroma demonstrating proliferation of Schwann cells. (From Yanoff M, Fine BS. *Ocular Pathology*, 5th ed. St Louis: Mosby; 2002.)

Slow-growing hamartoma derived from interstitial cells, astroglia, and oligodendroglia

Usually does not metastasize

Usually appears during 1st decade of life

Associated with NF-1 (25%–50%)

Findings: unilateral proptosis, loss of vision, strabismus, and papilledema; may develop retinal vascular occlusions, optociliary shunt vessels; orbital tumors may cause chorioretinal folds, optic disc swelling, or atrophy; chiasmal tumors may cause pituitary or hypothalamic dysfunction, and nystagmus and head nodding from compression of third ventricle

Pathology: circumscribed astrocytic tumor from neural crest tissue, glial hypercellularity, Rosenthal fibers, myxomatous, arachnoid hyperplasia; reactive meningothelial hyperplasia may occur, which can lead to a false diagnosis of meningioma

CT scan: fusiform enlargement of ON, enlargement of optic foramen, bony erosion

Treatment: observation; consider surgery if tumor spreads posteriorly into the chiasm; radiation alone for nonresectable lesions with neurologic symptoms; chemotherapy

Prognosis: in adults, tumor is malignant, with death occurring in 6-12 months; better prognosis in children or in adults with neurofibromatosis

Idiopathic Orbital Inflammation (IOI) (Orbital Pseudotumor)

Idiopathic inflammatory disorder of orbit

Commonly bilateral with episodic recurrence

Findings: decreased vision, diplopia, red eye, headache; acute, painful presentation in children; resembles orbital cellulitis

Other findings: constitutional symptoms in 50%

Treatment: systemic steroids

Graves' Disease

Occasionally occurs in adolescents (see Chapter 6, Orbit/Lids/Adnexa)

Malignant Neoplasms

Rhabdomyosarcoma

Most common primary orbital malignancy of children

Most common soft tissue malignancy of childhood

Most common mesenchymal tumor of orbit

Malignant spindle cell tumor with loose myxomatous matrix

Average age at diagnosis is 8 years old (90% before age 16)

Cell of origin is an undifferentiated, pluripotent cell of the soft tissue; does not originate from the extraocular muscles

Unilateral; tends to involve superonasal portion of orbit

More common in males (5:3)

Aggressive local spread through orbital bones; hematogenous spread to lungs and cervical lymph nodes; most common location for metastasis is chest

Findings: rapidly progressive proptosis, reddish discoloration of eyelid; may have ptosis; later develop tortuous retinal veins, choroidal folds, and ON edema

Types:
    Embryonal: most common (70%), usually occurs in children; tumor appears circumscribed, but often there is microscopic evidence of invasion of nearby structures
        PATHOLOGY: elongated spindle cell with central hyperchromatic nucleus, eosinophilic granular cytoplasm; cells arranged in parallel palisading bands; obvious cross-striations are rare (Fig. 5.4)
    Botryoid: subtype of embryonal; can occur in anterior orbit, embryonal rhabdomyosarcoma abutting a mucosal surface, multiple polypoid masses protruding from hollow viscera
    Pleomorphic: least common, usually occurs in adults, rare involvement of orbit, most differentiated, best prognosis
        PATHOLOGY: dense spindle cell arrangement with enlarged cells containing hyperchromatic nuclei, deeply eosinophilic cytoplasm; may see cross-striations on microscopic examination
    Alveolar: poorest prognosis, usually found in inferior orbit, generally arises in extremities (adolescents)
        PATHOLOGY: dense cellular proliferations of loosely cohesive small round cells separated by connective tissue septa; lack of cohesiveness may explain metastatic potential

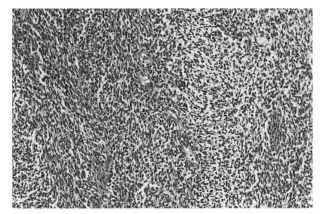

A

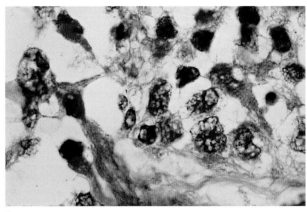

B

Figure 5.4 (A) Embryonal type demonstrating primitive rhabdomyoblasts. (B) Cross-striations in cytoplasm of some cells. (From Yanoff M, Fine BS. *Ocular Pathology*, 5th ed. St Louis: Mosby; 2002.)

CT scan: well-circumscribed orbital mass with possible extension into adjacent orbital bones or sinuses, bony destruction

A-scan ultrasound: orbital mass with medium internal reflectivity

Treatment: urgent biopsy, radiation (100% local control with 6000 cGy; 30% mortality as a result of metastases), chemotherapy for any microscopic metastases, surgical debulking

Prognosis: with chemotherapy and XRT, 3-year survival = 90%; cure rate close to 100% with localized orbital tumor; 60% if invasion of adjacent structures
Tumors arising in the orbit, bladder, and prostate: 77% disease-free survival at 2 years
Intrathoracic tumors: worst prognosis, 24% disease-free survival at 2 years

Neuroblastoma

Most common metastatic orbital tumor of childhood

Usually originates in the adrenal gland or sympathetic ganglion chain, also mediastinum or neck

40% develop orbital metastases

Average age of presentation with metastatic neuroblastoma to orbit is 2 years old

Spontaneous regression is rare

Findings: sudden proptosis and periorbital ecchymosis (raccoon eyes); may have ipsilateral Horner syndrome and opsoclonus (better prognosis)
Paraneoplastic syndrome associated with metastatic neuroblastoma: opsoclonus (saccadomania; random, rapid eye movements in all directions that disappear during sleep)

Pathology: sheets of indiscrete round cells with scant cytoplasm and high mitotic figures, areas of tumor necrosis; can have bony invasion; usually positive for neuronal markers (synaptophysin and neuron-specific enolase) (Fig. 5.5)

CT scan: bony destruction

Treatment: chemotherapy and local XRT

Prognosis: poor if age of onset is >1 year with metastases to bone; however, metastases to just liver, bone marrow, or spleen can be associated with a survival rate as high as 84%

15% of all childhood cancer deaths

In adults, neuroblastoma usually metastasizes to the uveal tract

Ewing Sarcoma

2nd most frequent metastatic tumor to the orbit

Primary intermedullary malignancy of bone; originates in long bones of extremities or axial skeleton

Frequently metastasizes to bone and lungs

Occurs in 2nd-3rd decade of life

Findings: acute proptosis, hemorrhage, and inflammation from tumor necrosis

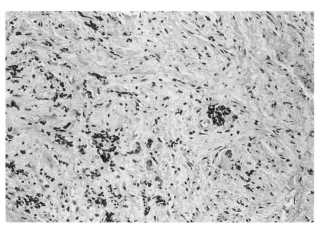

Figure 5.5 Neuroblastoma. (Case presented by Dr. E. Torcynski at the meeting of the Eastern Ophthalmic Society, 1994. From Yanoff M, Fine BS. *Ocular Pathology*, 5th ed. St Louis: Mosby; 2002.)

Treatment: chemotherapy

Granulocytic Sarcoma ("Chloroma")

Patients with myelogenous leukemia may present with orbital signs before hematologic evidence of leukemia

Findings: proptosis, may have subcutaneous periocular mass

Pathology: infiltration of involved tissues by leukemic cells

Treatment: radiotherapy, chemotherapy

Histiocytosis X (Langerhans Cell Histiocytosis)

Group of disorders resulting from abnormal proliferation of histiocytes (Langerhans cells) that may involve orbit

Spectrum of disease, from isolated bone lesions with excellent prognosis (eosinophilic granuloma) to systemic spread with rapid death (Letterer-Siwe disease)

Children age <2 with multifocal disease have a poor prognosis (50% survival rate)

Findings: most frequent orbital presentation is lytic defect of orbital roof causing progressive proptosis

Pathology: granulomatous histiocytic infiltrate, Birbeck granules (central, dense core, and thick outer shell), stains positively for S-100 and vimentin

Eosinophilic granuloma: benign, local, solitary bone lesion
Most likely to involve superior temporal bony orbit in childhood or adolescence
CT scan and X-ray: sharply demarcated osteolytic lesions
Treatment: incision and curettage, intralesional steroids, or radiotherapy

Hand-Schüller-Christian disease: triad of proptosis, lytic skull defects, and diabetes insipidus
More aggressive
Multifocal bony lesions; frequently involves orbit, usually superolaterally
Treatment: systemic steroids and chemotherapy
Prognosis: good

Letterer-Siwe disease: most severe and malignant
Progressive and fatal
Multisystem involvement
Rarely ocular/orbital involvement
Prognosis: systemic steroids and chemotherapy

Burkitt Lymphoma

Primarily affects the maxilla in black children, with secondary invasion of the orbit

Related to Epstein-Barr virus (EBV) infection

Findings: proptosis and bony destruction

Pathology: malignant B cells, "starry sky" appearance as a result of histiocytes interspersed among uniform background of lymphocytes

CRANIOFACIAL DISORDERS

Structural development of head and face occur during 4th-8th week of gestation

Ocular motility disturbances occur in 75% of patients with craniofacial disorders

Craniofacial cleft syndromes: ≥1 facial fissures fail to close during the 6th-7th week of gestation

Ocular complications: corneal exposure from proptosis or lid defects
Refractive errors from lid anomalies
Ocular motility disturbances, most commonly exotropia
Papilledema and optic atrophy from increased intracranial pressure (ICP) or fibrous dysplasia involving optic canal
Ocular anomalies from embryogenesis

Syndromes

Treacher-Collins Syndrome (Mandibulofacial Dysostosis)

Hypoplasia of the midface

Associated with dental and ear abnormalities, microtia, micrognathia, hypoplastic malar bones, and low sideburns

Findings: lateral lid defects, absent lateral canthal tendon, absent medial lashes, antimongoloid slant, ectropion, poorly developed puncta and meibomian glands

Goldenhar Syndrome (Oculoauriculovertebral Dysplasia)

Abnormalities of the 1st and 2nd brachial arches

Associated with Duane syndrome

Findings: limbal dermoids and dermolipomas; may have lower lid colobomas

Other findings: hypoplastic facial bones, pretragal auricular appendages, vertebral abnormalities; may have fistulas between the mouth and ear

Hypertelorism

Findings: increased interpupillary distance as a result of increased distance between medial orbital walls

Associated with blepharophimosis, frontal meningoceles, encephaloceles, meningoencephaloceles, and fibrous dysplasia

Craniosynostoses

Premature closure of bony sutures; inhibits growth of the cranium perpendicular to the axis of the suture; growth can continue parallel to the suture

Findings: hypertelorism; proptosis can also occur

Plagiocephaly: premature closure of one-half of the coronal sutures

Skull develops normally on one side and is underdeveloped on the other side (resulting in a flattened face)

Other findings: midfacial hypoplasia, proptosis, telecanthus, V-pattern exotropia (XT), oral and dental abnormalities, and respiratory problems

Crouzon Syndrome (Craniofacial Dysostosis) (Autosomal Dominant [AD] or Sporadic)

Absence of forward development of the cranium and midface

Multiple combinations of suture closure can occur

Findings: proptosis, V-pattern XT, nystagmus, hypertelorism; shallow orbits; optic atrophy (in 25%–50%; caused by narrowing of optic canal, kinking or stretching of ON)

Other findings: mental retardation, hypoplasia of maxilla, parrot's beak nose, high arched palate, external auditory canal atresia, anodontia

Apert Syndrome (AD)

Crouzon plus syndactyly

Anterior megalophthalmos

Associated with increased paternal age

Pfeiffer Syndrome (AD)

Findings: hypertelorism and pointy head; may have shallow orbits, syndactyly, and short digits

Carpenter Syndrome (Autosomal Recessive [AR])

Severe mental retardation

Involvement of sagittal, lambdoidal, and coronal sutures

Median Facial Cleft Syndrome

Findings: hypertelorism, exotropia

Other findings: medial cleft nose, lip, palate; widow's peak; cranium bifidum occultum

Waardenburg Syndrome (AD)

Findings: lateral displacement of inner canthi/puncta, confluent eyebrows, heterochromia iridis, fundus hypopigmentation

Other findings: sensorineural deafness, white forelock

Hemifacial Microsomia

Findings: upper lid coloboma, strabismus

Other findings: facial asymmetry with microtia, macrostomia, mandibular anomalies, orbital dystopia, ear tags, vertebral anomalies

Hallermann-Streiff Syndrome

Sporadic

Findings: bilateral cataracts, glaucoma, microphakia, microcornea

Other findings: mandibular hypoplasia, beaked nose

Pierre Robin Sequence

Findings: retinal detachment (RD), congenital glaucoma and/or cataracts, high myopia

Other findings: micrognathia, glossoptosis, cleft palate

Associated with Stickler syndrome

Fetal Alcohol Syndrome

Findings: short palpebral fissures, telecanthus, epicanthal folds, comitant strabismus, optic disc anomalies; may have high myopia, anterior segment anomalies

Other findings: thin vermilion border of upper lip, variable mental retardation, small birth weight and height, cardiovascular and skeletal abnormalities

LID DISORDERS

Ablepharon

Absence of lids

Ankyloblepharon

Partial or complete fusion of lid margins; usually temporal, often bilateral

Often AD

Associated with craniofacial abnormalities

Can be secondary to thermal or chemical burns, inflammation, ocular cicatricial pemphigoid, Stevens-Johnson syndrome

Blepharophimosis

Horizontally and vertically shortened palpebral fissures with poor levator function

Absent lid crease

May be part of AD syndrome (chromosome 3q) with ptosis, telecanthus, epicanthus inversus, lower lid ectropion, hypoplasia of nasal bridge and superior orbital rim, anteverted ears, hypertelorism

Treatment: surgical correction requires multiple procedures

Coloboma

Embryologic cleft involving lid margin; unilateral or bilateral; partial or full thickness

Ranges from notch to absence of entire lid

Upper lid: usually medial third, not associated with systemic abnormalities, usually full thickness

Lower lid: usually lateral third, associated with other abnormalities (Treacher-Collins, Goldenhar syndromes), usually partial thickness

May have exposure keratitis

Treatment: method of surgical repair depends on size of defect (see section on lid avulsion)

Congenital Blepharoptosis

Droopy eyelid; 75% unilateral; nonhereditary

Rarely causes amblyopia

Associated with blepharophimosis syndrome (AD)

Myogenic is most common

Etiology:
Myogenic:
    Dysgenesis of levator muscle
    Fibroadipose tissue in muscle belly
    Poor levator function, loss of lid crease, eyelid lag, sometimes lagophthalmos
Aponeurotic:
    Rare, possibly caused by birth trauma
    Good eyelid excursion, high or indistinct lid crease
Neurogenic:
    Congenital cranial nerve (CN) 3 palsy
    Marcus-Gunn jaw-winking (aberrant connections between motor division of CN V3 [to the external pterygoid muscle] and levator muscle; jaw movements cause elevation of ptotic lid)

Congenital Horner Syndrome

Ptosis, miosis, anhidrosis

May cause amblyopia

Treatment: surgical repair (levator resection), severe cases require frontalis sling

Congenital Ectropion

Eversion of eyelid margin caused by vertical shortening of anterior lamella

Etiology: inclusion conjunctivitis, anterior lamella inflammation, Down syndrome

Associated with blepharophimosis syndrome

Treatment: usually not required; otherwise, treat as the cicatricial form

Congenital Entropion

Inversion of eyelid margin

Etiology: lid retractor dysgenesis, tarsal plate defects, vertical shortening of posterior lamella

Usually involves lower eyelid

Treatment: may require surgical repair

Congenital Tarsal Kink

Upper eyelid bent back and open with complete fold of tarsal plate

May cause corneal abrasion and exposure keratopathy

Distichiasis

Partial or complete accessory row of eyelashes growing from or posterior to meibomian orifices

Results from improper differentiation of pilosebaceous units

Usually well tolerated, but trichiasis may develop

Treatment: lubrication, cryoepilation, surgical epilation

Epiblepharon

Pretarsal skin and orbicularis override the lid margin, causing a horizontal fold of tissue to push cilia vertically; no entropion

Most common among Asians

Usually occurs in lower lid and resolves spontaneously

Rarely requires surgery (excision of skin and muscle for significant trichiasis)

Epicanthus

Medial canthal vertical skin folds

Results from immature facial bones or redundant skin

Usually bilateral

Produces pseudoesotropia

Types:
Epicanthus tarsalis:
    Fold most prominent in upper eyelid
    Commonly associated with Asian eyelid
Epicanthus inversus:
    Fold most prominent in lower eyelid
    Associated with blepharophimosis syndrome

Epicanthus palpebralis:
Fold is equally distributed in upper and lower eyelids
Epicanthus supraciliaris:
Fold arises from eyebrow and extends to lacrimal sac

Euryblepharon

Horizontal widening of palpebral fissure as a result of inferior insertion of lateral canthal tendon

Associated with ectropion of lateral third of lid

Poor lid closure with exposure keratitis

Treatment: lubrication, may require surgical repair with resection of excess lid, lateral canthal tendon repositioning, and vertical eyelid lengthening

Microblepharon

Vertical shortening of lids

May have exposure keratitis

Telecanthus:

Widened intercanthal distance as a result of long medial canthal tendons

Associated with fetal alcohol, Waardenburg, and blepharophimosis syndromes

Treatment: surgery with transnasal wiring

LACRIMAL DISORDERS

Developmental Anomalies

Atresia of lacrimal puncta: ranges from thin membrane over punctal site to atresia of canaliculus

Supernumerary puncta: no treatment needed

Lacrimal fistula: usually located inferonasal to the medial canthus

Dacryocystocele

Cystic swelling of lacrimal sac accompanies obstruction of lacrimal drainage system above and below the sac

Presents at birth as bluish swelling inferior and nasal to medial canthus

Infection (dacryocystitis) develops if condition does not resolve spontaneously
Common organisms: Haemophilus influenzae, S. pneumoniae, Staphylococcus, Klebsiella, Pseudomonas

Treatment: digital massage, lacrimal probing, or surgical decompression (for dacryocystitis)

Nasolacrimal Duct Obstruction (NLDO)

Up to 5% of infants have obstruction of the nasolacrimal duct (NLD), usually as a result of membrane covering valve of Hasner

Most open spontaneously within 4-6 weeks of birth; ⅓ are bilateral

Increased risk in Down syndrome and craniofacial anomalies

Findings: tearing, discharge; may develop dacryocystitis or conjunctivitis

Digital pressure over lacrimal sac producing mucoid reflux indicates obstruction of NLD

May have a dacryocystocele (dilated lacrimal sac), or amniotic fluid or mucus trapped in tear sac; may be complicated by acute dacryocystitis

Treatment: lacrimal sac (Crigler) massage, topical antibiotic, probing and irrigation by 13 months of age (95% cure rate); consider turbinate infracture and silicone intubation if probing unsuccessful; dacryocystorhinostomy (DCR) after multiple failures, rarely needed

CONJUNCTIVAL DISORDERS

Ocular Melanocytosis

Unilateral excessive pigment in uvea, sclera, and episclera

Increase in number of normal melanocytes

More common among Caucasians

Findings: slate-gray appearance of sclera, darkened appearance of fundus

When associated with pigmentation of eyelid skin, called **nevus of Ota** (congenital oculodermal melanocytosis; more common among African Americans and Asians; malignant potential only in Caucasians)

Other findings: heterochromia iridis resulting from diffuse nevus of uvea; may develop glaucoma (caused by melanocytes in trabecular meshwork), rarely uveal, orbital, or meningeal melanoma

Pathology: spindle-shaped pigment cells in subepithelial tissue

Conjunctivitis

Ophthalmia Neonatorum

Conjunctivitis within first month of life

Papillary conjunctivitis (no follicular reaction in neonate because of immaturity of immune system)

Etiology:
Chemical/toxic: caused by silver nitrate 1% solution (Credé prophylaxis); occurs in first 24 hours, lasts 24-36 hours (therefore, prophylaxis is now with erythromycin or tetracycline ointment)
FINDINGS: usually bilateral, bulbar injection with clear watery discharge

No treatment necessary

Neisseria gonorrhoeae: days 1-2; can occur earlier with premature rupture of membranes

FINDINGS: severe purulent discharge, chemosis, eyelid edema; can be hemorrhagic; may develop corneal ulceration or perforation

DIAGNOSIS: Gram stain (gram-negative intracellular diplococci)

TREATMENT: IV ceftriaxone × 7 days; bacitracin ointment topically

High incidence of *Chlamydia* coinfection; therefore, also use oral erythromycin syrup and treat mother and sexual partners

Other bacteria: days 4-5; *Staphylococci, Streptococci, Haemophilus, Enterococci*

TREATMENT: bacitracin, erythromycin, or gentamicin ointment; fortified antibiotics for *Pseudomonas*

HSV: days 5-14; type 2 in 70%

FINDINGS: serous discharge, conjunctival injection, keratitis; may have vesicular lid lesions

Can have systemic herpetic infection

DIAGNOSIS: conjunctival scrapings with multinucleated giant cells; cultures take 5-7 days

TREATMENT: Zirgan 5 ×/d or Viroptic q2h × 1 week; acyclovir 10 mg/kg IV tid × 10 days

Chlamydia (neonatal inclusion conjunctivitis): days 5-14; most common infectious cause of neonatal conjunctivitis

FINDINGS: acute, mucopurulent, papillary (no follicles until 3 months of age); may have pseudomembranes

OTHER FINDINGS: pneumonitis, otitis, nasopharyngitis, gastritis

DIAGNOSIS: intracytoplasmic inclusions on Giemsa stain

TREATMENT: topical erythromycin, oral erythromycin syrup × 2–3 weeks (125 mg/kg/day qid) to prevent pneumonitis (onset 3–13 weeks later); treat mother and sexual partners with doxycycline100 mg bid × 1 week (do not use in nursing mothers)

Rule out concomitant *Gonococcus* infection

DDx: trauma, foreign body, corneal abrasion, congenital glaucoma, NLDO, dacryocystitis

Prophylaxis: tetracycline 1% or erythromycin 0.5% ointment at birth

Other Infections

Pediatric conjunctivitis is usually bacterial (50%–80%) vs. adult infectious conjunctivitis, which is usually viral

Age dependent; more common in younger children (<3 years old)

Organisms: *H. influenzae* (50%–65%), *S. pneumoniae* (20%–30%), *Moraxella catarrhalis* (10%); rarely *Streptococcus pyogenes* or *S. aureus*

Findings: purulent discharge (80%), red eye (50%)

Other findings: otitis media (30% in <3-year-olds; *H. influenzae*), preseptal cellulitis (>3-year-olds with sinusitis, fever, and elevated white blood cells [WBCs]; *S. pneumoniae*)

Diagnosis: culture refractory cases and neonates

Treatment: topical antibiotics; oral antibiotics (cefixime) for extraocular involvement (otitis media, sinusitis)

Vernal Keratoconjunctivitis

Form of seasonal (warm months), allergic conjunctivitis

Male > female (2:1); onset by age 10 years, lasts 2-10 years, usually resolves by puberty

Associated with atopic dermatitis (75%) or family history of atopy (66%)

Limbal vernal: more common among African Americans

Symptoms: intense itching, photophobia, pain

Findings: large upper tarsal papillae (cobblestones), minimal conjunctival hyperemia, Horner-Trantas dots (elevated white accumulations of eosinophils at limbus), limbal follicles (gelatinous nodules at limbus), copious ropy mucus; may have pseudomembrane, keratitis, micropannus, shield ulcer (central oval epithelial defect with white fibrin coating); high levels of histamine and immunoglobulin E (IgE) in tears

Pathology: chronic papillary hypertrophy, epithelial hypertrophy and then atrophy, conjunctiva contains many mast cells, eosinophils, and basophils

Treatment: topical allergy medication and steroids; consider topical cyclosporine or tacrolimus

Ligneous

Rare, bilateral, pseudomembranous conjunctivitis in children; commonly young girls

Acute onset, chronic course

Etiology: appears to be exaggerated response to tissue injury following infection, surgery, or trauma

Findings: unilateral or bilateral highly vascularized, raised, friable lesion; with continued inflammation, a white, thickened avascular woody (ligneous) mass appears above the neovascular membrane, usually on palpebral conjunctiva; easily removed but bleeds; may recur

Process affects all mucous membranes (mouth, vagina, etc.)

Pathology: acellular eosinophilic hyaline material (immunoglobulins, primarily immunoglobulin G [IgG]), granulation tissue, cellular infiltration (T cells, mast cells, eosinophils)

Treatment: complete excision (expect significant bleeding); any remaining portion of lesion results in rapid recurrence because retained lesion acts as physical barrier to topical medications; ENT evaluation before surgery to ensure respiratory tract not involved because many require general anesthesia

> *Postexcision:* topical steroids q1h; hyaluronidase, acetylcysteine, and α-chymotrypsin q4h; topical antibiotic; topical cyclosporine 2% (applied to surgical bed with sterile cotton-tipped applicator); oral prednisone (1 mg/kg/day); daily débridement of any recurrence

Kawasaki Disease (Mucocutaneous Lymph Node Syndrome)

Systemic childhood inflammatory disease/vasculitis with prominent mucocutaneous manifestations

Occurs in children <5 years old

More common among Asians and Pacific Islanders

Epidemics suggest exposure to causal agent; siblings have 10 × increased risk

>50% of familial cases occur within 10 days after onset of 1st case

Diagnostic criteria (requires 5 of 6): fever (≥5 days), bilateral conjunctivitis (90%), mild bilateral nongranulomatous uveitis (80%), rash, cervical lymphadenopathy, oral lesions (fissures, strawberry tongue), lesions of extremities (edema, erythema, desquamation)

Associated with polyarteritis, especially of coronary arteries (fatal in 1%–2%)

Findings: bilateral conjunctival injection, iridocyclitis, punctate keratitis, vitreous opacities, papilledema, and subconjunctival hemorrhages

Treatment: aspirin; systemic steroids contraindicated (increased risk of coronary artery aneurysm)

Prognosis: 0.3% mortality

Complications: 15% develop coronary arteritis (can lead to coronary artery aneurysm or myocardial infarction)

Tumors

Epibulbar Osseous Choristoma

Hard mass, composed of mature bone

Usually located on bulbar conjunctiva (superotemporal fornix)

Does not enlarge

Not associated with other osteomas

No malignant potential

Treatment: observe or excise

Complex Choristoma

May contain cartilage, ectopic lacrimal gland tissue, smooth muscle, sweat glands, sebaceous glands, hair

Isolated or associated with linear nevus sebaceous syndrome

Ectopic Lacrimal Gland

Fleshy, vascularized tumor with raised translucent nodules

Usually extends into corneal stroma

Mild growth during puberty

Pathology: lacrimal gland parenchyma

Treatment: excision

CORNEAL DISORDERS

Anterior Megalophthalmos

Large anterior segment of eye

Associations: Marfan syndrome, mucolipidosis type II, Apert syndrome

Findings: high myopia and astigmatism; enlarged cornea, lens, iris, and ciliary ring; iris transillumination defects, lens dislocation, cataract

Congenital Corneal Staphyloma

Protuberant corneal opacity as a result of intrauterine keratitis

Findings: atrophic iris adheres to back of markedly thickened, scarred, and vascularized cornea; lens may be adherent to posterior cornea; cornea may perforate

Cornea Plana (AD or AR)

Mapped to chromosome 12q

Associations: sclerocornea, microcornea, and angle-closure glaucoma

Findings: flat cornea with curvature equaling that of sclera (usually 20–30 D), diffuse scarring and vascularization; may have coloboma, cataract, sclerocornea, shallow anterior chamber (AC), refractive error

Pathology: thickened epithelium, absent basement membrane, very thin Descemet membrane, anterior 1/3 of stroma is scarred and vascularized

Megalocornea

Horizontal diameter of cornea >12 mm in newborns (>13 mm in adult)

Nonprogressive; most commonly X-linked (associated with anterior megalophthalmos), bilateral, 90% male; also AR

Associations: Marfan syndrome, Alport syndrome, Down syndrome, dwarfism, craniosynostosis, facial hemiatrophy

Findings: large cornea; may have weak zonules, lens subluxation, hypoplastic iris, and ectopic pupil

Complications: ectopia lentis (enlarged limbal ring stretches the zonular fibers), glaucoma (results from angle abnormalities), cataract (posterior subcapsular cataract [PSC])

Microcornea

Corneal diameter <9 mm in newborns (<10 mm in adult)

AD or sporadic; unilateral or bilateral

Etiology: arrested corneal growth after 5th month of fetal development

Associations: dwarfism, Ehlers-Danlos syndrome

Findings: small cornea; often hyperopic (relatively flat corneas); may have cataract, coloboma, persistent hyperplastic primary vitreous (PHPV), microphakia; may develop angle-closure glaucoma or primary open-angle glaucoma (POAG)

DDx: nanophthalmos (small but structurally normal eye), anterior microphthalmos (small anterior segment), microphthalmos (small malformed eye)

Posterior Keratoconus

Discrete posterior corneal indentation with stromal haze and thinning

Female > male

Nonprogressive, usually central and unilateral

Anterior corneal surface is normal

Vision usually good; causes irregular astigmatism

Pathology: loss of stromal substance; Descemet membrane may be thinned, but both it and endothelium are intact

Anterior Segment Dysgenesis (Mesodermal Dysgenesis Syndromes)

Bilateral, congenital, hereditary disorders affecting anterior segment structures

Axenfeld anomaly: posterior embryotoxon (anteriorly displaced Schwalbe line; found in 15% of healthy individuals) with iris processes to scleral spur; 50% develop glaucoma; AD; mapped to chromosomes 4q25 (*RIEG1*), 13q14 (*RIEG2*), 6p25(*FOXC1*), 11p13 (*PAX6*)

Alagille syndrome: Axenfeld plus pigmentary retinopathy, corectopia, esotropia, and systemic abnormalities (absent deep tendon reflexes, abnormal facies, pulmonic valvular stenosis, peripheral arterial stenosis, biliary hypoplasia, and skeletal abnormalities); mapped

to chromosome 20p12 (*JAG1 gene*); ERG and electro-oculogram (EOG) are abnormal

Rieger anomaly: Axenfeld plus iris hypoplasia with holes; glaucoma; mapped to chromosomes 4q25 (*RIEG1* or *PITX2*), 13q14 (*RIEG2*), 6p25 (*FOXC1*), 11p13 (*PAX6*), 13q14, and 16q24

Rieger syndrome: Rieger anomaly plus mental retardation and systemic abnormalities (dental, craniofacial, genitourinary [hypospadias], redundant periumbilical skin, and skeletal)

Peter anomaly: central corneal leukoma (opacity resulting from defect in posterior cornea stroma and Descemet membrane with absence of endothelium) with iris adhesions; lens involvement (cataract) may occur, and 50% develop glaucoma; may have microcornea, aniridia, microphthalmia, persistent hyperplastic primary vitreous; also associated with cardiac, craniofacial, and skeletal abnormalities; usually sporadic, bilateral (80%); AR or AD; mapped to chromosomes 11p13 (*PAX6*), 4q25-q26 (*PTX2*), 2p21-p22 (*CYP1B1*), and 6p25 (*FOXC1*); very poor prognosis as a result of glaucoma and corneal graft failure

DDx: mnemonic **STUMPED** (Box 5.1)

Sclerocornea

Scleralized (white vascularized opacification) cornea; peripheral or entire

Nonprogressive; sporadic (50%) or hereditary (50%; AD or AR), mapped to chromosome 14; 90% bilateral

Corneoscleral limbus indistinct

Associations: persistent pupillary membrane, congenital glaucoma, cornea plana (80%)

Poor prognosis for corneal transplant

Descemet Tear/Rupture

May be caused by forceps trauma (vertical or oblique) or glaucoma (horizontal or concentric to limbus; Haab striae)

Acutely, edema occurs, scarring develops later

May cause astigmatism and amblyopia

Box 5.1 DDx of congenital cloudy cornea: STUMPED
Sclerocornea
Tears in Descemet membrane
Ulcers
Metabolic disease
Peter anomaly
Edema (CHED)
Dermoid
Others: Congenital stromal corneal dystrophy (CSCD), rubella, posterior ulcer of von Hippel, posterior keratoconus, congenital corneal staphyloma
CHED, Congenital hereditary endothelial dystrophy.

Metabolic Disorders (Mucopolysaccharidoses, Mucolipidoses)

(See Table 5.3)

Brittle Cornea Syndrome (BCS) (AR)

Multisystem connective tissue disorder; 2 types: type 1 caused by defect in *ZNF469* gene, type 2 caused by defect in *PRDM5* gene

Findings: severe thinning of the cornea (<400 µm) and sclera with high risk of ocular rupture, early-onset keratoconus and/or keratoglobus, blue sclera, high myopia, RD

Other findings: deafness, hip dysplasia, scoliosis, arachnodactyly, joint hypermobility, pes planus, hallus valgus, and finger contractures; soft, doughy skin

Congenital Hereditary Endothelial Dystrophy (CHED; Formerly CHED2) (AR)

Rare, bilateral, nonprogressive mapped to chromosome 20p13 *(SLC4A11)*

Onset at or shortly after birth

Corneal clouding as a result of edema from defect of corneal endothelium and Descemet membrane

No association with other systemic abnormalities

Findings: cloudy corneas (often asymmetric), corneal edema, nystagmus, no pain or tearing

Pathology: thickened edematous stroma, massively thickened Descemet membrane, atrophic or nonfunctioning endothelium

X-Linked Endothelial Corneal Dystrophy (XECD) (X-Linked Dominant)

Rare, bilateral, minimally progressive (males), nonprogressive (females); mapped to chromosome X

Onset at or shortly after birth

Findings:
Males: cloudy corneas (diffuse haze to ground-glass, milky appearance), moon crater–like endothelial changes; decreased vision; may develop band keratopathy, may have nystagmus
Females: only moon crater–like endothelial changes

Pathology: moon crater–like endothelial changes, subepithelial keratopathy, thinning of epithelium and Bowman layer, thickening of Descemet membrane with pits, loss of endothelial cells

Congenital Stromal Corneal Dystrophy (CSCD) (AD)

Rare, bilateral nonprogressive, diffuse opacification of cornea; mapped to chromosome 12q21.33 *(DCN)*

Onset at or shortly after birth

Findings: flaky, feathery white stromal opacities clear peripherally; no corneal edema

May cause strabismus, nystagmus, and amblyopia

Dermoid

Smooth, solid, yellow-white choristoma that may extend into corneal stroma to cover visual axis or cause astigmatism

No hereditary pattern; 25% bilateral

Types:
Conjunctival (limbal) dermoid: straddles limbus, most commonly in inferotemporal quadrant
Isolated or associated with Goldenhar syndrome (30%; includes accessory auricular appendages, aural fistulas, vertebral body abnormalities)
May cause astigmatism and amblyopia
Also associated with linear sebaceous nevus syndrome
Dermolipoma of the conjunctiva: usually located in superotemporal fornix; can extend deep into orbit
Consists of adipose and connective tissue
High surgical complication rate, with risk of marked ptosis, lateral rectus muscle paresis, and dry eye

Findings: dermoid, layer of lipid at leading edge in cornea; may cause proptosis, astigmatism, restricted motility, amblyopia

Pathology: thickened collagen fibers covered by skinlike epithelium; contains hair, sebaceous and sweat glands, and fat; lined by squamous epithelium

Treatment: observation; excision for cosmesis or if visual axis is blocked (caution: may be full thickness; granulomatous reaction if ruptures)

Other Causes of Corneal Opacity

Interstitial keratitis: congenital syphilis causes keratitis with edema followed by stromal vascularization ("salmon patch"); blood flow stops and "ghost" vessels remain with corneal haze

Riley-Day syndrome (familial dysautonomia; AR): autonomic nervous system dysfunction resulting from block of norepinephrine (NE) production; Eastern European Jews
Findings: decreased corneal sensation, lack of tearing, poorly reactive pupils, light-near dissociation; may develop neurotrophic keratitis with risk of perforation
Other findings: poor pain, temperature, and taste sensation; spinal curvature; increased sweating; constipation; hypotension

Crisis (lasts 1–10 days): emotional lability, profuse sweating, postural hypotension, vomiting; treat with diazepam (Valium) and hydration

Increased risk with general anesthesia: exquisite sensitivity to thiopental sodium (Pentothal) (hypotension, cardiac arrest)

Diagnosis: high urinary homo-vanillic acid (HVA) and vanillylmandelic acid (VMA), low hexamethylphosphorous triamide (HMPT)

Infections

Syphilis

Congenital: maternal transmission after fourth month of gestation (50% for primary or secondary syphilis, 30% for untreated or late syphilis)

Findings: interstitial keratitis (33%), ectopia lentis, Argyll-Robertson pupil, optic atrophy, panuveitis with various retinal pigmentary changes (usually "salt-and-pepper" or pseudo–retinitis pigmentosa [RP] pattern)

Other findings:
Early (≤2 years old): stillbirth, low birth weight, failure to thrive, rhinitis ("snuffles"), osteochondritis, desquamative skin rash, pneumonia, hepatosplenomegaly, anemia
Late (≥3 years old): Hutchinson teeth (peg-shaped), mulberry molars, saber shins, frontal bossing, saddle nose, deafness (5%), tabes dorsalis, skin fissures (rhagades; especially corners of mouth and nose), neurosyphilis

Hutchinson triad: interstitial keratitis, deafness, and Hutchinson teeth
Interstitial keratitis (IK): immune response to treponemal antigens
Starts between ages of 5-20 years; triggered by minor corneal trauma
Bilateral with 2nd-eye involvement at 1-2 months in 50%, 12 months in 75%
3 STAGES:
PROGRESSIVE: pain, photophobia, poor vision; blepharospasm, fine keratic precipitates KP, perilimbal injection, diffuse or sectoral corneal haze (ground-glass appearance)
FLORID: acute inflammatory response; salmon patch of Hutchinson (cornea appears pink as a result of deep vascularization)
RETROGRESSIVE: vessels meet at center of cornea
LATE FINDINGS: ghost vessels, Descemet folds, guttata, secondary glaucoma (iris/angle damage)
PATHOLOGY: stromal blood vessels just anterior to Descemet
TREATMENT: steroids (do not prevent involvement of fellow eye); systemic penicillin

DDx: acquired syphilis (IK usually sectoral and less severe), leprosy (superficial avascular keratitis, usually superotemporal quadrant; later, leprous pannus of blood vessels, beading of corneal nerves)

Herpes Simplex Virus (HSV)

Often an asymptomatic primary infection before age of 5; 3- to 5-day incubation period

Congenital: ocular involvement in 10% of disseminated cases

Findings: vesicular skin eruption, conjunctivitis, epithelial keratitis, stromal immune reaction, cataracts, necrotizing chorioretinitis

IRIS DISORDERS

Aniridia

Bilateral absence of iris, commonly a rudimentary iris stump exists

Incidence 1 in 100,000

Hereditary or sporadic; mapped to chromosome 11p13 (*PAX6*)

Types:
AN1 (85%): AD, only eye involvement
AN2 (13%): sporadic, associated with Wilms tumor (Miller syndrome and WAGR [Wilms tumor, aniridia, genitourinary abnormalities, and mental retardation])
AN3 (2%): AR, associated with mental retardation and ataxia (Gillespie syndrome)

Findings: visual acuity usually <20/200 (60%), foveal and ON hypoplasia, nystagmus (90%), photophobia, amblyopia, strabismus

May have cataracts (anterior polar, 50%–85%), glaucoma (30%–50%), ectopia lentis, corneal pannus, microcornea, persistent pupillary membrane

Treatment: consider cosmetic/painted contact lenses for photophobia; peripherally painted intraocular lenses (IOLs), opaque polymethyl methacrylate (PMMA) rings, and artificial iris implants with cataract surgery

Coloboma

Iris sector defect resulting from incomplete closure of embryonic fissure; usually located inferonasal

May have other colobomas (lid, ciliary body, choroid, retina, and ON)

Associated with trisomy 13, 18, and 22; chromosome 18 deletion; Klinefelter syndrome, Turner syndrome, CHARGE, basal cell nevus syndrome, Goldenhar syndrome, Meckel syndrome, Rubinstein-Taybi syndrome, linear sebaceous nevus syndrome, congenital Zika syndrome

Treatment: consider surgical repair in symptomatic cases

Congenital Iris Ectropion

Ectropion uveae: ectropion of posterior pigment epithelium onto anterior surface of iris

Associated with neurofibromatosis, Prader-Willi syndrome

Congenital iris ectropion syndrome: unilateral congenital iris ectropion, high iris insertion, smooth and cryptless iris surface, dysgenesis of angle, and glaucoma

Congenital Iris Hypoplasia

Thin iris stroma with transillumination of entire iris

Associated with albinism

Congenital Miosis

May be associated with other anterior segment abnormalities

Etiology: absence or malformation of dilator pupillae muscle or contracture of fibrous material on pupil margin from tunica vasculosa lentis remnant or neural crest cell abnormalities

Congenital Mydriasis

Etiology: iris sphincter trauma, pharmacologic, neurologic disease

Corectopia

Displacement of pupil

Isolated or associated with ectopia lentis et pupillae, Axenfeld-Rieger syndrome, iridocorneal endothelial syndrome, uveitis, or trauma

Dyscoria

Abnormally shaped pupil

Isolated or associated with posterior synechiae, Axenfeld-Rieger syndrome, ectopia lentis et pupillae

Persistent Pupillary Membrane

Remnants of anterior tunica vasculosa lentis that appear as fine iris strands

Common congenital ocular anomaly

Rarely visually significant

Type I: iris to iris, bridging pupil

Type II: iris to lens; may have associated anterior polar cataract

Primary Iris Cysts

Caused by spontaneous separation of pigmented and nonpigmented epithelium

Occur anywhere between pupil and ciliary body

Miotics can cause cysts at pupillary border

Congenital stromal cysts occur in infants and young children from sequestration of epithelium during fetal development

Brushfield Spots

Focal areas of iris stromal hyperplasia surrounded by relative hypoplasia

Appear as ring of peripheral, elevated, white-gray spots (10–20/eye)

Occur in 85% of Down syndrome patients

May be found in normal individuals (Kunkmann-Wolffian bodies)

Lisch Nodules

Neural crest hamartomas

Associated with NF-1

Number and frequency increase with age

Appear as tan nodules, usually in inferior iris

Juvenile Xanthogranuloma (JXG; Nevoxanthoendothelioma)

Histiocytic proliferation usually of skin

Yellow-orange nodules appear before 1 year of age

Orange because of vascularity (red) combined with high lipid content (yellow)

May involve iris (may cause spontaneous hyphema)

May involve muscles, salivary glands, stomach, and other internal organs

Rarely associated with an orbital granuloma (which causes proptosis)

Lesions often spontaneously regress by 5 years of age

Pathology: diffuse nonnecrotizing proliferation of histiocytes with scattered Touton giant cells (ring of nuclei separating a central eosinophilic cytoplasm from peripheral foamy [or clear] cytoplasm)

Treatment: iris lesions are treated with steroids, XRT, and excision

Medulloepithelioma (Diktyoma)

Primary neoplasm of ciliary body neuroectoderm (arises in nonpigmented epithelium); arises from primitive medullary epithelium that lines neural tube; can also arise in retina and ON

Occurs in both benign and malignant forms (locally invasive but limited metastatic potential)

May have heterotopic elements; no calcification

Unilateral, unifocal, usually arises before 6 years of age; no hereditary pattern

Types:
> *Nonteratoid or simple:* pure proliferation of embryonic nonpigmented ciliary epithelium
> *Teratoid:* contains heterotopic elements such as cartilage, brain tissue, and rhabdomyoblasts

Findings: decreased vision, pain, strabismus, leukocoria, iris mass, fleshy pink to white peripheral fundus tumor; rubeosis, hyphema, glaucoma, lens coloboma occurs in some congenital cases

Pathology: undifferentiated round to oval cells containing little cytoplasm, organized into ribbon-like structures that have distinct cellular polarity; lined on one side by thin basement membrane; stratified sheets of cells are capable of forming mucinous cysts that are clinically characteristic; Flexner-Wintersteiner and Homer-Wright rosettes can be seen; called *teratoid medulloepithelioma* when composed of cells from 2 different embryonic germ layers; may contain cartilage, brain tissue, and rhabdomyoblasts

Treatment: resection (iridocyclectomy) or enucleation (not radiosensitive)

Prognosis: good if no extraocular extension; rarely metastasizes

LENS DISORDERS

Congenital Anomalies

Mittendorf dot: small white opacity on posterior lens capsule that represents a remnant of the posterior vascular capsule (tunica vasculosa lentis) where hyaloid artery is inserted

Chicken tracks (epicapsular star): brown or golden flecks on anterior lens capsule; remnant of anterior tunica vasculosa lentis

Lenticonus: cone-shaped lens deformity resulting from central bulge in area of thin capsule; causes irregular myopic astigmatism; "oil-droplet" sign on retinoscopy; associated with cataract
> *Anterior:* bilateral, male > female; associated with Alport syndrome (anterior lenticonus, hereditary nephritis, and deafness)
> *Posterior:* unilateral, sporadic, female > male, more common than anterior type, amblyopia common

Lens coloboma: focal flattening of lens edge resulting from absence of inferior zonules from ciliary body coloboma; not a true coloboma

Lentiglobus: generalized hemispherical deformity, very rare

Microphakia: small lens as a result of arrested development; associated with Lowe syndrome

Microspherophakia: small, spherical lens, usually bilateral; zonules visible on pupillary dilation; iridodonesis; zonule rupture is common, pupillary block may occur, especially with use of miotics (treat with cycloplegic to tighten zonules, flattening the lens and pulling it posteriorly)

Associated with Weill-Marchesani syndrome, hyperlysinemia, Lowe syndrome, Alport syndrome, congenital rubella, and Peter anomaly
> *Treatment:* cycloplegic (tightens zonules, flattening lens and pulling it posteriorly)

Congenital aphakia: rare, absence of lens

Ectopia Lentis

(See Chapter 10, Anterior Segment)

Congenital Cataracts

Characteristics:
> *Bilateral:* usually AD; consider diabetes, galactosemia, or Lowe syndrome; require metabolic workup and treatment by age 3 months, or irreversible nystagmus with poor visual acuity (≤20/200) occurs. Opacities >3 mm can be visually significant. Surgery often performed on the better-seeing eye first: lensectomy, anterior vitrectomy, and contact lens fitting for infants; posterior capsulotomy is necessary because of significant postoperative inflammation, which causes posterior capsular opacification
> *Unilateral:* generally not metabolic or genetic; therefore, laboratory testing is not needed. Usually local dysgenesis (PHPV, anterior polar or posterior lenticonus), often presents with leukocoria and strabismus. Requires treatment by 6-8 weeks of life

Types: classified by location or etiology
> *Polar* (subcapsular cortex and capsule): anterior or posterior, sporadic, or AD
>> **ANTERIOR:** usually small, bilateral, symmetric, nonprogressive; good visual prognosis; 90% are idiopathic. Remnant of the hyaloid system. Associated with microphthalmos and anterior lenticonus
>> PATHOLOGY: fibrous plaque beneath folded anterior capsule secreted by irritated metaplastic epithelial cells
>> **POSTERIOR:** larger, usually stable, but may progress; more visually significant; AD (bilateral) or sporadic (unilateral); often with associated weakness or defect of posterior capsule
>> Associated with remnants of the tunica vasculosa lentis, posterior lenticonus, or lentiglobus
>> PATHOLOGY: posterior migration of lens epithelium
> *Sutural* (AR): bilateral opacities of Y sutures; rarely affects vision. Occurs during development of fetal lens nucleus

Nuclear (usually AD): bilateral, opacification of embryonic fetal nucleus; typically axial, dense, bilateral, and >3 mm. Associated with small eye

Anterior pyramidal: congenital anterior subcapsular

Lamellar/zonular: bilateral, symmetric, appears like a sand dollar; circumscribed zone of opacity within lens, surrounding the nucleus. May be caused by transient toxic exposure during embryogenesis (neonatal tetany); can be AD. Usually does not interfere with vision

Complete: no red reflex; unilateral or bilateral

Membranous: lens proteins resorb following trauma; anterior and posterior capsules fuse into a dense white membrane

Crystalline: rare, bilateral congenital cataract, with refractile, rhomboid crystals (containing tyrosine and cysteine) radiating outward from the center of the lens into the juvenile nucleus

Anterior axial embryonic: most common type of congenital/infantile cataract. White, clustered, punctate opacities near the Y sutures; not visually significant

Pulverulent (AR): central, translucent, ovoid, and cluster of dotlike opacities in the fetal nucleus

Coronary (AR): wreath of peripheral cortical opacities that encircle the nucleus in a radial fashion; smaller punctate bluish opacities within the nucleus. Associated with Down syndrome

Etiology: 1/3 hereditary; 1/3 associated with systemic syndromes; 1/3 of unknown origin

Etiology of bilateral cataracts:

Idiopathic (60%)

Intrauterine infection (3%): TORCH syndrome; the alternate acronym is **TORCHES** (**TO**xoplasmosis, **R**ubella, **C**MV, **HE**rpes simplex, **S**yphilis)

Associated with ocular disorders: Leber congenital amaurosis, RP, PHPV, retinopathy of prematurity (ROP), aniridia, Peter anomaly, ectopia lentis, posterior lenticonus, uveitis, tumors (retinoblastoma, medulloepithelioma)

Metabolic: galactosemia, hypocalcemia, Lowe syndrome, congenital hemolytic jaundice, hypoglycemia, mannosidosis, Alport syndrome, Fabry disease

Hereditary (30%, usually AD):

WITHOUT SYSTEMIC ABNORMALITIES: AD, AR, X-linked

WITH CHROMOSOMAL ABNORMALITIES: trisomy 18, trisomy 21 (Down syndrome), Turner syndrome, trisomy 13 (Patau syndrome), "cri-du-chat" syndrome

CRANIOFACIAL SYNDROMES: Crouzon syndrome, Apert syndrome, Hallermann-Streiff syndrome, Pierre Robin sequence

CENTRAL NERVOUS SYSTEM (CNS) ABNORMALITIES: Zellweger syndrome, Torsten-Sjögren syndrome, Marinesco-Sjögren syndrome, Lawrence-Moon-Biedl-Bardet syndrome, Norrie disease, neurofibromatosis

SKIN ABNORMALITIES: Cockayne syndrome, Rothmund-Thomson syndrome, Werner syndrome, atopic dermatitis, ichthyosis, incontinentia pigmenti

Maternal drug ingestion/malnutrition

Trauma

Specific entities:

Galactosemia (AR): defect in 1 of 3 enzymes (galactose-1-P-uridyl transferase [most common], galactokinase, or uridine diphosphate [UDP] galactose-4-epimerase) causes inability to convert galactose into glucose; galactose is converted into galactitol, which serves as osmotic agent for influx of fluid; mapped to chromosomes 1p (*GALE*), 9p (*GALT*), and 17q (*GALK1*)

FINDINGS: oil-droplet cataract (reversible early on)

OTHER FINDINGS: mental retardation, hepatosplenomegaly, jaundice, diarrhea, cirrhosis, malnutrition, and failure to thrive

TREATMENT: eliminate lactose from diet; fatal if untreated

Mannosidosis: α-mannosidase deficiency causes Hurler-like syndrome

FINDINGS: posterior spokelike opacity; no corneal changes (unlike Hurler)

OTHER FINDINGS: mental retardation, short stature, skeletal changes, hepatosplenomegaly

Fabry disease: α-galactosidase A deficiency

FINDINGS: cornea verticillata; spokelike cataract in 25%

OTHER FINDINGS: angiokeratomas, cardiovascular abnormalities, renal disorders, bouts of pain in digits

Hypocalcemia: either idiopathic or following surgery of parathyroid glands

Punctate iridescent opacities in anterior and posterior cortex

Lowe (oculocerebrorenal) syndrome (X-linked): defect of amino acid metabolism, mapped to chromosome Xq25 (*OCRL*); male > female

FINDINGS: congenital cataract (100%), usually bilateral; small, thin, discoid lens (microphakic) associated with retained lens nuclei; glaucoma (50%); congenital cataract and glaucoma are very rare

Female carriers have white, punctate cortical opacities and subcapsular plaque-like opacities

OTHER FINDINGS: renal tubular acidosis, aminoaciduria, renal rickets, mental retardation, muscular hypotonia, failure to thrive

Alport syndrome (X-linked): triad of anterior lenticonus, deafness, and hemorrhagic nephropathy/renal failure; mapped to chromosome Xq22 (*COL4A5* [80%], also *COL4A3* and *COL4A4*)

FINDINGS: conjunctival calcium crystals, corneal endothelial pigment, juvenile arcus, spherophakia, anterior polar cataract, retinal changes similar to RP or fundus albipunctatus, ON drusen

Female carriers have lenticular changes

DIAGNOSIS: renal or skin biopsy (lack of α-5 type IV collagen in glomerular and epidermal basement membranes)

Hallermann-Streiff syndrome (mandibulo oculofacial dysmorphia): hypoplasia of mandible with birdlike facies; one of the few syndromes with combined cataract and glaucoma

FINDINGS: microphakia, microcornea, glaucoma, and cataract (can develop within first few weeks of life); spontaneous rupture of lens capsule with absorption of lens proteins can occur; immune response to lens proteins resembles phacoanaphylactic uveitis

Intrauterine infections: usually occur early in first trimester because lens capsule is formed during week 5 of embryogenesis; rubella, HSV, mumps, toxoplasmosis, vaccinia, CMV, EBV

Hypoglycemia during pregnancy: congenital lenticular opacities; associated with optic atrophy, mental retardation

Down syndrome: snowflake cataract, keratoconus

Diagnosis of bilateral cataracts: if AD pattern determined, no workup is necessary

Urinalysis: amino acids (Lowe syndrome), reducing substance after milk feeding (galactosemia)

Blood tests: calcium (hypocalcemia/hyperparathyroidism), glucose (hypoglycemia), red blood cell galactokinase, TORCH titers

Karyotyping: trisomy 13 (Patau syndrome), 18, and 21 (Down syndrome); Turner syndrome, "cri-du-chat" syndrome

Bilateral audiograms: congenital rubella, Alport syndrome

B-scan ultrasound: if no view of fundus

Etiology of unilateral cataracts:

Idiopathic (80%):

Ocular abnormalities (10%): PHPV, posterior lenticonus (90% unilateral), anterior segment dysgenesis, tumors (retinoblastoma, medulloepithelioma)

Trauma (9%)

Intrauterine infection: rubella; 33% unilateral

Diagnosis of unilateral cataracts: rule out non-accidental trauma (child abuse), TORCH titers

DDx of leukocoria (white pupil): cataract, retinoblastoma, toxoplasmosis, toxocariasis, RD, ROP, PHPV, Coats disease, coloboma, myelinated nerve fibers, retinal dysplasia, Norrie disease, incontinentia pigmenti, retinoschisis, cyclitic membrane, medulloepithelioma

DDx of congenital cataracts and glaucoma: Lowe syndrome, rubella, Hallermann-Streiff syndrome

Rubella: results from maternal infection late in the first trimester of pregnancy

FINDINGS (in 50%): cataract (usually bilateral, pearly white nuclear opacification; retention of lens nuclei in embryonic nucleus; virus remains viable in lens for years: viral shedding following cataract surgery can lead to intense and persistent AC inflammation), salt-and-pepper fundus (normal ERG) (see Fig. 5.24), glaucoma (usually either cataract or glaucoma, rarely both), microphthalmos (15%), necrotizing iridocyclitis, corneal clouding

OTHER FINDINGS (especially during first trimester): cardiac defects (patent ductus arteriosus), deafness (infection of the organ of Corti [90%]), and mental retardation

Complications of surgery: chronic aphakic glaucoma (15%). Usually discovered 5 to 6 years after surgery; increased risk with trauma, microcornea, PHPV, preexisting anterior segment abnormalities, and retained lens material

Prognosis:

Good: lamellar cataracts (later onset and less risk of glaucoma)

Intermediate: nuclear cataracts

Poor: total cataracts (high incidence of microcornea, poor pupillary dilation, and increased risk of glaucoma). Microphthalmos, strabismus, nystagmus, and amblyopia; 90% of patients with visually significant congenital bilateral cataracts will develop nystagmus if not treated by 2 months of age; nystagmus and amblyopia may not resolve even after cataract surgery

GLAUCOMA

Childhood Glaucoma

IOP-related damage to the eye

Classification: (Fig. 5.6)

Primary childhood glaucoma:

Primary congenital glaucoma (PCG): neonatal or newborn onset (age <1 month), infantile onset (age >1–24 months), late-onset (age >24 months); buphthalmos

EPIDEMIOLOGY: incidence ranges from 1 in 1250 to 1 in 68,000 births

ETIOLOGY: developmental abnormality of angle (goniodysgenesis) with faulty cleavage and abnormal insertion of ciliary muscle; 25% present at birth, >80% present during first year of life; 67% bilateral; 65% males. Hereditary in 10% to 40%, usually AR; mapped to chromosomes 2p21-p22 (*GLC3A, CYP1B1*), 1p36 (*GLC3B*), 14q24.3 (*GLC3C*), 14q24 (*GLC3D, LTBP2*), 9p21 (*GLC3E, TEK*); a mutation in the *CYP1B1* gene (member of cytochrome P450 gene family) accounts for ~85% of congenital glaucoma; 2% risk of affected parent with no family history having child with PCG

SYMPTOMS: tearing, photophobia, and blepharospasm (classic PCG triad); also red eye and eye rubbing. If age <3 months, usually presents with corneal clouding or tearing; if age >3 years, usually asymptomatic with progressive myopia and insidious visual field (VF) loss

FINDINGS: IOP >20 mm Hg (often 30–40 mm Hg); C/D ratio >0.3 (present in only 2.6% of normal infants; asymmetry >0.2 between the eyes also suggestive; cupping may be reversible in young children if IOP lowered); buphthalmos ("bull's-eye"; occurs in PCG, not in JOAG;

Primary infantile glaucoma (congenital glaucoma, trabeculodysgenesis)	
Secondary infantile glaucoma	
Associated with mesodermal neural crest dysgenesis	Iridocorneotrabeculodysgenesis • Rieger's anomaly or syndrome • Axenfeld's anomaly or syndrome • Peters' anomaly • systemic hypoplastic mesodermal dysgenesis (Marfan's syndrome) • systemic hyperplastic mesodermal dysgenesis (Weill–Marchesani syndrome)
	Iridotrabeculodysgenesis (aniridia)
Associated with phakomatoses and hamartomas	Neurofibromatosis (Von Recklinghausen's disease)
	Encephalotrigeminal angiomatosis (Sturge–Weber syndrome and variants, e.g., Klippel–Trénaunay–Weber syndrome)
	Angiomatosis retinae et cerebelli
	Oculodermal melanocytosis
Associated with metabolic disease	Oculocerebrorenal syndrome (Lowe's syndrome)
	Homocystinuria
Associated with inflammatory disease	Maternal rubella syndrome (congenital rubella)
	Herpes simplex iridocyclitis
Associated with mitotic disease	Juvenile xanthogranuloma (nevoxanthoendothelioma)
	Retinoblastoma
Associated with other congenital disease	Trisomy 13–15 syndrome (Patau's syndrome)
	Rubinstein–Taybi syndrome
	Persistent hyperplastic primary vitreous
	Congenital cataract • in phakic eyes • in aphakic eyes following surgery

Figure 5.6 Classification of the congenital and infantile glaucomas. (From Yanoff M, Duker JS, eds. *Ophthalmology*. London: Mosby; 1999.)

horizontal corneal diameter >13 mm [>11.5 in newborns, >12.5 in 1 year old]; limbal ectasia; stretching of zonules can lead to lens subluxation; irreversible); corneal clouding/edema/Haab striae (circumferential or horizontal Descemet ruptures [vs. oblique or vertical with forceps injury]; may result in chronic corneal edema, scarring, and astigmatism); myopia

Angle is of neural crest origin, as are facial bones, teeth, cartilage, and meninges; therefore, congenital glaucoma may be associated with malformation of these structures

Juvenile open-angle glaucoma (JOAG): AD, mapped to chromosome 1q21-q31 *(GLC1A, TIGR/MYOC);* onset after age 4 years; no buphthalmos, usually normal angles

Secondary childhood glaucoma: caused by other ocular anomalies (congenital or acquired) or associated with systemic disease

Associated with nonacquired ocular anomalies: microcornea, cornea plana, sclerocornea, Axenfeld/Rieger/Peter anomaly (50%), aniridia (50%–75% develop glaucoma by teens as a result of increased episcleral venous pressure, iris stump blocking trabecular meshwork [TM], or angle malformation or agenesis), microspherophakia, nanophthalmos,

iris/ciliary body/retina tumors, familial exudative vitreoretinopathy (FEVR), PHPV, ROP

Associated with nonacquired systemic disease or syndrome: Lowe (oculocerebrorenal) syndrome (50%); Sturge-Weber syndrome (50%, especially if nevus flammeus involves upper lid, results from primary defect in angle and increased episcleral venous pressure); NF-1 (25% if plexiform neurofibroma involves upper lid; may have hamartomatous infiltration of angle); congenital rubella (2%–15%); also Marfan syndrome, homocystinuria, Weill-Marchesani syndrome, Rubenstein-Taybi, Pierre Robin, nevus of Ota, trisomy 13 (Patau), Hallermann-Streiff, Stickler syndrome, mucopolysaccharidoses (Hurler and Hunter)

Associated with acquired conditions: inflammation, steroid-induced, lens-induced, trauma, tumors (retinoblastoma [RB], JXG, medulloepithelioma)

Following congenital cataract surgery: aphakic glaucoma develops in 15%-50% weeks, months, or years later (most within 3 years); mechanism unclear; increased risk if have surgery as infant, microcornea, PHPV

Diagnosis:

Examination under anesthesia (EUA): usually required for complete evaluation. Remember, ketamine and succinylcholine raise IOP; general anesthesia (halothane, thiopental, tranquilizers, and barbiturates) lowers IOP. Best time for IOP measurement is just as patient goes under and is not too deep

Gonioscopy: landmarks are often poorly recognized because of "Barkan membrane" covering TM (but no histologic evidence of such a structure)
1. Open-angle with anterior iris insertion above scleral spur (usual configuration is flat iris insertion into trabecular meshwork; less commonly, concave insertion with plane of iris posterior to scleral spur and anterior iris sweeping upward and inserting into TM)
2. Thickening of TM
3. Peripheral iris stromal hypoplasia

Treatment: definitive treatment is surgical; medication is a temporizing measure; treat refractive error and amblyopia if present

Topical medications: β-blockers most effective but can cause respiratory distress and bradycardia; carbonic anhydrase inhibitors (CAIs) less effective and can cause corneal edema; prostaglandin analogues effective but avoid in uveitis; miotics associated with paradoxical increase in intraocular pressure; α-agonists cause respiratory depression (especially brimonidine; associated with infant death, contraindicated in age <2 years)

Goniotomy: perform in child <1½ years of age; TM incised under direct gonioscopic visualization; requires clear cornea; 77% success rate

Trabeculotomy (ab externo): if cornea hazy, if <1½ years old, or if goniotomy fails twice; Schlemm canal is entered via an external incision, and the trabeculotome rotates into the AC and tears the TM; 77% success rate

If goniotomy and trabeculotomy fail, consider trabeculectomy with mitomycin C, drainage implant, cycloablation of ciliary body (CB) (laser or cryo)

Prognosis: variable; best for onset between 3-12 months (90% controlled with treatment), worse for neonatal (50% legal blindness), late onset, and corneal diameter >14 mm at diagnosis; overall, 50% of PCG have vision <20/50 and blindness in 2%-15%

UVEITIS

Anterior Uveitis

DDx: juvenile idiopathic arthritis (JIA), trauma, infection, tumor, sympathetic ophthalmia, sarcoidosis, familial juvenile systemic granulomatosis, phacoantigenic

Juvenile Idiopathic Arthritis (JIA)

Formerly Juvenile Rheumatoid Arthritis [JRA]
Arthritis in children <16 years old lasting ≥6 weeks with no identifiable cause

Associated with HLA-A2, B27, DR5, DR8, DR11, DRB1, DP2

Types:
I. Systemic (Still disease; 10%–15%): usually <5 years old; 60% male; small and large joints; negative rheumatoid factor (RF); negative antinuclear antibody (ANA); high fever, rash, lymphadenopathy, hepatosplenomegaly, polyserositis
II. Oligoarticular (pauciarticular; ≤4 joints in first 6 months; 40%–50%): most common type, mainly girls, anterior uveitis in 25%-35%; usually ANA+, almost always RF–
III. Polyarticular (>4 joints in first 6 months; 40%): 85% female, usually older, anterior uveitis in ~10%; may be ANA+ (increased risk uveitis), 75% RF–
IV. Spondyloarthritis: enthesitis-related arthritis (10%–20%), juvenile psoriatic arthritis, juvenile ankylosing spondylitis, enteropathic arthritis, reactive arthritis, undifferentiated spondyloarthritis; mainly boys, usually in adolescence, anterior uveitis in 25% (usually symptomatic), differentiated forms have enthesitis (inflammation of ligament, tendon, joint capsule insertion sites; especially patellar tendon, plantar fascia, Achilles tendon); HLA-B27 associated
V. Undifferentiated arthritis

Uveitis most common in pauciarticular (oligoarthritis), polyarticular RF– (rare in RF+), psoriatic arthritis, and enthesitis-related arthritis; average age 6 years old, 90% within 7 years of arthritis, usually asymptomatic; risk factors for chronic uveitis: female, oligoarticular, ANA+

Findings: chronic anterior uveitis (up to 34%, usually bilateral; eyes are white and quiet even with active ocular inflammation [visible flare]), fine KP, band keratopathy (40%), cataract (40%), glaucoma (20%), posterior synechiae, cyclitic membrane, hypotony, phthisis; rarely vitritis and macular edema

Other findings: arthritis, fever, lymphadenopathy, maculopapular rash, myocarditis, hepatosplenomegaly

Treatment: topical steroids and cycloplegic; consider systemic steroids or sub-Tenon steroid injection; treat complications. May require systemic immunomodulatory therapy, ethylenediaminetetraacetic acid (EDTA) chelation for band keratopathy, treatment of secondary glaucoma, cataract surgery (eyes should be without AC reaction for at least 3 months; intraoperatively, anterior vitrectomy, synechialysis, removal of cyclitic membranes; acrylic IOL only [may need to be explanted]; may be complicated by hypotony)

Intermediate Uveitis

Pars Planitis

(See Chapter 8, Uveitis)

Posterior Uveitis

DDx: toxoplasmosis, toxocariasis, presumed ocular histoplasmosis syndrome (POHS), HSV, syphilis, Lyme disease, sympathetic ophthalmia, sarcoidosis, familial juvenile systemic granulomatosis, masquerade syndromes (RB, leukemia, lymphoma, melanoma, JXG, intraocular foreign body, rhegmatogenous retinal detachment [RRD], RP, multiple sclerosis [MS])

Familial Juvenile Systemic Granulomatosis (Blau Syndrome)

Mapped to chromosome 16 *(NOD2)*; AD

Similar to early onset sarcoidosis with granulomatous arthritis, uveitis, rash but no lymphadenopathy or pulmonary involvement

Causes chronic panuveitis with multifocal choroiditis; may have only anterior uveitis; often develop cataract, glaucoma, band keratopathy

Toxoplasmosis

Caused by infection with *Toxoplasma gondii* (obligate intracellular parasitic protozoan)

Cats are definitive host, humans are intermediate host

Life cycle has 3 major forms:
Oocyst: soil form, contains sporozoites; reproduce in cat intestine, shed in feces, ingested by intermediate host
Tachyzoite: infectious form; hematogenous spread to most tissues in host
Tissue cyst: latent form, contains bradyzoites

Congenital: transplacental transmission of *T. gondii*; 40% chance if maternal infection during pregnancy; highest risk during 3rd trimester; severity inversely proportional to gestational age; retinochoroiditis in 80%, usually bilateral (85%)
1st-trimester infection: spontaneous abortion, stillbirth, neonatal convulsions, intracerebral calcifications, retinochoroiditis
Later infection: may be asymptomatic or have retinochoroiditis only

Sabin's tetrad (<10%): hydrocephalus/microcephaly, retinochoroiditis, intracranial calcifications, mental retardation

Acquired: more common than previously thought; occurs via ingestion of undercooked infected meat or contaminated water, fruit, vegetables; contact with oocysts in cat feces, litter, or soil; blood transfusion or organ transplant

90% of women are seronegative (and therefore susceptible); ~11% US population ≥6 years old is infected (2% may have ocular involvement)

Primary retinal infection with coagulative necrosis and secondary granulomatous choroiditis with vitritis; intraretinal cysts cause recurrent disease

Most common cause of posterior uveitis (25%); most common cause of pediatric uveitis (50% of posterior uveitis in children)

Findings: inactive pigmented chorioretinal scar in posterior pole, often in macula (Fig. 5.7); active focal white fluffy lesion with overlying vitritis ("headlight in fog" appearance) occurs adjacent to old scar, often have granulomatous anterior uveitis, increased IOP (20%); may have perivasculitis with venous sheathing and white spots along arterioles (Kyrieleis plaques); may develop vascular occlusions, cystoid macular edema (CME), RD, epiretinal membrane (ERM), choroidal neovascularization (CNV), optic atrophy, cataract; may also have microphthalmia, nystagmus, strabismus. May have atypical presentation: punctate outer retinal toxoplasmosis (PORT), neuroretinitis, unilateral pigmentary retinopathy (similar to RP), retinal necrosis (similar to acute retinal necrosis [ARN])

In AIDS: head CT may show ring-enhancing lesions; minimal AC reaction and vitritis because immunocompromised host is unable to mount normal immune response

Other findings:

Congenital toxoplasmosis: stillbirth, mental retardation, seizures, hydrocephalus, microcephaly, intracranial calcifications, hepatosplenomegaly, vomiting, diarrhea

Acquired toxoplasmosis: rash, meningoencephalitis, flu-like syndrome

Pathology: round *Toxoplasma* cysts (Fig. 5.8); chronic granulomatous choroiditis

Diagnosis: enzyme-linked immunoassay (ELISA) or immunofluorescence assay (IFA) for *Toxoplasma* IgG or immunoglobulin M (IgM)

Treatment:

Indications: retinochoroiditis with decreased vision, moderate to severe vitreous inflammation, lesions that threaten macula or ON, lesion size >1 disc diameter, multiple active lesions, or active disease >1 month; small peripheral lesions may be observed (heal spontaneously)

Antibiotics: kill tachyzoites in retina during active retinitis but do not affect cysts

PYRIMETHAMINE (DARAPRIM): 50-100 mg loading dose, then 25-50 mg qd × 4-8 weeks (bone marrow suppression; prevent with folinic acid [Leucovorin 5–10 mg qd]; check complete blood count [CBC] q 2 weeks)

SULFADIAZINE: 2 g loading dose, then 1 g qid

CLINDAMYCIN: 300 mg qid (risk of pseudomembranous colitis)

ALTERNATIVES: trimethoprim-sulfamethoxazole (Bactrim), azithromycin, atovaquone

Steroids: systemic (0.25–0.75 mg/kg x 3–5 weeks; consider after 48 hours of antibiotic therapy, never without concomitant antibiotics), topical for anterior uveitis; long-acting periocular and intraocular contraindicated (risk of panophthalmitis and loss of eye)

Other treatment indications: pregnant woman with newly acquired infection (spiramycin, azithromycin, clindamycin, or atovaquone; or intravitreal injection of clindamycin and short-acting periocular steroid), newborns with congenital infection (pyrimethamine

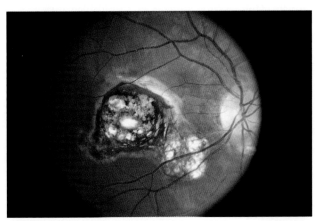

Figure 5.7 Congenital toxoplasmic retinitis. Note inactive satellite scars at the macula, the inferior juxtapapillary scar, and the temporal pallor of the disc. (From Khanna A, Goldstein DA, Tessler HH. Protozoal posterior uveitis. In: Yanoff M, Duker JS, eds. *Ophthalmology*. London: Mosby; 1999.)

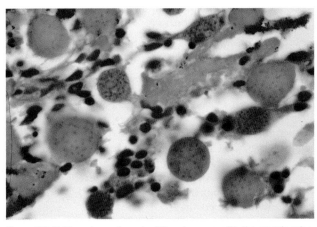

Figure 5.8 Viable and necrotic cysts of *Toxoplasma gondii* in the necrotic retina. (From Khanna A, Goldstein DA, Tessler HH. Protozoal posterior uveitis. In: Yanoff M, Duker JS, eds. *Ophthalmology*. London: Mosby; 1999.)

and sulfonamides × 1 year), immunocompromised patients (extended treatment)

Toxocariasis

Caused by infection with nematode larvae of dog and cat roundworm *Toxocara canis* (30% of puppies) and *Toxocara cati* (25% of cats)

Acquired by ingestion of contaminated soil or food, or fecal-oral transmission

5% of US population is seropositive

Larvae grow in small intestine, hematogenous spread to liver, heart, lung, brain, muscle, eye; does not complete life cycle (stool examination unnecessary)

Ocular larva migrans: usually unilateral, solitary lesion

Visceral larva migrans: usually in children age <3 years; fever, rash, malaise, lymphadenopathy, hepatomegaly, pneumonitis, eosinophilia, meningoencephalitis, no eye involvement

Findings: 3 clinical presentations depending on patient age (chronic endophthalmitis [25%], posterior pole granuloma [25%], or peripheral granuloma [50%; may have fibrous vitreous bands with macular traction]) (Table 5.2); vitreous abscess; dragging of macula temporally owing to peripheral lesion results in apparent XT; often presents with leukocoria; traction RD can occur (Fig. 5.9). Rare presentations: pars planitis, ON granuloma, diffuse unilateral subacute neuroretinitis

DDx: as for leukocoria

Diagnosis: clinical; consider AC tap for eosinophils, ELISA for *Toxocara* antibody titers, no ova/parasites in stool

Treatment: topical steroids and cycloplegic for active uveitis, periocular or systemic steroids for posterior lesion and endophthalmitis; vitrectomy, may require surgical repair of RD; albendazole for visceral larva migrans

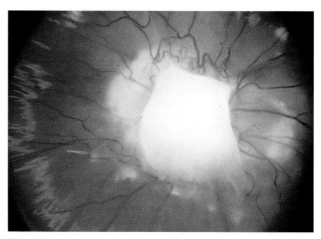

Figure 5.9 Typical toxocara granuloma located over the optic nerve. (From Yanoff M, Duker JS, eds. *Ophthalmology*. London: Mosby; 1999, chapter 173.)

METABOLIC DISORDERS

See Table 5.3, Box 5.2

RETINAL DISORDERS

Persistent Hyperplastic Primary Vitreous (PHPV; Persistent Fetal Vasculature [PFV])

Unilateral microphthalmia with spectrum of findings from prominent hyaloid vessel remnant with large Mittendorf dot and Bergmeister papillae to angle-closure from fibrovascular invasion of lens through posterior lens capsule

Caused by incomplete regression of tunica vasculosa lentis and primary vitreous

Sporadic, 90% unilateral

Findings: microphthalmia, vascularized retrolental plaque (may contain cartilage), elongated ciliary processes, prominent radial vessels on iris surface, shallow AC, iris vascularization; may have cataract, angle-closure glaucoma, vitreous hemorrhage, RD

DDx of intraocular cartilage: PHPV, medulloepithelioma, teratoma, trisomy 13

Treatment: observation, lensectomy with or without vitrectomy

Prognosis: depends on degree of amblyopia; visual prognosis variable after surgery, often depends on status of posterior segment

Coloboma

Yellow-white lesion with pigmented margins resulting from incomplete closure of embryonic fissure; usually located inferonasal

Retina is reduced to glial tissue; no retinal pigment epithelium (RPE); may have colobomas of other ocular structures

Table 5.2	Clinical presentations of toxocariasis		
	Chronic endophthalmitis	**Posterior pole granuloma**	**Peripheral granuloma**
Age range	2–9 years	6–14 years	6–40 years
Lesion	Exudation filling vitreous cavity, cyclitic membrane	Single localized granuloma in macula or peripapillary region	Peripheral granuloma with dense fibrotic strand, often to disc
Symptoms	Pain, photophobia, lacrimation, decreased vision, acute inflammation	Quiet eye, decreased vision, strabismus	Decreased vision, strabismus
Course	Often leads to destruction of globe	Nonprogressive	Nonprogressive

Table 5.3 Metabolic diseases with eye findings

Disease	Enzyme deficiency	Inheritance	Findings	Other findings
Sphingolipidoses				
GM2 gangliosidoses				
Type I (Tay-Sachs disease)	Hexosaminidase A	Autosomal recessive	Cherry red spot, optic atrophy, blindness, nystagmus, ophthalmoplegia	Normal at birth, motor deterioration starts at 3–5 months of age, rapid after 10 months; Death by 2–3 years
Type I (Sandhoff disease)	Hexosaminidase B	Autosomal recessive	Cherry red spot, optic atrophy, blindness	Death by 2–12 years
Type III (Bernheimer-Seitelberger disease)	Hexosaminidase A (partial)	Autosomal recessive	Optic atrophy, pigmentary retinopathy	Death by 15 years of age
GM1 gangliosidoses				
Type I (Landing disease)	β-Galactosidase A, B, and C	Autosomal recessive	Cherry red spots in 50%, optic atrophy, high myopia, blindness, subtle corneal clouding, nystagmus	Psychomotor delay present at birth with rapid neurologic deterioration and death by 2 years
Type II (Derry disease)	β-Galactosidase B and C	Autosomal recessive	RPE degeneration, possible optic atrophy, nystagmus, esotropia	Neurologic deterioration in first or second year of life, seizures, death between 3 and 10 years
Mucopolysaccharidoses (MPSs)				
MPS type I-H (Hurler)	α-Iduronidase	Autosomal recessive	Corneal clouding, RPE degeneration, optic atrophy, glaucoma	Onset between 6 and 24 months of age, gargoyles facies, mental retardation, dwarfism, skeletal dysplasia
MPS type I-S (Scheie)				Coarse facial features, clawlike hands, aortic valve disease
MPS type II (Hunter)	Iduronate sulfatase	X-linked recessive	RPE degeneration, optic atrophy	Similar to 1-H, less skeletal deformity
MPS type III (Sanfilippo)	4 types: A, B, C, D Heparan N-sulfatase; acetyl-CoA-glucosaminidase-N,N-acetyltransferase; N-acetylglucosamine-6-sulfate sulfatase	Autosomal recessive	RPE degeneration, optic atrophy	Mild dysmorphism, progressive dementia
MPS type IV (Morquio)	2 types: A, B galactose-6-sulfatase; β-galactosidase	Autosomal recessive	Corneal clouding, optic atrophy	Short trunk, dwarfism, skeletal deformities, aortic valve disease, normal mental development
MPS type VI (Maroteaux-Lamy)	Arylsulfatase B	Autosomal recessive	Corneal clouding, RPE degeneration, optic atrophy	Normal mental development, similar to 1-H
MPS type VII (Sly)	β-Glucuronidase	Autosomal recessive	Corneal clouding	Onset after 4 years of age, similar to 1-H
MPS type VIII (Diferrante)	Glucosamine-S-sulfate sulfatase	Autosomal recessive	Clear cornea	
Lipidoses				
Fabry disease	α-Galactosidase A	X-linked recessive	Whorl-like corneal changes, granular opacities of lens, tortuosity of retinal and conjunctival vessels	Systemic ischemia and infarction (cerebrovascular, cardiac, skin)
Metachromatic leukodystrophy	Arylsulfatase A	Autosomal recessive	Nystagmus, cherry red spot, optic atrophy	Weakness, mental deterioration, developmental delay, may be infantile, juvenile, or adult onset
Krabbe disease	Galactocerebrosidase	Autosomal recessive	Optic atrophy, blindness	Rapidly progressive and fatal, usually with infantile onset
Gaucher disease	β-Galactosidase	Autosomal recessive	RPE degeneration, EOM abnormalities	Hepatosplenomegaly, bone complications, neurologic deterioration
Niemann-Pick disease	Sphingomyelinase	Autosomal recessive	Corneal opacities, cherry red spot, lens opacities	Severity of disease varies depending on type, loss of motor and cognitive skills, splenomegaly
Others				
Cystinosis	Defective transport of cystine	Autosomal recessive	Corneal crystals, secondary photophobia and blepharospasm, RPE degeneration	Infantile and late-onset forms; renal failure (Fanconi syndrome), CNS damage
Galactosemia	Gal-1-UDP transferase	Autosomal recessive	Cataract (oil-drop)	Failure to thrive, hepatomegaly and liver dysfunction, developmental delay
Mannosidosis	α-Mannosidase	Autosomal recessive	Corneal clouding, lens opacification	Coarse features, hepatosplenomegaly, mental deterioration, hearing loss
Mucolipidoses II and III	Multiple lysosomal enzymes	Autosomal recessive	Corneal clouding	Coarse features, psychomotor retardation, organomegaly, cardiorespiratory problems
Refsum disease	Phytanic acid oxidase	Autosomal recessive	Retinal degeneration, optic disc pallor, cataracts	Peripheral neuropathy, cerebellar ataxia, elevated CSF protein
Adrenoleukodystrophy	Peroxisomal disorder	X-linked, autosomal recessive	Optic atrophy, RPE degeneration, strabismus	CNS demyelination, adrenal insufficiency, high long-chain fatty acid levels
Homocystinuria	Cystathionine synthase	Autosomal recessive	Dislocated lenses, optic atrophy, glaucoma	Osteoporosis, thromboembolic disease, seizures

CNS, Central nervous system; CSF, cerebrospinal fluid; EOM, extraocular muscle; RPE, retinal pigment epithelium.

Conjunctival telangiectasia: ataxia telangiectasia, Fabry disease

Glaucoma: MPS I-Scheie, Zellweger disease (rare)

Corneal opacity: MPS I, III, IV, VI; mucolipidoses III, IV; Fabry disease, sialidosis with chondrodystrophy, Cockayne disease, xeroderma pigmentosum, Zellweger disease (occasionally), Wilson disease (Kayser-Fleischer ring)

Lens opacity: Wilson disease, galactosemia, Marinesco-Sjögren syndrome, Lowe disease, cerebrocutaneous xanthomatosis, sialidosis, mannosidosis

Cherry red spot: Tay-Sachs disease, sialidosis, Niemann-Pick disease (50%), GM1 gangliosidosis (50%), Farber disease, multiple sulfatase deficiency (metachromatic leukodystrophy variant)

Macular and pigmentary degeneration: ceroid lipofuscinosis, MPS 1-H, 1-S, II, III; mucolipidoses IV, Refsum disease (phytanic acid lipidosis), Bassen-Kornzweig (abetalipoproteinemia), Kearns-Sayre syndrome

Optic atrophy: Krabbe disease, metachromatic leukodystrophy, sphingolipidoses, adrenoleukodystrophy, Alexander disease, spongy degeneration, Pelizaeus-Merzbacher disease, neuraxonal dystrophy, Alpers disease, spinocerebellar degeneration, diseases with retinal pigmentary degeneration

Nystagmus: diseases with poor vision (searching nystagmus), Pelizaeus-Merzbacher disease, metachromatic leukodystrophy, Friedreich ataxia, other spinocerebellar degenerations and cerebellar atrophies, neuraxonal dystrophy, ataxia telangiectasia, Leigh syndrome, Marinesco-Sjögren syndrome, opsoclonus-myoclonus syndrome, Chédiak-Higashi disease

Ophthalmoplegia: Leigh syndrome, Kearns-Sayre syndrome, Niemann-Pick variant with vertical ophthalmoplegia, Gaucher disease, Bassen-Kornzweig syndrome, ataxia-telangiectasia, Tangier disease

MPS, Mucopolysaccharidosis.

Retinopathy of Prematurity (Retrolental Fibroplasia)

Vasoproliferative retinopathy occurring almost exclusively in premature infants; occasionally in full-term infants

Risk factors: low birth weight (<1.5 kg; if <1.25 kg, 65% develop some degree of ROP) early gestational age (<33 weeks' gestation), supplemental oxygen (>50 days; controversial), complicated hospital course

Risk increases exponentially the more premature and the smaller the infant: <2 kg (4 pounds, 7 ounces), <36 weeks (at 36 weeks, nasal retina is completely vascularized; at 40 weeks, temporal retina is fully vascularized)

2 phases:

Acute: abnormal vessels develop in association with fibrous proliferation; >85%-90% spontaneously regress

Late: retinal detachment, temporal displacement of macula, severe vision loss; occurs in 15%

Classification: International Classification of ROP, Third Edition (ICROP 3); for each eye based on fundus examinationn

Zone: location of disease; 3 retinal zones centered on optic disc, disease location based on most posterior lesion (Fig. 5.10)

I: posterior pole, area enclosed by 60° diameter circle centered on optic disc

II: area between edge of zone I and circle centered on optic disc and tangent to nasal ora serrata

Posterior zone II is the region from edge of zone I extending 2 disc diameters into zone II

III: remaining crescent of temporal peripheral retina anterior to zone II

Notch: 1-2 clock hour lesion extending into more posterior zone

Stage: appearance of acute disease at avascular/vascular junction

1: demarcation line (flat, white) (Fig. 5.11)

2: ridge (elevated, pink/white) (Fig. 5.12)

3: extraretinal neovascular proliferation (Figs. 5.13 and 5.14)

4: partial RD (Fig. 5.15)

4A: fovea attached

4B: fovea detached

5: total RD

5A: optic disc visible; open-funnel detachment

5B: optic cisc not visible; closed-funnel detachment

5C: 5B with anterior segment changes (anterior lens displacement, marked AC shallowing, iridocorneolenticular adhesions, corneal opacification)

Extent: circumferential involvement in clock hours (30° sectors)

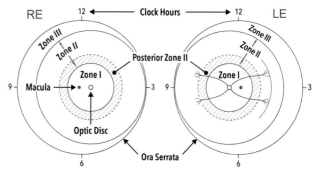

Figure 5.10 Schema of right eye (RE) and left eye (LE) showing zone borders and clock hour sectors used to describe the location of vascularization and extent of retinopathy. Solid circles represent borders of zones I through III, and dotted circles represent borders of posterior zone II (2 disc diameters beyond zone I). A hypothetical example of examination findings is shown in LE, representing approximately 3 clock hours of stage 1 disease in zone II (note single line on drawing to document presence of stage 1 disease). (Reproduced from Ophthalmology 2021;128:e51–e68)

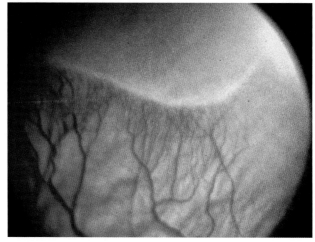

Figure 5.11 Stage 1 retinopathy of prematurity. The flat, white border between the avascular and vascular retina seen superiorly is called a *demarcation line.* (Reproduced from Earl A. Palmer, MD, and the Multicenter Trial of Cryotherapy for Retinopathy of Prematurity. From Yanoff M, Duker JS, eds. *Ophthalmology.* London: Mosby; 1999.)

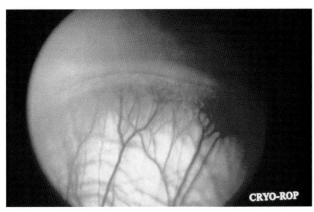

Figure 5.12 Stage 2 retinopathy of prematurity. The elevated mesenchymal ridge has height. Highly arborized blood vessels from the vascularized retina dive into the ridge. (Reproduced from Palmer EA, MD, and the Multicenter Trial of Cryotherapy for Retinopathy of Prematurity. From Yanoff M, Duker JS, eds. *Ophthalmology*. London: Mosby; 1999.)

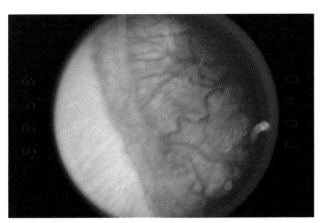

Figure 5.13 Stage 3 retinopathy of prematurity. Vessels on top of the ridge project into the vitreous cavity. The extraretinal proliferation carries with it a fibrovascular membrane. Note the opalescent avascular retina anterior to the ridge. (From Sears J, Capone A. Retinopathy of prematurity. In: Yanoff M, Duker JS, eds. *Ophthalmology*. London: Mosby; 1999.)

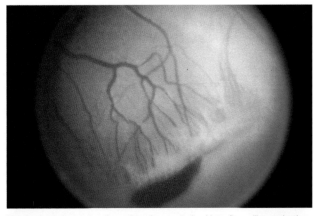

Figure 5.14 Stage 3 retinopathy of prematurity. Note finger-like projections of extraretinal vessels into the vitreous cavity. Hemorrhage on the ridge is not uncommon. (From Sears J, Capone A. Retinopathy of prematurity. In: Yanoff M, Duker JS, eds. *Ophthalmology*. London: Mosby; 1999.)

Acute disease represents continuous spectrum of vascular changes from normal to plus disease

No ROP: incomplete vascularization (specify zone)

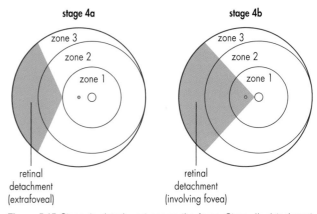

Figure 5.15 Stage 4a detachment spares the fovea. Stage 4b detachment involves the fovea. (From Sears J, Capone A. Retinopathy of prematurity. In: Yanoff M, Duker JS, eds. *Ophthalmology*. London: Mosby; 1999.)

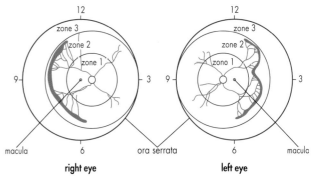

Figure 5.16 Definition of "threshold" retinopathy of prematurity. (From Sears J, Capone A. Retinopathy of prematurity. In: Yanoff M, Duker JS, eds. *Ophthalmology*. London: Mosby; 1999.)

Plus disease: severe vascular dilation and tortuosity in zone I; engorged, tortuous vessels around disc, vitreous haze, and iris vascular congestion; progressive vascular incompetence throughout eye; poor prognostic sign

Preplus disease: abnormal vascular dilation and/or tortuosity less severe than plus disease

Threshold disease: level at which 50% go blind without treatment = stage 3 in zone I or II with plus disease and at least 5 contiguous or 8 cumulative clock hours of involvement; usually develops at 27 weeks' gestational age (Fig. 5.16)

Prethreshold: approximately 1/3 progress to threshold disease
1. Zone I, any stage
2. Zone II, stage 2+ or 3
3. Zone II, stage 3+ for >5 clock hours

Aggressive ROP (A-ROP): previously termed aggressive-posterior ROP or rush disease; severe, rapidly progressive ROP; also occurs in larger preterm infants beyond posterior retina

Late phase:
Regression: disease involution and resolution; 1st signs are vascular (decreased plus disease, vascularization into peripheral avascular retina, tunica vasculosa lentis regression, better pupillary dilation, clearer ocular media, intraretinal hemorrhage resolution)

then ROP lesion regresses (thinning and whitening of neovascular tissue); can occur spontaneously or after treatment (laser photocoagulation or anti-VEGF injection), can begin as soon as 1-3 days following anti-VEGF injection, ~7-14 days after laser or spontaneous regression. Complete or incomplete (persistent avascular retina [PAR]): note location and extent. After spontaneous regression, PAR usually peripheral; after anti-VEGF treatment, PAR more frequent and extensive

Reactivation: recurrence of acute disease lesions and vascular changes after regression (incomplete or complete); note stage. Frequency after anti-VEGF rx > spontaneous regression >> laser (very rare) Usually occurs at 37-60 weeks postmenstrual age

Sequelae: late RD (tractional, rhegmatogenous, rarely exudative), retinoschisis (after chronic traction from regressed stage 3 ROP), PAR (with increased risk of retinal thinning, holes, lattice-like changes, and late RD), macular abnormalities (small foveal avascular zone, shallow or absent foveal depression), retinal vascular changes (tortuosity, straightening of arcades and macular dragging, falciform retinal fold, abnormal vessel branching, circumferential vascular arcades, telangiectasia, vitreous hemorrhage), secondary angle-closure glaucoma; can also occur in premature infants without acute ROP

DDx of peripheral vascular changes and retinal dragging: FEVR, incontinentia pigmenti (Bloch-Sulzberger syndrome), X-linked retinoschisis

DDx of temporally dragged disc: FEVR, *Toxocara*, congenital falciform fold

Diagnosis: screen infants <1500 g, on supplemental oxygen during first 7 days of life, or <30 weeks' gestation

Treatment: observation, laser, cryotherapy, anti–vascular endothelial growth factor (VEGF) injections, surgery

Cryotherapy for ROP (Cryo-ROP) Study: determined whether treatment for ROP would prevent poor outcomes (see accompanying box)

Treat with laser to peripheral avascular retina: when patient reaches type 1 ROP, defined as:
Zone I, any stage with plus disease
Zone I, stage 3 without plus disease
Zone II, stage 2 or 3 with plus disease
(Early Treatment for ROP [ETROP] Study)

Indirect argon green or diode laser photocoagulation: 500-μm spots to entire avascular retina in zone I and peripheral zone II (at least as effective as cryotherapy; Laser-ROP study)

Cryotherapy: to entire avascular retina in zone II, but not ridge (cryo-ROP study)

Anti-VEGF agents: intravitreal injection of 0.625 mg bevacizumab (Avastin; BEAT-ROP Study) or 0.1-0.25 mg ranibizumab (Lucentis; RAINBOW Study) for zone I, stage 3 plus disease. Aflibercept is being evaluated (Eylea; FIREFLEYE Study)

Serial exams: with type 2 ROP, defined as:
Zone I, stage 1 or 2
Zone II, stage 3

Surgery: vitrectomy with or without lensectomy, membrane peel, and possible scleral buckle for tractional retinal detachment (TRD) or RRD (cicatricial ROP, stages 4 and 5)

Complications:
Grade I-II: myopia (80%; caused by forward displacement of lens–iris diaphragm), anisometropia, strabismus, amblyopia, macular heterotopia, pseudo-XT (change in angle κ as a result of macular dragging from peripheral cicatrization), increased risk of retinal tear or RD

Grade III-V: nystagmus, glaucoma, cataracts, heterochromia irides, rubeosis iridis, anterior uveitis, RD, band keratopathy, phthisis bulbi

Prognosis: depends on extent of disease; most cases resolve spontaneously without visible residua

Some develop cicatricial changes: retrolental fibroplasia
GRADE I: myopia and peripheral glial scar (visual acuity [VA] >20/40)
GRADE II: dragged retina, macular heterotopia (VA 20/50–20/200)
GRADE III: retinal fold (VA <20/200)
GRADE IV: partial retrolental membrane and RD (VA = hand motion [HM] or light perception [LP])
GRADE V: complete retrolental membrane and RD (VA = LP or no light perception [NLP])

MAJOR CLINICAL STUDY

The Bevacizumab Eliminates the Angiogenic Threat of Retinopathy of Prematurity (BEAT-ROP) Study

Objective: To compare intravitreal bevacizumab to conventional laser therapy in cases of stage 3+ retinopathy of prematurity (ROP) with zone I or II posterior disease

Results: 150 infants (300 eyes) were enrolled; 143 infants survived to 54 weeks' postmenstrual age. Significantly higher rate of recurrence in zone I disease with conventional laser therapy compared with bevacizumab (42% vs. 6%). However, the rate of recurrence in zone II posterior disease did not differ significantly between the 2 groups (12% vs. 5%). There was also a difference in the timeline for recurrence between the 2 groups (16.0 ± 4.6 weeks for bevacizumab vs. 6.2 ± 5.7 weeks for laser therapy). There was no evidence of systemic or local toxicity

Conclusions: Intravitreal bevacizumab had a lower recurrence rate in infants with stage 3+ retinopathy of prematurity for zone I but not zone II disease compared with conventional laser therapy

131

Cryotherapy for ROP (Cryo-ROP) Study

Objective

To evaluate whether cryotherapy for ROP in preterm infants with birth weights <1251 g prevents unfavorable outcomes (posterior retinal fold, stage 4B or 5 retinal detachment, or VA of ≤20/200)

Results

The more posterior the zone and the greater the extent of stage 3+ ROP, the poorer the outcome

All unfavorable fundus structural outcomes and almost all unfavorable visual acuity outcomes occurred in eyes with zone I or II ROP and >6 sectors of stage 3+ disease

Fewer unfavorable outcomes occurred in treated versus control eyes (44.4% vs. 62.1% for VA; 27.2% vs. 47.9% for fundus status)

Retinal detachments remained stable in treated eyes (22%) but continued to occur in control eyes (from 38.6% at 5.5 years to 41.4% at 10 years)

After 10 years, treated eyes were much less likely than control eyes to be blind

Conclusions

Cryotherapy preserves visual acuity in eyes with threshold disease
Initial examination: 4-6 weeks after birth or at 30 weeks' gestational age (whichever is later), then every 2 weeks until vessels reach zone III
Prethreshold disease: examine every week until regression or threshold disease develops
Threshold disease: perform cryotherapy within 72 hours of diagnosis
Laser photocoagulation or cryotherapy to avascular retina, 90% regression rate
After 1 week, plus disease is usually less if treatment will work, fibrovascular proliferation often takes 2 weeks to begin regressing; consider retreatment if ROP is worse after 1 week; retreat untreated areas
Stage 4 disease: 60% reattachment rate with scleral buckle; 5% obtain useful vision
Stage 5 disease: vitrectomy (very poor success rate)

Early Treatment for Retinopathy of Prematurity (ETROP) Randomized Trial

Objective

To determine if early treatment with laser to avascular retina in high-risk prethreshold ROP results in better vision and anatomic outcomes vs conventional laser treatment

Results

307 eyes were randomized. "Unfavorable" visual outcomes were reduced by early treatment (19.5% vs. 14.5%); "unfavorable" anatomic outcomes were reduced with early treatment (15.6% vs. 9.1%) at 9 months

Conclusions

Early laser therapy for type1 ROP defined as zone I, any stage ROP with plus disease; zone I, stage 3 without plus; or zone II, stage 2 or 3 without plus disease. Observation for type 2 ROP defined as zone I, stage 1 or 2 without plus or zone II, stage 3 without plus disease

Familial Exudative Vitreoretinopathy (FEVR) (AD, AR, or X-Linked Recessive)

AD mapped to chromosome 11q13-q23 (*EVR1, FZD4, LRP5*), 11p13-p12 (*EVR3*); X-linked (*NDP*); AR (most severe form) gene not identified

Most are unaware that they have this disorder

Rare, progressive developmental abnormality of peripheral retinal vasculature (especially temporally)

Findings: similar to ROP (Figs. 5.17 and 5.18)
Stage 1: avascular peripheral retina, white without pressure, vitreous bands, peripheral cystoid degeneration, microaneurysms, telangiectasia, straightened vessels, vascular engorgement; may have strabismus or nystagmus; most asymptomatic; may progress to stage 2
Stage 2: fibrovascular proliferation with neovascularization, exudates, dragging of disc and macula, retinal folds and detachments; visual loss after 2nd or 3rd decade of life rare unless progression to stage 3
Stage 3: cicatrization with rhegmatogenous retinal detachments (10%–20%; usually in 3rd-4th decade of life), may develop proliferative vitreoretinopathy; prognosis poor

Treatment: prophylactic laser treatment to avascular retina (controversial); may require RD repair

Coats Disease (Leber Miliary Aneurysms)

Nonhereditary, proliferative exudative vascular disease

Spectrum of disease:
Leber miliary aneurysm: mild form, older patients, male = female, often bilateral
Coats disease: more severe form, males (10:1), bimodal distribution (peak in 1st decade of life and small peak in young adulthood [associated with hypercholesterolemia]), 80%-95% unilateral; 50% progressive

Findings: usually presents with leukocoria and strabismus; telangiectatic blood vessels leak (with large amount of

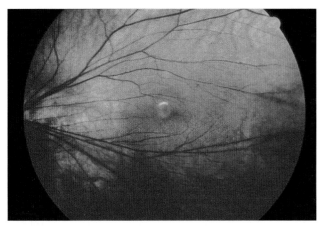

Figure 5.17 Fundus view of a patient who has familial exudative vitreoretinopathy. Note abnormally straightened retinal vasculature. (From Kimura AJ. Hereditary vitreoretinopathies. In: Yanoff M, Duker JS, eds. *Ophthalmology*. London: Mosby; 1999.)

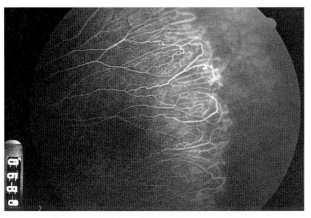

Figure 5.18 Fluorescein angiogram of a patient who has familial exudative vitreoretinopathy. (From Kimura AJ. Hereditary vitreoretinopathies. In: Yanoff M, Duker JS, eds. *Ophthalmology*. London: Mosby; 1999.)

subretinal lipid in outer plexiform layer), noncalcified yellow subretinal lesions, exudative RD in 66% (especially in patients <4 years old), microaneurysms, capillary nonperfusion

Staging: 2 methods
Gomez-Morales Staging:
Stage I: focal exudates
Stage II: massive exudation
Stage III: partial exudative RD
Stage IV: total RD
Stage V: complications
Spigelman Staging:
Stage I: telangiectasia only
Stage II: focal exudates
Stage III: partial exudative RD
Stage IV: total RD
Stage V: complications

Pathology: triad of retinal vascular anomalies, subretinal and intraretinal cholesterol deposits, and intraretinal periodic acid-Schiff (PAS)–positive deposits; loss of vascular endothelium and pericytes; gliotic retina over subretinal fluid with cholesterol clefts and hemosiderin-laden macrophages. Aspiration of subretinal exudates reveals cholesterol and pigment-laden macrophages

DDx: retinoblastoma, angiomatosis retinae (von Hippel–Lindau syndrome), PHPV

B-scan ultrasound: consider ruling out retinoblastoma

Fluorescein angiogram (FA): blood-fluid levels; saccular aneurysms ("light bulb" dilatations) of retinal arterioles and venules (Fig. 5.19)

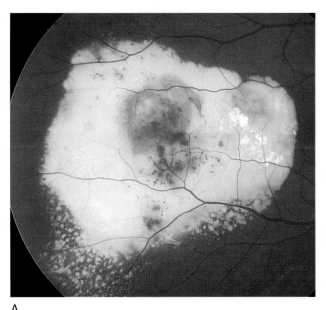

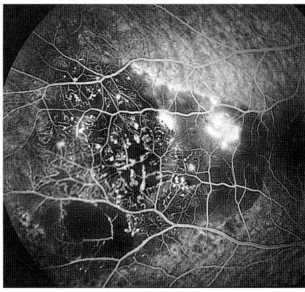

A   B

Figure 5.19 (A) The classic fundus picture of Coats disease with massive lipid exudation that causes an exudative retinal detachment. (B) Fluorescein angiogram from the same patient with large telangiectatic vessels and numerous leaking aneurysms. (From Mittra RA, Mieler WF, Pollack JS. Retinal arterial macroaneurysms. In: Yanoff M, Duker JS, eds. *Ophthalmology*. London: Mosby; 1999.)

Treatment: cryotherapy or laser to stop leaking blood vessels, intravitreal anti-VEGF agents for CME and massive exudation, consider surgery in severe cases

Prognosis: depends on stage; better for older age of presentation, poor if present before age 3 years

Norrie Disease (X-Linked Recessive)

Defect of retinal development

Mapped to chromosome Xp11.4-p11.3 *(NDP)*

Findings: bilateral leukocoria (white, often hemorrhagic retrolental mass), retinal dysplasia, peripheral neovascularization (NV), hemorrhagic RD, and retinal necrosis

Other findings: deafness, mental retardation

Shaken Baby Syndrome

30%-40% of children subjected to child abuse (non-accidental trauma) will have ophthalmic sequelae

Most common in children <3 years old

Findings: diffuse retinal hemorrhages, papilledema, vitreous hemorrhage, retinal tissue disruption (retinoschisis, retinal breaks, folds); may resemble central retinal vein occlusion (CRVO), Terson syndrome, or Purtscher retinopathy

Associated with other injuries: subdural hematoma, subarachnoid hemorrhage, bruises, fracture of long bones or ribs

Prognosis: poor because of macular scarring, vitreous hemorrhage, RD

Inherited Retinal Diseases

Fundus Flavimaculatus (AR)

Mapped to chromosome 1p21-p13 *(ABCA4)*

Findings: bilateral pisiform, yellow-white flecks at level of RPE

Predominantly involves peripheral retina with macula involved to a lesser degree; flecks, then macular degeneration

Central vision preserved until macula involved

Pathology: lipofuscin deposits within hypertrophied RPE cells

ERG: degree of abnormality correlates with amount of fundus involvement

Stargardt Disease

AR or less often AD; mapped to chromosomes 1p21-p22 *(STGD1; ABCA4,* typical form, AR), 4p *(STGD4,* AD), 6q14 *(STGD3, Stargardt-like macular dystrophy)*

Juvenile macular degeneration with flecks

Most common hereditary macular dystrophy

Onset in first 2 decades of life with decreased vision

Symptoms: decreased vision, nyctalopia

Findings: bilateral pisiform, yellow-white flecks at level of RPE; change with time (new ones appear, others disappear); beaten-metal appearance of fundus; foveal atrophy; bull's-eye maculopathy; may have salt-and-pepper pigmentary changes of peripheral retina (Fig. 5.20)

Pathology: RPE massively thickened by accumulation of lipofuscin, *ABCA4* localizes to the disc membranes in cone and rod outer segments; part of the retinoid cycle

FA: dark choroid (85%) resulting from accumulation of lipofuscin in RPE; areas of hyperfluorescence do not directly correspond to flecks; pigmentary changes in macula appear as window defects (Fig. 5.21)

Fundus autofluorescence (FAF): hyper-autofluorescence as a result of excessive lipofuscin accumulation in RPE; hypo in areas of RPE atrophy

ERG and EOG: normal or subnormal in widespread disease; delayed dark adaptation

Treatment: gene therapy being tested; vitamin A supplementation accelerates accumulation of lipofuscin

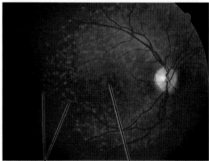

pisciform flecks   "bull's-eye" maculopathy

Figure 5.20 Stargardt disease. (From Kaiser PK, Friedman NJ, Pineda R II. *Massachusetts Eye and Ear Infirmary Illustrated Manual of Ophthalmology,* 2nd ed. Philadelphia: WB Saunders; 2004.)

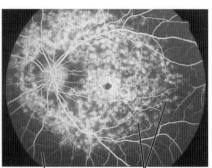

"silent" choroid   pisciform flecks

Figure 5.21 Fluorescein angiogram of Stargardt disease demonstrating dark choroid and hyperfluorescent pisiform flecks. (From Kaiser PK, Friedman NJ, Pineda R II. *Massachusetts Eye and Ear Infirmary Illustrated Manual of Ophthalmology,* 2nd ed. Philadelphia: WB Saunders; 2004.)

pigments in RPE. Long-term vitamin supplementation increases formation of vitamin A dimers, which favor lipofuscin synthesis and deposition. Therefore, avoid vitamin A supplementation

Prognosis: 50% have at least 20/40 vision in one eye by age 19; only 22% have 20/40 vision by age 39; rapid progression to 20/200—counting fingers (CF)

Best Disease (Vitelliform Dystrophy) (AD)

Variable penetrance; hereditary dystrophy mapped to chromosome 11q13 (*VMD2* [BEST1], encodes bestrophin1 located on basolateral aspect of RPE)

Second most common hereditary macular dystrophy

Progressive with onset in 1st decade of life

Macular dystrophy in which RPE is primarily affected; form of exudative central macular detachment in which pigmentation can occur in end stages with atrophic scarring and/or CNV

Associated with strabismus and hyperopia

Symptoms: none or mild decreased vision initially; later decreases to 20/30-20/100; better vision than expected by clinical appearance

Findings: progressive macular changes; can get CNV
Stage 1—Previtelliform stage: small round submacular yellow dot, subtle RPE changes; normal vision
Stage II—Vitelliform stage: yellow-orange egg yolk/fried egg appearance; can be multiple; usually between ages 3-15 (Fig. 5.22)
Stage III—Pseudohypopyon stage: layering of lipofuscin, RPE atrophy
Stage IV—Scrambled egg stage: irregular subretinal spots; vision usually still good
Stage V—Round chorioretinal atrophy stage: atrophic scar; vision usually stabilizes at 20/100
Stage VI—CNV stage: occurs in 20%

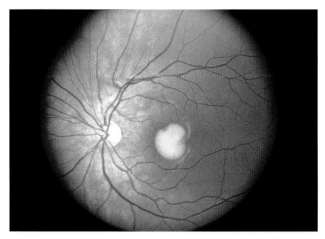

Figure 5.22 Best disease. Vitelliform stage. (Courtesy of Ola Sandgren, University Hospital of Umea, Sweden. From Parnell JR, Small KW. Macular dystrophies. In: Yanoff M, Duker JS, eds. *Ophthalmology*. London: Mosby; 1999.)

DDx: central serous chorioretinopathy, retinal pigment epithelial dystrophy (RPED), toxoplasmosis, macular coloboma, solar retinopathy, old foveal hemorrhage, adult foveomacular vitelliform dystrophy, syphilis, North Carolina dystrophy, AR bestrophinopathy, dominant drusen, age-related macular degeneration (AMD), macular hole, myopic degeneration

FA: blockage by egg yolk lesion; window defect when cyst ruptures

Optical coherence tomography (OCT): localizes vitelliform lesion, thickening of outer segments, evaluate for CNV

FAF: hyper-autofluorescence of lesion in early stages; mottled hypo during later stages; hypo in atrophic stage

ERG: normal

EOG: abnormal (Arden ratio ≤1.5; also in carriers)

Dark adaptation: normal

Prognosis: good vision (20/30–20/100 range)

Familial Drusen (Doyne Honeycomb Dystrophy) (AD)

Mapped to chromosome 2p16-p21 *(EFEMP1)*

Small yellow-white, round to oval deposits on Bruch membrane; decreased vision after age 40

Complications: macular edema, hemorrhage, CNV

Maternal Inherited Diabetes and Deafness (MIDD)

Mitochondrial disease (maternal inheritance); point mutation at position 3243 of maternal mtDNA

Eye findings occur in 5th decade of life with ptosis, external ophthalmoplegia, ragged red fibers in extraocular muscles, chorioretinal atrophy, iris atrophy, pigmentary retinopathy (annular perifoveal RPE atrophy in macula or pattern-type dystrophy appearance); associated with pattern dystrophies

VF: annular defect

FA: autofluorescence around dark pigment atrophy area

OCT: photoreceptor dropout

ERG: normal

North Carolina Macular Dystrophy (AD)

Mapped to chromosome 6q14-q16 *(MCDR1)*

Onset in 1st decade of life with drusen progressing to chorioretinal atrophy with staphyloma of macula (Fig. 5.23)

May develop CNV

ERG, EOG, and dark adaptation: normal

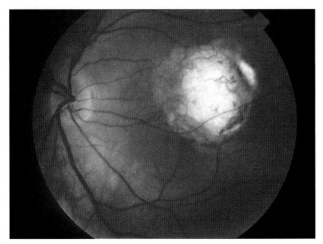

Figure 5.23 North Carolina macular dystrophy. (From Parnell JR, Small KW. Macular dystrophies. In: Yanoff M, Duker JS, eds. *Ophthalmology*. London: Mosby; 1999.)

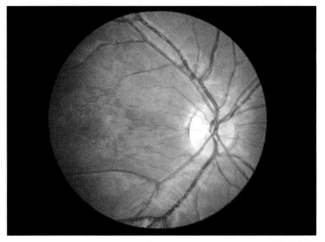

Figure 5.24 The "bull's-eye" maculopathy in this 5-year-old male who has a cone–rod dystrophy is not found in all cases of this entity. (From Sieving PA. Retinitis pigmentosa and related disorders. In: Yanoff M, Duker JS, eds. *Ophthalmology*. London: Mosby; 1999.)

Pseudoinflammatory Macular Dystrophy (Sorsby) (AD)

Mapped to chromosome 22q12-q13 *(SFD [TIMP-3])*

Atrophy, edema, hemorrhage, and exudate

Decreased acuity and color vision occurs between ages 40-50 years

ERG and EOG: subnormal late

Dark adaptation: delayed

Pattern Dystrophies (Usually AD)

Group of diseases with central pigmentary disturbance, good central vision, normal ERG, abnormal EOG

May develop CNV

Sjögren reticular dystrophy: fishnet configuration; fishnet is hypofluorescent on FA

Butterfly-shaped dystrophy: bilateral gray–yellow butterfly wing–shaped lesion with surrounding depigmentation; onset between ages 20-50 years with slightly reduced vision; mapped to chromosome 6p21 *(RDS [peripherin])*; butterfly lesion is hypofluorescent on FA

Adult onset foveomacular vitelliform dystrophy: onset between ages 30-50 years; early ringlike area of RPE clumping that develops into symmetric, solitary yellow macula lesions (like Best egg yolk lesions but smaller [½ DD in central fovea] and do not break up); often have central area of pigment; CNV is more common than in Best disease; normal EOG

Fundus pulverulentus: rarest form, coarse pigment mottling in macula; associated with pseudoxanthoma elasticum

Progressive cone dystrophy: AD or less often X-linked; mapped to chromosomes 6p21 *(COD3)*, Xp21 *(COD1 [RPGR])*, Xq27 *(COD2)*

Progressive dysfunction of cones with normal rod function

Onset during first 3 decades of life with decreased vision, dyschromatopsia, photophobia

Symptoms: visual loss, photophobia (usually precede visible macular changes)

Findings: decreased vision (to 20/200), decreased color vision, central scotoma, nystagmus (25%), nerve fiber layer (NFL) loss, optic atrophy, macular degeneration (granular appearance early, then beaten-metal appearance); can have fine, golden subretinal deposits, bull's-eye maculopathy (Fig. 5.24); can develop a pattern that mimics Stargardt or fundus flavimaculatus

VF: normal

FA: may show window defects early

ERG: absent photopic, normal scotopic

EOG: normal

Dark adaptation: rod phase only

Prognosis: poor vision (20/200 level) by 4th decade of life

Stationary Cone Disorders

Present at birth; nonprogressive

Complete rod monochromatism (congenital achromatopsia) (AR): mapped to chromosome 14 *(ACHM1)*; absent or abnormal cones; nonprogressive
> *Findings:* decreased vision (~20/200), complete color blindness, photophobia, nystagmus, normal retinal examination
> *VF:* central scotoma
> *ERG:* normal scotopic, abnormal photopic

Blue cone monochromatism (X-linked recessive): have only blue-sensitive cones
> *Findings:* decreased vision (20/40–20/200), photoaversion, nystagmus
> *ERG:* absent cone response, normal rod response

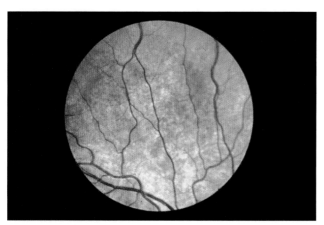

Figure 5.25 Rubella retinopathy. (Courtesy of George S. Novalis, MD. From Hudson HL, Boyer DS, Martin DF, et al. Viral posterior uveitis. In: Yanoff M, Duker JS, eds. *Ophthalmology*. London: Mosby; 1999.)

Infections

Congenital Rubella Syndrome

Fetus infected from maternal viremia; may cause spontaneous abortion, stillbirth, severe malformations

Congenital defects include deafness, cardiac and ocular abnormalities

Findings: pigmentary retinopathy (25%–50%; salt-and-pepper fundus, unilateral or bilateral), cataracts (15%), glaucoma (10%), microphthalmia, strabismus, corneal opacity; rare to have both cataract and glaucoma (Fig. 5.25)

Other findings: sensorineural hearing loss, patent ductus arteriosus, interventricular septal defects, pulmonary stenosis

Vision and electrophysiologic testing are usually normal

Live virus in an infant is found in the lens, as well as conjunctival swab, pharyngeal swab, and urine cultures

Rubella (German measles): acquired infection causes fever, malaise, rash, and eye findings including conjunctivitis (most common), keratitis, and retinitis (acute decreased vision, multifocal chorioretinitis with exudative RDs, AC, and vitreous cells)

Measles

Pigmentary retinopathy resulting from infection with rubeola virus acquired in utero

Acute blindness 6-12 days after measles rash appears

Findings:
Congenital infection: bilateral pigmentary retinopathy with retinal edema, vascular attenuation, macular star, no hemorrhages, cataract, ON head drusen
Acquired infection: fever, cough, runny nose, conjunctivitis, and Koplik spots (small gray-white spots on buccal mucosa opposite lower molars during prodromal phase); 3-5 days later, develop rash. Most infants recover, *may* develop keratitis or severe visual loss 6-12 days after the rash caused by retinopathy (similar to

congenital but also with acute retinal hemorrhages and optic disc edema, then late pigmentary changes [bone spicule or salt-and-pepper appearance]) and optic atrophy. Vision may improve over weeks to months as retinopathy resolves.

Complications: hearing loss, pneumonia, seizures, hepatitis, encephalitis
Subacute sclerosing panencephalitis (SSPE): rare complication of acquired measles occurring in late childhood/adolescence (~6–8 years after infection) with decreased vision, behavior and cognitive changes, seizures, myoclonus, paresis, dementia, and death within 3 years. Eye findings in 50% including focal retinitis with macular edema and RPE changes (36%), optic disc edema, papilledema, optic atrophy, exudative RD, drusen, epiretinal membrane, macular hole, cortical blindness, hemianopia, nystagmus, ptosis. Pathology shows eosinophilic nuclear inclusionns in neuronal and glial cells

Labs: usually not necessary, but virus detected from nasopharynx, conjunctiva, mucous membranes, urine, and blood before and several days after rash; serology tests (complement fixation, ELISA, immunofluorescent and hemagglutination inhibition assays)

VF: may have constriction, ring scotoma, peripheral islands

ERG: extinguished in acute retinopathy, may improve as inflammation resolves

Treatment: supportive; may require treatment of conjunctivitis or keratitis; consider systemic steroids for acute retinopathy. Consider prophylactic treatment with gamma globulin (0.25 mL/kg) for high-risk individuals (pregnant women, children age <1 year old, immunocompromised patients) within 5 days of exposure.

Zika Virus

Congenital Zika syndrome from Zika virus (ZIKV) causes neurologic, skeletal, ocular, and hearing abnormalities

Findings: usually bilateral and more common in infants with severe microcephaly; focal pigment mottling and chorioretinal atrophy, may also have retinal hemorrhages, microphthalmia, iris coloboma, lens subluxation, cataracts, glaucoma, ON hypoplasia, optic atrophy. Severe visual loss is common, and many develop strabismus and nystagmus

Metabolic Diseases

Mucopolysaccharidoses (AR Except Hunter [X-Linked Recessive])

Accumulation of acid mucopolysaccharides as a result of lysosomal enzyme defects

Syndromes in which heparin sulfate accumulates are associated with pigmentary retinopathy

Findings: may have corneal clouding (stromal; progressive), retinopathy (RPE degeneration), and/or optic atrophy (see Table 5.3)

> *Corneal clouding and retinopathy:* Hurler (type Ia), Scheie (type Ib), Maroteaux-Lamy (type VI)
> *Retinopathy only:* Hunter (type II), Sanfilippo (type III)
> *Corneal clouding only:* Morquio (type IV), Sly (type VII)
> *No corneal clouding or retinopathy:* Sly (type VII)

Sphingolipidoses (AR)

Accumulation of sphingolipids as a result of lysosomal enzyme defects

Sphingolipids accumulate in retinal ganglion cells; result in cherry red spot (macula has highest concentration of ganglion cells) (see Table 5.3)

Cherry red spot: Tay-Sachs, Sandhoff, Niemann-Pick, and Gaucher disease

> *Tay-Sachs:* most common; hexosaminidase A deficiency; death by 3 years of age; cherry red spot and mental retardation
> *Sandhoff:* similar to Tay-Sachs; extensive visceral involvement
> *Niemann-Pick:* cherry red spot, macular halo, optic atrophy; hepatosplenomegaly, infiltration of lungs, foam cells in bone marrow, no mental retardation

DDx of cherry red spot: CRAO, commotio retinae, macular hole, macular hemorrhage, ocular ischemic syndrome, subacute sclerosing panencephalitis, quinine toxicity, methanol toxicity

No cherry red spot: Fabry and Krabbe diseases

> *Fabry* (X-linked dominant): α-galactosidase A deficiency; accumulation of trihexosylceramide in smooth muscle of blood vessels
> > **FINDINGS:** cornea verticillata (whorl-like opacities in basal epithelium), tortuous conjunctival and retinal vessels, cataracts (posterior lenticular spokelike changes); manifest in heterozygous females (carriers) and 90% of affected males
> > **OTHER FINDINGS:** paresthesias in extremities, cutaneous telangiectases, angiokeratomas, poor temperature regulation, abdominal pain, anemia, renal failure, hypertension; vascular anomalies of heart, kidney, and brain; renal failure is leading cause of death
> > **DIAGNOSIS:** failure to detect α-galactosidase in tears

Cystinosis

Mapped to chromosome 17p13

Amino acid disorder; lysosomes cannot excrete cystine

Findings: iridescent fusiform cystine crystals in conjunctiva, cornea, iris, lens, and retina; photophobia

> *Infantile form* (nephropathic form) (AR): Fanconi syndrome: polyuria, growth retardation, rickets, progressive renal failure, salt-and-pepper fundus

changes (but no visual disturbance); the only form with retinopathy; most die before puberty

> *Adolescent form* (AR): less severe nephropathy than in Fanconi syndrome
> *Adult form:* benign; no renal problems; deposits limited to anterior segment

Treatment: cysteamine (systemically for renal disease, topically for corneal crystals)

Long-Chain 3-Hydroxyacyl-CoA Dehydrogenase (LCHAD) Deficiency

Disorder of mitochondrial fatty acid beta-oxidation resulting from mutation of guanine to cytosine at position 1528

Findings: normal fundus at birth, followed by RPE pigment dispersion; eventually develop chorioretinal atrophy and occlusion of choroidal vessels; deterioration of central vision; may have posterior staphylomas, developmental cataracts, progressive myopia

Treatment: low-fat, high-carbohydrate diet with carnitine supplementation

Prognosis: usually fatal by 2 years of age (hepatic or cardiorespiratory failure) unless dietary treatment is started

Tapetoretinal Degeneration

Processes that involve the outer half of the retina (photoreceptor/RPE); RPE = tapetum nigran (black carpet)

Leber Congenital Amaurosis (AR)

Group of hereditary disorders, LCA 1–17 mapped to multiple chromosomes and genes:

LCA 1 (17p13.1, *GUCY2D*), LCA 2 (1p31, *RPE65*), LCA 3 (14q31.1, *SPATA7*), LCA 4 (17p13.1, *AILP1*), LCA 5 (6q11-q16, *LCA5*), LCA 6 (14q11, *RPGRIP1*), LCA 7 (19q13.3, *CRX*), LCA 8 (1q13.1, *CRB1*), LCA 9 (1p36), LCA 10 (6q21.3, *CEP290*), LCA 11 (7q31.3-q32, *IMPDH1*), LCA 12 (1q32.3, *RD3*), LCA 13 (14q23.3, *RDH12*), LCA 14 (4q32.1, *LRAT*), LCA 15 (6p21.31, *TULP1*), LCA 16 (2q37.1, *KCNJ13*), LCA 17 (8q22.1, *GDF6*; 14q22.3, *OTX2*; 1p36.22, *NMNAT1*; 11q13, *CABP4*; 3q, *IQCB1*, *MERTK1*)

Blind or severe visual impairment in infancy or early childhood; responsible for ~10% of childhood blindness

Associations: keratoconus, hyperopia, cataract, macular coloboma, mental retardation, deafness, seizures, renal and musculoskeletal abnormalities

Findings: decreased vision (20/40 to NLP, most have 20/200 to CF), nystagmus, hyperopia, poorly reactive pupils, nyctalopia, photophobia (50%), range of fundus appearance from normal (most common) to variety of pigmentary changes (granular, fleck, salt and pepper, sheen, RP-like, or atrophic)

Oculodigital sign: child rubs eyes to elicit entopic stimulation of retina

Pathology: diffuse absence of photoreceptors

VF: severely constricted

FAF: macular hypo-autofluorescence

OCT: retinal thinning with loss of outer nuclear layers, photoreceptors, and outer segments

ERG: low or completely flat

EOG: abnormal

Treatment: for patients with *RPE65* mutations consider gene replacement therapy with subretinal injection of voretigene neparvovec (Luxturna)

Retinitis Pigmentosa (RP)

Group of progressive dystrophies caused by abnormal photo-receptor protein production

Most common hereditary degeneration, incidence 1:5000

RP type I (rod–cone):
Inheritance patterns:
    AR (37%): most common form; may result from defects in 2 RPE genes (which provide instructions for vitamin A transport proteins): *RPE 65, CRALBP*
    X-LINKED RECESSIVE (4%): rarest and most severe form; poor prognosis; vision <20/100 by 3rd decade of life; carriers may have fundus changes
    AD (20%): least severe form, later onset; most likely to retain good vision
    SPORADIC (30%–50%)
Associations: keratoconus, macular cystoid degeneration, Coats disease, optic disc drusen, astrocytic hamartoma of ON, myopia
Symptoms: nyctalopia, "blue blindness," decreased vision late
Findings: pigmentary retinal changes (bone spicules), attenuated arteries, waxy pallor of ON (resulting from glial membrane formation over disc), retinal atrophy with increased visibility of choroidal vessels, vitreous cells, cataract; some forms can have prominent subretinal exudation (Coats-like disease) (Fig. 5.26)
Pathology: photoreceptor atrophy including outer nuclear layer; inner retina well preserved; RPE cells invade retina and surround retinal vessels (bone spicules)
VF: inferotemporal scotoma, enlarges to form ring/annular scotoma; constricted
ERG: early, increased rod threshold with normal cone response and decreased scotopic b-wave; late, nonrecordable; abnormalities precede retinal changes and visual complaints
EOG: abnormal
Dark adaptation: prolonged

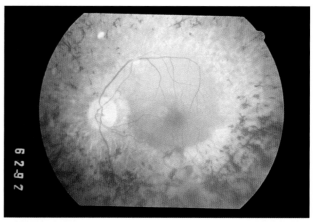

Figure 5.26 "Typical" retinitis pigmentosa changes. (From Sieving PA. Retinitis pigmentosa and related disorders. In: Yanoff M, Duker JS, eds. *Ophthalmology*. London: Mosby; 1999.)

RP carriers:
    FUNDUS: bone spicules, salt-and-pepper changes, bronze sheen in macula
    ERG: decreased scotopic amplitude and delayed cone b-wave implicit time in X-linked carriers
    VITREOUS FLUOROPHOTOMETRY: abnormal in X-linked carriers
DDx of tunnel vision: glaucoma, functional, gyrate atrophy, vitamin A toxicity, occipital lobe stroke
DDx of nyctalopia: uncorrected myopia, vitamin A deficiency, zinc deficiency, choroideremia, gyrate atrophy, CSNB, Goldman-Favre disease
DDx of salt-and-pepper fundus: rubella retinopathy, Leber congenital amaurosis, carrier states (albinism, RP, choroideremia), syphilis, cystinosis, phenothiazine toxicity, pattern dystrophy, following resolution of an exudative RD
Macular complications: CME (no leakage on FA), epiretinal membrane, atrophy

RP type II (cone–rod): AD, AR, or X-linked
Findings: less pigment deposition; 50% are sine pigmento
ERG: cones more affected than rods

Treatment: low-vision aids, dark glasses; vitamin A slows reduction of ERG (controversial)

Prognosis: poor

RP Variants

Treatable RP: Bassen-Kornzweig (abetalipoproteinemia), Refsum (elevated phytanic acid), gyrate atrophy (elevated ornithine)

Sector RP (AD or AR): retinal changes limited to focal area, usually inferonasal quadrant
    VF: abnormal
    ERG: abnormal; normal b-wave implicit time reflects nonprogression
    Prognosis: good

Unilateral RP: very rare

Inverse RP: posterior pole affected (rather than midperiphery): bone spicules in macula, normal periphery
FA: dark choroid (probably a variant of Stargardt)

Retinitis punctata albescens (AR): small white spots in midperiphery of retina, no bone spicules

RP sine pigmento: no retinal pigmentary changes

Pseudoretinitis pigmentosa: migration of RPE melanin into sensory retina leading to bone spicule pattern
Etiology: trauma, drug toxicity (chloroquine, chlorpromazine), infection/inflammation (syphilis, toxoplasmosis, measles, rubella), post–CRVO, resolved exudative RD, ophthalmic artery occlusion

RP Syndromes

Usher syndrome (AR): most common syndrome associated with RP; mapped to multiple chromosomes and genes: USH1A (14q32), USH1B (11Q13.5, *MYO7A*), USH1C (11p15.1, *USH1C*), USH1D (10q22.1, *CDH23*), USH1E (21q21), USH1F (10q21.1, *PCDH15*), USH1G (17q25.1, *USH1G*), USH1J (15q25.1, *CIB2*), USH2A (1q41, *USH2A*), USH2B (3p24.2-p23), USH2C (5q14.3, *GPR98*), USH2D (9q32, *DFNB31*), USH3A (3q25.1, *CLRN1*), USH3B (20q), USH3-like (2p11.21, *ABHD12*; 5q31.3, *HARS*)
Findings: RP and deafness; ataxia, low phosphate (rickets), muscle wasting, 10%-20% of patients with RP are deaf; 5% of congenitally deaf individuals have Usher type I; most develop cataracts by age 40; 25% have mental retardation or psychosis
TYPE I (75%): night blindness (1st-2nd decade of life), profound deafness, unintelligible speech, ataxia
TYPE II (23%): night blindness (2nd-4th decade of life), partial deafness, intelligible speech, no ataxia
TYPE III (2%; Hallgren syndrome): night blindness, progressive deafness, ataxia; 42% of Usher in Finland
TYPE IV: deafness and mental retardation
Note: controversial if types III and IV are forms of Usher syndrome or separate entities
DDx of deafness and RP: Usher, Hallgren, Alstrom, Laurence-Moon-Biedl-Bardet, and Cockayne syndromes
Other eye syndromes associated with hearing loss: Cogan (IK plus hearing loss), Stickler (vitreous changes, joint and orofacial abnormalities, hearing loss), Waardenburg-Klein (iris heterochromia, white forelock), Duane (15% have hearing loss)

Refsum disease (AR): deficiency of phytanic acid oxidase interferes with fatty acid metabolism

Phytanic acid accumulates in RPE cells, sensory retina deteriorates; onset in childhood

Mapped to chromosomes 7q21-q22 (*PEX1*), 10p15-p12 (*PNYH*)
Findings: atypical RP (often sine pigmento or starts in macula), cataracts, prominent corneal nerves

Other findings: ataxia, peripheral neuropathy, deafness, anosmia, ichthyosis, cardiac abnormalities, hypotonia, hepatomegaly, mental retardation
Diagnosis: increased serum copper and ceruloplasmin; increased cerebrospinal fluid (CSF) protein without pleocytosis
Treatment: dietary restriction of animal fats, milk products, leafy green vegetables

Bassen-Kornzweig syndrome (AR): hereditary abetalipoproteinemia; mapped to chromosome 4q24 *(MTP)*

Inability to transport and absorb lipids because apolipoprotein B is a major protein of chylomicrons; deficiency in fat-soluble vitamins (A, D, E, and K)
Findings: RP (usually without bone spicules); may have Bitot spots on conjunctiva
Other findings: ataxic neuropathy, growth retardation, coagulopathy
Diagnosis: CBC, cholesterol (low), stool sample; elevated CSF protein; no apolipoprotein B-48 (low chylomicrons) or apolipoprotein B-100 (low low-density lipoprotein [LDL] and very low-density lipoprotein [VLDL])
Treatment: vitamin A and E supplements
Other causes of treatable RP resulting from vitamin A deficiency: chronic pancreatitis, cirrhosis, bowel resection

Bardet-Biedl syndrome (AR): types 1-18 mapped to multiple chromosomes and genes; 2 syndromes:
Bardet-Biedl: polydactyly (75%), syndactyly (14%) (Fig. 5.27)
Lawrence-Moon: spastic paraplegia, no polydactyly/ syndactyly
Findings: both have pigmentary retinopathy (flat ERG), short stature, congenital obesity (above 95th percentile), hypogenitalism (74%–96%; sterility in males), partial deafness (5%), renal abnormalities (46%–95%), and mental retardation (41%–85%); nystagmus in 5% of patients with Bardet-Biedl syndrome, may also have posterior cortical and precapsular cataracts, myopia, gaze limitation, short and narrow palpebral fissures,

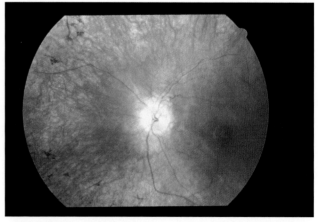

Figure 5.27 Bardet-Biedl syndrome with extensive peripheral retinal pigment epithelium and parafoveal retinal pigment epithelium atrophy. (From Sieving PA. Retinitis pigmentosa and related disorders. In: Yanoff M, Duker JS, eds. *Ophthalmology*. London: Mosby; 1999.)

pigmentary vitreous syneresis, macular edema, and diffuse secondary optic atrophy

Chronic progressive external ophthalmoplegia (CPEO): mitochondrial inheritance; 50% with positive family history

Findings: pigmentary retinopathy (salt-and-pepper changes with normal retinal function; progresses to RP-like disease), ptosis, ophthalmoplegia, strabismus

Other findings: facial weakness, dysphagia, small stature, limb girdle myopathy, cardiac conduction defects (Kearns-Sayre syndrome)

Olivopontocerebellar atrophy: retinal degeneration; tremors, ataxia, dysarthria

Alstrom disease: mapped to chromosome 2p13 *(ALMS1)*

RP with profound visual loss in 1st decade of life; diabetes, obesity, deafness, renal failure, baldness, acanthosis nigricans, hypogenitalism

Cockayne syndrome: RP with profound visual loss by 2nd decade of life; dwarfism, deafness, mental retardation, premature aging, psychosis, intracranial calcifications

Neuronal ceroid lipofuscinoses (AR): pigmentary retinopathy associated with seizures, dementia, ataxia, mental retardation; mapped to chromosomes 1p32 *(CLN1)*, 11p15.5 *(CLN2)*, 16p12.1 *(CLN3)*. 4 types:

Infantile (onset 6 months to 2 years): Hagberg-Santavuori syndrome; usually death in infancy or early childhood; blindness, may have cataracts; seizures, rapid mental and physical decline

Late infantile (onset 2–4 years): Jansky Bielschowsky; usually death in 1st decade of life or early teenage years

Juvenile (onset before 40 years): Vogt-Spielmeyer and Batten; most die in 3rd decade of life; blindness, amaurotic pupils, bull's-eye macular lesion, and retinal vessel attenuation; seizures, dementia, loss of speech and motor skills

Adult (onset after 40 years): Kufs; variable life expectancy; no blindness; milder and slower mental and physical decline

Central Areolar Choroidal Dystrophy (AD)

Mapped to chromosome 6p *(PRPH2)*, and less commonly 17p13 *(CACD)*

Decreased vision in 4th decade of life

Findings: RPE mottling in macula progressing to geographic atrophy (choroidal vessels visible) (Figs. 5.28 and 5.29)

FA: window defect of central lesion

ERG: normal or subnormal

EOG, dark adaptation: normal

Bietti Crystalline Retinopathy (AR)

Decreased vision in 5th decade of life

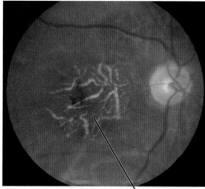

central areolar choroidal dystrophy

Figure 5.28 Central geographic atrophy in a patient with central areolar choroidal dystrophy. (From Kaiser PK, Friedman NJ, Pineda R II. *Massachusetts Eye and Ear Infirmary Illustrated Manual of Ophthalmology*, 2nd ed. Philadelphia: WB Saunders; 2004.)

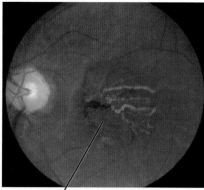

central areolar choroidal dystrophy

Figure 5.29 Left eye of same patient as shown in Figure 5.27 demonstrating similar central geographic atrophy. (From Kaiser PK, Friedman NJ, Pineda R II. *Massachusetts Eye and Ear Infirmary Illustrated Manual of Ophthalmology*, 2nd ed. Philadelphia: WB Saunders; 2004.)

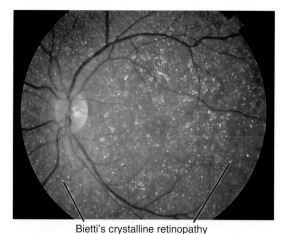

Bietti's crystalline retinopathy

Figure 5.30 Bietti crystalline retinopathy. (From Kaiser PK, Friedman NJ, Pineda R II. *Massachusetts Eye and Ear Infirmary Illustrated Manual of Ophthalmology*, 2nd ed. Philadelphia: WB Saunders; 2004.)

Findings: yellow-white refractile spots throughout fundus, geographic atrophy; may have crystals in peripheral corneal stroma (Fig. 5.30)

FA: crystals hyperfluoresce, window defects and areas of blockage

ERG: reduced

Congenital Stationary Night Blindness (CSNB)

Poor night vision (nyctalopia)

Group of nonprogressive rod disorders classified by fundus appearance

Findings: normal vision, VF, and color vision; may show paradoxical pupillary dilation to light; no Purkinje shift (always most sensitive to 550 nm)

ERG: scotopic and photopic implicit times are identical; decreased scotopic ERG; photopic ERG almost normal

Normal fundus:

Nougaret type (AD): no rod function; mapped to chromosome 3p21 *(GNAT1)*
Riggs type (AR): some rod function
Schubert-Bornschein type (X-linked or AR): some or no rod function, myopia

Abnormal fundus:

Fundus albipunctatus (AR): mapped to chromosome 12q13-q14
    FINDINGS: midperipheral deep yellow-white spots spare macula (Fig. 5.31)
    ERG: normalization of scotopic after 4 to 8 hours of dark adaptation
    ALPORT SYNDROME (AD): kidney failure, deafness, anterior lenticonus with anterior polar cataract; may have retinal appearance similar to fundus albipunctatus
Oguchi disease: mapped to chromosomes 2q37 *(Oguchi 1, Arrestin, SAG),* 13q34 *(Oguchi 2 [RHOK])*

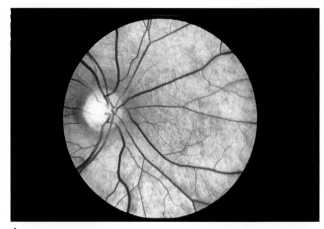

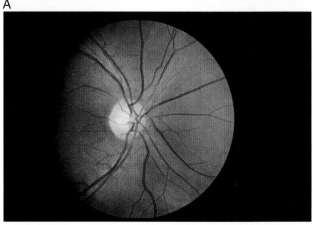

A

B

Figure 5.32 Oguchi disease. (A) The yellowish metallic sheen is apparent nasal to the optic disc. (B) After 3 hours of dark. (From Noble KG. Congenital stationary night blindness. In: Yanoff M, Duker JS, eds. *Ophthalmology*. London: Mosby; 1999.)

    MIZUO-NAKAMURA PHENOMENON: golden-brown fundus (yellow/gray sheen) in light-adapted state, normal-colored fundus in dark-adapted state (takes around 12 hours) (Fig. 5.32)
    ERG: absent b-wave; only scotopic a-wave
Kandori flecked retina (AR): yellow-white spots scattered in equatorial region; spares macula

Choroideremia (X-Linked Recessive)

Mapped to chromosome Xq21 *(CHM);* basic defect localized to the RPE (*not* the choriocapillaris as previously believed)

Progressive degeneration of the RPE and choriocapillaris; considered a form of rod–cone degeneration

Onset during late childhood with nyctalopia, photophobia, constricted visual fields in affected males

Findings: early—degeneration of RPE and choriocapillaris in periphery (scalloped RPE atrophy); late—absence of RPE and choriocapillaris except in macula (Fig. 5.33) Female carriers have salt-and-pepper fundus

Pathology: defect in choroidal vasculature

ERG: markedly reduced; undetectable late

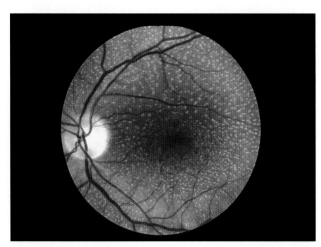

Figure 5.31 Fundus albipunctatus. This posterior pole and beyond show multiple small, discrete, round, white dots that spare the fovea. (From Noble KG. Congenital stationary night blindness. In: Yanoff M, Duker JS, eds. *Ophthalmology*. London: Mosby; 1999.)

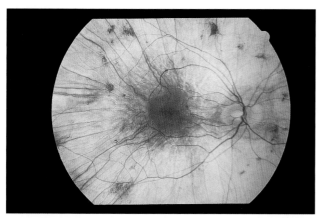

Figure 5.33 Fundus changes in the right eye from a patient with late-stage choroideremia. (From Grover S, Fishman GA. Choroidal dystrophies. In: Yanoff M, Duker JS, eds. *Ophthalmology*. London: Mosby; 1999.)

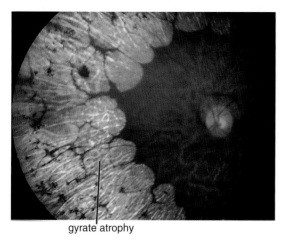

gyrate atrophy

Figure 5.34 Gyrate atrophy. (From Kaiser PK, Friedman NJ, Pineda R II. *Massachusetts Eye and Ear Infirmary Illustrated Manual of Ophthalmology*, 2nd ed. Philadelphia: WB Saunders; 2004.)

Gyrate Atrophy (AR)

Mapped to chromosome 10q26

Deficiency of ornithine aminotransferase; elevated ornithine levels (10–20 × normal), low lysine levels; chorioretinal dystrophy itself is not caused by high ornithine levels

Progressive retinal degeneration; starts peripherally and spreads toward posterior pole

Onset by 2nd decade of life with decreased vision, nyctalopia, and constricted visual fields

Findings: scalloped areas of absent choriocapillaris and RPE in periphery with abrupt transition between normal and atrophic areas (Fig. 5.34); generalized *hyperpigmentation* of remaining RPE (vs. choroideremia); eventually lose choriocapillaris and medium-size choroidal vessels; myopia (90%), cataracts, vitreous degeneration, CME

Other findings: seizures, structural changes in muscle and hair fibers

Diagnosis: blood tests (increased ornithine, decreased lysine), urinalysis (increased ornithine)

Carrier: decreased levels of ornithine ketoacid transaminase

ERG and ECG: abnormal

Dark adaptation: prolonged

Treatment: restrict arginine and protein in diet; consider vitamin B_6 supplementation (pyridoxine; reduces ornithine)

Vitreoretinal Dystrophies

Vitreous abnormalities associated with schisis cavity at level of NFL and ganglion cell layer

Juvenile Retinoschisis (X-Linked Recessive)

Mapped to chromosome Xp22 (*XLRS1* [retinoschisin])

Males; bilateral; present at birth; progresses rapidly during first 5 years of life; stable by age 20

Cleavage of retina at NFL (in senile retinoschisis, cleavage is at outer plexiform layer)

Findings: foveal retinoschisis (only abnormality in 50%, pathognomonic; earliest change is radial, spoke-like inner limiting membrane (ILM) folds centered on fovea because of dehiscence of NFL; appears like CME; later, cystoid structure appears in fovea with round microcysts in perifoveal area and marked pigmentary degeneration; bullous schisis cavities develop; retinal vessels are only remaining structure within inner layer and may bleed causing vitreous hemorrhage; also have marked sclerosis/sheathing of blood vessels with appearance of vitreous veils, vitreous cells (30%), true retinoschisis (NFL) in periphery in 50% (usually inferotemporal; does not extend to ora), vitreous syneresis, hyperopia, decreased vision (20/50–20/100)
Carriers have normal retinal appearance and function

VF: absolute scotoma

FA: microcysts with no leakage

ERG: normal a-wave until late, reduced b-wave (especially scotopic) in proportion to amount of retinoschisis, markedly reduced oscillatory potentials

EOG: normal

Complications: RD and vitreous hemorrhage (VH) (uncommon)

Goldmann-Favre disease (AR)

Mapped to chromosome 15q23 (*PNR*)

Rare, vitreotapetoretinal degeneration with nyctalopia and constricted visual fields (like RP plus juvenile retinoschisis)

Findings: decreased vision, nyctalopia, optically empty vitreous with strands and veils, bilateral central and peripheral retinoschisis, attenuated retinal vessels, peripheral bone–spicule retinal pigmentary changes, lattice degeneration, optic disc pallor, cataracts

ERG: markedly reduced

EOG: abnormal (distinguishes from juvenile retinoschisis)

Treatment: may require retinal surgery for retinal tears or detachments

Vitreoretinal Degenerations

Wagner Syndrome (AD)

Mapped to chromosomes 5q13-q14 *(WGN1)*, 12q13 *(COL2A1)*; also mutations in *VCAN* gene (encodes versican)

Findings: optically empty vitreous (abnormal vitreous structure; vitreous liquefaction and fibrillar condensation result in a clear vitreous space with membranes, veils, and strands), no RD, equatorial and perivascular pigmented lattice-like changes, peripheral vessel sheathing, RPE atrophy, cataract (wedge and fleck opacities between ages 20-40), moderate myopia, optic atrophy

ERG: may be abnormal

Treatment: cataract extraction; genetic counseling

Jansen Syndrome (AD)

Wagner syndrome + RD

Stickler Syndrome (AD)

Mapped to chromosomes 1p21 *(COL11A1)*, 6p21 *(COL11A2)*, 12q13 *(COL2A1)*

Progressive arthro-ophthalmopathy; Wagner-like ocular changes with severe myopia and marfanoid habitus

Findings: optically empty vitreous, lattice degeneration, RD (50%), optic atrophy, cataract, glaucoma, high degree of myopia (Fig. 5.35)

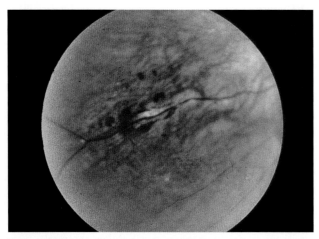

Figure 5.35 Fundus view of the eye of a Stickler syndrome patient. Note the radial perivascular pigmentary changes. (From Kimura AJ. Hereditary vitreoretinopathies. In: Yanoff M, Duker JS, eds. *Ophthalmology*. London: Mosby; 1999.)

Other findings: orofacial abnormalities (Pierre Robin anomaly: midfacial flattening and cleft palate), marfanoid habitus, hearing loss, mitral valve prolapse, joint abnormalities (hyperextensibility, enlargement, arthritis)

ERG: decreased b wave

Hereditary Arthro-Ophthalmopathy (Weill-Marchesani-Like Variety)

Similar to Stickler but short stature with stubby hands and feet; increased risk of ectopia lentis

Snowflake Degeneration (AD)

Very rare, progressive vitreoretinal degeneration

Manifests after 25 years of age

Findings: optically empty vitreous; associated with peripheral NV, increased risk of RD, early cataracts
  Stage 1: extensive white without pressure
  Stage 2: snowflakes (white dots in superficial retina) within white without pressure
  Stage 3: sheathing of retinal vessels and early peripheral pigmentation
  Stage 4: disappearance of retinal vessels in periphery and increased retinal pigmentation

ERG: decreased scotopic b-wave amplitude

EOG: normal

Dark adaptation: elevated rod threshold later in disease

Miscellaneous Retinal Disorders

Albinism

Albinoidism: only minimal reduction in vision; no nystagmus

Albinism: AR or less frequently AD disorder characterized by decreased melanin and congenitally subnormal vision (foveal hypoplasia and nystagmus)
  Oculocutaneous: lack of pigmentation of skin, hair, and eyes; increased risk of skin cancer
    TYROSINASE-NEGATIVE (OCULOCUTANEOUS ALBINISM [OCA] TYPE 1A; no pigmentation): mapped to chromosome 11q14.3 *(TYR)*
      FINDINGS: decreased vision (~20/200), iris transillumination, foveal hypoplasia, hypopigmented fundus, nystagmus, photophobia, high myopia, strabismus
      OTHER FINDINGS: hypopigmentation of skin and hair (white hair, pink skin)
    TYROSINASE-POSITIVE (OCA TYPE 2; some pigmentation): mapped to chromosome 15q12-q13.1 *(OCA2)* and 11q14-q21 *(TYR)* (paternal = Prader-Willi syndrome; maternal = Angelman syndrome)
      Ocular and systemic characteristics less severe (vision 20/40–20/200)

POTENTIALLY LETHAL VARIANTS:

CHÉDIAK-HIGASHI SYNDROME: large melanosomes on skin biopsy, reticuloendothelial dysfunction with pancytopenia, recurrent infections, and malignancies (leukemia, lymphoma)

HERMANSKY-PUDLAK SYNDROME: clotting disorder resulting from abnormal platelets, pulmonary fibrosis, commonly of Puerto Rican descent

Ocular: abnormal melanogenesis limited to eye (decreased number of melanosomes); X-linked recessive with variable phenotypic expression. Giant melanosomes in skin, normal pigmentation of skin, associated with deafness

FINDINGS: may have decreased vision (normal to 20/400), reduced or absent stereoacuity, and photophobia; congenital nystagmus, strabismus, high myopia, diffuse iris transillumination, foveal hypoplasia, fundus hypopigmentation, lack of retinal vessels wreathing the fovea, and abnormal decussation of ON fibers at the chiasm (only 10%–20% remain uncrossed); female carriers with variable retinal pigmentation (mosaic or "mud-splattered" pattern)

OCT: may have shallow or absent foveal pit and absent photoreceptor differentiation

ERG and EOG: supranormal

Table 5.4	Color vision abnormalities		
Type	**Genetics**	**Male**	**Female**
Deuteranomaly	X-linked recessive	5%	0.35%
Deuteranopia	X-linked recessive	1%	0.01%
Protonanomaly	X-linked recessive	1%	0.03%
Protonanopia	X-linked recessive	1%	0.01%
Tritanomaly	Autosomal dominant	0.0001%	0.0001%
Tritanopia	Autosomal recessive	0.001%	0.001%

Color Blindness/Deficiency (Tables 5.4 and 5.5)

Classification: normal individuals are trichromats, can match any color by mixing three primary colors (red, green, and blue)

3 types of cones: L (long-wavelength sensitive; red), M (middle-wavelength sensitive; green), S (short-wavelength sensitive; blue)

Congenital color blindness/deficiency caused by absence or abnormality of ≥1 photopigments

Prot = red; deuter = green; trit = blue (Greek for *first, second, third*; order in which these deficits were described)

Anopia = absent; anomaly = abnormal; An = unspecified

Congenital color vision defect is typically red–green; acquired color vision defect is typically blue–yellow (depends on location of lesion: outer retinal layer lesions and ocular media changes produce blue–yellow defect; inner retinal layer, ON, and visual pathways lesions produce red–green defect, main exception is glaucoma (blue–yellow defect); S cones most susceptible to sensitivity loss (occurs with increased blood glucose levels (diabetes) and glaucoma (test with SWAP [short-wavelength automated perimetry with blue flash on yellow background])

Congenital color vision defects do not cause decreased vision, except for red and blue cone monochromatism

Genetics: red–green disorders are X-linked recessive (male preponderance; chromosome Xq28 *OPN1LW* [opsin 1 long wave; encoding red sensitive pigment] and *OPN1MW* [opsin 1 middle wave; encoding green sensitive pigment]); incidence: 8% males, 0.5% females (Northern European ancestry); 3%-4% African males; 3%-6% Asian males; men and women can have tritan disorders (AD)

Blue–yellow disorders are linked to chromosome 7

Table 5.5	Comparison of dyschromatopsias	
Congenital dyschromatopsia	**Acquired dyschromatopsia**
Deuteranomalous trichromats are most common (5% of male population)	Ocular pathology, intracranial injury, medication
Usually red–green axis (protan or deutan)	Usually blue–yellow axis (tritan)
	Type 1 (red–green; similar to protan): progressive cone dystrophies, RPE dystrophies
	Type 2 (red–green; similar to deutan): optic neuritis, Leber optic atrophy, tobacco/toxic amblyopia, lesions of optic nerve and visual pathway, papillitis
	Type 3 (tritan): glaucoma, AMD, CSR, rod and rod–cone dystrophies, retinal detachment, retinal vascular occlusion, diabetic retinopathy, myopic degeneration, papilledema, autosomal dominant optic atrophy
Males > females	Females = males
Nonprogressive	May be slowly progressive
Bilateral and symmetric	Unilateral or a asymmetric
Normal eye examination (normal visual acuity and visual fields)	Associated with abnormality on eye examination (usually have decreased visual acuity and visual field defects)
X-linked recessive	No heritability
Deep blue is perceived as purple	Deep blue is perceived as gray

AMD, Age-related macular degeneration; *CSR,* central serous retinopathy; *RPE,* retinal pigment epithelium.

Anomalous trichromatism: all 3 cones present but one with abnormal proportions; photopigment (altered spectral sensitivity causing slight shift in maxima of absorption curve); difficulty distinguishing shades of colors, especially colors of low saturation

According to which pigment is abnormal, the disorders are called:

Protanomaly: abnormal red-sensitive pigment
Deuteranomaly: abnormal green-sensitive pigment
Tritanomaly: abnormal blue-sensitive pigment

Congenital dichromatism: absence of 1 type of color photopigment; severe color defects

Protanopia: absence of red-sensitive pigment (no functional L [red] cones)
Deuteranopia: absence of green-sensitive pigment (no functional M [green] cones)
Tritanopia: absence of blue-sensitive pigment (no functional S [blue] cones)

Monochromatism (achromatism): absence of 2 or 3 types of color photopigment; unable to distinguish colors; 2 forms of congenital dyschromatopsia associated with low vision:

Cone monochromatism (atypical achromatopsia; X-linked recessive): failure of 2 of the 3 cone cell photopigments to work; only one type of functional cone; can be red cone monochromatism, green cone monochromatism, or blue cone monochromatism (atypical achromatopsia; most severe form; nystagmus, decreased vision, photophobia, myopia; vision helped by magenta filter)
Rod monochromatism (achromatopsia; AR): no cones have functional photopigment and therefore complete achromatopsia. Linked to 5 genes: *CNGA3/ACHM2* on chromosome 2q11.2, *CNGB3/ACHM3* on chromosome 8q21.3, *GNAT2/ACHM4* on chromosome 1p13.3, *PDE6C/ACHM5/COD4* on chromosome 10q23.33, and *PDE6H* on chromosome 12p12.3; most cases from *CNGB3* mutations. Poor vision (<20/200 in complete form; as high as 20/80 in incomplete form) and nystagmus in infants, macular pigmentary changes (light fundus, granularity, bull's-eye maculopathy); vision helped by red filter
ERG: normal under scotopic conditions; reduced during photopic conditions

Tritan color defect and slightly subnormal vision: consider Kjer dominant optic atrophy

Diagnosis: color vision testing
Farnsworth-Munsell 100-hue test: consists of 85 hue caps contained in 4 separate racks with 2 end caps fixed; patient arranges caps between fixed ends in order of hue; tests for both red–green and blue–yellow defects
Farnsworth panel D-15: derived from 100-hue test, but uses only 15 caps
City university test: derived from 100-hue test, but uses 10 charts with a central color and 4 peripheral colors; select outer color that matches central color
Pseudoisochromatic plates: Ishihara plates (for protanopes and deuteranopes; detect only red–green defects), and

Hardy-Rand-Ritter (HRR) polychromatic plates (test for both red–green and blue–yellow defects)
Anomaloscope: tests severity of color blindness and distinguishes between dichromats and anomalous trichromats; based on Rayleigh match (adjust mixture of red and green light to match yellow light source) and may also include Moreland match (blue-green test for tritan defects)

Köllner's rule: errors made by persons with ON disease tend to resemble those made by protans and deutans (red and green), whereas errors made by individuals with retinal disease resemble those made by tritans (blue)

Retinal Tumors

Congenital Hypertrophy of the RPE (CHRPE)

Usually unilateral, congenital, asymptomatic

Findings: flat, well-circumscribed dark brown-black pigmented lesion with surrounding halo; larger lesions often contain depigmented lacunae (choroid visible through lacunae); multiple patches with sector distribution called "bear tracks" (Figs. 5.36 to 5.38)

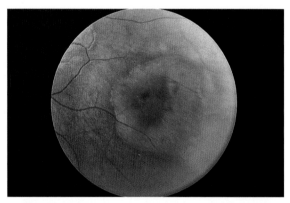

Figure 5.36 Typical congenital hypertrophy of retinal pigment epithelium. (From Augsburger JJ, Bolling JJ. Hypertrophy of retinal pigment epithelium. In: Yanoff M, Duker JS, eds. *Ophthalmology*. London: Mosby; 1999.)

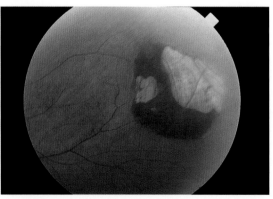

Figure 5.37 Congenital hypertrophy of retinal pigment epithelium with prominent depigmented lacunae. (From Augsburger JJ, Bolling JJ. Hypertrophy of retinal pigment epithelium. In: Yanoff M, Duker JS, eds. *Ophthalmology*. London: Mosby; 1999.)

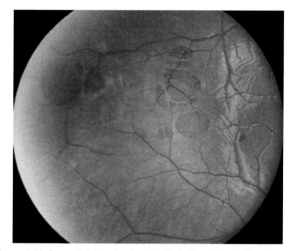

Figure 5.38 Congenital hypertrophy of retinal pigment epithelium (grouped by pigmentation of retina). (From Augsburger JJ, Bolling JJ. Hypertrophy of retinal pigment epithelium. In: Yanoff M, Duker JS, eds. *Ophthalmology*, 2nd ed. Philadelphia: WB Saunders; 2004.)

Pathology: melanosomes in RPE cells are larger and more spherical than normal; densely packed round melanocytes and increased thickness of RPE; focal areas of RPE loss (lacunae)

Atypical multifocal bilateral variant: >4 lesions; occurs in 75% of patients with **familial adenomatous polyposis** (FAP: AD, mapped to chromosome 5q; high incidence of multiple adenomas of colon and rectum; eventually undergo malignant transformation; Gardner syndrome [variant of FAP]: combination of colonic polyps and extracolonic manifestations [osteomas, dermoid tumors])

DDx: (Box 5.3)

Retinoblastoma (RB)

Most common intraocular malignancy in children

Box 5.3 DDx of congenital hypertrophy of the retinal pigment epithelium
Reactive hyperplasia of retinal pigment epithelium
Massive gliosis of retina
Combined hamartoma of retina
Melanotic choroidal nevus or melanoma
Bilateral diffuse uveal melanocytic proliferation associated with systemic carcinoma syndrome
Adenoma or adenocarcinoma of retinal pigment epithelium
Metastatic melanoma to retina
(From Augsburger JJ, Bolling JJ. Hypertrophy of retinal pigment epithelium. In: Yanoff M, Duker JS, eds. Ophthalmology. London: Mosby; 1999.)

Incidence 1 in 15,000-20,000; no sex or race predilection

90% diagnosed by 5 years of age; 30% bilateral, 30% multifocal

Genetics: (Table 5.6)

Mapped to chromosome 13q14 *(RB1)*, must have gene defect on both chromosomes

Sporadic in 96% (75% somatic, 25% germinal mutation); familial in 4% (AD)

Heritable in 40%, 90% penetrance

Most occur sporadically in infants with no family history; bilateral cases are usually familial (risk that additional offspring will have retinoblastoma is 40%)

75% are caused by mutation (inactivation of both RB genes) in a single retinal cell; these tumors are unilateral and unifocal; the chance of inactivation of both RB genes is very small

  Parents with 1 affected child: 6% risk of producing more affected children
  Parents with ≥2 affected children: 40% risk (because only 90% penetrance)
  Retinoblastoma survivor with hereditary form: 50% chance of transferring to children (but children have only 40% chance of manifesting a tumor)

Presentation: leukocoria (60%), strabismus (20%), decreased vision (5%)

Findings: yellow-white retinal mass, rubeosis, pseudohypopyon, hyphema, angle-closure glaucoma, uveitis; tumor necrosis occurs when outgrows blood supply, then calcification (seen on CT and ultrasound); may develop NV glaucoma (17%); no macular tumors after 1.5 months of age

Types:
  Endophytic: arises from inner retina and grows toward vitreous; can simulate endophthalmitis; can have pseudohypopyon (Fig. 5.39)
  Exophytic: arises from outer retina and grows toward choroid causing solid RD; can extend through sclera; can simulate Coats disease or traumatic RD

ON involvement: present in 29% of enucleated eyes

Risk for ON invasion: exophytic tumors >15 mm, and eyes that have secondary glaucoma

Second tumors: commonly present around age 17; osteogenic sarcoma of femur (most common), malignant melanoma of eye or orbit, leiomyosarcoma of eye or orbit, lymphoma, leukemia, rhabdomyosarcoma, medulloblastoma

Table 5.6 Chances of having a baby with retinoblastoma				
	Negative family history		**Positive family history**	
Offspring of	Unilateral (%)	Bilateral (%)	Unilateral (%)	Bilateral (%)
Parents with an affected child	1	6	40	40
Affected patient	8	40	40	40
Normal sibling of affected patient	1	<1	7	7

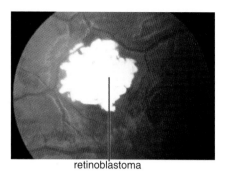

retinoblastoma

Figure 5.39 Retinoblastoma demonstrating discrete round tumor. (From Kaiser PK, Friedman NJ, Pineda R II. *Massachusetts Eye and Ear Infirmary Illustrated Manual of Ophthalmology*, 2nd ed. Philadelphia: WB Saunders; 2004.)

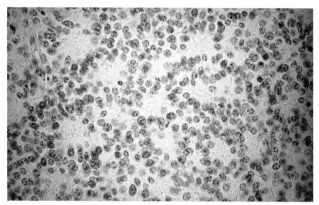

Figure 5.40 Homer-Wright rosettes. (From Augsburger JJ, Bornfeld M, Giblin ME. Retinoblastoma. In: Yanoff M, Duker JS, eds. *Ophthalmology*. London: Mosby; 1999.)

Trilateral retinoblastoma: bilateral RB with a pinealoblastoma or parasellar neuroblastoma; occurs in 3% of children with unilateral RB and 8% with bilateral RB; 95% have a positive family history and/or other tumors; spontaneous regression occurs with subsequent necrosis and phthisis

Pathology: rosettes are histologic markers for tumor differentiation

In order of increasing differentiation:

Homer-Wright rosette: no lumen; nuclei surround tangle of neural filaments; reflects low-grade neuroblastic differentiation; can be found in other types of neuroblastic tumors (adrenal neuroblastoma, medulloblastoma) (Fig. 5.40)

Flexner-Wintersteiner rosette: ring of single row of columnar cells around central lumen; cells have eosinophilic cytoplasm and peripheral nuclei; photoreceptors contain cilia with a 9 + 0 pattern; represent early retinal differentiation; attempt of outer photoreceptor production; special stains show hyaluronidase-resistant acid mucopolysaccharides in lumen; also present in medulloepitheliomas (Fig. 5.41)

Fleurettes: bouquet of pink bulbous neoplastic photoreceptor inner segments; highest degree of differentiation in retinoblastoma; found in relatively eosinophilic areas of tumor (photoreceptor differentiation)

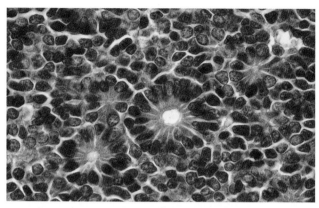

Figure 5.41 Flexner-Wintersteiner rosettes. (From Augsburger JJ, Bornfeld M, Giblin ME. Retinoblastoma. In: Yanoff M, Duker JS, eds. *Ophthalmology*. London: Mosby; 1999.)

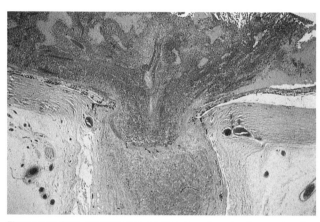

Figure 5.42 Retinoblastoma demonstrating necrosis and optic nerve invasion. (From Yanoff M, Fine BS. *Ocular pathology*, 5th ed. St Louis: Mosby; 2002.)

Pseudorosettes: circumferential arrangements of viable tumor cells surrounding a central vessel

Cells have round, spindle-shaped hyperchromatic nuclei and very little cytoplasm; high mitotic activity; as tumor grows, outgrows blood supply, creating necrosis with areas of calcification (80%)

H&E stain:

BLUE AREAS: represent viable tumor; differentiated cells that have basophilic nuclei and little cytoplasm

PINK AREAS: represent necrotic tumor; lose basophilic nuclei and appear eosinophilic (pink)

PURPLE AREAS: represent calcified tumor; occur in necrotic areas; calcium stains purple (Fig. 5.42)

DDx (leukocoria): cataract, retrolental mass (PHPV, ROP, Norrie disease, RD), tumor (choroidal metastases, retinal astrocytoma), exudates (FEVR, Coats disease, Eales disease), change in retinal pigment (incontinentia pigmenti, high myopia, myelinated nerve fiber, retinal dysplasia, choroideremia, coloboma), infections (toxoplasmosis, toxocariasis, endophthalmitis)

Diagnosis:

LDH levels: ratio of aqueous:plasma lactate dehydrogenase (LDH) >1.0

Ultrasound: acoustic solidity and high internal reflectivity; calcium appears as dense echoes

FA: early hyperfluorescence with late leakage of lesions

MRI: look for pineal tumor, ON involvement

CT scan (less preferred because of radiation exposure): calcification;

Metastatic workup: bone scan, bone marrow aspirate, lumbar puncture (LP) (cytology)

Treatment:

Chemotherapy: systemic chemotherapy often indicated for bilateral disease, intra-arterial chemotherapy for unilateral disease, intravitreal chemotherapy for vitreous seeds

Photocoagulation/cryotherapy: eyes with one or a few small tumors, not involving ON or macula, tumors that have been reduced by chemotherapy

Enucleation: all blind and painful eyes; affected eye in many unilateral cases; worse eye in most asymmetric cases; both eyes in many symmetric cases; excise at least 10 mm of ON to prevent spread

External beam radiation: salvageable eyes with vitreous seeding or large tumor; most eyes with multifocal tumors; eyes that have failed coagulation therapy; RB is very radiosensitive; used to treat most 2nd tumors

Episcleral plaque radiation: salvageable eyes with single medium-size tumor that does not involve ON or macula, even with localized vitreous seeding

Prognosis: 90%-95% of children with retinoblastoma survive (same with either growth pattern); 3% spontaneously regress; fatal in 2-4 years if untreated

Metastases: most commonly to CNS along ON; 50% to bone

Familial RB: location related to age, earliest in macula, later in periphery; second eye tumor develops up to 44 months later; 45% mortality by age 35 (vs. 19% long-term survival for all patients with RB by age 35); multiple primary tumors in an eye does not worsen prognosis

Increased risk of second unrelated malignancy in 25%-30% of children with heritable retinoblastoma

Poor prognostic signs: ON invasion, uveal invasion, extrascleral extension, multifocal tumors (represent seeding); delay in diagnosis, degree of differentiation, prior inadvertent surgical intervention (biopsy, vitrectomy)

Bilateral involvement does not worsen prognosis; prognosis depends on status of tumor in worse eye; degree of necrosis and calcification does not influence prognosis

Reese-Ellsworth classification: predicts visual prognosis (not survival) in eyes treated with radiation

International Classification of Retinoblastoma (ICRB): better predicts outcomes:

GROUP A: small intraretinal tumors (<3 mm) not located near macula or disc

GROUP B: tumors >3 mm, macular or juxtapapillary location, or with subretinal fluid

GROUP C: tumor with focal subretinal or vitreous seeding within 3 mm of tumor

GROUP D: tumor with diffuse subretinal or vitreous seeding >3 mm from tumor

GROUP E: extensive tumor occupying >50% of the globe with or without neovascular glaucoma (NVG), hemorrhage, extension of tumor to ON or anterior chamber

Retinocytoma/Retinoma

Benign tumor with same appearance and genetics as RB

Pathology: numerous fleurettes among cells with varying degrees of photoreceptor differentiation

Differentiation from RB: more cytoplasm, more evenly dispersed nuclear chromatin, no mitoses, calcification may be present, and necrosis is usually absent in retinocytoma

13q Deletion Syndrome

Associated with retinoblastoma, microcephaly, hypertelorism, microphthalmos, ptosis, and epicanthus

Leukemia

Most common malignancy of childhood

Usually affects choroid with retinal hemorrhages; usually unilateral

Symptoms: blurred vision, floaters

Findings (Figs. 5.43 and 5.44): cellular infiltration of vitreous; infiltrative lesions of retina, ON, or uvea; multiple hemorrhages, Roth spots, cotton wool spots (CWS); heterochromia irides, pseudohypopyon, spontaneous hyphema, uveitic glaucoma, cataract

Optic nerve infiltration causes loss of vision and papilledema

Orbital infiltration (rare) causes proptosis, lid swelling, ecchymosis (1%–2% of patients)

Treatment: emergent XRT for ON infiltration; patient is more susceptible to developing radiation optic neuropathy when chemotherapy is used concurrently

Prognosis: poor; high mortality; can be rapidly fatal if untreated

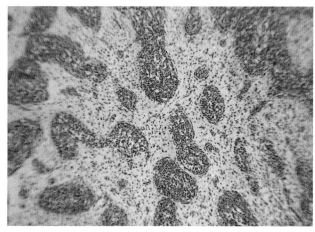

Figure 5.43 Leukemic infiltrate in optic nerve. (From Yanoff M, Fine BS. *Ocular Pathology*, 5th ed. St Louis: Mosby; 2002.)

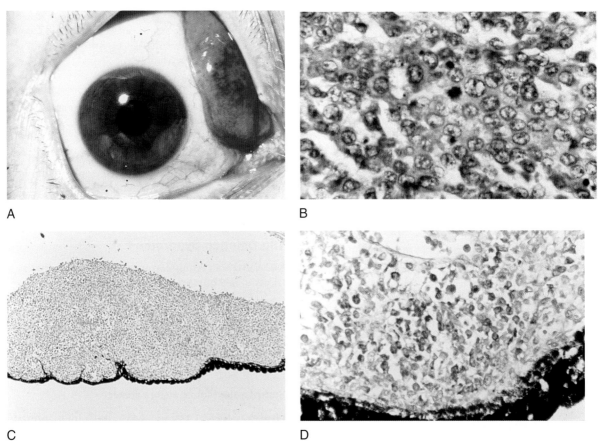

Figure 5.44 Acute leukemia. (A) A patient presented with a large infiltrate of leukemic cells positioned nasally within the conjunctiva of the right eye, giving this characteristic clinical picture. These lesions look similar to those caused by benign lymphoid hyperplasia, lymphoma, or amyloidosis. (B) A biopsy of the lesion shows primitive blastic leukocytes. (C) In another case, the iris is infiltrated by leukemic cells. A special stain (Lader stain) shows that some of the cells stain red, better seen when viewed under increased magnification in (D). This red positiveness is characteristic of myelogenous leukemic cells. (From Augsburger JJ, Tsiaras WG. Lymphoma and leukemia. In: Yanoff M, Duker JS, eds. *Ophthalmology*. London: Mosby; 1999.)

PHAKOMATOSES

Group of disorders (neurocutaneous syndromes) characterized by ocular and systemic hamartomas. Most are AD with variable penetrance except Sturge-Weber and Wyburn-Mason (no hereditary pattern) and ataxia-telangiectasia (AR) (Table 5.7)

Treatment: often requires CT scans and medical consultations; may require treatment of elevated IOP

Table 5.7 Genetics of the phakomatoses

Disorder	Chromosome
Neurofibromatosis:	
Type 1	17
Type 2	22
Sturge-Weber	None
von Hippel–Lindau	3
Tuberous sclerosis	9
Ataxia-telangiectasia	11
Wyburn-Mason	None

Neurofibromatosis (AD)

Variable expressivity

Disorder of Schwann cells and melanocytes with hamartomas of nervous system, skin, and eye

Types:

NF-1 (von Recklinghausen syndrome): mapped to chromosome 17q11 (neurofibromin), 50% caused by new mutation; 80% penetrance

More common form (prevalence 1 in 3000-5000)

    CRITERIA (>2 of the following): ≥6 café au lait spots >5 mm in diameter in prepubescent or >15 mm in postpubescent individuals

    ≥2 neurofibromas or 1 plexiform neurofibroma

    Freckling of intertriginous areas

    Optic nerve glioma

    ≥2 Lisch nodules

    Osseous lesion (sphenoid bone dysplasia, thinning of long bone cortex)

    1st degree relative with NF-1

    FINDINGS: plexiform neurofibroma (plexus of abnormal markedly enlarged nerves; occurs in 25%; 10% involve face, often upper eyelid or orbit; "bag of worms" appearance and S-shaped upper lid; congenital glaucoma in ipsilateral eye in up to 50%), fibroma molluscum, plexiform neurofibroma of conjunctiva, prominent corneal nerves, Lisch nodules (glial/melanocytic iris hamartomas), diffuse uveal thickening as a result of excess melanocytes and neurons (similar to ocular melanocytosis), ectropion uveae, retinal astrocytic hamartoma (less likely to be calcified than in tuberous sclerosis), increased incidence of myelinated nerve fibers and choroidal nevi (33%), ON glioma (juvenile pilocytic astrocytoma in >30%; may cause visual loss, hypothalamic dysfunction or hydrocephalus; neuroimaging shows fusiform enlargement of nerve with kinking; if have glioma, 25% have NF), meningioma, orbital plexiform neurofibroma, schwannoma, absence of sphenoid wing (pulsating exophthalmos)

OTHER FINDINGS: café au lait spots, intertriginous (axillary) freckling, cutaneous peripheral nerve sheath tumors

Neurofibromatosis type 2 (NF-2): mapped to chromosome 22q

Prevalence 1 in 50,000

CRITERIA: bilateral cerebellar–pontine angle tumors (acoustic neuromas; cause hearing loss, ataxia, headache)

1st degree relative with NF-2 and either a unilateral acoustic neuroma or two of the following: meningioma, schwannoma, neurofibroma, glioma, posterior subcapsular cataract

May have pheochromocytoma and other malignant tumors

No Lisch nodules

Encephalotrigeminal Angiomatosis (Sturge-Weber Syndrome)

Nonhereditary

No racial or sex predilection

Facial hemangioma: nevus flammeus (port wine stain) limited to first 2 divisions of CN 5; 5%-10% bilateral

Findings: dilated tortuous vessels of the conjunctiva and episclera, congenital or juvenile glaucoma (25% risk, especially if upper lid is involved), heterochromia irides (as a result of angiomas of iris), angiomas of episclera and CB, diffuse cavernous choroidal hemangioma ("tomato-ketchup" fundus [50%]), peripheral retinal AV malformations, may get RD or severe RPE alterations (pseudo-RP)

Mechanism of glaucoma: neovascular, increased episcleral venous pressure, immature angle structures

Other findings: leptomeningeal vascular malformations (ipsilateral to port wine stain), central calcifications, mental retardation, seizures, pheochromocytoma

Klippel-Trénaunay-Weber: variant of Sturge-Weber with cutaneous nevus flammeus, hemangiomas, varicosities, intracranial angiomas, and hemihypertrophy of limbs

Findings (uncommon): congenital glaucoma, conjunctival telangiectasia; can have AV malformation similar to Wyburn-Mason

Angiomatosis Retinae (von Hippel–Lindau Disease) (AD)

Incomplete penetrance; mapped to chromosome 3p26-p25 (*VHL*)

Prevalence 1 in 100,000

Bilateral in 50%

Hamartomas of eye, brain (cerebellum), kidney/adrenal gland

(Note: disease has 3 names, 3 locations for tumors, and defect on chromosome 3)

Findings: retinal angioma (hemangioma or hemangioblastoma; round orange-red mass fed by dilated tortuous retinal artery and drained by engorged vein; may be multifocal as well as bilateral; often in midperiphery, may be near disc; leaks heavily causing serous RD and/or macular edema; treat with yellow dye laser if enlarges)

Other findings: 25% of retinal capillary hemangiomas associated with CNS tumor (hemangioblastoma of cerebellum [60%]; pons, medulla, and/or spinal cord is less common); visceral lesions (cysts and tumors of kidney, pancreas, liver, adrenal glands, including renal cell carcinoma [25%], pheochromocytoma [10%–20%])

Von Hippel disease: only ocular involvement

Treatment: observation, cryotherapy, or laser photocoagulation

Tuberous Sclerosis (Bourneville disease) (AD or sporadic)

Mapped to chromosomes 9q34 (*TSC1* [hamartin]), 16p13 (*TSC2* [tuberin])

Prevalence 1 in 10,000-100,000

Triad of adenoma sebaceum, mental retardation, and epilepsy

Findings: astrocytic hamartoma of the retina (flat or mulberry-shaped with calcifications; usually in posterior pole; consists of nerve fibers and undifferentiated glial cells; occurs in 50%; bilateral in 15%), astrocytic hamartoma of the ON ("giant drusen"; benign)

Other findings:

Cutaneous: facial angiofibroma (adenoma sebaceum; vascularized red papules in butterfly distribution, not present at birth, become visible between ages 2-5), ash leaf spots (hypopigmented spots that fluoresce under Wood's light, considered pathognomonic), shagreen patches (25%; areas of fibromatous infiltration, usually on trunk), periungual fibromas, may have café au lait spots

CNS: subependymal hamartomas (calcify, forming "brain stones" with rootlike appearance; concentrated in periventricular area), mental retardation (60%), seizures (80%), cerebral calcification

Other: cardiac rhabdomyoma, spontaneous pneumothorax (from pleural cyst), renal angiomyolipomas, pheochromocytoma

Early mortality

Ataxia-Telangiectasia (Louis-Bar Syndrome) (AR)

Mapped to chromosome 11q22 *(ATM)*

Prevalence 1 in 40,000

Findings: prominent dilated conjunctival vessels, impaired convergence, nystagmus, oculomotor apraxia

Other findings: cutaneous telangiectasia in butterfly distribution during 1st decade of life, mental retardation, cerebellar ataxia (as a result of cerebellar atrophy), thymic hypoplasia with defective T-cell function and immunoglobulin A (IgA) deficiency with increased risk of infections, malignancy (leukemia/lymphoma)

Racemose Hemangiomatosis (Wyburn-Mason Syndrome)

Nonhereditary, usually unilateral

Findings: racemose hemangioma of retina (arteriovenous malformation with markedly dilated and tortuous shunt vessels); may have intraocular hemorrhage or glaucoma

Other findings: arteriovenous malformations in brain (may cause seizures, paresis, mental changes, VF defects), orbit and facial bones; may have small facial hemangiomas

Others

Retinal Cavernous Hemangioma

Cluster of intraretinal aneurysms filled with venous blood

Appears as "cluster of grapes"

Vitreous hemorrhage is rare

May be associated with cutaneous and CNS hemangiomas

FA: fluid levels without leakage within lesions

Incontinentia Pigmenti (Bloch-Sulzberger Syndrome) (X-Linked Dominant)

Occurs exclusively in females (lethal in males)

Mapped to chromosome Xq28 *(IKBKG;* encodes NEMO protein, which protects cells against tumor necrosis factor-α [TNF-α]–induced apoptosis)

Findings: proliferative retinal vasculopathy (resembles ROP); may have VH, traction RDs, retrolental membrane (Fig. 5.45)

Other findings:
Skin lesions:
STAGE 1 (AT BIRTH): erythematous macules, papules, and bullae on trunk and extremities (intraepithelial vesicles containing eosinophils)

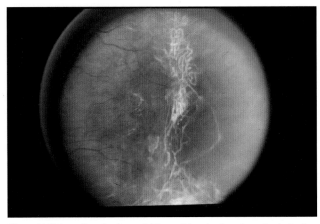

Figure 5.45 Incontinentia pigmenti. The peripheral retina of a patient who has incontinentia pigmenti demonstrates somewhat elevated vessels with vessel walls. A majority of these vessels show nonperfusion. The more posterior retina was perfused, and the anterior retina was ischemic. (From Ebroom DA, Jampol JM. Proliferation retinopathies. In: Yanoff M, Duker JS, eds. *Ophthalmology.* London: Mosby; 1999.)

STAGE 2 (2 MONTHS OF AGE): vesicles are replaced by verrucous lesions
STAGE 3 (3–6 MONTHS OF AGE): lesions take form of pigmented whorls on trunk
STAGE 4: skin is atrophic with hypopigmented patches
Hair abnormalities: alopecia
CNS abnormalities: microcephaly, hydrocephalus, seizures, mental deficiency
Dental abnormalities: missing and cone-shaped teeth

Treatment: photocoagulation (variable results)

OPTIC NERVE DISORDERS

Aplasia

Complete absence of ON; very rare; may occur with anencephaly or major cerebral maldevelopment

Hypoplasia

Variable visual compromise

No sex predilection

Unilateral cases usually idiopathic

Bilateral cases associated with midline anomalies, endocrine dysfunction, congenital intracranial tumors (craniopharyngioma, optic glioma), maternal diabetes or drug ingestion during pregnancy (alcohol, LSD, quinine, dilantin), sepsis, congenital Zika syndrome

Findings: small discs, "double ring" sign (thin ring of pigment surrounding nerve tissue; halo of retina and RPE partially covering lamina cribrosa), strabismus, amblyopia, nystagmus, positive RAPD, VF defects

Other findings: CNS abnormalities (45%), growth retardation, seizures, endocrine abnormalities

De Morsier syndrome (septo-optic dysplasia):

bilateral ON hypoplasia, septum pellucidum abnormality, pituitary and hypothalamus deficiency; associated with agenesis of the corpus callosum; may have chiasmal developmental anomalies with VF defects; may have see-saw nystagmus. Associated with mutations in the *HESX-1* gene. At risk for sudden death; obtain MRI and pediatric neurologic evaluation

Treatment: brain MRI, endocrine workup

Coloboma

Caused by incomplete closure of embryonic fissure; usually located inferonasal

Mutations in *CHD7* gene in 67% of cases, AD inheritance

Unilateral or bilateral

Variable visual acuity and visual field defects

Associated with other ocular colobomas

Findings: large anomalous discs, deep excavation with abnormal vascular pattern (ranges from complete chorioretinal coloboma to involvement of proximal portion of embryonic fissure causing only ON deformity); may resemble physiologic cupping if mild; systemic defects include congenital heart defects, double aortic arch, transposition of the great vessels, coarctation of the aorta, and intracranial carotid anomalies; sometimes accompanied by microphthalmia

Aicardi Syndrome (X-Linked Dominant)

Only females, lethal in males

Occurs in 1 in 105,000 newborns

Findings: widespread depigmented lacunar chorioretinal defects, ON head coloboma, microphthalmos, nystagmus

Other findings: infantile spasms, severe mental retardation, agenesis of corpus collosum, sparse lateral eyebrows, hand malformations, scoliosis

Morning Glory Disc Anomaly

Probably represents a dysplastic coloboma

Generally unilateral

Female > male (2:1)

Often seen with high myopia

Findings: enlarged, excavated disc often with central, white, glial tissue surrounded by pigment ring, adjacent retinal folds common; vessels radiate in spokelike fashion; usually poor vision; present with leukocoria or strabismus; may develop peripapillary serous RD; systemic associations include midline facial defects and forebrain anomalies, basal encephalocele, renal defects, Moyamoya disease, oculo-renal syndrome (autosomal dominant *PAX2* gene mutation that is required for closure of optic fissure and neural tube)

Optic Disc Pit

Gray-white depression in optic disc, usually in inferotemporal area, 0.1-0.7 disc diameter

85% unilateral

Associated with peripapillary RPE disturbances

May develop serous retinal detachment extending from pit (40%)

Tilted Disc

Findings (any of the following may occur, alone or in combination): apparent tilting (usually inferiorly with superior pole of disc elevated), scleral crescent, situs inversus arteriosus (vessels emerge temporally from ON [rather than nasally] and course nasally before sweeping temporally), high myopia and/or astigmatism, reduced visual acuity, visual field defects (usually bitemporal and do not respect vertical midline)

Myelinated Nerve Fibers

Myelination begins at lateral geniculate body and usually ceases at lamina cribrosa; however, some retinal fibers may acquire myelin sheath during 1st month of life

Unilateral or bilateral (20%)

Male > female

Vision generally good unless macula involved; increased risk of amblyopia

Findings: superficial white flame–shaped patches with feathery margins; usually peripapillary; can be extensive

Relative or absolute scotoma corresponds to area of myelination

Persistence of Hyaloid System

Common; ranges from tuft of glial tissue on disc (Bergmeister papillae) to patent artery extending from disc to lens

Megalopapilla

Enlarged optic disc

Peripapillary Staphyloma

Posterior bulging of sclera in which optic disc occupies bottom of bulge

Optic Nerve Drusen

Superficial or buried hyaline bodies in prelaminar portion of ON

Sporadic or AD; 75% bilateral

Incidence 0.3%-1% clinically; 2% histopathologically

More common in Caucasians; no sex predilection

Most common cause of pseudopapilledema

Associations: angioid streaks, retinitis pigmentosa, Alagille syndrome (familial intrahepatic cholestasis, posterior embryotoxin, bilateral optic disc drusen [80%])

Findings: disc margins may show irregular outline, bumpy nodular chunky appearance to nerve head (pseudopapilledema); VF defects (especially with deep drusen; enlarged blind spot, arcuate scotoma, sectoral scotoma); may have transient visual obscurations, positive RAPD (unilateral ON drusen); often calcify with age

Pathology: hyaline bodies that become calcified; stain positively for amino acids, calcium, acid mucopolysaccharides, and hemosiderin; stain negatively for amyloid

Diagnosis: B-scan ultrasound, CT scan, autofluorescence

Complications: rarely visual loss as a result of axonal compression, anterior ischemic optic neuropathy (AION), CNV, subretinal or vitreous hemorrhage, vascular occlusion

Melanocytoma (Magnocellular Nevus of the Optic Disc)

Deeply pigmented tumor with feathery border located over ON

Derived from uveal dendritic melanocytes

May have choroidal and NFL involvement

15% show minimal enlargement over 5 years

Findings: VF defect; may have positive RAPD (even with good vision)

Pathology: benign, plump, round polyhedral melanocytes

Malignant transformation very rare

Hereditary Optic Neuropathy

Group of disorders with ON dysfunction (isolated or part of systemic disease)

Most common are:

Isolated

Leber hereditary optic neuropathy (LHON): maternal mitochondrial DNA; point mutations in mitochondrial gene for reduced nicotinamide adenine dinucleotide (NADH) subunit 4 (position 11778 [most common], 3460, 14484); male > female (9:1); maternal transmission to all sons (50% affected) and all daughters (15% of daughters affected, 85% are carriers); onset between ages of 15-30; subacute sequential bilateral vision loss (≤20/200) over days; tobacco or alcohol can trigger decompensation

> *Findings:* disc hyperemia, peripapillary telangiectatic vessels (do not leak fluorescein, also found in 60% of asymptomatic family members), tortuous vessels, peripapillary NFL edema, late optic disc pallor; may have cardiac conduction abnormalities

Autosomal dominant optic atrophy (AD)**:** dominant optic atrophy, formerly Kjer of juvenile optic atrophy; most common form of heritable optic atrophy; mapped to

chromosome 3q28-q29 (*OPA1*), 18q12.2-q12.3 (*OPA4*), and 22q12-q13 (*OPA5*); insidious onset between ages of 4-8; bilateral and symmetric; decreased vision (20/40–20/200), blue–yellow dyschromatopsia, temporal wedge of disc pallor

Recessive optic atrophy (Costeff syndrome, AR): mapped to chromosome 8q21-q22 (*OPA6*)

X-linked optic atrophy: mapped to chromosome Xp11.4-p11.2 (*OPA2*)

Syndromic

DIDMOAD (Wolfram syndrome): Diabetes insipidus, diabetes mellitus, optic atrophy, deafness; mitochondrial DNA inheritance; mapped to chromosome 4p16.1 (*WFS1*) and 4q22-q24 (*WFS2*); onset between ages of 5-21; slowly progressive; decreased vision (<20/400), diffuse optic atrophy; ataxia, seizures, mental retardation

Complicated hereditary infantile optic atrophy (Behr syndrome, AR): onset before age 10, male > female, nonprogressive; mapped to chromosome 19q13 (*OPA3*); moderate to severe decreased vision, nystagmus (50%), diffuse optic atrophy; ataxia, spasticity, hypotonia, urinary incontinence, mental retardation

DDx: acquired optic neuropathies: compressive (tumors [craniopharyngioma, ON/chiasmal gliomas], hydrocephalus), toxic (anoxia at birth or in neonatal period), traumatic, infiltrative (leukemia, metabolic storage diseases)

Treatment: no treatment; genetic counseling; consider idebenone (co-enzyme Q10 derivative) 900 mg/day for LHON (gene therapy with mitochondrial ND4 protein is investigational)

Mitochondrial Diseases

Maternal inheritance; children of both sexes affected; only female offspring can pass on

Findings: optic atrophy, CPEO, pigmentary retinopathy, retrochiasmal visual loss

Disorders:

> *Maternal inherited diabetes and deafness (MIDD):* see above
> *Leber hereditary optic neuropathy (LHON):* see above
> *Kearns-Sayre syndrome:* onset before age 20; gene deletion impairs oxidative phosphorylation
>> **FINDINGS:** chronic progressive external ophthalmoplegia with ptosis, pigmentary retinopathy (salt and pepper, bone spicules, and/or RPE atrophy), mild visual loss (50%)
>> **OTHER FINDINGS:** neck and limb weakness, cardiac conduction defects (arrhythmias, heart block, cardiomyopathy), cerebellar ataxia
>> **PATHOLOGY:** ragged red fibers (contain degenerated mitochondria) on muscle biopsy
>> **EKG:** heart block
>> **CSF:** elevated protein
> *MELAS:* **M**itochondrial **E**ncephalopathy, **L**actic **A**cidosis, and **S**trokelike episodes
>> Onset before age 15; 80% caused by mutations in *MT-TL1* gene (impair ability of mitochondria to make proteins, use oxygen, and produce energy)

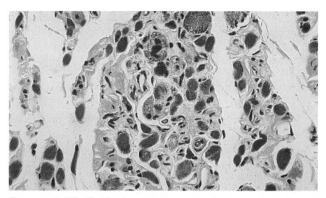

Figure 5.46 MELAS (**M**itochondrial **E**ncephalopathy, **L**actic **A**cidosis, and **S**trokelike episodes) syndrome demonstrating degenerated extraocular muscle (EOM) with trichome stain shows "ragged red" fibers. (Case presented by Dr. R. Folberg to the meeting of the Verhoeff Society, 1993, and reported by Rummelt V, Folberg R, Ionasescu V, et al. Ocular pathology of MELAS syndrome with mitochondrial DNA nucleotide 3243 point mutation. *Ophthalmology*. 1993;100:1757–1766.)

FINDINGS: retrochiasmal visual loss; recurrent attacks of headache, vomiting, seizures; transient focal neurologic deficits (hemiplegia, hemianopia/cortical blindness), CPEO, optic neuropathy; pigmentary retinopathy, dementia, hearing loss, short stature, muscle weakness

PATHOLOGY: ragged red fibers on muscle biopsy, abnormal mitochondria in blood vessels (Fig. 5.46)

DIAGNOSIS: Elevated serum and CSF lactate
   CT SCAN: basal ganglia calcification
   MRI: posterior cortex lesions, spare deep white matter; can resolve

MERRF: **M**yoclonus, **E**pilepsy, and **R**agged **R**ed **F**ibers
   Onset in 1st or 2nd decade of life; majority caused by mutations in *MT-TK* gene

FINDINGS: encephalopathy with myoclonus, seizures, ataxia, spasticity, dementia; may have dysarthria, optic neuropathy, nystagmus, short stature, hearing loss

PATHOLOGY: ragged red fibers on muscle biopsy (Gomori trichrome stain)

STRABISMUS

ANATOMY AND PHYSIOLOGY

Subconjunctival Fascia (Fig. 5.47)

Tenon capsule: thin elastic connective tissue sheath surrounding globe from ON to limbus, allows free movement of globe
   Anterior: fuses with conjunctiva and intermuscular septum 3 mm behind limbus
   Posterior: fuses with ON sheath, separates orbital fat from muscles and globe

Intermuscular septum: extension of Tenon, connects muscles

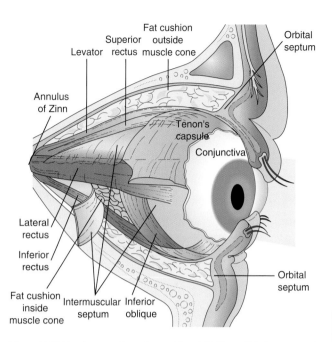

Figure 5.47 Muscle cone. (From Campolattaro BN, Wang FM. Anatomy and physiology of the extraocular muscles and surrounding tissues. In: Yanoff M, Duker JS, eds. *Ophthalmology*, 2nd ed. St Louis: Mosby; 2004.)

Check ligaments: connect muscles to overlying Tenon and inserts on orbital walls to support globe

Lockwood ligament: fusion of sheaths of inferior rectus and inferior oblique; attaches to medial and lateral retinaculi and supports globe

Extraocular Muscles (Table 5.8, Figs. 5.48 to 5.50)

Vascular supply: muscular branches of ophthalmic artery (lateral [superior] and medial [inferior] anterior ciliary arteries) to rectus muscles (1-4 to each); infraorbital artery to inferior rectus and inferior oblique; lacrimal artery to lateral rectus

All rectus muscles have two accompanying ciliary arteries except lateral rectus, which has one

Annulus of Zinn: Superior and inferior orbital tendons, which are the origin of the rectus muscles

Spiral of Tillaux: imaginary spiral line that passes through insertions of rectus muscles; the temporal aspect of vertical muscles lies farther from limbus than the nasal aspect (Fig. 5.51)

Medial rectus (MR):
1. Pure adductor
2. Closest to limbus
3. Hardest to find if slipped because no fascial attachment to an oblique muscle

Lateral rectus (LR):
1. Pure abductor
2. Easiest exposure
3. Connected to inferior oblique

Superior rectus (SR):
1. Elevates, adducts, and incyclotorts

155

Table 5.8 Extraocular muscles

Muscle	Muscle length (mm)	Tendon length / width (mm)	Arc of contact (mm)	Anatomic insertion from limbus	Action from primary position	Origin	Innervation
Medial rectus (MR)	40.8	3.7/10.3	7	5.5 mm	Adduction	Annulus of Zinn	Cranial nerve (CN) 3 (inferior division)
Lateral rectus (LR)	40.6	8/9.2	12	6.9 mm	Abduction	Annulus of Zinn	CN 6
Superior rectus (SR)	41.8	5.8/10.6	6.5	7.7 mm	Elevation Intorsion Adduction	Annulus of Zinn	CN 3 (superior division)
Inferior rectus (IR)	40	5.5/9.8	6.5	6.5 mm	Depression Extorsion Adduction	Annulus of Zinn	CN 3 (inferior division)
Superior oblique (SO)	40	20/10.8	7–8	Posterior to equator in superotemporal quadrant	Intorsion Depression Abduction	Orbital apex above annulus of Zinn	CN 4
Inferior oblique (IO)	37	1/9.6	15	Posterior to equator in inferotemporal quadrant	Extorsion Elevation Abduction	Behind lacrimal fossa	CN 3 (inferior division)
Levator palpebrae	40	14-20	—	Septa of pretarsal orbicularis and anterior surface of tarsus	Lid elevation	Orbital apex above annulus of Zinn	CN 3 (superior division)

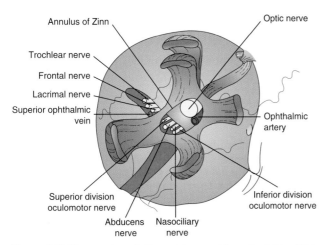

Figure 5.48 The annulus of Zinn and surrounding structures. (From Campolattaro BN, Wang FM. Anatomy and physiology of the extraocular muscles and surrounding tissues. In: Yanoff M, Duker JS, eds. *Ophthalmology*, 2nd ed. St Louis: Mosby; 2004.)

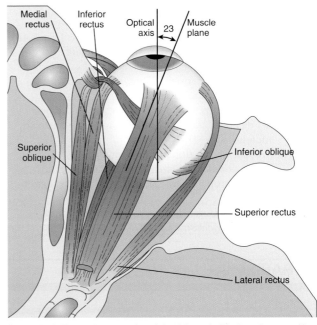

Figure 5.49 The extrinsic muscles of the right eyeball in the primary position, seen from above. The muscles are shown as partially transparent. (From Campolattaro BN, Wang FM. Anatomy and physiology of the extraocular muscles and surrounding tissues. In: Yanoff M, Duker JS, eds. *Ophthalmology*, 2nd ed. St Louis: Mosby; 2004.)

2. Inserts 23° temporal to visual axis in primary position; pure elevator only in 23° abduction
3. Fascial connections: superior oblique (SO), upper eyelid elevators. Therefore, superior rectus (SR) recession may cause lid retraction, and resection may cause fissure narrowing
4. Passes over SO

Inferior rectus (IR):

1. Depresses, adducts, and excyclotorts
2. Inserts 23° temporal to visual axis in primary position; pure depressor only in 23° abduction
3. Fascial connections: IO, lower eyelid retractors (Lockwood ligament). Therefore, IR recession may cause lid retraction, and resection may cause fissure narrowing

Superior oblique (SO):

1. Incyclotorts, abducts, and depresses
2. Inserts 51° to visual axis; pure depressor only in 51° adduction
3. Passes inferior to SR
4. Arises from orbital apex above annulus of Zinn (lesser wing of sphenoid)

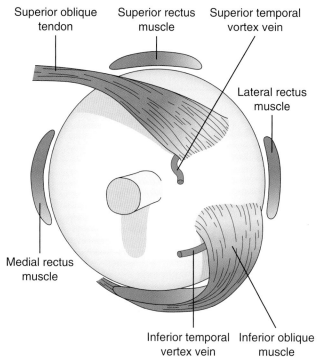

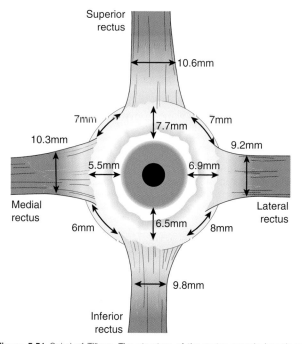

Figure 5.50 Posterior view of the eye with Tenon capsule removed. (From Campolattaro BN, Wang FM. Anatomy and physiology of the extraocular muscles and surrounding tissues. In: Yanoff M, Duker JS, eds. *Ophthalmology*, 2nd ed. St Louis: Mosby; 2004.)

Figure 5.51 Spiral of Tillaux. The structure of the rectus muscle insertions. (From Campolattaro BN, Wang FM. Anatomy and physiology of the extraocular muscles and surrounding tissues. In: Yanoff M, Duker JS, eds. *Ophthalmology*, 2nd ed. St Louis: Mosby; 2004.)

Inferior oblique (IO):

1. Excyclotorts, abducts, and elevates
2. Inserts 51° to visual axis; pure elevator only in 51° adduction

3. Passes inferior to IR
4. Originates from periosteum of maxillary bone
5. Inserts near macula
6. Avoid inferotemporal vortex vein during surgery
7. The inferior division of CN 3 up to the inferior oblique carries parasympathetic supply to iris constrictor; injury to these fibers results in mydriasis

Pediatric Eye Examination

Visual development:

At birth: blinking response to bright light
At 7 days: vestibulo-ocular response
At 2 months: fixation well developed
At 6 months: VER acuity at adult level
At 2 years: Snellen acuity at adult level
At 7 years: stereoacuity at adult level

Hyperopia (average of 2 D) increases during 1st year of life; 50% have >1 D with-the-rule astigmatism; decreases after age 7 years

Vision testing:

Infancy: optokinetic (OKN) response, forced preferential looking (Teller acuity cards), visual evoked response (VER)
Older children: Allen pictures, HOTV (letter symbols used in pediatric visual acuity testing), tumbling E, Snellen acuity

Sensory Testing

Binocular vision:

Horopter: the set of object points imaged on corresponding retinal points
Panum's fusional space: region around horopter in which binocular vision exists (Fig. 5.52)

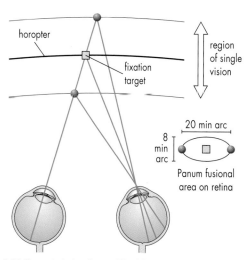

Figure 5.52 Panum's fusional area. The left eye fixates a square target, and a search object visible only to the right eye is moved before and behind this target. The ellipse of retinal area, for which typical dimensions are given for the parafoveal area, is the projection of Panum's fusional area. Diplopia is not perceived for two targets within this area. (From Diamond GR. Sensory status in strabismus. In: Yanoff M, Duker JS, eds. *Ophthalmology*. London: Mosby; 1999.)

Table 5.9 Normal fusional amplitudes (prism diopters [Δ])

Testing distance	Convergence (Δ)	Divergence (Δ)	Vertical (Δ)
6 m	14	6	2.5
25 cm	38	16	2.6

Types of binocularity:

SIMULTANEOUS PERCEPTION: ability to see two images, one on each retina (superimposed, not blended)

FUSION: simultaneous perception of two similar images blended as one (Table 5.9)

STEREOPSIS: perception of two slightly dissimilar images blended as one with appreciation of depth

STEREOACUITY: occurs when retinal disparity is too small to cause diplopia but too great to allow superimposition of fusion of the two visual directions. Normal is 20-50 seconds of arc

TITMUS STEREOTEST: readily available, monocular clues present. Determines normal retinal correspondence (NRC) in binocular patient.

Example: Fly = 3000 arc seconds; animals = 400, 200, 100 arc seconds; circles = 800-40 arc seconds

RANDOM DOT STEREOGRAMS: monocular clues absent but more difficult for children to understand

Sensory phenomena associated with strabismus:

Diplopia: simultaneous perception of similar images falling on noncorresponding retinal points

Visual confusion: simultaneous perception of dissimilar images falling on corresponding retinal points

Sensory adaptations to diplopia and visual confusion:

Suppression **(scotoma):** image from one eye is inhibited or does not reach consciousness (Fig. 5.53)

CENTRAL: adaptation to avoid confusion

PERIPHERAL: adaptation to avoid diplopia

OBLIGATORY: present all the time

FACULTATIVE: present only when eyes are deviated

TESTS:

WORTH 4-DOT: with red lens over one eye and green lens over other eye, patient views red, green, and white lights. Green light is visible to eye under green lens, red light visible to eye under red lens, and white light visible to both eyes. Determines binocularity (Figs. 5.54

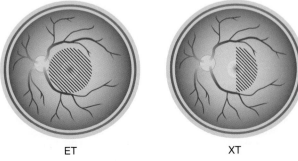

Figure 5.53 Suppression scotomas for esotropia (ET) and exotropia (XT).

Esotropic left eye with ARC and suppression or with monofixation syndrome, fixing with right eye

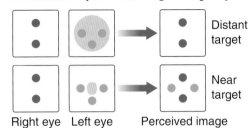

Right eye   Left eye   Perceived image

Esotropic right eye with ARC and suppression or with monofixation syndrome, fixing with left eye

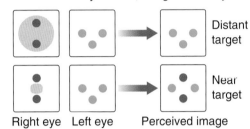

Right eye   Left eye   Perceived image

Figure 5.54 Possible Worth 4-Dot test percepts in binocular patients. Note the similar distant responses in patients who have esotropia with abnormal retinal correspondence (ARC) and suppression and in those who have monofixation syndrome. Patients who have exotropia with ARC and suppression give the same responses, but the suppression scotoma is larger and shaped somewhat differently. The red lens is over the right eye, and the green lens is over the left eye. (From Diamond GR. Sensory status in strabismus. In: Yanoff M, Duker JS, eds. *Ophthalmology*, 2nd ed. St Louis: Mosby; 2004.)

Any strabismus in patient fixing right eye

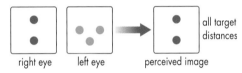

right eye   left eye   perceived image

Any strabismus in patient fixing left eye

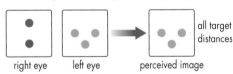

right eye   left eye   perceived image

Figure 5.55 Possible Worth 4-Dot test responses in patients who do not have binocularity. The red lens is over the right eye, and the green lens is over the left eye. (From Diamond GR. Sensory status in strabismus. In: Yanoff M, Duker JS, eds. *Ophthalmology*. London: Mosby; 1999.)

and 5.55). May be used to define the size and location of a suppression scotoma in patients with strabismus

Performed at distance (central fusion) and at near (peripheral fusion)

Results:

Suppression: 2 red or 3 green lights seen

Fusion: 4 lights seen

Diplopia: 5 lights seen

4-PRISM DIOPTER BASE-OUT PRISM TEST: for small suppression scotomas; 4-prism diopter (Δ) prism placed base-out over one eye; if suppression scotoma is present, eye will not move

HORROR FUSIONIS: intractable diplopia with absence of central suppression

Abnormal retinal correspondence (ARC): (see below)

Monofixation syndrome: binocular sensory state in patients with small-angle strabismus (≤8 Δ; microtropia)

CHARACTERISTICS: central scotoma and peripheral fusion present with binocular viewing

Usually esotropic (ET), may appear exotropic (XT) or orthophoric

Amblyopia common, usually mild

Stereoacuity reduced

Central or eccentric fixation

Typically occurs when preexisting strabismus is controlled nonoperatively or after surgery, but may occur in nonstrabismic patients, also from macular lesions and anisometropia

Decompensation occurs when the deviation changes from a latent to a manifest one

DIAGNOSIS: 4 Δ base-out prism test (used to shift image outside scotoma to cause eye movement). In normal patient, when prism is placed in front of one eye, eyes turn and then refixate

In monofixation syndrome, when prism is placed in front of normal eye, there is no refixation movement, and when prism is placed in front of eye with scotoma, there is no initial eye turn

Retinal correspondence: the ability of the sensory system to appreciate the perceived direction of the fovea and other retinal elements in each eye relative to each other

Corresponding retinal points: 2 retinal points (1 in each eye) that, when stimulated simultaneously, result in the subjective sensation that the stimulating target comes from the same direction in space. If diplopia occurs, then the 2 points are noncorresponding

Normal retinal correspondence (NRC): corresponding areas of the retina that have identical relationships to the fovea of each eye

CHARACTERISTICS: occurs in straight eyes under binocular conditions

Occurs in eyes in which the objective and subjective angles of strabismus are the same; measured with amblyoscope (patient superimposes dissimilar targets)

OBJECTIVE ANGLE: measured angle

SUBJECTIVE ANGLE: the amount of prism required to superimpose the images or promote fusion

Other dissimilar target tests: Lancaster red–green test and Hess screen; require NRC; used to measure paretic strabismus

Abnormal retinal correspondence (ARC): corresponding areas of the retina that have dissimilar relationships to their respective foveas. Sensory adaptation eliminates peripheral diplopia and confusion by permitting fusion of similar images projecting onto noncorresponding retinal areas

CHARACTERISTICS: change in visual direction of retinal points

Manifests only during binocular viewing

Objective and subjective angles are not equal

Sensory adaptation of immature visual system to strabismus

Prevents diplopia

Accompanied by scotoma

No fusional amplitudes and no stereopsis

Fovea in deviating eye and fovea in fixing eye do not have the same visual direction

Fovea of fixing eye shares common visual direction with peripheral area of the nonfixing eye

HARMONIOUS ARC: subjective angle = 0

UNHARMONIOUS ARC: subjective angle is >0 but less than objective angle

TESTS FOR ARC:

AFTERIMAGE TEST: label fovea of each eye with a linear light afterimage (vertical image for deviating eye and horizontal image for fixing eye). Each eye is stimulated individually (monocular), then patient draws perceived afterimages (Fig. 5.56):

NRC: cross with central gap

ET with ARC: afterimages crossed

XT with ARC: afterimages uncrossed

BAGOLINI LENSES: glasses have no dioptric power but have narrow striations running at

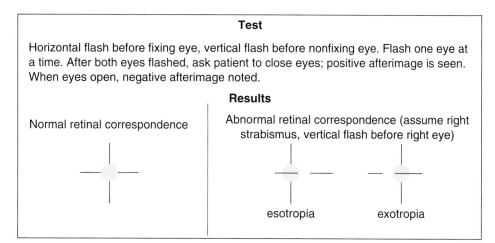

Test

Horizontal flash before fixing eye, vertical flash before nonfixing eye. Flash one eye at a time. After both eyes flashed, ask patient to close eyes; positive afterimage is seen. When eyes open, negative afterimage noted.

Results

Normal retinal correspondence

Abnormal retinal correspondence (assume right strabismus, vertical flash before right eye)

esotropia   exotropia

Figure 5.56 Afterimage test percepts, central fixation. Shown are those possible in patients who have central fixation and binocular vision. (From Diamond GR. Sensory status in strabismus. In: Yanoff M, Duker JS, eds. *Ophthalmology*, 2nd ed. St Louis: Mosby; 2004.)

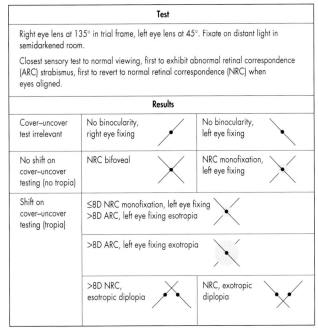

Figure 5.57 Possible Bagolini lens percepts, central fixation. (From Diamond GR. Sensory status in strabismus. In: Yanoff M, Duker JS, eds. *Ophthalmology*. London: Mosby; 1999.)

45° and 135°. With glasses on, patient fixes on a light and draws perceived image. Allows determination of strabismus as well as retinal correspondence. Break in line is proportional to size of suppression scotoma (Fig. 5.57)

RED GLASS TEST: with red glass in front of deviating eye, patient fixes on light; angular deviation can be measured with a Maddox rod to determine retinal correspondence

ET: uncrossed images

XT: crossed images

Harmonious ARC: patient sees pink light

AMBLYOSCOPE: device with which patient views two dissimilar targets and attempts to superimpose them

NRC: objective and subjective angles of strabismus are equal

Harmonious ARC: subjective angle equals zero (arms of amblyoscope are parallel)

Unharmonious ARC: subjective angle is between zero and objective angle

Amblyopia

Unilateral or bilateral reduction of visual acuity that cannot be attributed directly to any structural abnormality of the eye or visual system. Results from disuse of fovea

Characteristics: prevalence 2%-4%; preventable or reversible with appropriately timed intervention

Types:

Strabismic: crowding phenomenon (letters or symbols are more difficult to recognize if closely surrounded by similar forms; therefore, visual acuity may substantially improve with isolate letters); neutral density filters do not reduce acuity as much in the amblyopic eye as in the normal eye

Refractive: high ametropia (hyperopia of +5 D, myopia of −8 D, astigmatism of 2.5 D) or anisometropia (1 D for hyperopia, 3 D for myopia, 1.5 D for astigmatism)

Deprivation: media opacity, ptosis, occlusion

Diagnosis: reduced visual acuity that cannot be entirely explained by physical abnormalities

Treatment: treat amblyopia before strabismus surgery (eliminate any obstacle to vision, remove significant congenital lens opacity by 2 months of age). Force use of poorer eye by limiting use of better eye (full-time occlusion, part-time occlusion, optical degradation of better eye, atropinization of better eye). Full-time occlusion for 1 week per year of age at most before reexamination; continue until no further improvement. Reevaluate until 10 years of age

Prognosis: good for strabismic, poor for deprivation

Motor Testing

Ductions: monocular rotations of eye

Versions: conjugate binocular eye movements

Vergence: disconjugate binocular eye movement

Agonist: primary muscle moving eye in given direction (Table 5.10)

Synergist: secondary muscle that acts with agonist to move eye in given direction

Antagonist: muscle that acts to move eye in opposite direction as agonist

Yoke muscles: 2 muscles, 1 in each eye, that act to move respective eyes into a cardinal position

Cardinal positions: 6 positions of gaze in which 1 muscle of the eye is the prime mover (Fig. 5.58)

Midline positions: straight up and straight down from primary position

Hering's law (equal innervation): equal and simultaneous innervation to synergistic muscles; amount of innervation to eyes is determined by the fixating eye; therefore, the amount of deviation depends on which eye is fixating:

Primary deviation (paralytic strabismus): deviation measured with normal eye fixing

Table 5.10	Agonists, synergists, and antagonists	
Agonist	**Synergists**	**Antagonists**
Medial rectus (MR)	SR, IR	LR, SO, IO
Lateral rectus (LR)	SO, IO	MR, SR, IR
Superior rectus (SR)	IO, MR	IR, SO
Inferior rectus (IR)	SO, MR	SR, IO
Superior oblique (SO)	IR, LR	IO, SR
Inferior oblique (IO)	SR, LR	SO, IR

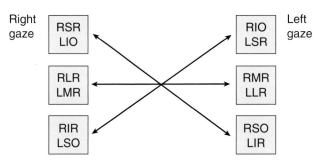

Right gaze

Left gaze

Figure 5.58 Cardinal positions and yoke muscles.

Secondary deviation (paralytic strabismus): deviation measured with paretic eye fixing; larger than primary deviation

Hering's law also explains the term "inhibitional paresis of the contralateral antagonist"

This is the incorrect impression that a muscle in the normal eye is responsible for the ocular misalignment and may occur in an SO palsy when the paretic eye fixes (e.g., in SO palsy, less innervation is required by the antagonist [IO], and therefore less innervation is directed to the yoke [contralateral SR]). The contralateral antagonist is actually the antagonist of the yoke of the paretic muscle

Sherrington's law (reciprocal innervation): innervation to ipsilateral antagonist decreases while innervation to the agonist increases

Optic/Optical axis: extends from anterior to posterior pole of eye through nodal point and geometric centers of lens and cornea

Visual axis: extends from fovea through nodal point of eye to object of fixation

Angle alpha (α): angle between visual axis and optic axis as they cross at the nodal point of the eye, measure of tilt of eye, approximately 5.2° horizontally; important for pseudophakic IOL centration

Angle kappa (κ): angle between visual axis and center of the pupil (Fig. 5.59); approximately 2.6° horizontally, measured as distance between center of pupil and corneal light reflex (near visual axis); important for centration of corneal refractive procedures

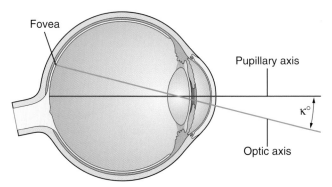

Figure 5.59 The angle κ. This is the displacement in degrees of the pupillary axis from the visual axis. The positive-angle κ provides the illusion of exotropia in the left eye. (Adapted from Diamond GR. Sensory status in strabismus. In: Yanoff M, Duker JS, eds. *Ophthalmology*, 2nd ed. St Louis: Mosby; 2004.)

Positive-angle κ: temporal position of fovea relative to pupillary axis; causes slight temporal rotation of globe to keep image in focus; light reflex appears nasal. May cause a pseudoexotropia or increase the apparent degree of an XT, and lessen or mask an ET

Example: ROP, *Toxocara*

Negative-angle κ: nasal position of fovea relative to pupillary axis; causes slight nasal rotation of globe to keep image in focus; light reflex appears temporal. May cause a pseudoesotropia or increase the apparent degree of an ET, and lessen or mask an XT

Eccentric fixation: consistent use of a nonfoveal region of retina for monocular viewing in an amblyopic eye; a monocular phenomenon

Detecting deviations:

Corneal light reflex: if equal, no manifest deviation (tropia) but may have latent deviation (phoria); if unequal, tropia is present

Monocular cover–uncover test: tests for phoria or tropia by detecting movement of eyes when one eye is covered and then uncovered (Fig. 5.60)

Measuring deviations:

Modified Krimsky method: place prism over fixating eye to center the corneal light reflex over the pupil; place over deviating eye in incomitant or paralytic deviations (Fig. 5.61)

Hirschberg method: estimate each millimeter of decentration of corneal light reflex from the center of the pupil (1 mm = 7° or 15 Λ of deviation) (Fig. 5.62)

Simultaneous prism cover test or cover–uncover test: measures tropia

Alternate cover testing: measures tropia and phoria

Measurements are affected by corrective lenses: minus (concave lenses; myopia) measures more, and plus (convex lenses; hyperopia) measures less, because of the prismatic effect of the lenses. Difference = 2.5% × D

Other tests:

Double Maddox rod test: measures torsion

Parks-Bielschowsky 3-step test: identifies cyclovertical palsy

1. Which eye has hyperdeviation?
   Identify weak depressors in higher eye (IR, SO) and elevators in lower eye (IO, SR)
2. Is hyperdeviation greater in right or left gaze?
   Identify muscles that act in direction as hyperdeviation increases
   Right gaze: SR and IR of right eye, IO and SO of left eye
   Left gaze: IO and SO of right eye, SR and IR of left eye
3. Is hyperdeviation greater with right or left head tilt?
   Identify torting muscles that act in direction as hyperdeviation increases
   Right head tilt:
   Intorsion of right eye (SR and SO)
   Extorsion of left eye (IO and IR)
   Left head tilt is reversed
   (Remember: supinate–superiors intort)
   Circle involved muscles at each step described previously. Muscle with 3 circles is the one with palsy

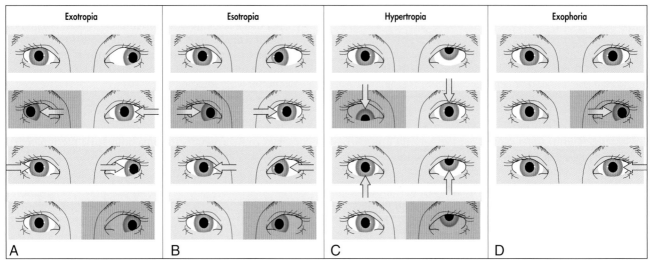

Figure 5.60 Cover test for tropias and phorias. (A) For exotropia, covering the right eye drives inward movement of the left eye to take up fixation; uncovering the right eye shows recovery of fixation by the right eye and leftward movement of both eyes; covering the left eye discloses no shift of the preferred right eye. (B) For esotropia, covering the right eye drives outward movement of the left eye to take up fixation; uncovering the right eye shows recovery of fixation by the right eye and rightward movement of both eyes; covering the left eye discloses no shift of the preferred right eye. (C) For hypertropia, covering the right eye drives downward movement of the left eye to take up fixation; uncovering the right eye shows recovery of fixation by the right eye and upward movement of both eyes; covering the left eye shows no shift of the preferred right eye. (D) For exophoria, the left eye deviates outward behind a cover and returns to primary position when the cover is removed. An immediate inward movement denotes a phoria, a delayed inward movement denotes an intermittent exotropia. (From Diamond G, Eggers H. *Strabismus and Pediatric Ophthalmology.* London: Mosby; 1993.)

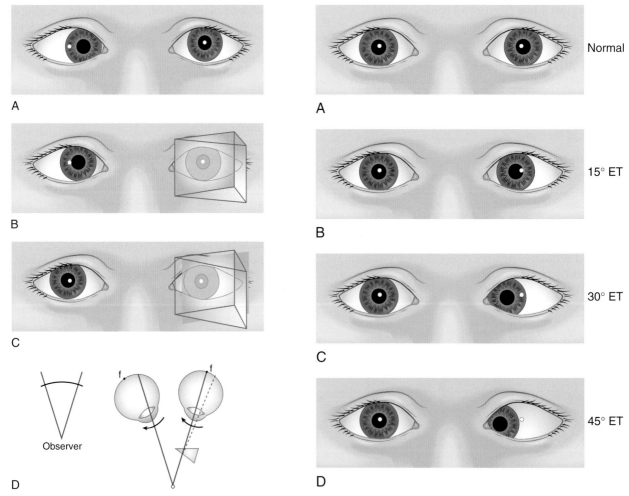

Figure 5.61 Modified Krimsky method of estimating deviation. (From von Noorden GK. *Von Noorden-Maumenee's Atlas of Strabismus,* 3rd ed. St Louis: Mosby; 1977.)

Figure 5.62 Hirschberg method of estimating deviation. (From von Noorden GK. *Von Noorden-Maumenee's Atlas of Strabismus,* 3rd ed. St Louis: Mosby; 1977.)

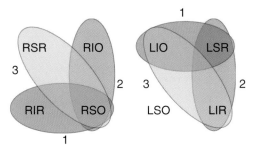

Figure 5.63 Parks-Bielschowsky 3-step test for right superior oblique (RSO) palsy.

Example: RSO palsy (Fig. 5.62)

Forced duction test: determines deviation as a result of muscle restriction

Forced generation test: measures muscle strength

NYSTAGMUS

Oscillation of eyes

Childhood Nystagmus

Most commonly congenital, latent, sensory, and spasmus nutans

Congenital

Benign disorder of eye movement calibration system (between sensory and motor systems)

Characteristics: long-standing, horizontal in all positions, may have rotary component, increases intensity with fixation, null point, no oscillopsia, may have head posture, dampened by convergence (better near than distance vision), exponentially increasing velocity of slow phase, OKN reversal in 60%, strabismus in 33%, similar monocular and binocular vision (20/20–20/70), absent during sleeping, latent nystagmus can be present (cover one eye, nystagmus converts to jerk away from covered eye), may develop head oscillations at 3 months of age, wide-swinging eye movements; at 1 year, small pendular movements; at 2 years, jerk nystagmus with null zone, discover convergence dampens nystagmus and may develop nystagmus blockage syndrome

Waveform: exponentially increasing velocity of slow phase

Associations: albinism, aniridia, Leber congenital amaurosis, ON hypoplasia, congenital cataracts, achromatopsia

Treatment: base-out prisms in glasses dampen nystagmus by forcing patient to converge (only fusional convergence [overcoming exophoria] diminishes the nystagmus; therefore, minus lenses that stimulate accommodative convergence do not dampen nystagmus); if head posture >50% of time, surgical correction (Kestenbaum procedure)

Distinguish congenital nystagmus from latent nystagmus:

Cover one eye: latent nystagmus worsens

Reversal of normal OKN response: congenital nystagmus
Dampens with convergence: congenital nystagmus
Examine slow-phase velocity: increases (congenital), decreases (latent)

Latent

Jerk nystagmus during monocular viewing away from covered eye

Associated with congenital esotropia and dissociated vertical deviation (DVD)

Pure form is rare

Etiology: abnormal cortical binocularity, proprioceptive imbalance, defective egocentric localization

Characteristics: cover one eye and uncovered eye, fast phase to side of fixing eye develops nystagmus; long-standing; normal OKN response; nulls with adduction; normal vision when both eyes open, vision decreases when each eye is tested separately; may have strabismus, especially infantile esotropia, DVD (50%)

Waveform: exponentially decreasing velocity of slow phase

Alexander's rule: intensity increases when looking toward fast phase and decreases when looking toward slow phase (i.e., adduction nulls; therefore, no head posture)

Treatment: surgery for strabismus or head turn

Sensory

Pendular nystagmus caused by visual loss; more common than congenital nystagmus

Etiology: aniridia, albinism, rod monochromatism (achromatopsia), CSNB, ON coloboma, cataracts, ON hypoplasia, Leber congenital amaurosis, bilateral macular coloboma

Spasmus Nutans

Benign form of nystagmus consisting of fine, rapid, often monocular or markedly asymmetric eye movements

Diagnosis of exclusion

Onset during first year of life with spontaneous resolution by age 3 years

Triad of findings: eye movements, head nodding/bobbing, and torticollis (diagnosis can be made in absence of head nodding)

Waveform: high frequency, low amplitude, pendular, asymmetric (dissociated form of nystagmus)

DDx: chiasmal glioma, subacute necrotizing encephalomyopathy

Neuroimaging: rule out tumor

Acquired Nystagmus

(See Chapter 4, Neuro-Ophthalmology)

OCULAR ALIGNMENT

Horizontal Deviations

At birth, 1/3 of babies are orthophoric and 2/3 are slightly XT

Orthophoria: normal alignment; eyes are straight; no latent or manifest deviation

Comitant: deviation is equal in all positions of gaze

Incomitant: deviation varies in different positions of gaze (paralytic or restrictive etiologies)

Esodeviations: latent or manifest convergence of the visual axes

Most common deviation (50%–75%)

Types:

PSEUDOESOTROPIA: patient is orthophoric but has appearance of esotropia. Results from broad nasal bridge, prominent medial epicanthal folds, or negative-angle κ

ESOPHORIA (E): latent deviation controlled by fusional mechanisms; may manifest under certain conditions (fatigue, illness, stress, or tests that dissociate eyes [alternate cover test])

INTERMITTENT ESOTROPIA (E(T)): deviation that is sometimes latent and sometimes manifest; partially controlled by fusional mechanisms

ESOTROPIA (ET): manifest deviation (Box 5.4)

Exodeviations: latent or manifest divergence of the visual axes

Less common than ET

25% of strabismus in children

In neonates, up to 60% have a constant, transient exodeviation

Most common form is intermittent exotropia

Types:

PSEUDOEXOTROPIA: patient is orthophoric but has appearance of exotropia. Results from positive-angle κ without other abnormalities, macular heterotopia (temporally dragged macula [PHPV, ROP, toxocariasis] with large-angle κ), wide interpupillary distance

EXOPHORIA (X): latent deviation; detected by alternate cover testing; may be related to asthenopia

INTERMITTENT EXOTROPIA (X(T)): deviation that is sometimes latent and sometimes manifest; partially controlled by fusional mechanisms

EXOTROPIA (XT): manifest deviation

BASIC: exodeviation equal at distance and near

DIVERGENCE EXCESS: exodeviation greater at distance than near by at least 10 Δ

Types:

Simulated (pseudodivergence excess): enhanced fusional convergence at near related to accommodation 30-minute patch test: binocular fusional impulses suspended and exodeviation becomes equal at distance

Box 5.4 Classification of esotropia

Infantile

Classic congenital

Early-onset accommodative

Duane syndrome type I

Abducens paralysis from birth trauma

Nystagmus blockage syndrome

Möbius syndrome

Acquired

Accommodative

Refractive

Nonrefractive

Mixed (partially accommodative and partially basic)

Decompensated

Nonaccommodative

Stress-induced acquired

Cyclic

Acute comitant

Sensory deprivation

Divergence insufficiency

Divergence paralysis

Spasm of near synkinetic reflex

Restrictive (thyroid eye disease, medial orbital wall fracture, overresected medial rectus [MR])

Lateral rectus (LR) weakness (cranial nerve [CN] 6 palsy, iatrogenic/surgical [slipped, detached, overrecessed LR])

and near. If near deviation increases to close to distance deviation with +3.00 D lenses, then high AC/A ratio exists

True: after 30-minute patch test, still has divergence excess at distance

CONVERGENCE INSUFFICIENCY: near exotropia is greater than distance exotropia

Congenital Esotropia

1%–2% of all strabismus

Equal sex distribution

Present by 6 months of age

Family history of strabismus is common

Increased frequency in cerebral palsy or hydrocephalus

Findings: deviation usually ≥30 Δ, low amounts of hyperopia, often cross-fixation with equal visual acuity in each eye, rarely develop normal binocular vision (even with surgery)

Associations: DVD in 70%

Overaction of inferior obliques in 70%

Involved eye elevates with adduction

Onset usually in second year of life; greatest occurrence between ages 3-7 years

Treat with IO weakening procedure

Latent nystagmus

Congenital, conjugate, horizontal jerk nystagmus that occurs under monocular conditions

When one eye is occluded, nystagmus develops in both eyes with fast phase toward the fixing eye and slow phase toward the occluded eye

MANIFEST LATENT NYSTAGMUS: nystagmus present when both eyes are open

Because of induced nystagmus in the uncovered eye with latent nystagmus, binocular visual acuity is better than when each eye is tested individually

NYSTAGMUS BLOCKAGE SYNDROME: overaccommodation to dampen nystagmus results in ET at near (usually large). Can differentiate from essential infantile esotropia (EIE) with manifest latent nystagmus because nystagmus does not increase with occlusion of one eye. Nystagmus dampens in convergence or adduction and increases in primary or lateral gaze. Adduction continues even when one eye is occluded, and head turn occurs toward the uncovered eye when the fellow eye is occluded. With adduction effort, the pupil constricts, demonstrating that accommodative mechanisms are present. May treat with large (≥6 mm) bimedial resections using a Faden suture

Asymmetry of the monocular, optokinetic motion–processing response

Nasal to temporal smooth pursuit less well developed than temporal to nasal pursuit

Can establish congenital nature of ET in an older patient

Asymmetry also seen in healthy newborns and disappears by 6 months of age

Diagnosis: demonstrate potential for full abduction with vestibular ocular reflex and doll's head maneuver to rule out congenital CN 6 palsy

Look for synkinetic lid or eye movements with attempted horizontal gaze to rule out Duane syndrome

Rule out accommodative component with glasses if older than age 1 year or phospholine iodide 0.125%

Treatment:

Nonsurgical: correct amblyopia before surgery; cross fixation suggests equal visual acuity of both eyes

Early surgery (as early as 6 months): potential for sensory binocular fusion; aim for alignment within 10 Δ of orthophoria

PROCEDURES:

Bilateral medial rectus recession

Recess medial rectus muscle and resect lateral rectus muscle of 1 eye

Associated surgery of inferior obliques if overaction present

3- or 4-muscle surgery for large deviation

Accommodative Esotropia

Onset 6 months to 7 years

May be intermittent at onset

Table 5.11 Types of accommodative esotropia

Type	Characteristics	Treatment
Refractive accommodative (normal AC/A ratio)	Esotropia at distance and near within 10 Δ	Full cycloplegic refraction
	High hyperopia (range +3.00 to +10.00 D, average = +4.00 D)	Treat amblyopia
Nonrefractive accommodative (high AC/A ratio)	Lower amount of hyperopia (average = +2.25 D)	Consider bifocal when esotropia at near exceeds distance by 10 Δ (executive type)
	Esotropia greater at near than at distance (may resolve with age)	Consider miotics (phospholine iodide 0.125%)
	Esotropia reduced at near with plus lens	Surgery if needed for residual esotropia
Mixed mechanism	Partially accommodative	Full cycloplegic refraction
	Angle of deviation reduced but not eliminated with spectacles	Surgery for nonaccommodative component
Decompensated accommodative	Residual esotropia after correction with full cycloplegic refraction	Full cycloplegic refraction
	Occurs more commonly with high AC/A ratio	Surgery

AC/A, Accommodative convergence to accommodation.

Often, positive family history

Associated with amblyopia (generally from anisometropia)

May be precipitated by trauma or illness

Types: (Table 5.11)

Accommodative convergence to accommodation (AC/A) ratio: normally between 3:1 and 5:1 prism diopters per diopter of accommodation

High AC/A ratio: usually present when near deviation exceeds distance deviation by >10-15 Δ

Calculation (two methods):

HETEROPHORIA METHOD: AC/A = IPD + [(N − D)/Diopt]

IPD = interpupillary distance (cm)

N = near deviation

D = distance deviation

Diopt = accommodative demand at fixation distance

Example: near deviation = 35 Δ; distance deviation = 10 Δ; accommodative demand = 20 cm (5 D); IPD = 60 mm (6 cm). Therefore, AC/A = 6 + [(35 − 10)/5] = 11:1

LENS GRADIENT METHOD: AC/A = (WL − NL)/D

WL = deviation with lens in front of eye

NL = deviation without lens in front of eye

D = dioptric power of lens used

Example: near deviation with a + 1.00 lens is 50 Δ and without a lens is 35 Δ. Therefore, AC/A = (50 − 35)/1.00 = 15:1

Natural history: hyperopia may decrease with age, AC/A ratio may normalize, and fusional divergence can improve; may begin to reduce strength of glasses and bifocals slowly as child gets older

Treatment: correct refractive error and treat amblyopia; consider surgery for residual component
Satisfactory: residual esotropia <10 Δ; peripheral fusion and expansion of fusional amplitudes possible
Unsatisfactory: try atropine with glasses or long-acting cholinesterase inhibitors; recheck refraction for increased or latent hyperopia
Echothiophate (phospholine iodide) causes accommodation that removes convergence with accommodative effort

Nonaccommodative Acquired Esotropia

Stress-induced acquired ET: breakdown of fusional divergence that occurs after illness, emotional trauma, or injury; requires surgery

Cyclic ET: intermittent, usually present every other day (48-hour cycle) and becomes constant with time
Findings: V-pattern ET is common; amblyopia can develop; on days when ET is not present, normal binocular visual acuity with good stereovision
Treatment: prescribe full hyperopic correction; may also require surgery if glasses do not fully correct deviation; phenobarbital and amphetamines can alter the frequency of the cycles

Sensory ET: results from loss of vision (sensory deprivation) in one or both eyes, usually during childhood (age <6 years); identify and treat obstruction to vision

Divergence insufficiency: ET greater at distance than near; fusional divergence is reduced
Treat with base-out prisms (to correct diplopia) or surgery
Rule out divergence paralysis (associated with pontine tumors, head trauma, or other neurologic abnormalities; may mimic bilateral CN 6 paralysis)

Spasm of near synkinetic reflex (ciliary spasm): intermittent episodes of sustained convergence with accommodative spasm and miosis
Findings: headache, blurred distance visual acuity (recent onset of myopia is present in history [pseudomyopia]), abnormally close near point, and fluctuating visual acuity; variable angle of deviation; monocular abduction is normal; large difference between manifest and cycloplegic refraction
Treatment: cycloplegia may break spasm; on postcycloplegic refraction push plus

Incomitant ET:
Etiology: MR restriction: thyroid, orbital wall fractures, or excessively resected MR muscle
Slipped muscle following strabismus surgery
Neurogenic: CN 6 palsy (spontaneous or results from intracranial lesions [33%], infections, or birth trauma)
Myasthenia gravis

Consecutive esotropia: follows surgery for exotropia; rule out slipped muscle

Prism adaptation test: prisms are used to help patients obtain binocular fusion while awaiting surgical alignment of the eyes. Used to preoperatively predict which patients will develop residual esotropia after surgery. Patients who respond with increasing deviation are given stronger prism until orthophoria is obtained. The largest angle is the target for surgical correction

Intermittent Exotropia

Most common form of XT

Onset varies from infancy to age 4 years

May be progressive

Often have reflex closure of one eye in bright light

Suppression only when eyes are deviated (facultative suppression)

Amblyopia is uncommon

Natural history:
Phase 1: X(T) at distance and straight at near
Present when fatigued
May see double
Most maintain excellent stereovision
Phase 2: X(T) becomes more constant at distance with X(T) at near
Suppression increases
Phase 3: XT at distance and near
Often no diplopia because of suppression
Most common cause of a constant XT

Treatment: treat amblyopia, alternate occlusion therapy, induce accommodative convergence by prescribing overminus spectacles (also for consecutive exotropia), prism therapy with base-in prisms, fusional convergence training (progressive base-out prism to induce convergence)
Surgery for increased tropic phase, poor recovery of fusion once tropic, increasing ease of dissociation, XT >50% of time at home
PROCEDURES:
Bilateral lateral rectus recession
Recess lateral rectus and resect medial rectus of 1 eye
3- or 4-muscle surgery for large deviation

Congenital Exotropia

Rare

May be primary (otherwise-healthy patients) or secondary (from ocular or systemic abnormalities)

Usually large angle of deviation (average >35 Δ)

Amblyopia is uncommon; similar refractive error to general population

Most resolve by age 6 months; if not, consider surgery

Associations: DVD and oblique muscle overaction; orbital or skull defects, neurologic disease, or other ocular, genetic, or systemic conditions

Convergence Insufficiency

Exophoria greater at near than at distance (not exotropic at near)

Remote near point of convergence and reduced fusional convergence amplitudes at near

Female > male

Common in teenagers and young adults; incidence increases with age; prevalence 2%-8%

Associations: can be exacerbated by fatigue, drugs, uveitis, or Adie tonic pupil; may also follow head trauma. Also associated with systemic illnesses, or as a conversion reaction

Findings: asthenopia, diplopia; reduced fusional convergence amplitudes and remote near point of convergence, may have exophoria at near

Treatment: observation; orthoptic exercises to improve fusional amplitudes, base-out prisms; rarely surgery (medial rectus resection)

Convergence Paralysis Secondary to Intracranial Lesion

Normal adduction and accommodation

XT and diplopia on attempted near fixation

Associations: Parinaud syndrome

Treatment: base-in prisms or occlusion of 1 eye to relieve diplopia

Sensory Exotropia

Caused by loss of vision or long-standing poor vision in 1 eye

Children age <6 years with unilateral vision loss; may develop ET or XT; adults usually develop XT

Angle of deviation may be variable and usually increases with time

Consecutive Exotropia

Follows previous strabismus surgery for esotropia

Vertical Deviations

Dissociated Vertical Deviation (DVD; Dissociated Horizontal Deviation [DHD]; Dissociated Torsional Deviation [DTD])

Intermittent deviation of nonfixing eye consisting of upward excursion, extorsion, excyclotorsion, abduction, or lateral deviation

Exact etiology unknown but associated with early disruption of binocular development

Usually asymptomatic because of poor fusion and suppression

Often asymmetric

Does not obey Hering's law (fellow eye does not exhibit refixation movement in opposite direction)

Occurs with eye occlusion or visual inattention

May be latent or manifest

Usually presents before 12 months of age

Usually more marked when patient is fatigued, daydreaming, under stress, or sick

Associations: nystagmus (latent or manifest latent), inferior oblique overaction, often occurs in patients with history of congenital ET; isolated in 40% of patients

Findings: slow movement of eye in the characteristic direction, amount of deviation variable (accurate measurements difficult to obtain), dissociated deviation occurs in all directions of gaze

Diagnosis:
  Bielschowsky's phenomenon: occurs in 50% of patients with DVD
    Elevated eye will drift downward when light in fixing eye is reduced; conversely, increased illumination in an eye with DVD will cause it to drift up
  Red lens phenomenon: place red lens over either eye while patient fixates on light source
    Red image is always seen below the white image
    In patients with a true hypertropia, the red image is seen above or below the primary image, depending on whether the red filter is placed in front of the hyperdeviated or hypodeviated eye

Treatment:
  Increase fusional mechanisms: give optimal spectacle correction; switch fixation to nonpreferred eye
  Surgery:
    INDICATIONS: increasing size or frequency of manifest DVD, abnormal head position
    PROCEDURES: SR recession, IR resection, IO weakening or anterior transposition (in patients with inferior oblique overaction [IOOA] and DVD)
    CAUTIONS: perform bilateral surgery (unilateral surgery often reveals occult contralateral DVD); often recurs or persists after surgery

Inferior Oblique Overaction (IOOA)

Occurs in 2/3 of patients with congenital ET

Usually bilateral and asymmetric

Early surgery for ET is important for development of binocular vision but does not reduce incidence of IO dysfunction

May be primary (resulting from paralysis of the antagonist [SO]) or secondary

Findings: when fixing eye is abducted, adducting eye is elevated; when fixing eye is adducted, abducted eye is depressed; V-pattern deviation; primary position extorsion of fundus on indirect ophthalmoscopy

Treatment: IO weakening procedure (recession, myectomy, anteriorization)

167

Inferior Oblique Palsy

Rare

Usually idiopathic but may follow orbital trauma, viral illness, or other neurologic problems

May be bilateral

Findings: eye is hypotrophic when fixing with normal eye, hypertropia of normal eye when fixing with involved eye, deviation worsens with gaze into field of action of involved inferior oblique, deviation is worse with head tilt opposite of paretic eye, poor elevation in adduction, normal forced duction (distinguishes from Brown syndrome), A-pattern

Treatment:
  With associated SO overaction: SO-weakening procedure. If hyperdeviation develops in downgaze, then weaken contralateral IR
  IO palsy with hypotropia in primary gaze and no SO overaction: IR recession (2.5 Δ per mm of recession)

Superior Oblique Overaction

Less common than IO overaction or DVD

Findings: A-pattern; associated with depression on attempted adduction if fixing with uninvolved eye; may have associated horizontal deviation

Treatment: weaken overacting SO with tenotomy (uncontrolled) or silicone spacer (controlled)

Superior Oblique Palsy

Most common isolated cyclovertical muscle palsy

Congenital (75%): large fusional amplitudes (≥15 Δ)
  SO tendon often long or floppy; sometimes absent
  Long-standing CN 4 palsy results in ocular torticollis, which may lead to facial asymmetry
  Examine old photographs to determine duration of head tilt
  Can mimic a double elevator palsy (if fixation preference is for the affected eye, the contralateral SR muscle can appear to underact [inhibitional palsy of the contralateral antagonist] and the contralateral IR can undergo contracture, leading to double elevator palsy)

Acquired: often a result of trauma (long course of fourth nerve makes it especially vulnerable)

Findings: diplopia (vertical, horizontal, or torsional). In long-standing cases of SO palsy, comitance develops, and the deviation becomes more difficult to localize (hypertropia can be present in all fields of gaze)

Bilateral: objective torsion is often >10° of excyclotorsion (measure with double Maddox rod), often have inferior oblique overaction with V-pattern ET and chin-down head posture, alternate hypertropia with head tilt

Diagnosis: Parks-Bielschowsky 3-step test (i.e., right superior oblique palsy produces right hypertropia in primary gaze, worsens in left gaze and in right head tilt)

Treatment: surgery
  Indications: significant head tilt, large hypertropia in primary gaze, diplopia
  Procedures:
    If deviation in primary gaze is ≤15 Δ, operate on 1 muscle; if deviation >15 Δ, operate on ≥2 muscles
    With IO overaction, weaken ipsilateral IO (corrects approximately 15 Δ of vertical deviation)
    If hyperdeviation is >15 Δ in primary gaze, strengthen ipsilateral IR or weaken contralateral SR
    With no inferior oblique overaction, consider weakening ipsilateral SR or recessing contralateral IR; SO tuck may also be considered if there is laxity of the tendon
    Knapp classification for treatment of superior oblique palsy offers guidance
    General principle is to match the fields of greatest deviation to the muscles that work most in those fields to guide surgical approach
    Check traction test in operating room to assess laxity of superior oblique tendon
  Torsional symptoms: most people can tolerate 7° of torsion
    Consider Harada-Ito procedure: lateral transposition of anterior portion of SO tendon; corrects excyclotorsion only; no effect on vertical deviation or fusion

Inferior Rectus Palsy

Results from trauma to CN 3 or IR

May occur at time of injury or repair of an orbital fracture

May resolve with time

Double-Elevator Palsy (Monocular Elevation Deficiency)

Sporadic, unilateral defect of upgaze associated with ipsilateral ptosis

There are two elevators of the eye: the SR (provides most of elevation) and the IO

May be supranuclear (may not involve both elevators)

May be congenital or acquired (cerebrovascular disease, tumor, or infection)

Types:
  IR restriction: unilateral fibrosis syndrome
    Positive forced ductions to elevation
    Positive force generation (no muscle paralysis)
    Normal saccades of SR
  Elevator weakness: (SR and IO)
    Free forced ductions to elevation
    Reduced force generation (muscle paralysis)
    Reduced velocities of upgaze movements
  Combination: IR restriction plus weak elevators
    Positive forced ductions to elevation
    Reduced force generation (muscle paralysis)
    Reduced velocities of upgaze movements

Findings: unilateral limitation of upgaze above midline with accompanying ptosis in both adduction and abduction, variable head position (normal or chin-up), hypotropia increases on upgaze, fixing with involved eye causes large secondary hypotropia in nonparetic eye

Treatment: surgery
 Indications: chin-up head position, large vertical deviation in primary position, poor fusion in primary position
 Procedures:
  DOUBLE-ELEVATOR PALSY WITH TIGHT IR: IR recession
  DOUBLE-ELEVATOR PALSY WITH SR WEAKNESS: Knapp procedure (elevation and transposition of MR and LR to the side of SR)
  DOUBLE-ELEVATOR PALSY WITH PTOSIS: correct strabismus then residual ptosis

Brown Syndrome (SO Tendon Sheath Syndrome)

Inability to elevate the eye in adduction, both actively and passively on forced duction testing

May be congenital or acquired (traumatic, inflammatory, iatrogenic [following SO tuck, glaucoma drainage implant, scleral buckle])

Findings: limitation of elevation in adduction, less elevation deficiency in midline, minimal or no elevation deficiency in abduction, V-pattern divergence in upgaze, restricted forced ductions, minimal or no superior oblique overaction, "clicking" may occur and suggests a trochlear problem, anomalous head posture or hypotropia in primary position may be present

Treatment:
 Observation: spontaneous improvement may occur
 Surgery:
  INDICATIONS: abnormal head position, large hypotropia in primary position, constant deviation causing amblyopia and threatening binocularity
  PROCEDURE: superior weakening procedure (SO tenectomy, tenotomy, or silicone spacer)
  COMPLICATION: SO palsy

A- and V-Patterns

Change in horizontal deviation as eyes move between upgaze and downgaze

Up to 50% of all strabismus has an associated A- or V-pattern

May present as compensatory head posture (chin-up or chin-down) in child with binocular function

A-pattern: increasing convergence or decreasing divergence in upgaze, increasing divergence in downgaze

Clinically significant when eyes diverge >10 Δ from upgaze to downgaze

V-pattern: increasing convergence or decreasing divergence in downgaze, increasing divergence in upgaze

Clinically significant when eyes converge >15 Δ from upgaze to downgaze

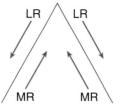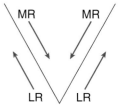

Figure 5.64 Direction of muscle transposition for A- and V-patterns.

Etiology: oblique muscle dysfunction (obliques are abductors, IO overaction creates a V-pattern), horizontal rectus muscle dysfunction, vertical rectus muscle dysfunction, structural factors (e.g., craniosynostosis is associated with a V-pattern, abnormal insertions of rectus muscles, absence of SO tendon)

Diagnosis: measure deviation in primary position, then with eyes directed 25° in upgaze and downgaze

Treatment: surgery
 Indications: abnormal head position; to improve motor alignment
 Procedures:
  If no oblique muscle overaction is present, vertical transposition of horizontal muscles (Fig. 5.64)
  Corrects about 15 Δ of the A- and V-patterns, muscles are transposed ½ to 1 tendon width up or down, transposition is in the direction of the desired weakening
  Mnemonic: **MALE** (**M**edial rectus to **A**pex of pattern; **L**ateral rectus to the **E**mpty space)
  If oblique muscle overaction present, oblique muscle weakening
  IO WEAKENING: corrects ≥15 Δ of eso shift in upgaze, with no effect on horizontal alignment in primary gaze
  BILATERAL SO TENOTOMIES: corrects up to 30-40 Δ of eso shift in downgaze; torsional symptoms may occur in patients with good fusion

SPECIAL FORMS OF STRABISMUS

Duane Retraction Syndrome

Usually sporadic, may be inherited, female > male (3:2)

Cocontraction of medial and lateral rectus muscles causes retraction of the globe with secondary narrowing of the palpebral fissure

Vertical deviations may be present with characteristic upshoot or downshoot (leash phenomenon)

Bilateral in 15%-20%, affects OS > OD (3:1), type 1 > type 3 > type 2

Head turn common (for fusion), amblyopia rare

Etiology: abnormal innervation of lateral rectus by a branch of CN 3; electromyography shows decreased firing of lateral rectus during abduction and paradoxical innervation of the lateral rectus during adduction

Exact etiology unclear, proposed mechanisms include hypoplasia of sixth nerve nucleus, midbrain pathology, fibrosis of lateral rectus

Types:
  Type 1 (most common): limitation of abduction, retraction and narrowing of palpebral fissures in adduction; appears esotropic
  Type 2: limitation of adduction; appears exotropic
  Type 3: limitation of abduction and adduction

Associations (rare): deafness, crocodile tears, syndromes (Goldenhar syndrome, Klippel-Feil syndrome, Wildervanck syndrome [Duane syndrome associated with Klippel-Feil], thalidomide toxicity, fetal alcohol syndrome, cat-eye syndrome)

Treatment: correct any refractive error, treat amblyopia
  Surgery
  Indications: abnormal head position or deviation in primary gaze
  Procedures: for esotropia: recession of medial rectus muscle
  For globe retraction: simultaneous lateral rectus recession
  For upshoot or downshoot: splitting of lateral rectus or Faden procedure
  Avoid muscle resection (increases globe retraction, upshoots and downshoots)

Möbius Syndrome

CN 6 and 7 palsies

Results from aplasia of involved brainstem nuclei

Associations: congenital facial diplegia (mask facies); combined CN 6, 7, 9, and 12 palsies; gaze palsy (PPRF involvement); chest, limb, tongue defects

Findings: esotropia with limitation of abduction, exposure keratitis from poor lid closure

Congenital Fibrosis Syndrome

Group of congenital anomalies characterized by variable amounts of restriction of extraocular muscles and replacement of the muscles with fibrous tissue

Nonprogressive

≥1 muscles may be involved

Positive forced duction testing

Types:
  Generalized fibrosis:
    Most severe
    Usually autosomal dominant, may be recessive
    All extraocular muscles involved, including levator (with ptosis)
  Congenital fibrosis of inferior rectus:
    Sporadic or familial
    Levator may be involved
  Strabismus fixus:

Severe esotropia
Horizontal rectus muscles involved (usually MR, occasionally LR)
Vertical retraction syndrome:
  SR fibrosis (inability to depress eye)
Congenital unilateral fibrosis:
  Enophthalmos and ptosis
  Fibrosis of all muscles, including levator

Chronic Progressive External Ophthalmoplegia (CPEO)

Sporadic or maternal inheritance (mitochondrial DNA)

May present at any age

Associations:
  Kearns-Sayre syndrome: triad of CPEO, retinal pigmentary changes, and cardiac conduction defects
  Bassen Kornzweig syndrome (abetalipoproteinemia): retinal pigmentary changes similar to RP, diarrhea, ataxia, and other neurologic signs
  Refsum disease: RP-like syndrome with elevated phytanic acid levels
  Oculopharyngeal dystrophy (AR and AD): difficulty swallowing atrophy of tongue, and proximal muscle (hips and upper legs) weakness

Findings: severe ptosis with complete ophthalmoplegia, absent Bell's phenomenon, no restrictions on forced ductions, large-angle strabismus (often XT)

Orbital Floor Fracture

Findings: ecchymosis, diplopia in some or all positions of gaze immediately after injury, paresthesia or hypesthesia in distribution of infraorbital nerve, entrapment of inferior rectus muscle or inferior oblique muscle; may have associated ocular damage, may have associated wall fractures (e.g., medial wall with medial rectus entrapment)

Diagnosis: forced duction testing orbital imaging

Treatment: observation (usually 5–10 days until edema and hematoma resolve, then reevaluate), surgery

Following Surgery

Commonly after cataract, scleral buckle, and glaucoma drainage implant procedures

May be transient and resolve spontaneously

Horizontal, vertical, or torsional

Etiology:
  Mechanical: adhesions, mass effect (implant or buckle)
  Motor: trauma, ischemia, slipped or disinserted muscle, toxicity (local anesthetic; most commonly IR fibrosis with hypotropia in primary gaze that worsens in abduction; positive forced ductions)
  Sensory: fusion breakdown, anisometropia, aniseikonia, image distortion

Treatment: observation, prism spectacles, surgery

Other Forms of Strabismus

Myasthenia gravis, thyroid eye disease, CN 3 palsy, skew deviation

STRABISMUS SURGERY

Indications: establish binocularity, improve fusion, improve symptoms or appearance

Anesthesia:
Topical: may consider for recession procedures
Retrobulbar: use shorter-acting anesthetic for adjustable sutures
General: for children; consider in adults undergoing bilateral surgery

Incisions:
Fornix: in superior or inferior cul-de-sac on bulbar conjunctiva
Limbal: conjunctival/Tenon flap at limbus
Swan: over the muscle (causes more scarring)

Weakening Procedures

Recession: most common technique used to weaken rectus muscles by moving muscle posteriorly; also used to weaken inferior oblique

Myotomy (cutting across muscle) **or myectomy** (excising a portion of muscle): used to weaken inferior oblique

Denervation and extirpation: used to weaken inferior oblique by ablating all muscle within Tenon capsule

Tenotomy (cutting across tendon) **or tenectomy** (excising a portion of tendon): most commonly used to weaken superior oblique

Posterior fixation suture (Faden procedure): suture placed 11-18 mm from insertion through belly of muscle and sclera to weaken muscle only in its field of action; decreases mechanical advantage of muscle acting on globe; often combined with recession

Strengthening Procedures

Resection: used to strengthen rectus muscles by excising portion of muscle and reattaching muscle at its insertion site

Advancement (moving muscle forward): often used for muscles previously recessed, also in Harada-Ito procedure

Tuck: technique used to strengthen superior oblique by shortening the tendon (may produce iatrogenic Brown syndrome)

Other Techniques

Adjustable suture: slipknot or noose suture to enable muscle adjustment postoperatively under topical anesthesia

Transposition: moving muscle out of original plane of action; used in cases of paralysis, double-elevator palsy, or A- and V-patterns

Harada-Ito procedure: anterior temporal displacement of anterior half of superior oblique tendon; used to correct excyclotorsion

Kestenbaum procedure: bilateral resection/recession to dampen nystagmus in patients with nystagmus and head turn; eyes are surgically moved toward direction of head turn

Botulinum toxin (Botox): interferes with release of acetylcholine to paralyze muscle into which it is injected. When an extraocular muscle is paralyzed by Botox, the antagonist contracts to change the alignment of the eyes

Used in cases of paralytic strabismus to prevent contracture of muscles or postoperative residual strabismus, and when surgery is inappropriate

General Principles

Needles: use spatulated needles (cutting surface on the side) to decrease risk of perforation (sclera is thinnest just posterior to insertion of rectus muscles [0.3 mm])

Vertical deviations: in general, surgery should be performed on muscles whose field of action is in same field as the vertical deviation (e.g., left hypertropia that is greatest down and to patient's right might be addressed by either weakening right inferior rectus or strengthening left superior oblique)

Horizontal incomitancy: can be treated by adjusting amount of surgery performed on each muscle (i.e., if exotropia increases from right gaze to primary gaze to left gaze, consider larger recession on left lateral rectus to have a greater effect on exotropia to left [in field of action of that muscle])

Distance–near disparity: perform surgery on lateral rectus muscles if exodeviation is greater at distance than at near. Perform surgery on medial rectus muscles if esodeviation is greater at near than at distance

Complications of Strabismus Surgery

Residual strabismus (most common): alignment in postoperative period can change owing to poor fusion, poor vision, altered accommodation, and contracture of scar tissue

Scleral perforation: usually creates only a chorioretinal scar but can also lead to vitreous hemorrhage, retinal tear, retinal detachment, or endophthalmitis. If suspected during surgery, perform indirect ophthalmoscopy to determine whether a perforation is present; consider retinal laser treatment, cryotherapy, or observation

Infection: uncommon; includes endophthalmitis, cellulitis, and subconjunctival abscess

Foreign body granuloma: may develop weeks after surgery, often at suture site. Localized, elevated, slightly hyperemic, tender mass, usually <1 cm; may require surgical excision

Conjunctival inclusion cyst: may occur when conjunctiva is buried during closure of incision. Appears days to weeks later as noninflamed, translucent mass under conjunctiva. May resolve spontaneously or require excision if symptomatic

Conjunctival scarring: can occur with orbital fat encroaching under bulbar conjunctiva because of inadvertent openings through Tenon capsule

Fat adherence syndrome: violation of Tenon capsule with prolapsed orbital fat into sub-Tenon space can lead to fibrofatty scar. May have positive traction test and restricted motility

Delle: thin, dehydrated area of cornea caused by elevated limbal conjunctiva that prevents adequate corneal lubrication during blinking

Anterior segment ischemia: most blood to anterior segment supplied by anterior ciliary arteries that travel in rectus muscles. Usually occurs with surgery on ≥3 muscles. Corneal edema and anterior uveitis are present. Treat with topical steroids

Diplopia

Change in eyelid position: most commonly with surgery of vertical rectus muscles

Lost or slipped muscle: when only the capsule is sutured to insertion site, muscle can slip back; prevented with locking bites during suturing

Oculocardiac reflex: slowing of heart rate with traction on extraocular muscles

Malignant hyperthermia: acute metabolic disorder that may be fatal if diagnosis or treatment is delayed. Triggered by inhalation agents and succinylcholine. Signs include tachycardia, unstable blood pressure, arrhythmias, increased temperature, muscle rigidity, cyanosis, dark urine

REVIEW QUESTIONS (Answers start on page 415)

1. The approximate age of onset for accommodative ET is closest to
   a. 1 year old
   b. 3 years old
   c. 5 years old
   d. 7 years old
2. A 15-year-old girl with strabismus is examined, and the following measurements are recorded: distance deviation of 10 Δ, near deviation of 35 Δ at 20 cm, and interpupillary distance of 60 mm. Her AC/A ratio is
   a. 11:1
   b. 10:1
   c. 5:1
   d. 3:1
3. Duane syndrome is thought to result from a developmental abnormality of the
   a. trochlear nucleus
   b. motor endplate
   c. oculomotor nucleus
   d. abducens nucleus
4. The most helpful test in a patient with aniridia is
   a. electrocardiogram
   b. abdominal ultrasound
   c. chest X-ray
   d. CBC

5. The best test for an infant with a normal fundus and searching eye movements is
   a. VER
   b. ERG
   c. EOG
   d. OKN
6. The most common congenital infection is
   a. toxoplasmosis.
   b. HSV
   c. CMV
   d. rubella
7. ARC is most likely to develop in a child with
   a. congenital esotropia
   b. amblyopia and suppression
   c. alternating exotropia
   d. small-angle esotropia
8. Which of the following most accurately reflects what a patient with harmonious ARC reports when the angle of anomaly is equal to the objective angle?
   a. fusion
   b. crossed diplopia
   c. simultaneous macular perception
   d. uncrossed diplopia
9. The inferior oblique muscle is weakened most by which procedure?
   a. disinsertion
   b. recession
   c. myotomy
   d. anteriorization
10. The test that gives the best dissociation is
    a. Maddox rod
    b. Worth 4-Dot
    c. Bagolini glasses
    d. red glass
11. The 3-step test shows a left hypertropia in primary position that worsens on right gaze and with left head tilt. The best surgical procedure is
    a. RIR resection
    b. RSO tuck
    c. LIR recession
    d. LIO weakening
12. In the treatment of a superior oblique palsy, Knapp recommended all of the following, *except*
    a. SO plication
    b. recession of the contralateral IR
    c. IO weakening
    d. resection of the contralateral SR
13. The best results of cryotherapy for ROP occur for treatment of disease in which location?
    a. zone I
    b. anterior zone II
    c. posterior zone II
    d. zone III
14. The *least* common finding of congenital ET is
    a. dissociated vertical deviation
    b. cross fixation
    c. amblyopia
    d. inferior oblique overaction

15. The contralateral antagonist of the right superior rectus
    a. passes under another muscle
    b. causes incyclotorsion when paretic
    c. adducts the eye
    d. is innervated by the inferior division of CN 3
16. With respect to Panum's area, physiologic diplopia occurs at what point?
    a. on the horopter
    b. within Panum's area
    c. in front of Panum's area
    d. none of the above
17. The best treatment of an A-pattern ET with muscle transposition is
    a. MR resection with upward transposition
    b. LR resection with upward transposition
    c. MR recession with downward transposition
    d. LR resection with downward transposition
18. A superior rectus Faden suture is used for the treatment of which condition?
    a. Duane syndrome
    b. dissociated vertical deviation
    c. Brown syndrome
    d. double-elevator palsy
19. Which medication should be administered to a child who develops trismus under general anesthesia?
    a. atropine
    b. edrophonium chloride
    c. lidocaine
    d. dantrolene
20. Congenital superior oblique palsy is characterized by all of the following, *except*
    a. excyclotorsion <10°
    b. head tilt
    c. facial asymmetry
    d. <10 D of vertical vergence amplitudes
21. Which of the following statements regarding monofixation syndrome is *false*?
    a. there is no diplopia with the 4 Δ base-out prism test.
    b. fusion with the Worth 4-Dot test is absent at distance
    c. fusional vergence amplitudes are absent
    d. titmus test for fly is normal
22. Iridocyclitis is most commonly associated with which form of JIA?
    a. systemic
    b. polyarticular
    c. spondyloarthritis
    d. pauciarticular
23. Congenital rubella is most commonly associated with
    a. retinal pigment epitheliopathy
    b. cataracts
    c. glaucoma
    d. strabismus
24. The most common cause of proptosis in a child is
    a. idiopathic orbital inflammation
    b. orbital cellulitis
    c. cavernous hemangioma
    d. Graves' disease

25. Which form of rhabdomyosarcoma has the worst prognosis?
    a. botryoid
    b. pleomorphic
    c. alveolar
    d. embryonal
26. Which of the following conditions is the *least* common cause of childhood proptosis?
    a. cavernous hemangioma
    b. rhabdomyosarcoma
    c. lymphangioma
    d. mucocele
27. A child with retinoblastoma is born to healthy parents with no family history of RB. The chance of RB occurring in a second child is approximately
    a. 5%
    b. 25%
    c. 40%
    d. 50%
28. The best chronologic age to examine a baby for ROP is
    a. 28 weeks
    b. 32 weeks
    c. 36 weeks
    d. 40 weeks
29. All of the following are associated with trisomy 13, *except*
    a. anophthalmos
    b. retinal dysplasia
    c. epiblepharon
    d. intraocular cartilage
30. Paradoxical pupillary response does *not* occur in
    a. achromatopsia
    b. CSNB
    c. Leber congenital amaurosis
    d. albinism
31. An infant with bilateral cataracts is diagnosed with galactosemia. Which enzyme is most likely to be defective?
    a. galactokinase
    b. galactose-1-P-uridyl transferase
    c. galactose-6-sulfatase
    d. UDP galactose-4-epimerase
32. All of the following are associated with ON drusen, *except*
    a. peripapillary hemorrhage
    b. inferior nasal VF loss
    c. increased risk of intracranial tumors
    d. AD inheritance
33. Which is the most likely etiology of torticollis and intermittent, fine, rapid, pendular nystagmus of the right eye in a 10-month-old baby?
    a. metastatic neuroblastoma
    b. posterior fossa tumor
    c. optic nerve meningioma
    d. none of the above
34. The most common malignant tumor of the orbit in a 6-year-old boy is
    a. neuroblastoma
    b. rhabdomyosarcoma
    c. optic nerve glioma
    d. lymphosarcoma

35. RP and deafness occur in all of the following disorders, *except*
    a. Usher syndrome
    b. Alstrom syndrome
    c. Refsum disease
    d. Cockayne syndrome
36. α-Galactosidase A deficiency is associated with
    a. cornea verticillata
    b. corneal clouding
    c. corneal vascularization
    d. no corneal changes
37. Congenital cataracts and glaucoma may occur in all of the following disorders, *except*
    a. Hallermann-Streiff syndrome
    b. Alport syndrome
    c. rubella
    d. Lowe syndrome
38. RPE degeneration and optic atrophy are found in all of the following mucopolysaccharidoses, *except*
    a. MPS type I
    b. MPS type II
    c. MPS type III
    d. MPS type IV
39. Which vitamin is *not* deficient in a patient with abetalipoproteinemia (Bassen-Kornzweig syndrome)?
    a. A
    b. C
    c. D
    d. E
40. Hearing loss is *not* found in
    a. Cogan syndrome
    b. Refsum disease
    c. Duane syndrome
    d. Stickler syndrome
41. Pheochromocytoma may occur in all of the following phakomatoses, *except*
    a. Louis-Bar syndrome
    b. von Hippel–Lindau disease
    c. Sturge-Weber syndrome
    d. Bourneville disease
42. Maternal ingestion of LSD is most likely to result in which congenital ON disorder?
    a. coloboma
    b. optic pit
    c. hypoplasia
    d. morning glory disc
43. A patient with strabismus wearing −6 D glasses is measured with prism and cover test. Compared with the actual amount of deviation, the measurement would find
    a. more esotropia and less exotropia
    b. more esotropia and more exotropia
    c. less esotropia and more exotropia
    d. less esotropia and less exotropia
44. Prism glasses are *least* helpful for treating
    a. incomitant esotropia
    b. divergence insufficiency
    c. sensory esotropia
    d. intermittent exotropia
45. A 4-year-old boy has bilateral lateral rectus recessions for exotropia. Two days after surgery, he has an esotropia measuring 50 Δ. The most appropriate treatment is
    a. atropinization
    b. prism glasses
    c. alternate patching
    d. surgery
46. The most common cause of a vitreous hemorrhage in a child is
    a. ROP
    b. shaken baby syndrome
    c. FEVR
    d. Coat disease
47. A 5-year-old girl with 20/20 vision OD and 20/50 vision OS is diagnosed with an anterior polar cataract OS. Which is the most appropriate treatment?
    a. start occlusion therapy
    b. observe and reexamine in 6 months
    c. perform cataract surgery and use aphakic contact lens
    d. perform cataract surgery with lens implant
48. Chronic iritis in a child is most commonly caused by
    a. JIA
    b. trauma
    c. sarcoidosis
    d. Lyme disease
49. All are features of ataxia-telangiectasia, *except*
    a. sinopulmonary infections
    b. thymic hyperplasia
    c. IgA deficiency
    d. AR inheritance
50. All of the following vitreoretinal disorders are inherited in an AD pattern, *except*
    a. familial exudative vitreoretinopathy
    b. Wagner syndrome
    c. Stickler syndrome
    d. Goldmann-Favre disease
51. The most common location for an iris coloboma is
    a. superotemporal
    b. superonasal
    c. inferotemporal
    d. inferonasal
52. Von Hippel–Lindau disease has been mapped to which chromosome?
    a. 3
    b. 9
    c. 11
    d. 17
53. Which X-linked disorder is *not* associated with an ocular abnormality in the female carrier?
    a. choroideremia
    b. albinism
    c. juvenile retinoschisis
    d. retinitis pigmentosa
54. Which tumor is *not* associated with von Hippel–Lindau disease?
    a. hepatocellular carcinoma
    b. pheochromocytoma
    c. renal cell carcinoma
    d. cerebellar hemangioblastoma

55. The most useful diagnostic test in an infant with an oil-droplet cataract is
    a. urine amino acids
    b. calcium
    c. TORCH titers
    d. urine-reducing substances
56. The genetics of aniridia are best summarized as
    a. 1/4 AR, 3/4 AD
    b. 1/4 sporadic, 3/4 AR
    c. 1/4 AD, 3/4 sporadic
    d. 1/4 sporadic, 3/4 AD
57. A pigmentary retinopathy occurs in which mesodermal dysgenesis syndrome?
    a. Axenfeld anomaly
    b. Alagille syndrome
    c. Rieger syndrome
    d. Peter anomaly
58. Which of the following laboratory tests is most commonly found in JIA-related iritis?
    a. RF−, ANA−
    b. RF+, ANA−
    c. RF−, ANA+
    d. RF+, ANA+
59. The size of an esodeviation is measured with the
    a. cover–uncover test
    b. double Maddox rod test
    c. alternate prism and cover test
    d. Worth 4-Dot test
60. Toxoplasmosis is most likely to be acquired from
    a. cat scratch
    b. undercooked meat
    c. needle stick
    d. eating dirt
61. A 10-day-old infant develops an acute papillary conjunctivitis with mucoid discharge. Which of the following is the most likely cause?
    a. *Neisseria gonorrhoeae*
    b. *Escherichia coli*
    c. *Chlamydia*
    d. Herpes simplex
62. An infant is brought to the emergency department after a fall. There is a bruise on the forehead and numerous retinal hemorrhages. There are also bruises on the back. An X-ray shows previous rib fractures. The most likely diagnosis is
    a. Coats disease
    b. malnutrition
    c. anemia
    d. nonaccidental trauma
63. A child undergoes uncomplicated cataract surgery with phacoemulsification and insertion of an acrylic posterior chamber intraocular lens. What is the most likely complication to develop in the future?
    a. capsular opacification
    b. cystoid macular edema
    c. hyperopia
    d. retinal detachment
64. On a routine eye exam, a 5-year-old girl is found to have mild iritis in both eyes. What is the most helpful test to order?
    a. ANA
    b. ANCA
    c. HLA
    d. PPD
65. The most common color vision defect is
    a. protanomaly
    b. protanopia
    c. deuteranomaly
    d. deuteranopia
66. Corneal clouding does *not* occur in which mucopolysaccharidosis?
    a. Hunter
    b. Hurler
    c. Scheie
    d. Sly
67. Which combination of findings is *least* likely to occur in congenital rubella syndrome?
    a. retinopathy and cataract
    b. glaucoma and cataract
    c. glaucoma and retinopathy
    d. cataract and deafness
68. Which is *least* helpful for the diagnosis of toxocariasis?
    a. ELISA test
    b. AC tap
    c. vitrectomy
    d. stool examination
69. What is the chance that a child of a patient with Best disease will inherit the disorder?
    a. 25%
    b. 50%
    c. 75%
    d. 100%
70. The inheritance of gyrate atrophy is
    a. sporadic
    b. X-linked recessive
    c. autosomal dominant
    d. autosomal recessive
71. An 8-year-old boy has new-onset ptosis and proptosis. His CT scan shows a superior orbital mass. The most appropriate treatment is
    a. steroids
    b. chemotherapy
    c. radiation
    d. biopsy

Please visit the eBook for an interactive version of the review questions. See front cover for activation details.

SUGGESTED READINGS

Basic and Clinical Sciences Course. (2021). *Section 6: Pediatric ophthalmology and strabismus*. San Francisco: AAO.

Burian, H. M., & von Noorden, G. K. (1974). *Binocular vision and ocular motility: Theory and treatment of strabismus*. St Louis: Mosby.

Del Monte, M. A., & Archer, S. M. (1991). *Atlas of pediatric ophthalmology and strabismus surgery*. Philadelphia: Butterworth-Heinemann.

Lambert, S., & Lyons, C. (2016). *Taylor and Hoyt's pediatric ophthalmology and strabismus* (5th ed.). Philadelphia: Elsevier.

Nelson, L. B., & Catalano, R. A. (1997). *Atlas of ocular motility*. Philadelphia: WB Saunders.

Nelson, L. B., & Olitsky, S. E. (2013). *Harley's pediatric ophthalmology* (6th ed.). Philadelphia: Lippincott Williams & Wilkins.

Netland, P. A., & Mandal, A. K. (2006). *Pediatric glaucoma*. Philadelphia: Elsevier Butterworth-Heinemann.

Von Noorden, G. K. (1983). *Atlas of strabismus* (4th ed.). St Louis: Mosby.

Von Noorden, G. K., & Campos, E. C. (2002). *Binocular vision and ocular motility: Theory and treatment of strabismus* (6th ed.). St Louis: Mosby.

Wright, K. W., & Strube, Y. N. J. (2012). *Pediatric ophthalmology and strabismus* (3rd ed.). New York: Oxford University Press.

6

Orbit/Lids/Adnexa

ANATOMY
IMAGING
ORBITAL DISORDERS
EYELID DISORDERS
NASOLACRIMAL SYSTEM DISORDERS
ORBITAL SURGERY

ANATOMY

Dimensions

Orbit: pear shaped (widest diameter is 1 cm posterior to orbital rim); 45 mm wide, 35 mm high, 40-45 mm deep, volume ~30 mL (Table 6.1)

Mnemonics (bones of the orbital walls):

Roof: **Frontless** (**Front**al, **less**er wing of sphenoid)

Lateral wall: **Great Z** (**Great**er wing of sphenoid, **Z**ygomatic)

Floor: **Zip My Pants** (**Z**ygomatic, **M**axilla, **P**alatine)

Medial wall: **My Little Eye Sits in the orbit** (**M**axilla, **L**acrimal, **E**thmoid, **S**phenoid)

Optic nerve: orbital length = 25-30 mm; width = 1.8 mm in globe, 3.5 mm posterior to lamina cribrosa (as a result of myelin), 5.0 mm with the addition of the optic nerve sheath (see Fig. 4.2). Most direct access to nerve is along medial wall of orbit.

Proptosis: measure with Hertel exophthalmometer (Table 6.2)

Apertures

(Figs. 6.1–6.3)

Superior orbital fissure:

Separates greater and lesser sphenoid wings: 20 mm long

Spanned by annulus of Zinn

Between roof and lateral wall

Transmits: cranial nerve (CN) 3, 4, V$_1$, and 6; superior ophthalmic vein; and sympathetic fibers to iris dilator

Mnemonics:

Nerves passing through superior orbital fissure:

Live **F**ree **T**o **S**ee **N**o **I**nsult at **A**ll (**L**acrimal, **F**rontal, **T**rochlear, **S**uperior division oculomotor, **N**asociliary, **I**nferior division oculomotor, **A**bducens)

Structures passing above annulus of Zinn: **LOFT** (**L**acrimal nerve, **O**phthalmic vein, **F**rontal nerve, **T**rochlear nerve)

Structures passing through annulus of Zinn: **3N3** is **6** (CN **3** superior branch, **N**asociliary nerve, CN **3** inferior branch, CN **6**)

Optic canal:

Within lesser wing of sphenoid: 10 mm long

Enlarged with optic nerve glioma

Transmits: Optic nerve (CN 2), ophthalmic artery, and sympathetic nerves to ocular and orbital blood vessels

Inferior orbital fissure:

Bordered medially by maxillary bone, anteriorly by zygomatic bone, and laterally by greater wing of sphenoid

Transmits: CN V$_2$, zygomatic nerve, inferior ophthalmic vein, venous communication between ophthalmic vein and pterygoid plexus, sphenopalatine ganglion branches

Nasolacrimal canal:

Runs from lacrimal sac fossa to inferior meatus under the inferior turbinate

Contains the nasolacrimal duct

Lateral wall = maxillary bone

Medial wall = lacrimal bone and inferior turbinate

Zygomaticofacial and zygomaticotemporal canals:

Transmit: vessels and branches of the zygomatic nerve through the lateral wall to cheek and temporal fossa

Ethmoidal foramina:

Transmit: anterior and posterior ethmoid arteries

Table 6.1 Osteology

Orbit	Bones	Related structures/miscellaneous
Roof	Sphenoid (lesser wing)	Lacrimal gland fossa
	Frontal	Trochlea
		Supraorbital notch (medial)
Lateral wall	Sphenoid (greater wing)	Lateral orbital tubercle of Whitnall
	Zygomatic	Strongest orbital wall
		Lateral orbital rim at equator of globe
Floor	Maxilla	Contains infraorbital nerve and canal
	Palatine	Forms roof of maxillary sinus
	Zygomatic	
Medial wall	Sphenoid (lesser wing)	Lacrimal sac fossa
	Maxilla	Adjacent to ethmoid and sphenoid sinuses
	Ethmoid	Posterior ethmoidal foramen
	Lacrimal	Weakest orbital wall

Table 6.2 Hertel exophthalmometry measurements

	Mean (mm)	Upper limit of normal (mm)
Caucasian male	16.5	21.7
Caucasian female	15.4	20
African American male	18.5	24.7
African American female	17.8	23.0

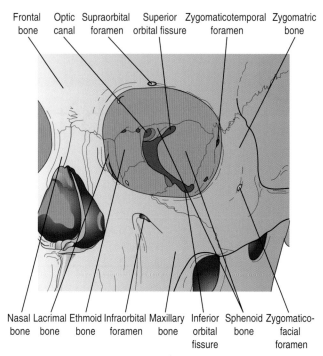

Figure 6.1 Bony anatomy of the orbit in frontal view. (From Dutton JJ. *Atlas of Clinical and Surgical Orbital Anatomy*. Philadelphia: WB Saunders; 1994.)

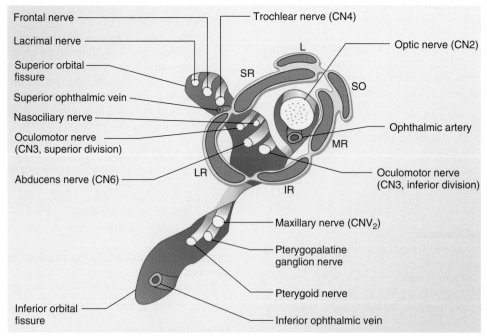

Figure 6.2 Orbital apex, superior and inferior orbital fissure. *IR*, inferior rectus; *L*, levator; *LR*, lateral rectus; *MR*, medial rectus; *SO*, superior oblique; *SR*, superior rectus. Note that the trochlear nerve lies outside the muscle cone.

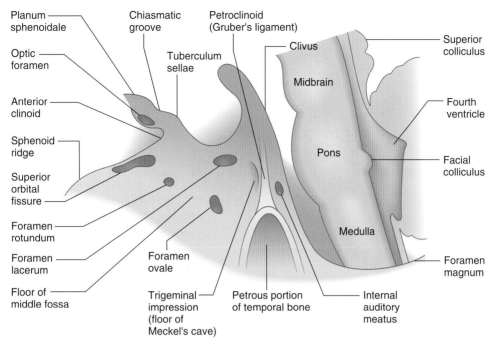

Figure 6.3 Schematic representation of the landmarks, temporal view. (From Bajandas FJ, Kline BK. *Neuro-Ophthalmology Review Manual*. Thorofare, NJ: Slack; 1988.)

Potential route for spread of infectious sinusitis

Frontosphenoidal foramina:

Transmit: anastomosis between the middle meningeal and lacrimal arteries, which provides collateral blood supply to the orbit

Foramen ovale:

Transmits: CN V$_3$

Foramen rotundum:

Transmits: CN V$_2$

Foramen lacerum:

Transmits: internal carotid artery

Vascular Supply to Eye

(Figs. 6.4–6.6)

Ophthalmic artery: first branch of internal carotid within skull

Central retinal artery:
Enters optic nerve 13 mm posterior to globe
Supplies blood to inner 2/3 of retina

Posterior ciliary arteries:
Long posterior ciliary arteries (2) supply anterior segment
Short posterior ciliary arteries (16–20) supply choroid
Optic nerve head is primarily supplied by blood from the vascular **circle of Zinn-Haller** (collection of anastomotic arteries arising from the short posterior ciliary arteries)

Venous system: orbital veins do not have valves

Vortex veins:
4-8 per eye; 1-2 per quadrant
Exit posterior to the equator
Drain choroid and merge into the superior or inferior ophthalmic veins

Superior ophthalmic vein:
Exits via superior orbital fissure into the cavernous sinus
2 superior vortex veins

Interior ophthalmic vein:
Exits via inferior orbital fissure
2 inferior vortex veins

Central retinal vein:
Joins superior or inferior ophthalmic vein
Leaves nerve 10 mm behind globe

Innervation of Eye

Sensory innervation provided by ophthalmic and maxillary division of trigeminal nerve (CN 5) (Fig. 6.7)

Ophthalmic division (V$_1$):

Nasociliary nerve:
Enters orbit within the annulus of Zinn
Short ciliary nerves (6–10) pass through ciliary ganglion
Long ciliary nerves (2) supply iris, cornea, and ciliary muscle

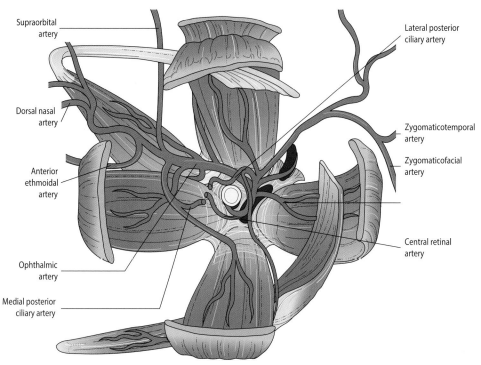

Figure 6.4 Arterial supply to the orbit, in coronal view. (From Dutton JJ. *Atlas of Clinical and Surgical Orbital Anatomy*. Philadelphia: WB Saunders; 1994.)

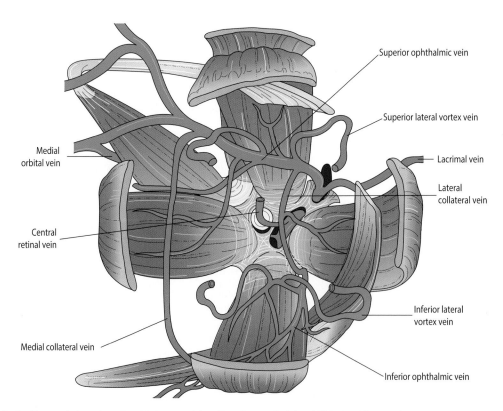

Figure 6.5 Orbital veins. Venous drainage from the orbit, in coronal view. (From Dutton JJ. *Atlas of Clinical and Surgical Orbital Anatomy*. Philadelphia: WB Saunders; 1994.)

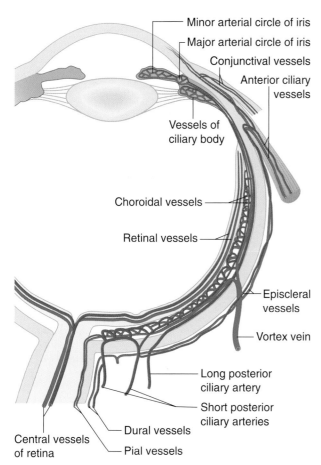

Figure 6.6 Vascular supply to the eye. All arterial branches originate with the ophthalmic artery. Venous drainage is through the cavernous sinus and the pterygoid plexus.

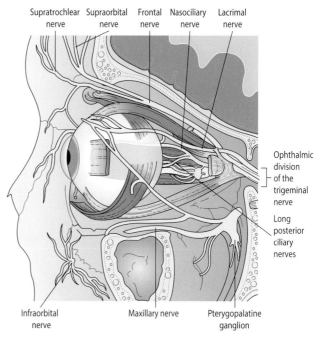

Figure 6.7 Sensory nerves of the orbit, in lateral view. (From Dutton JJ. *Atlas of Clinical and Surgical Orbital Anatomy*. Philadelphia: WB Saunders; 1994.)

Frontal nerve:
    Enters orbit above annulus of Zinn
    Divides into supraorbital nerve and supratrochlear nerve
    Innervates medial canthus, upper lid, and forehead
Lacrimal nerve:
    Enters orbit above annulus of Zinn
    Innervates upper eyelid and lacrimal gland

Maxillary nerve (V_2):
    Passes through foramen rotundum, then passes through inferior orbital fissure
    Divides into infraorbital nerve, zygomatic nerve, and superior alveolar nerve

Parasympathetic innervation:
    Controls accommodation, pupillary constriction, and lacrimal gland stimulation
    Enters eye as short posterior ciliary nerves after synapsing in the ciliary ganglion

Sympathetic innervation:
    Controls pupillary dilation, vasoconstriction, and smooth muscle function of eyelids and orbit, and hidrosis
    Dysfunction: Horner syndrome (ptosis, miosis, anhidrosis, and vasodilation)
        Nerve fibers follow arterial supply as well as long ciliary nerves

Sinuses

(Fig. 6.8)

Frontal:
    Not radiographically visible before age 6
    Drains into anterior portion of the middle meatus

Ethmoid:
    Multiple thin-walled cavities
    1st sinus to aerate
    Anterior and middle air cells drain into the middle meatus
    Posterior air cells drain into the superior meatus
    Ethmoidal sinusitis is the most common source of infection that leads to orbital cellulitis

Sphenoid:
    Rudimentary at birth
    Reaches full size after puberty
    Optic canal is superior and lateral to sphenoid sinus
    Drains into sphenoethmoid recess of each nasal fossa

Maxillary:
    Largest sinus
    Roof contains the infraorbital nerve
    Drains into middle meatus

Soft Tissues

(Fig. 6.9)

Periorbita:
    Periosteum is attached firmly at the orbital rim and suture

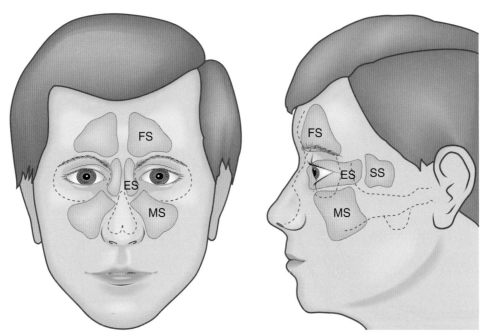

Figure 6.8 Relationship of the orbits to the paranasal sinuses. *FS,* Frontal sinus; *ES,* ethmoid sinus; *MS,* maxillary sinus; *SS,* sphenoid sinus. (Reprinted with permission from Slamovits TL. *Basic and Clinical Science Course, Section 7: Orbit, Eyelids and Lacrimal System.* San Francisco: American Academy of Ophthalmology, 1993.)

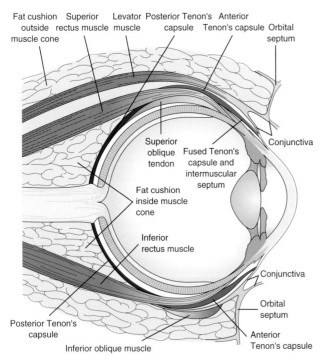

Figure 6.9 Sagittal section of orbital tissues through the vertical recti. (Adapted from Parks MM. Extraocular muscles. In: Duane TD. *Clinical Ophthalmology.* Philadelphia: Harper and Row; 1982.)

lines

Arcus marginalis: fusion of periosteum and orbital septum at orbital rim

Fuses with the dura covering the optic nerve

Annulus of Zinn:

Fibrous tissue ring (superior and inferior orbital tendons) arising from periorbita that surrounds the optic canal

Origin of the 4 recti muscles

Fuses with dura covering optic nerve at apex

Adipose tissue:

Surrounds most of orbital contents; divided by fine fibrous septa

Preaponeurotic fat pads: lie immediately posterior to orbital septum

   2 FAT PADS IN UPPER LID: anterior to levator aponeurosis; medial pad smaller and paler than central pad; with aging, medial pad moves anteriorly and may cause bulging of upper nasal orbit

   3 FAT PADS IN LOWER LID: anterior to capsulopalpebral fascia; inferior oblique muscle separates the medial and central pads; lateral pad is small and more inferior

Lacrimal gland:

2 lobes: orbital (larger) and palpebral, separated by levator aponeurosis

Ducts from both lobes pass through the palpebral lobe and empty into the superior fornix

Innervation: secretomotor from superior salivary nucleus via CN 7; sensory (afferent) from CN 5; sympathetic from superior cervical ganglion via deep petrosal nerve, pterygopalatine ganglion, and zygomatic nerve

Blood supply: lacrimal artery

Accessory lacrimal glands: glands of Wolfring located in tarsus and glands of Krause located in the conjunctival fornices (10% of production)

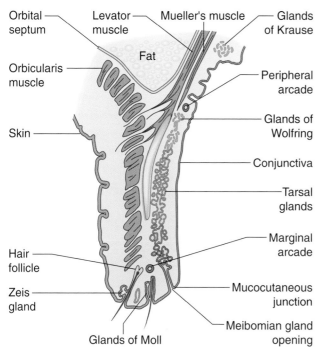

Figure 6.10 Cross-section of upper eyelid. Note position of cilia, tarsal gland orifices, and mucocutaneous junction. (Reprinted with permission from Grand MG. *Basic and Clinical Science Course, Section 2: Fundamentals and Principles of Ophthalmology*. San Francisco: American Academy of Ophthalmology;1993.)

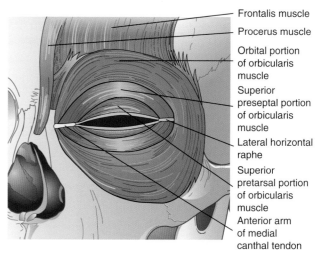

Figure 6.11 The orbicularis and frontalis muscles. (From Dutton JJ. *Atlas of Clinical and Surgical Orbital Anatomy*. Philadelphia: WB Saunders; 1994.)

Eyelid

Lamellae of upper eyelid: (Fig. 6.10)

Anterior: skin, orbicularis

Posterior: tarsus, levator aponeurosis, Müller muscle, palpebral conjunctiva

Skin:

Thinnest skin of the body, no subcutaneous fat layer

Upper eyelid crease approximates attachments of the levator aponeurosis to the pretarsal orbicularis and skin

Histology of epidermis:

BASILAR LAYER (stratum basalis): cuboidal cells with scant cytoplasm; responsible for generating superficial layers

PRICKLE CELL LAYER: multiple layers of cells with abundant cytoplasm attached to each other by desmosomes

GRANULAR CELL LAYER (stratum granulosum): cells contain granular material that stains blue with hematoxylin and eosin (H&E)

KERATIN LAYER: superficial, acellular keratin devoid of nuclei; stains pink with H&E

Orbicularis oculi: (Fig. 6.11)

Main protractor of the eyelid; acts as lacrimal pump; innervated by CN 7

3 anatomic parts: palpebral portion (pretarsal and preseptal) involved with involuntary blinking; orbital portion involved with voluntary, forced lid closure

PRETARSAL: overlies tarsus, originates from lateral orbital tubercle, forms muscle of Riolan (seen as gray line at lid margin)

SUPERFICIAL HEAD: medially inserts into anterior lacrimal crest, contributes to medial canthal tendon, laterally inserts into zygomatic bone

DEEP HEAD: medially inserts into posterior lacrimal crest, called *Horner muscle*, surrounds canaliculi facilitating tear drainage, laterally inserts into lateral orbital tubercle, contributes to lateral canthal tendon

PRESEPTAL: overlies orbital septum

Originates from anterior limb of the medial canthal tendon and from posterior lacrimal crest and lacrimal sac fascia

Forms lateral palpebral raphe overlying the lateral orbital rim

ORBITAL: lies beneath skin

Thickest portion of orbicularis

Inserts at medial canthal tendon

Interdigitates with the frontalis muscle superiorly at eyebrow

Other muscles of forehead and eyebrow:

Frontalis: moves scalp anteriorly and posteriorly; raises eyebrows; innervated by CN 7

Corrugator: pulls medial eyebrow inferiorly and medially, producing vertical glabellar wrinkle; originates from nasal process of frontal bone; inserts laterally into subcutaneous tissue; innervated by CN 7

Procerus: pulls forehead and medial eyebrow inferiorly producing horizontal lines in nose; interdigitates with inferior edge of frontalis; innervated by CN 7

Orbital septum: (Fig. 6.12)

Dense fibrous sheath that acts as barrier between the orbit and eyelid; stops spread of infection

Originates from periosteum of the superior and inferior orbital rims

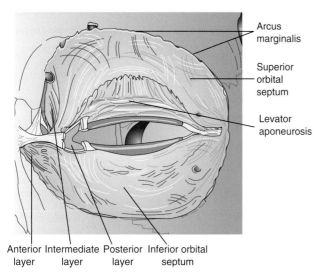

Figure 6.12 The orbital septum. (From Dutton JJ. *Atlas of Clinical and Surgical Orbital Anatomy*. Philadelphia: WB Saunders; 1994.)

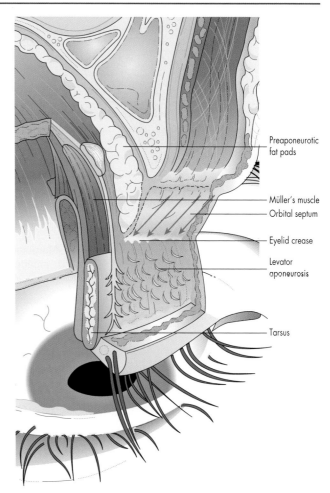

Figure 6.13 The orbital septum inserts into the levator aponeurosis *(arrows)*. The preaponeurotic fat pads are located posterior to the septum. In downgaze, the lid crease becomes attenuated (weakened), and in a normal young eyelid, the fold is absent. (From Zide BW, Jelks BW. *Surgical Anatomy of the Orbit*. New York: Raven Press; 1985.)

Inserts into levator aponeurosis superiorly (2–5 mm above superior tarsal border in non-Asians) and into lower eyelid retractors inferiorly (capsulopalpebral fascia just below inferior tarsal border)

Medially inserts into lacrimal crest

Structures posterior to the septum: palpebral lobe of lacrimal gland, lateral canthal tendon, trochlea of superior oblique muscle

In Asians, orbital septum fuses with levator aponeurosis between the eyelid margin and the superior border of the tarsus

Upper eyelid retractors: (Fig. 6.13)

Levator palpebrae:

Originates from lesser wing of sphenoid above annulus of Zinn

Innervated by CN 3

MUSCULAR PORTION: 40 mm

APONEUROTIC PORTION: 14-20 mm and has lateral and medial extensions (horns) (Fig. 6.14)

LATERAL HORN:

Inserts onto lateral orbital tubercle

Divides lacrimal gland into orbital and palpebral portions

MEDIAL HORN:

Inserts onto posterior lacrimal crest

More delicate and weaker than lateral horn

Anterior portion inserts into septa between pretarsal orbicularis muscle bundles

Posterior portion inserts onto anterior surface of lower half of tarsus; forms eyelid crease

Disinsertion of aponeurosis results in loss of eyelid crease

Whitnall ligament (superior transverse ligament):

condensation of levator muscle sheath

Visible as horizontal white line 10 mm above superior edge of tarsus

Arises from the sheath of anterior portion of levator muscle

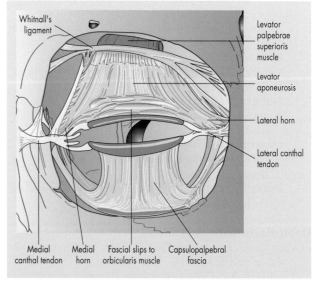

Figure 6.14 The levator aponeurosis and the medial and lateral canthal tendons. (From Dutton JJ. *Atlas of Clinical and Surgical Orbital Anatomy*. Philadelphia: WB Saunders; 1994.)

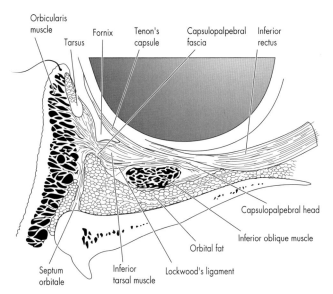

Orbicularis muscle
Tarsus
Fornix
Tenon's capsule
Capsulopalpebral fascia
Inferior rectus
Capsulopalpebral head
Inferior oblique muscle
Orbital fat
Lockwood's ligament
Inferior tarsal muscle
Septum orbitale

Figure 6.15 Anatomy of the lower eyelid retractors. (Adapted from Hawes MJ, Dortzbach RK. The microscopic anatomy of the lower eyelid retractors. *Arch Ophthalmol*. 1982;100:1313–1318.)

Medially attaches to trochlea

Laterally forms septa through stroma of lacrimal gland and attaches to inner aspect of lateral orbital wall at the frontozygomatic suture (10 mm above orbital tubercle [tubercle of Whitnall]) and at the orbital tubercle

Acts to change direction of pull of levator and serves as check ligament to prevent excessive lid elevation

Müller muscle (superior tarsal muscle):

Posterior to levator aponeurosis

Sympathetic innervation

Originates from undersurface of levator approximately at level of Whitnall ligament

Inserts into upper border of tarsus

Length of 12-15 mm; raises eyelid 2 mm

Peripheral arterial arcade found between aponeurosis and Müller muscle

Lower eyelid retractors: (Fig. 6.15)

Capsulopalpebral fascia: analogous to levator aponeurosis

Originates from inferior rectus (IR) muscle sheath, divides as it encircles inferior oblique muscle, and then joins to form Lockwood ligament

Fuses with septum and inserts into inferior tarsus

Lockwood suspensory ligament: analogous to Whitnall ligament

Arises posteriorly from fibrous attachments to inferior side of the IR muscle and continues anteriorly as capsulopalpebral fascia

Medial and lateral horns attach to retinacula forming a suspensory hammock for the globe

Inferior tarsal muscle: analogous to Müller muscle

Sympathetic innervation

Arises from capsulopalpebral fascia

Tarsus:

Dense connective tissue plate in each eyelid; not cartilage

Contains meibomian glands (tarsal glands), 30-40 in upper lid, 20-30 in lower lid

Length of 29 mm; 1 mm thick; tapered at ends

Rigid attachments to periosteum medially and laterally

Superior tarsal plate: 10 mm in maximal height centrally

Inferior tarsal plate: 4 mm in maximal height

Medial canthal tendon:

Fusion of tendinous insertions of pretarsal and preseptal orbicularis muscles

Attaches to tarsal plates

Anterior limb: attaches to frontal process of maxillary bone and serves as origin of superficial head of pretarsal orbicularis; passes in front of lacrimal sac and attaches to anterior lacrimal crest

Posterior limb: attaches to posterior lacrimal crest; passes behind lacrimal sac; more important than anterior limb for normal medial canthal appearance and function (maintaining apposition of lids to globe)

Lateral canthal tendon:

Broad band of connective tissue from lateral borders of upper and lower tarsal plates

Inserts onto lateral orbital tubercle of Whitnall; 3 mm superior to medial canthal tendon insertion

Eyelid margin: 3 distinguishing landmarks

Lash line: 2-3 rows of lashes; 100 in upper lid, 50 in lower lid; 10-week growth, 5-month resting phase

Gray line: border of pretarsal orbicularis (muscle of Riolan); junction of anterior and posterior lamellae; vascular watershed

Meibomian gland orifices: 30 in upper lid, 20 in lower lid

Vascular supply: (Fig. 6.16)

Upper lid: internal carotid artery → ophthalmic artery → superior marginal arcade (deep to orbicularis and anterior surface of tarsus)

Lower lid: external carotid artery → facial artery → angular artery → inferior marginal arcade

Angular artery is 6-8 mm medial to medial canthus, posterior to orbicularis, 5 mm anterior to lacrimal sac

Marginal arcades are 3 mm from lid margin

Peripheral and marginal arcades allow for anastomosis between the internal carotid artery (ICA) and external carotid artery (ECA)

Venous drainage:

SUPERFICIAL (PRETARSAL): angular vein medially, superficial temporal vein temporally, drains into internal and external jugular veins

DEEP (POSTTARSAL): orbital vein, anterior facial vein, and pterygoid plexus, drains into cavernous sinus

Innervation:

Sensory: CN V_1 (upper lid), CN V_2 (lower lid)

Motor: CN 3, CN 7, sympathetics

Lymphatic drainage:

Submandibular nodes: drain medial 1/3 of upper lid, medial 2/3 of lower lid

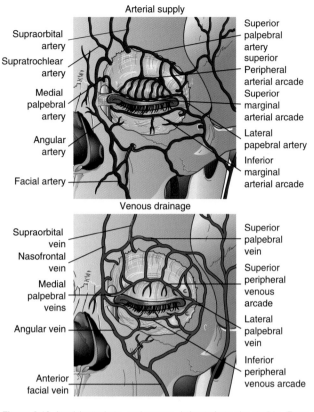

Arterial supply

Supraorbital artery
Supratrochlear artery
Medial palpebral artery
Angular artery
Facial artery

Superior palpebral artery superior
Peripheral arterial arcade
Superior marginal arterial arcade
Lateral papebral artery
Inferior marginal arterial arcade

Venous drainage

Supraorbital vein
Nasofrontal vein
Medial palpebral veins
Angular vein
Anterior facial vein

Superior palpebral vein
Superior peripheral venous arcade
Lateral palpebral vein
Inferior peripheral venous arcade

Figure 6.16 Arterial supply to, and venous drainage from, the eyelids. (From Dutton JJ. *Atlas of Clinical and Surgical Orbital Anatomy*. Philadelphia: WB Saunders; 1994.)

Preauricular nodes: drain lateral 2/3 of upper lid, lateral 1/3 of lower lid

No lymphatic vessels or nodes are found within the orbit

Lymphatic vessels are found in the conjunctiva

Glands of the eyelids: (Table 6.3)

Eccrine: secretion by simple exocytosis

Holocrine: secretion by release of entire cellular contents (disruption of cell)

Apocrine: secretion by pinching or budding off of a portion of cellular cytoplasm

Nasolacrimal System

(Fig. 6.17)

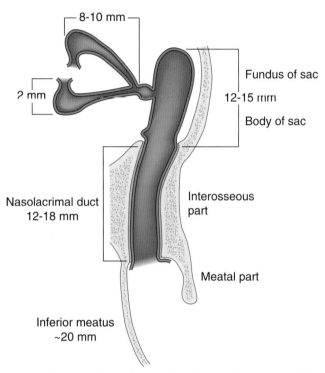

8-10 mm

2 mm

Fundus of sac
12-15 mm
Body of sac

Nasolacrimal duct 12-18 mm

Interosseous part

Meatal part

Inferior meatus ~20 mm

Figure 6.17 Excretory lacrimal system. (From Grand MG. *Basic and Clinical Science Course, Section 2: Fundamentals and Principles of Ophthalmology*. San Francisco: American Academy of Ophthalmology; 1993.)

Table 6.3 Glands of the eyelids				
Gland	**Location**	**Type**	**Function**	**Pathology**
Lacrimal	Superotemporal orbit	Eccrine	Reflex tear (aqueous) secretion	Dacryoadenitis Tumors
Accessory lacrimal: Krause Wolfring	Fornix Just above tarsus	Eccrine	Basal tear (aqueous) secretion	Sjögren syndrome GVH disease Rare tumors (BMT)
Meibomian	Within tarsus	Holocrine	Lipid secretion Retards tear evaporation	Chalazion Sebaceous carcinoma
Zeis	Near lid margin Caruncle Associated with cilia	Holocrine	Lipid secretion Lubricates cilia	External hordeolum Sebaceous carcinoma
Moll	Near lid margin	Apocrine	Modified sweat glands Lubricates cilia	Ductal cyst Apocrine carcinoma
Sweat		Eccrine	Electrolyte balance	Ductal cyst Syringoma Sweat gland carcinoma
Goblet cells	Conjunctiva Plica Caruncle	Holocrine	Mucin secretion Enhances corneal wetting	Dry eye

BMT, Bone marrow transplant; *GVH,* graft-versus-host disease.

Puncta:

Upper and lower; 6 mm from medial canthus, lower is slightly more temporal

Slightly inverted against globe

Open into ampulla (2 mm long) oriented perpendicular to eyelid margin

Canaliculi:

Length of 10 mm (2 mm vertical segment [ampulla] and 8 mm horizontal portion parallel to lid margin)

Combine to form single common canaliculus in 90% of individuals

Valve of Rosenmüller prevents reflux from lacrimal sac into canaliculi

Nasolacrimal sac:

Length of 12-15 mm, occupies the lacrimal fossa

Lies between anterior and posterior crura of the medial canthal tendon, anterior to orbital septum

Lateral to middle meatus of nose

Nasolacrimal duct:

Length of 12-18 mm

Passes inferiorly, posteriorly, and laterally within canal formed by maxillary and lacrimal bones

Extends into inferior meatus, which opens under inferior turbinate (2.5 cm posterior to naris)

Partially covered by valve of Hasner

Lacrimal pump:

Lids close: pretarsal orbicularis contracts, compresses ampulla, shortens canaliculus; punctum moves medially; lacrimal sac expands, creates negative pressure, draws fluid from canaliculus into sac

Lids open: muscles relax, lacrimal sac collapses, tears forced into nose, punctum moves laterally, tears enter canaliculus

IMAGING

Ultrasound

Optimal sound wave frequency is 10 MHz

Higher frequencies give better resolution; lower frequencies provide better penetration (Table 6.4)

Magnetic resonance imaging (MRI)

Strong magnetic field results in alignment of nuclei of atoms with odd numbers of protons or neutrons

Radiofrequency pulse disturbs the alignment by energizing protons or neutrons

When pulse terminates, protons return to previous alignment and emit absorbed energy as radiofrequency signal, generating an image

Axial, coronal, and sagittal views

Table 6.4 Ultrasound characteristics of lesions	
Good sound transmission	**Poor sound transmission**
Cavernous hemangioma	Metastatic cancer
Lymphangioma	Orbital pseudotumor
Mucocele	Glioma
Dermoid	Neurofibroma
High Reflectivity	**Low Reflectivity**
Neurofibroma	Metastatic cancer
Fresh hemorrhage	Orbital pseudotumor
Hemangioma	Cyst
Thyroid eye disease	Mucocele
	Varix
	Dermoid
	Lymphoma

Relaxation times:

Longitudinal relaxation time (T1): time required for net bulk magnetization to realign itself along original axis

Blood, orbital fat, melanin, and mucus appear bright

Acute hemorrhage, vitreous, optic nerve sheath, and extraocular muscles appear dark

Most orbital tumors are hypointense to fat on T1-weighted images

EXCEPTIONS: mucinous lesions (orbital dermoid cyst, mucocele), lipoma, liposarcoma, melanoma, subacute hemorrhage

Gadolinium: bright white on T1-weighted images

Must perform fat suppression on T1-weighted images when gadolinium is used

Fat suppression renders orbital fat hypointense and permits better visualization of optic nerve and extraocular muscles

Transverse relaxation time (T2): mean relaxation time

Based on interaction of hydrogen nuclei within a given tissue

Provides more information about pathologic processes

Helps differentiate melanotic lesions from hemorrhagic process

Vitreous is bright on T2-weighted images

Blood and fat appear dark

Demyelinating plaques of multiple sclerosis (MS) are best seen with T2-weighted images (hyperintense foci, usually in periventricular white matter)

Advantages: better for soft tissues, posterior fossa, and distinguishing gray from white matter, sagittal sections, better resolution, no artifacts from bone or teeth, no ionizing radiation; modality of choice for central nervous system (CNS) evaluation

Disadvantages: poor bony detail, longer imaging time, more expensive, contrast reactions (gadolinium based), certain contraindications

Contraindications: metallic foreign body/implant, pacemaker, aneurysm clip, cochlear implant, renal insufficiency

Computed Tomography (CT)

For orbital trauma, to detect foreign body or calcification, or for evaluation of orbital soft tissue lesion with suspicion of bony erosion

Bone and metal appear bright

Cross-sectional axial slices (thin-section 0.5 mm for high resolution); reconstructions for coronal and sagittal views

Advantages: better bony detail and for acute hemorrhage, sinuses, and trauma; shorter imaging time; less expensive

Disadvantages: poor posterior fossa detail (decreased by skull base streak artifact); no direct sagittal sections, ionizing radiation, contrast dye reactions (iodine based) (Table 6.5)

Table 6.5 CT and MRI characteristics of lesions

Most common orbital lesions with well-circumscribed appearance on CT and MRI	Most common orbital lesions with Ill-defined appearance on CT and MRI
Children:	Children:
Dermoid cyst	Capillary hemangioma
Lymphangioma	Orbital pseudotumor
Rhabdomyosarcoma	Plexiform neurofibroma
Optic nerve glioma	Leukemic infiltrate
	Eosinophilic granuloma
Adults:	Adults:
Cavernous hemangioma	Orbital pseudotumor
Neurofibroma	Metastasis
Neurilemmoma	Leukemic infiltrate
Fibrous histiocytoma	Primary malignant tumor
(Lymphoproliferative disorders)	Lymphoproliferative disorders

CT, Computed tomography; *MRI*, magnetic resonance imaging.

Contrast Agents

Improve sensitivity and specificity of MRI and CT scans

Angiography and Combined Modalities

Magnetic resonance angiography (MRA) and CT angiography and venography used to evaluate vascular lesions; less invasive than traditional catheter angiography but resolution limited

CT also combined with nuclear medicine imaging (radiolabeled molecules): single-photon emission CT (SPECT) for evaluation of cardiac and brain perfusion and positron emission tomography (PET-CT) for evaluation

of tumors, degenerative brain disease, sarcoidosis, and screening for uveal melanoma metastases

Radiographs

Specific views can be helpful, especially when CT is unavailable or to quickly rule out a metallic foreign body

Plain-film radiography also detects sinus pathology, calcification, hyperostosis, and lytic lesions

Canthomeatal line: radiographic baseline of skull (line between lateral canthal angle and tragus of ear)

Waters view: occipitomental; head extended until canthomeatal line lies at 37° to the central beam; best view of orbital roof and floor

Caldwell view: posteroanterior view with central beam tilted 25° toward feet; best view of superior and lateral orbital rim, medial wall, and ethmoid and frontal sinuses

Lateral view: best for evaluation of sella turcica

Submental vertex view: basal or Hirtz view with head tilted back until canthomeatal line is perpendicular to central beam; best view of sphenoid and ethmoid sinuses, nasal cavities, and zygomatic arch

Oblique (×2) views: posteroanterior (PA) view with central beam tilted 32° toward feet and 37° from perpendicular; best views of optic foramina

ORBITAL DISORDERS

Congenital and Developmental Anomalies

(See Chapter 5, Pediatrics/Strabismus)

Trauma

Orbital Contusion

Bruising from blunt trauma

Pain, decreased vision

Often have associated lid, orbit, and ocular injuries

Treatment: ice compresses, systemic nonsteroidal anti-inflammatory drugs (NSAIDs)

Orbital Fractures

Fractures of orbital bones, often associated with ocular or intracranial injuries

Orbital floor (blow-out): Maxillary bone
　　Posterior medial floor is weakest area

Findings: may have enophthalmos, diplopia, infraorbital hypesthesia, orbit or lid emphysema, and medial wall fracture

Complications: orbital contents may become entrapped in maxillary sinus, with resultant restriction of ocular motility, diplopia, and globe ptosis. Entrapment is common in children with a "white-eyed blow-out fracture" in which the pliable bone creates a "trapdoor" with ensnarement of the inferior rectus or perimuscular tissue, resulting in positive forced ductions and nausea and bradycardia (oculocardiac reflex); this requires urgent surgery

Medial wall:

Maxillary, lacrimal, and ethmoid bones

Direct (naso-orbito-ethmoidal). Type I: central bone fragment, tendon attached; Type II: comminuted fracture of bones; Type III: avulsed tendon (miniplate fixation, transnasal wiring)

Indirect (blow-out)

Findings: may have depressed nasal bridge, telecanthus, medial canthal rounding, floor fracture, enophthalmos

Complications: epistaxis from injury of anterior ethmoidal artery, cerebrospinal fluid (CSF) rhinorrhea, lacrimal drainage injury, orbit or lid emphysema

Orbital apex:

Can involve optic canal and superior orbital fissure

Complications: CSF rhinorrhea, carotid-cavernous fistula, direct damage to the optic nerve with vision loss

Orbital roof:

Uncommon, entrapment rare

May affect frontal sinus, cribriform plate, and brain

Complications: CSF rhinorrhea, pneumocephalus, pulsating exophthalmos (delayed complication)

Zygomatic (tripod):

Fracture of zygoma at 3 sites (zygomaticomaxillary suture, zygomaticofrontal suture, and zygomatic arch) and orbital floor

Findings: discontinuity of orbital rim, flattening of malar eminence, enophthalmos, infraorbital hypesthesia, trismus, orbit or lid emphysema, downward displacement of lateral canthus

Le Fort 3 types:

I: low transverse fracture of maxillary bone above teeth; no orbital involvement

II: pyramidal fracture of nasal, lacrimal, and maxillary bones; involves medial orbital floors

III: craniofacial dysjunction; involves orbital floor, lateral and medial walls; may involve optic canal

CT scan: identify and localize fracture and coexisting injuries

Treatment: systemic steroids and antibiotics; surgical repair depends on type, location, and severity of fracture and associated findings

Intraorbital Foreign Bodies

Commonly associated with intraocular and/or optic nerve injury

Inert material can be well tolerated and may be observed

Copper and organic material are poorly tolerated and must be removed

Often asymptomatic but may have pain or decreased vision

CT scan (MRI is contraindicated for metallic foreign bodies)

Treatment: systemic antibiotics, tetanus booster, consider surgical removal

Orbital (Retrobulbar) Hemorrhage

Compartment syndrome resulting from bleeding in orbit with globe and nerve compression

Ocular emergency

Findings: pain, decreased vision, subconjunctival hemorrhage, proptosis, restriction of ocular motility, increased intraocular pressure (IOP), tense orbit

Treatment: lateral canthotomy, inferior and possibly superior cantholysis

Degeneration

Atrophia Bulbi

Progressive degeneration and decompensation of globe following severe injury

3 stages: atrophia bulbi without shrinkage, atrophia bulbi with shrinkage, atrophia bulbi with disorganization (phthisis bulbi)

Increased risk of intraocular malignancy

Annual B scan to rule out malignancy

Findings: cataract, retinal detachment, hypotony, corneal edema, globe shrinkage, intraocular hemorrhage, inflammation, calcification, and disorganization

Treatment: topical steroid and cycloplegic for pain; consider retrobulbar alcohol injection or enucleation for severe pain

Infections

Bacterial

Preseptal cellulitis/orbital cellulitis

(See Chapter 5, Pediatrics/Strabismus.) In adults, preseptal most commonly caused by cutaneous trauma, dacryocystitis

Necrotizing fasciitis

Superficial and deep fascia; rapid evolution, potentially fatal

Organisms: group A β-hemolytic *Streptococcus* most common

Findings: anesthesia, disproportionate pain, rose to blue-gray skin discoloration, cutaneous necrosis, systemic shock

Treatment: early débridement, intravenous (IV) antibiotics (clindamycin has activity against group A *Streptococcus* toxins), adjuvant steroid therapy

Fungal

Most commonly *Phycomycetes*

Mucormycosis

Most common and virulent fungal orbital disease
Nonseptated, large, branching hyphae, with invasion of
    blood vessels, thrombosis, and necrosis
Black eschar may be visible in nose or palate
Intracranial spread is hematogenous via ophthalmic artery

Risk factors: diabetes mellitus (70%), immunosuppression (18%), renal disease (5%), leukemia (3%)

Findings: painful orbital apex syndrome, proptosis, ptosis, ophthalmoplegia, decreased vision, corneal anesthesia; may develop retinal vascular occlusions; stains with H&E

Treatment: requires immediate and emergent management
    Surgical débridement, IV amphotericin B; control
        underlying illness

Complications: intracranial involvement, death

Aspergillosis

Septated branching hyphae

Disseminated form: occurs in immunosuppressed hosts; widespread necrotizing angiitis, thrombosis, endophthalmitis

Local form: sclerosing granulomatous infiltrative mass that originates in the sinus; proptosis, periorbital pain, visual loss

Treatment: surgical débridement, amphotericin B, flucytosine, rifampin (IV and oral)

Viral

Dengue Fever

Caused by infection with flavivirus
Ocular soreness and pain on eye movement in 75%

Parasitic

Trichinosis

Caused by infection with *Trichinella spiralis*
Larvae from ingestion of raw meat migrate to muscle and
    brain and become encysted
Associated with fever, myalgia, diarrhea, eosinophilia, and
    periorbital edema

Cysticercosis

Caused by infection with *Taenia solium*

Larvae penetrate intestinal wall, enter bloodstream, and migrate to eyes, lungs, brain, muscle, and connective tissue; become encysted

Inflammation

Idiopathic Orbital Inflammation (Orbital Pseudotumor)

Idiopathic inflammatory disease of orbital tissues

Findings: acute orbital pain, lid erythema and edema, lacrimal gland enlargement, restricted eye movements, proptosis, diplopia, increased IOP; may have impaired vision from optic nerve involvement

Adults: usually unilateral; bilateral cases need workup for systemic vasculitis and lymphoproliferative disorders

Children: bilateral in 33%; commonly have headache, fever, vomiting, and lethargy; may have associated papillitis or iritis; workup usually not needed (see Chapter 5, Pediatrics/Strabismus)

Pathology: enlargement of extraocular muscles and tendons; patchy infiltrate of lymphocytes, plasma cells, and eosinophils

Differential diagnosis (DDx): thyroid eye disease, orbital cellulitis, tumor, vasculitis, trauma, atrioventricular (AV) fistula, cavernous sinus thrombosis, CN palsy

Diagnosis:
    Lab tests: eosinophilia, elevated erythrocyte sedimentation rate
        (ESR), positive antinuclear antibody (ANA), CSF pleocytosis
    CT scan: enlargement of extraocular muscles and tendons, ring
        sign (contrast-enhanced sclera), enlarged lacrimal gland
    B-scan ultrasound: may show acoustically hollow area
        corresponding to edematous Tenon capsule

Treatment: systemic NSAIDs, systemic steroids (1 mg/kg oral prednisone, taper slowly over months); biopsy for atypical presentation, poor therapeutic response, recurrence; consider radiation if unresponsive to steroids, chemotherapy (cyclophosphamide)

Orbital myositis: localized to extraocular muscles, medial rectus (MR) and lateral rectus (LR) most commonly involved (33% each), inferior rectus (IR) 10%
    Findings: diplopia, pain, proptosis, ptosis, conjunctival
        injection, and chemosis
    Complications: fibrosis with strabismus

Tolosa-Hunt syndrome: localized to superior orbital fissure, optic canal, and cavernous sinus
    Findings: painful ophthalmoplegia, decreased vision

Sclerosing orbital pseudotumor: fibrosis of orbit and lacrimal gland
    Insidious onset
    More steroid resistant; typically requires
        immunomodulating therapy

Pain is less common, and eye is often white and quiet
Associated with retroperitoneal fibrosis
A-scan ultrasound: low reflectivity (seen with both orbital pseudotumor and lymphoma)

Thyroid Eye Disease

Also called *thyroid-related ophthalmopathy, dysthyroid ophthalmopathy,* or *Graves' ophthalmopathy*

Autoimmune disease with spectrum of ocular manifestations

Most common cause of unilateral or bilateral proptosis in adults

Most common cause of acquired diplopia in adults

Women affected 8-10 × more often than men

Patient can be hyperthyroid (~90%), hypothyroid (~5%), or euthyroid (~5%); most commonly associated with Graves' disease; increased incidence in patients with Graves' who smoke (7 × more likely)

Associated with myasthenia gravis (in 5% of patients with Graves' disease)

Usually asymptomatic

Findings: eyelid retraction (90%), proptosis (63%), restrictive myopathy with diplopia; overaction of levator (secondary to restrictive myopathy of inferior rectus muscle); pseudoretraction (secondary to proptosis); lagophthalmos; lid lag on downgaze (von Graefe's sign); dry eye (resulting from corneal exposure and infiltration of lacrimal glands); conjunctival injection and chemosis; corneal exposure (from combination of eyelid retraction, proptosis, and lagophthalmos); increased IOP on upgaze; choroidal folds or disc hyperemia; compressive optic neuropathy (<5%) with decreased acuity and color vision, relative afferent pupillary defect (RAPD), and visual field (VF) defect

Werner Classification of Eye Findings in Graves' Disease (mnemonic **NO SPECS**):
  No signs or symptoms
  Only signs
  Soft tissue involvement (signs and symptoms)
  Proptosis
  Extraocular muscle involvement
  Corneal involvement
  Sight loss (optic nerve compression)

Pathology: enlargement of extraocular muscles; patchy infiltrates of lymphocytes, monocytes, mast cells, and fibroblasts; fibroblasts produce mucopolysaccharides, which leads to increased water content of muscles; inflammation spares tendons (Fig. 6.18)

CT scan: enlargement of extraocular muscles, sparing tendons; Inferior rectus > Medial rectus > Superior rectus > Lateral rectus > Obliques (mnemonic **IMSLO**)

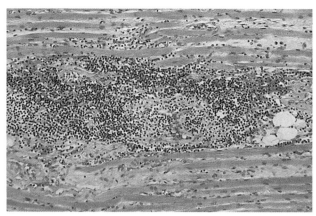

Figure 6.18 Thyroid eye disease demonstrating thickened extraocular muscles with inflammatory cell infiltrate and fluid. (Courtesy of Dr. RC Eagle, Jr. Reported in Hufnagel TJ, Hickey WF, Cobbs WH, et al. Immunohistochemical and ultrastructural studies on the exenterated orbital tissues of a patient with Graves' disease. *Ophthalmology.* 1984;91:1411–1419.)

Treatment: control underlying thyroid abnormality; ocular lubrication; consider lid taping or tarsorrhaphy; teprotumumab (Tepezza), systemic steroids; radiation (effects take 2–4 weeks)
  Surgery:
    ORBITAL DECOMPRESSION: perform before strabismus surgery; 2-4 walls; 80% will experience postoperative diplopia
    STRABISMUS SURGERY: perform before lid surgery
      INDICATIONS: diplopia, abnormal head position, large-angle strabismus
      Strabismus must be stable for at least 6 months
      Avoid if anterior inflammatory signs present
      Recession of affected muscles is mainstay of treatment, avoid resections (can exacerbate restrictions already present)
      Vertical muscle surgery can affect eyelid position (recession of IR can cause increased lid retraction as a result of connection of IR to lower lid retractors; recession of IR can decrease upper lid retraction in that the superior rectus [SR] now has to work less against the tight IR [thus, the associated levator muscle is less stimulated, causing less eyelid retraction])
      Beware late slippage of inferior rectus
      Consider adjustable sutures
    LID SURGERY: eyelid retraction repair; perform after orbital decompression and strabismus surgery

Sarcoidosis

(See Chapter 8, Uveitis)

Chronic, idiopathic, multisystem, granulomatous disease primarily affecting lung, skin, eye

More common among young African Americans or Scandinavians

Findings: bilateral panuveitis, corneal abnormalities (thickening of Descemet membrane, calcific band keratopathy, nummular keratitis, and deep stromal vacuolation), pars planitis, chorioretinitis, optic nerve involvement, orbital apex syndrome, ptosis, conjunctival nodules, dacryoadenitis; most frequently involves lacrimal gland

Pathology: noncaseating granulomas and Langhans giant cells

Diagnosis: chest X-ray (CXR), purified protein derivative (PPD) and controls, angiotensin-converting enzyme (ACE), serum lysozyme, gallium scan, pulmonary function tests

Treatment: systemic steroids, chemotherapy; treat ocular complications

Granulomatosis With Polyangiitis

Formerly Wegener granulomatosis

Systemic disease of necrotizing vasculitis and granulomatous inflammation involving sinuses, respiratory system, kidneys, and orbit

Findings: painful proptosis, reduced ocular motility, chemosis, scleritis (25%), keratitis, optic nerve edema, nasolacrimal duct obstruction

Pathology: triad of vasculitis, granulomatous inflammation, and tissue necrosis

Diagnosis: antineutrophil cytoplasmic antibodies (ANCA) (positive in 67%)

Treatment: systemic steroids, immunosuppressive therapy

Complications: fatal if untreated

Vascular Abnormalities

Varix

(See Chapter 5, Pediatrics/Strabismus)

AV Fistula

Direct or indirect communication between previously normal carotid artery and venous structures of the cavernous sinus

Direct carotid-cavernous sinus fistula: high flow; associated with head trauma, especially basal skull fracture; caused by spontaneous rupture of aneurysm
  Findings: dilated corkscrew scleral/episcleral vessels, conjunctival injection and chemosis, elevated IOP on involved side, proptosis (may be pulsatile), orbital bruit that may be abolished by ipsilateral carotid compression, dilated tortuous retinal veins; may develop ischemic maculopathy or retinal artery occlusion, enlarged cup-to-disc ratio, ophthalmoplegia

(often CN 6), anterior segment ischemia, blood in Schlemm canal
  CT/MRI scan: dilated superior ophthalmic vein
  Treatment (for severely affected patients): embolization, surgical ligation

Dural-sinus fistula: low-flow communication between meningeal branches of carotid artery and dural walls of cavernous sinus; often asymptomatic; associated with hypertension, atherosclerosis, and connective tissue diseases; may close spontaneously; need MRI/MRA

Tumors

See Table 6.6

Hamartomas: growth arising from tissue normally found at that site (e.g., nevus, neurofibroma, neurilemmoma, schwannoma, glioma, hemangioma, hemangiopericytoma, lymphangioma, trichoepithelioma)

Choristomas: growth arising from tissue not normally found at that site (e.g., dermoid cyst, dermatolipoma, ectopic lacrimal gland)

Table 6.6 Common orbital tumors	
In children[a]	**In adults**
90% are benign; 10% are malignant	Mucocele
Rhabdomyosarcoma (most common primary orbital malignancy)	Cavernous hemangioma
Capillary hemangioma (most common benign orbital tumor)	Meningioma
Lymphangioma	Fibrous histiocytoma
Neuroblastoma (most common metastatic orbital tumor)	Neurilemmoma
Dermoid (most common orbital mass)	Pleomorphic adenoma benign mixed tumor (BMT)
Teratoma	Lymphoid tumors
Optic nerve glioma	Metastatic tumors
Granulocytic sarcoma ("chloroma")	
Burkitt lymphoma	
Histiocytic tumors	
[a]See Chapter 5, Pediatrics/Strabismus. *BMT,* Bone marrow transplant.	

Cystic Tumors

(See Chapter 5, Pediatrics/Strabismus)

Vascular Tumors

Lymphangioma

(See Chapter 5, Pediatrics/Strabismus)

Capillary Hemangioma

(See Chapter 5, Pediatrics/Strabismus)

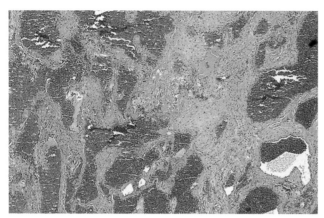

Figure 6.19 Cavernous hemangioma demonstrating large, blood-filled spaces and fibrous septa. (Case presented by Dr. WC Frayer to the meeting of the Verhoeff Society, 1989. From Yanoff M, Fine BS. *Ocular Pathology*, 5th ed. St Louis: Mosby; 2002.)

Cavernous Hemangioma

Most common benign orbital tumor in adults (usually middle-aged women)

Findings: slowly progressive proptosis; may induce hyperopia, may also have retinal striae, IOP elevation, strabismus, or optic nerve compression

Growth may accelerate during pregnancy

Pathology: encapsulated lesion composed of blood-filled cavernous spaces, lined by endothelial cells (Fig. 6.19)

CT scan: well-demarcated, encapsulated, intraconal mass

MRI: hypointense to fat on T1-weighted images, hyperintense to fat and equivalent to vitreous on T2-weighted images

A-scan ultrasound: high internal reflectivity

Treatment: observation, surgical excision

Hemangiopericytoma

Rare tumor of abnormal pericytes surrounding blood vessels

Occurs in middle-aged adults

More common in women

Often located in superior orbit

Can metastasize to lung, bone, liver

Findings: slowly progressive proptosis, pain, decreased vision, diplopia

CT scan: well-circumscribed, encapsulated mass

A-scan ultrasound: low to medium internal reflectivity

Treatment: complete surgical excision because it may metastasize

Neural Tumors

Optic Nerve Glioma

(See Chapter 5, Pediatrics/Strabismus)

Neurofibroma

(See Chapter 5, Pediatrics/Strabismus)

Neurilemmoma (Schwannoma)

Encapsulated tumor consisting of benign proliferation of Schwann cells

No malignant potential

Occurs in middle-aged individuals

Lesion can be painful as a result of perineural spread and compression of nerve

Usually located in the superior orbit, causing gradual proptosis and globe dystopia

Schwannomas can grow along any peripheral or cranial nerve, most commonly CN 8 (acoustic neuroma)

Rarely associated with neurofibromatosis

Pathology: stains with S-100
Antoni A: spindle cells arranged in interlacing cords, whorls, or palisades; contains Verocay bodies (collections of cells resembling sensory corpuscles) (Fig. 6.20)
Antoni B: loose, myxoid; stellate cells with a mucoid stroma (Fig. 6.21)

CT scan: well-circumscribed, fusiform mass

Treatment: complete surgical excision; can recur after complete surgical removal

Meningioma

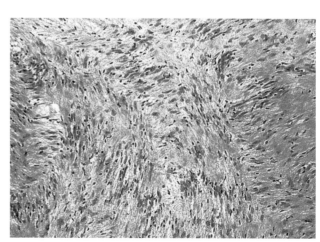

Figure 6.20 Antoni A pattern demonstrating palisading spindle cells with Verocay bodies (areas that appear acellular). (From Yanoff M, Fine BS. *Ocular Pathology*, 5th ed. St Louis: Mosby; 2002.)

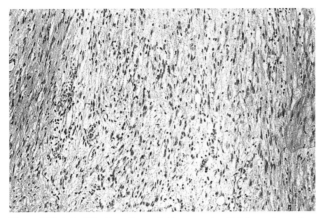

Figure 6.21 Antoni B pattern demonstrating necrosis with inflammatory cells. (From Yanoff M, Fine BS. *Ocular Pathology*, 5th ed. St Louis: Mosby; 2002.)

Optic nerve sheath meningioma:

More common in women

33% of all primary optic nerve tumors

Increased incidence in neurofibromatosis

Arises from arachnoid cells in the meninges

Findings: decreased visual acuity and color vision, visual field loss, proptosis, disc edema or pallor, optociliary shunt vessels

Spencer's triad: optociliary shunts, optic atrophy, optic nerve meningioma

Pathology: sheets of cells or whorls; psammoma bodies (calcified) in the center of whorls

CT scan: tubular enlargement of optic nerve that enhances (railroad track sign); optic foramen enlargement

Treatment: observation, surgical excision to prevent involvement of optic nerve or chiasm

Sphenoid wing meningioma:

Most common tumor to spread to orbit from intracranial space

Findings: temporal fullness, proptosis, lid edema

CT scan: hyperostosis and calcifications

Treatment: observation, surgical excision

Rhabdomyosarcoma

(See Chapter 5, Pediatrics/Strabismus)

Lymphoid Tumors

Spectrum of disorders characterized by abnormal proliferation of lymphoid tissue

10% of all orbital tumors; 90% are non-Hodgkin's low-grade B-cell lymphoma

Usually occur in adults 50-70 years old; rare in children

Women > men (3:2)

Frequency of periocular involvement: orbit (up to 75%), conjunctiva (20%–33%), eyelid (5%–20%)

Cause painless proptosis

Tissue biopsy with immunohistochemical studies required for diagnosis

All lymphoid lesions of orbit must have a workup for systemic lymphoma, including complete blood count (CBC) with differential, serum protein electrophoresis (SPEP), physical examination for lymphadenopathy, CT of thoracic and abdominal viscera, and bone scan

Perform every 6 months for 2 years

Bone marrow biopsy (better than bone marrow aspirate)

Benign Reactive Lymphoid Hyperplasia

Findings: bilateral painless lacrimal gland enlargement, limitation of ocular motility, visual disturbances

Pathology: mature lymphocytes with reactive germinal centers; T cells, 60%-80% with scattered polyclonal B cells; high degree of endothelial cell proliferation

Atypical Lymphoid Hyperplasia

Low-grade lymphoma, no mitotic activity

Pathology: follicles and polymorphous response consistent with benign process

40% develop systemic disease within 5 years

Orbital Lymphoma

Primary orbital lymphoma and usually involves superior orbit (only Burkitt occurs in children)

50% are mucosa-associated lymphoid tissue (MALT) 15%-20% of MALT transform to more aggressive form

Secondary orbital lymphoma is typically intermediate of high grade

17% bilateral

Findings: limitation of ocular motility, painless lacrimal gland swelling, conjunctival salmon patches, visual changes;

Pathology: atypical immature lymphocytes with mitoses; diffuse or follicular growth; monoclonal B-cell proliferations in 60%-90% with scattered or reactive T cells; involves reticuloendothelial system, including retroperitoneal lymph nodes (Fig. 6.22)

CT scan: putty-like molding of tumor; orbital tissues not displaced

Treatment: radiotherapy for localized orbital disease, chemotherapy for systemic involvement

Prognosis: 50% risk of systemic involvement; lower for MALT; location appears more important than histopathology for determining systemic involvement: lymphoma of eyelids (67% have systemic involvement) > orbit (35%) > conjunctiva (20%); 90% 5-year survival

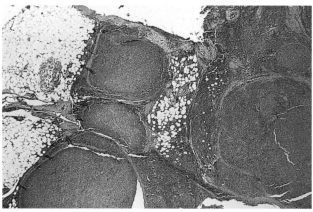

A

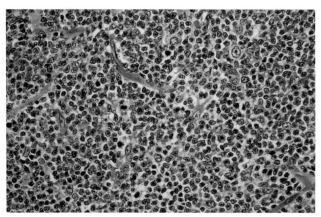

B

Figure 6.22 (A) Nodular lymphoid infiltrate. (B) Higher magnification shows uniform lymphocyte infiltrate with mitotic figures. (From Yanoff M, Scheie HG. Malignant lymphoma of the orbit—difficulties in diagnosis. *Surv Ophthalmol.* 1967;12:133–140.)

Plasmacytoma

Tumor composed of plasma cells

Pathology: plasmacytoid lymphocytes, immunoblasts, mature plasma cells

DDx: Waldenström macroglobulinemia, multiple myeloma, lymphoma with immunoglobulin production

Granulocytic Sarcoma ("Chloroma")

(See Chapter 5, Pediatrics/Strabismus)

Burkitt Lymphoma

(See Chapter 5, Pediatrics/Strabismus)

Systemic Lymphoma and Waldenström Macroglobulinemia

Solid infiltrating tumor with putty-like molding of tumor to preexisting structures

Pathology: Dutcher bodies (intranuclear PAS-positive inclusions of immunoglobulin)

Fibro-Osseous Tumors

Fibrous Dysplasia

(See Chapter 5, Pediatrics/Strabismus)

Ossifying Fibroma

Variant of fibrous dysplasia

Occurs in 2nd and 3rd decades of life

More common in women

Well-circumscribed, slow-growing, monostotic lesion

Pathology: vascular stroma containing lamellar bone with a rim of osteoid and osteoblasts

Osteoma

Dense bony lesions originating in the frontal and ethmoid sinus

Well-circumscribed, slow-growing mass

Symptoms secondary to sinus obstruction and intracranial or intraorbital extension

Pathology: lamellar bone with variable amounts of fibrous stroma

Fibrous Histiocytoma

Firm orbital mass composed of fibroblasts and histiocytes

Usually benign; 10% malignant

Distinguished from hemangiopericytoma only on biopsy

Most common mesenchymal orbital lesion of adults

Pathology: storiform (cartwheel or spiral), nebular pattern of tumor cells (fibroblasts); both fibrous histiocytoma and hemangiopericytoma are spindle cell tumors, and they can be difficult to differentiate (Fig. 6.23)

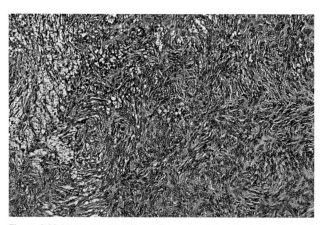

Figure 6.23 Histiocytes (*on left*) and fibrous (*on right*, with storiform [matted] appearance) components. (From Jones WD 3rd, Yanoff M, Katowitz JA. Recurrent facial fibrous histiocytoma. *Br J Plast Surg.* 1979;32:46–51.)

CT scan: well-circumscribed mass anywhere in the orbit (upper nasal most common)

Treatment: surgical excision; Moderate risk of recurrence

Histiocytosis X (Langerhans Cell Histiocytosis)

(See Chapter 5, Pediatrics/Strabismus)

Juvenile Xanthogranuloma (JXG; Nevoxanthoendothelioma)

(See Chapter 5, Pediatrics/Strabismus)

Adult-Onset Xanthogranuloma

Often associated with systemic manifestations

4 syndromes (in order of frequency):
1. Necrobiotic xanthogranuloma (NBX)
2. Adult-onset asthma with periocular xanthogranuloma (AAPOX)
3. Erdheim-Chester disease (ECD)
4. Adult-onset xanthogranuloma (AOX)

Epithelial Lacrimal Gland Tumors

50% of lacrimal gland lesions are inflammatory and lymphoproliferative; contour around the globe

50% of lacrimal gland tumors are of epithelial origin

50% of epithelial tumors are benign pleomorphic adenomas

50% of malignant tumors are adenoid cystic carcinomas

Pleomorphic Adenoma (Benign Mixed Tumor)

Most common epithelial tumor of the lacrimal gland

Occurs in 4th or 5th decade of life

More common in men

Slow onset (6–12 months)

Firm mass in lacrimal fossa with painless proptosis; globe often displaced medially and downward

Progressive expansile growth may indent bone of lacrimal fossa

Tumor growth stimulates periosteum to deposit a thin layer of new bone (cortication)

Pathology: proliferation of epithelial cells into a double layer, forming lumina with ductal and secretory elements; ductal inner cells secrete mucus; outer stromal cells give rise to fibrous stroma and osteoid and cartilaginous metaplasia, pseudoencapsulated with surface bosselations (Fig. 6.24)

CT scan: well circumscribed but may have nodular configuration

Treatment: complete en bloc excision without biopsy; incomplete excision may result in recurrence and malignant transformation into pleomorphic adenocarcinoma

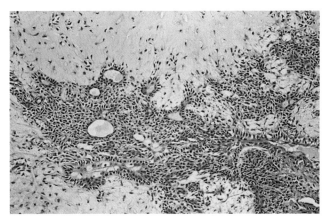

Figure 6.24 Benign mixed tumor (BMT) demonstrating ductal structures in a myxoid stroma. (From Yanoff M, Fine BS. *Ocular Pathology*, 5th ed. St Louis: Mosby; 2002.)

Pleomorphic Adenocarcinoma (Malignant Mixed Tumor)

Long history of mass in lacrimal fossa

Occurs in elderly individuals

Findings: rapid, progressive, painful proptosis

Pathology: similar to benign mixed tumor but with foci of malignant change

Treatment: radical orbitectomy and bone removal

Adenoid Cystic Carcinoma

Most common malignant tumor of the lacrimal gland

Highly malignant

Presents in 4th decade of life

Rapidly progressive proptosis, pain and paresthesia result from perineural invasion and bony destruction

Pathology: small, benign-appearing cells arranged in nests, tubules, or in a "Swiss-cheese" (cribriform) pattern (Fig. 6.25)

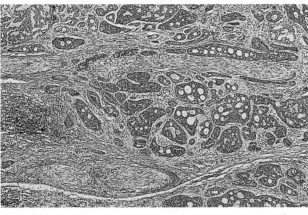

Figure 6.25 Adenoid cystic carcinoma demonstrating characteristic "Swiss-cheese" appearance. (From Yanoff M, Fine BS. *Ocular Pathology*, 5th ed. St Louis: Mosby; 2002.)

CT scan: poorly circumscribed mass, bony destruction, calcifications

Treatment: removal of any bone that is involved, exenteration, adjunctive radiation and chemotherapy

Prognosis: poor; survival rate = 20%-70%

Sinus Tumors

Sinus Mucocele

Cystic, slowly expanding sinus lesion

Entrapment of mucus in aerated space as a result of obstruction of sinus ostia

Exerts pressure on surrounding bony structures

May become infected (mucopyocele)

Causes of ostial obstruction: inflammation with scarring, congenital narrowing of ostia, trauma, osteomas, polyps, septal deviation, mucus retention cysts

Associated with cystic fibrosis

Must rule out encephalocele and meningocele

Findings:
Frontoethmoid sinus (most common location): outward and downward displacement of globe, fullness in superonasal and medial canthal regions, above the medial canthal tendon
Sphenoid and posterior ethmoid sinus: visual symptoms, retrobulbar pain; may have cranial nerve palsies; 50% have nasal symptoms
Maxillary sinus (rare): upward displacement of globe, erosion of orbital floor may cause enophthalmos

CT scan: homogeneous opacified cyst with bowing of sinus wall and attenuation/erosion of bone

MRI: highly variable signal intensities

Treatment: surgical excision with IV antibiotics; reestablish normal drainage; obliteration of sinus (only if frontal)

Sinus Carcinoma

Usually squamous cell

Most commonly from maxillary sinus

No early signs except for sinusitis

Late findings: nonaxial proptosis, epiphora, epistaxis, infraorbital anesthesia

Metastatic Tumors

In contrast to adults, pediatric tumors metastasize to the orbit more frequently than to the uvea

Orbital metastases produce rapid painful proptosis with restricted ocular motility

Neuroblastoma

(See Chapter 5, Pediatrics/Strabismus)

Leukemia

(See Chapter 5, Pediatrics/Strabismus)

Ewing Sarcoma

(See Chapter 5, Pediatrics/Strabismus)

Breast Carcinoma

Most common primary source of orbital metastasis in women

May occur many years after primary diagnosis

May elicit a fibrous response and cause enophthalmos and ophthalmoplegia

May respond to hormonal manipulation

Lung Carcinoma

Most common primary source of orbital metastasis in men

Very aggressive

Prostate carcinoma

May present similarly to acute pseudotumor

Less aggressive than lung carcinoma

EYELID DISORDERS

Congenital Anomalies

(See Chapter 5, Pediatrics/Strabismus)

Trauma

Lid Laceration

Partial- or full-thickness cut in eyelid that may involve the lid margin, canthus, or canaliculus

Treatment: antibiotics, tetanus booster; surgical repair; technique depends on severity and location of injury

Lid Avulsion

Complete or partial tearing of eyelid with or without tissue loss

Treatment: technique of repair depends on severity and location of injury
Small defect (<25%): direct closure
Moderate defect (25%–50%): Tenzel flap
Large defect (>50%): bridge flap reconstruction (Cutler-Beard [for upper lid] or Hughes [for lower lid] procedure with flap advancement)

Inflammation

Hordeolum

Obstruction and infection of Zeiss (external hordeolum, stye) or meibomian (internal hordeolum, chalazion) glands

Painful erythematous eyelid swelling

Accumulation of secretions causes acute inflammatory response

Lipogranuloma formation (chalazion) often evolves from internal hordeolum

Pathology: epithelioid and giant cells surrounding empty lipid vacuoles, zonal granulomatous inflammation (zonal lipogranuloma) (Fig. 6.26)

Treatment: warm compresses, topical antibiotic ointment, lid scrubs (for associated blepharitis); if no response, consider local steroid injection, or incision and curettage (submit specimen to pathology, especially for atypical or recurrent lesions)

Blepharitis and Meibomian Gland Dysfunction

Inflammation of lid margin (blepharitis) and obstruction of oil-producing sebaceous glands (meibomian gland dysfunction [MGD], meibomitis); often occur together

Ocular surface disease results from disruption of the tear film (from bacterial lipolytic exoenzymes and abnormal meibum), epithelial cell death, and inflammation

~86% of patients with dry eye have signs of MGD

58% of patients have collarettes (pathognomonic for Demodex), increases with age (84% in those ≥60 years old, 100% in those >70 years old)

Blepharitis classified by location or etiology:

Anterior lid margin disease: seborrheic or chronic *Staphylococcus* or *Demodex* infection

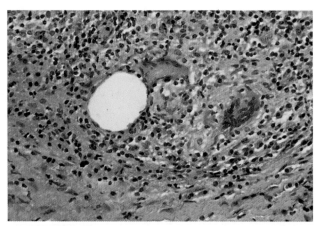

Figure 6.26 Chalazion demonstrating epithelioid and giant cells surrounding clear areas that contained lipid. (From Yanoff M, Fine BS. *Ocular Pathology*, 5th ed. St Louis: Mosby; 2002.)

Posterior lid margin disease: meibomitis, meibomian gland dysfunction (MGD)

Angular blepharitis: at lateral canthus; associated with *Moraxella*

Symptoms: burning, itching, redness, tearing, photophobia

Findings:
Anterior blepharitis: crusting/scales along eyelashes ("scurf" [scale fragments] and "collarettes" [scales that encircle base of lash; represents debris and waste of *Demodex* mites, pathognomonic for *Demodex* infestation]), loss of eyelashes (madarosis), lid margin redness, conjunctival injection; may develop pannus, phlyctenules, corneal infiltrates, and ulceration
MGD: thickened, erythematous lid margins with telangiectatic blood vessels; atrophic, swollen, pitted, or blocked meibomian glands; turbid, thickened meibum (graded on a scale from 0 to 3: 0 = clear; 1 = cloudy; 2 = cloudy with debris [granular]; 3 = thick [toothpaste]); may have meibomian gland inclusions (visible under the tarsal conjunctiva as yellow bumps), decreased tear breakup time (<10 seconds), tear film debris and foam, conjunctival injection, corneal staining (typically inferiorly); may develop recurrent chalazia/hordeola, trichiasis

Treatment:
Anterior blepharitis: lid hygiene (hot compresses, hypochlorous acid spray, and/or lid scrubs), topical antibiotic ointment (bacitracin or erythromycin qhs), mechanical scrubbing (in-office treatment to remove biofilm, scurf, debris), consider tea tree oil scrubs for *Demodex*
MGD: hot compresses, lid massage, lid scrubs, hypochlorous acid spray, lubrication (for associated dry eye), oral supplements (omega-3 fatty acids); consider oral tetracycline/doxycycline, topical azithromycin, topical steroid; consider in-office heat/expression treatments, intense pulsed light (IPL), meibomian gland probing

Acne Rosacea

Idiopathic, chronic skin disorder affecting sebaceous glands of face (including meibomian glands)

Type IV hypersensitivity may play a role

Common between ages 40-60 years

Ocular involvement in >50%

Findings: chronic blepharitis, meibomitis, lid margin telangiectasia, conjunctival injection, abnormal tear film (foam, mucin particles, excess oil), decreased tear breakup time, meibomian gland plugging, recurrent chalazions; may develop keratitis with peripheral corneal infiltrates, vascularization, scarring, thinning, ulceration, and rarely perforation

Other findings: acne-like skin changes, telangiectatic vessels, papules, and rhinophyma

Pathology: granulomatous inflammation

Treatment: warm compresses and lid scrubs, oral doxycycline or erythromycin, oral fish oil (omega-3 fatty acids), topical azithromycin, lubrication (for associated dry eye); topical metronidazole to facial skin; consider topical steroid

Treatment: Lid scrubs, oral tetracycline/doxycycline, oral fish oil (omega-3 fatty acids), lubrication (for associated dry eye), topical metronidazole to facial skin

Contact Dermatitis

Inflammation of lid skin as a result of exogenous irritant or allergic hypersensitivity reaction

Symptoms: red, swollen, itchy periorbital skin

Findings: erythematous, scaling lesions; may have vesicles or weeping areas

Treatment: eliminate inciting agent; use mild steroid cream or tropical tacrolimus 0.1% (Protopic)

Infections

Molluscum Contagiosum

Shiny, white-yellow papule with central umbilication

Infection by the poxvirus molluscum contagiosum virus (MCV)

Spread by direct contact; consider HIV in healthy adult

Usually asymptomatic

Can cause follicular conjunctivitis and punctate keratitis

Pathology: lobular acanthosis, large basophilic poxviral intracytoplasmic inclusions composed of nucleic acids from DNA virus (Fig. 6.27)

Treatment: surgical excision, cryo, incision, and curettage

Phthiriasis Palpebrarum/Pediculosis

Lice infection of lashes

Spread by direct contact, usually sexually transmitted

Produces blepharoconjunctivitis

Findings: follicles, injection, small white eggs (nits) and lice attached to lashes

Treatment: remove nits and lice, topical ointment to suffocate lice, delousing creams and shampoo

Verruca Vulgaris (Papilloma)

Pink, pedunculated or sessile mass

Associated with human papillomavirus (HPV)

Usually asymptomatic

Often multiple and resolve spontaneously

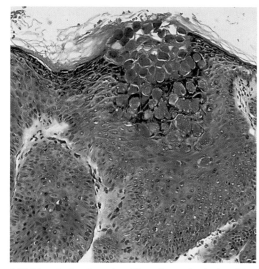

Figure 6.27 Intracytoplasmic, eosinophilic molluscum bodies in epidermis; they become larger and more basophilic near the surface. (Courtesy of Dr. WC Frayer. From Yanoff M, Fine BS. Skin and lacrimal drainage system. In: Yanoff M, Fine BS. *Ocular Pathology*, 5th ed. St Louis: Mosby; 2002.)

Herpes Infection

Herpes simplex virus (HSV):
Primary infection causes vesicular dermatitis
May be associated with follicular conjunctivitis and keratitis
Treatment: cold compresses, antibiotic ointment to skin lesions, systemic antiviral; topical antiviral if eye involved

Varicella zoster virus (VZV):
Vesicular dermatitis with ulceration, crusting, and scarring
Reactivation of latent infection along distribution of trigeminal nerve (most often V_1)
Dermatomal distribution, does not cross midline
May have constitutional symptoms and ocular involvement
Treatment: cold compresses, antibiotic ointment to skin lesions, systemic antiviral; (see Chapter 7, Cornea/External Disease, for ocular involvement), may require treatment of postherpetic neuralgia (PHN)

Leprosy

Caused by infection with acid-fast bacillus *Mycobacterium leprae*

Tuberculoid and lepromatous leprosy can affect lids

Findings: loss of lashes, trichiasis, ectropion, and exposure keratitis

Treatment: systemic antibiotics (dapsone, rifampin)

Malposition and Other Disorders

Blepharospasm

Bilateral, intermittent, involuntary contractions of orbicularis and facial muscles causing uncontrolled blinking; may cause functional blindness

Etiology unknown but may be caused by an abnormality of basal ganglia

Usually occurs in 5th-7th decade of life; female > male (3:1); associated with Parkinson disease

Absent during sleep

Meige syndrome: blepharospasm, cervical dystonia, and facial oromandibular dystonia (involuntary jaw and tongue contractions)

DDx: secondary blepharospasm (resulting from ocular irritation), hemifacial spasm (usually unilateral, caused by compression of CN 7, can be caused by cerebellopontine-angle [CPA] tumor, present during sleep), myokymia, Tourette syndrome, trigeminal neuralgia, basal ganglia disease, tardive dyskinesia

Consider CT/MRI scan to rule out posterior fossa lesion

Treatment: Botox (botulinum toxin type A) injections, surgery (excision of lid protractors or differential section of CN 7), medications (tetrabenazine, lithium, carbidopa, clonazepam); also deep brain stimulation for Meige syndrome
> *Botox:* derived from *Clostridium botulinum*, freeze-dried solution; subcutaneous injection, no more than 200 units/month
> > MECHANISM: blocks neuromuscular conduction by binding to receptors on nerve terminals and stops release of acetylcholine (ACh) by disrupting calcium metabolism; does not cross blood–brain barrier
> > INDICATIONS: blepharospasm (effective in 90%, lasts 3 months), hemifacial spasm (lasts 4 months), strabismus (lasts 1–8 weeks)
> > ADVERSE EFFECTS (NO SYSTEMIC TOXICITY): exposure keratopathy, ptosis, diplopia, flaccid lower lid ectropion

Blepharochalasis

Idiopathic inflammatory edema of the eyelids

Familial, most often in young women

Recurrent attacks of transient, painless eyelid edema resulting in atrophy, wrinkling, and redundancy of eyelid skin

May develop ptosis and herniation of orbital lacrimal gland

Dermatochalasis

Redundancy of eyelid skin with orbital fat prolapse as a result of involutional changes

Blepharoptosis (Acquired)

Eyelid malposition characterized by drooping upper eyelid

Myogenic: uncommon; caused by local or systemic muscular disease (e.g., myotonic dystrophy, chronic progressive external ophthalmoplegia, myasthenia gravis)

Treat underlying condition; usually requires frontalis sling

Involutional (aponeurotic): most common form of ptosis; disinsertion of levator aponeurosis

Caused by aging or chronic inflammation; may be exacerbated by eye surgery or trauma

High eyelid crease with good levator function; ptotic lid in all positions of gaze (no lid lag on downgaze as in congenital cases); may have thinning of eyelid above tarsal plate

Neurogenic: caused by CN 3 palsy, aberrant regeneration of CN 3 (Marcus-Gunn jaw-winking ptosis), Horner syndrome, multiple sclerosis, ophthalmoplegic migraine
> *Treatment for Horner:* shorten Müller muscle (Putterman [conjunctival-Müller muscle resection]) or Fasanella-Servat [tarsoconjunctival resection] procedure)

Mechanical: caused by mass effect of orbital or eyelid tumors, dermatochalasis, blepharochalasis, cicatrix

Traumatic: caused by trauma to levator aponeurosis; may have lagophthalmos from cicatricial changes

May improve spontaneously; therefore observe for 6 months

Examination:
> *Palpebral fissure height (PF):* normally 10-11 mm in primary gaze
> *Marginal reflex distance (MRD):* MRD1 is distance between corneal light reflex and upper lid margin in primary gaze; normally 4 mm MRD2 is distance to lower lid margin
> *Levator function (LF):* distance of upper lid excursion while frontalis is immobilized; normal >12 mm, f air if 6-11 mm, poor if <5 mm
> *2.5% phenylephrine test:* activates sympathetic fibers of Müller muscle; resulting lid elevation simulates position after Müller muscle resection

DDx: pseudoptosis (nanophthalmos, microphthalmos, phthisis bulbi, hypotropia, dermatochalasis, enophthalmos, contralateral eyelid retraction or proptosis)

Treatment: eyelid crutches, levator aponeurosis advancement, levator muscle resection, Müller muscle resection, frontalis suspension with autogenous fascia lata, banked fascia lata, or synthetic materials

Surgical complications: overcorrection or undercorrection, lid lag, lagophthalmos, exposure keratopathy

Eyelid Retraction

Upper eyelid at or above superior limbus

Lower eyelid exposing sclera

DDx: thyroid eye disease (most common, lateral upper eyelid more retracted than medial eyelid, fibrous contraction of eyelid retractors), orbital pseudotumor (idiopathic orbital inflammation [IOI]), pharmacologic (phenylephrine, α-agonists, cocaine), resection of superior rectus, overcorrection of ptosis, contralateral ptosis (Hering's law)

Treatment: lubrication; surgical repair (levator aponeurosis recession, levator myotomy, spacer insertion, full-thickness skin graft for lower eyelid, hard palate grafts for lower eyelid)

Ectropion

Eversion of eyelid margin; may cause keratinization and hypertrophy of conjunctiva

Symptoms: tearing, foreign body sensation, redness

Involutional: most common cause of ectropion; often in lower eyelid
  Etiology: horizontal laxity, disinsertion of lower eyelid retractors
  Diagnosis: snap-back test, distraction test
  Treatment: horizontal eyelid shortening (lateral tarsal strip), lateral canthoplasty, repair of lower eyelid retractors

Paralytic: occurs after CN 7 palsy
  Frequent complaints of tearing from chronic reflex secretion
  Treatment: lubrication, taping of temporal lower eyelid, moisture chamber goggles, lateral tarsorrhaphy, horizontal tightening procedure, hard palate mucosal graft for lower eyelid elevation, gold weight implantation to aid in closure of upper eyelid

Cicatricial: shortening of anterior lamella
  Etiology: burns, trauma, tumor, infection, chronic inflammation causing secondary anterior lamellar contraction (acne rosacea, atopic dermatitis, eczema, herpes zoster dermatitis, scleroderma, epidermolysis bullosa, porphyria, xeroderma pigmentosum)
  Treatment: revision and relaxation of cicatrix, horizontal tightening procedure, may require vertical lengthening with full-thickness graft

Mechanical:
  Etiology: tumors of eyelid, herniated orbital fat, poorly fitted spectacles, chronic edema
  Treat underlying condition

Entropion

Inversion of eyelid margin

Lower eyelid entropion usually involutional

Upper eyelid entropion usually cicatricial

Symptoms: tearing, foreign body sensation, redness

Congenital:
  Very rare; caused by epiblepharon or tarsal kink (see Chapter 5, Pediatrics/Strabismus)
  Usually does not require treatment

Spastic:
  Associated with ocular inflammation, trauma, and prolonged patching
  Squeezing of eyelids causes inward rolling of eyelid margin; ocular surface irritation perpetuates cycle
  Treatment: taping of eyelid, cautery, Botox injection, Quickert suture, lateral tightening with transconjunctival advancement of lid retractors

Involutional:
  Etiology: canthal tendon laxity (horizontal lid laxity, diagnose with snap-back test), eyelid retractor dehiscence (vertical lid laxity), overriding preseptal orbicularis muscle, involutional enophthalmos
  Treatment: Quickert suture, horizontal lid-shortening procedure (Bick, lateral tarsal strip, marginal wedge resection), vertical lid-shortening procedure (Jones, Hotz, Wies marginal rotation), retractor advancement, excision of preseptal orbicularis

Cicatricial: Shortening of posterior lamella
  Etiology: ocular cicatricial pemphigoid, Stevens-Johnson syndrome, trachoma, herpes zoster dermatitis, surgery, trauma, chemical burns, miotics
  Digital pressure on inferior border of tarsus corrects eyelid position in involutional entropion but not cicatricial entropion
  Treatment: lubrication, avoid surgery during acute phase of autoimmune disease, remove lashes in contact with cornea, use tarsal fracture operation, apply tarsoconjunctival grafts or hard palate mucosal grafts to replace scarred tarsus; may require symblepharon ring and amniotic membrane graft to prevent recurrent scarring

Trichiasis

Misdirection of eyelashes and contact with ocular surface

Etiology: trauma (injury, thermal burn, surgery), infection (trachoma, herpes zoster), autoimmune disease (ocular cicatricial pemphigoid, Steven-Johnson syndrome), inflammation (chronic blepharitis, vernal keratoconjunctivitis)

DDx: pseudotrichiasis (entropion, epiblepharon) or distichiasis (abnormal growth of lashes from meibomian gland orifices)

Symptoms: tearing, foreign body sensation, redness

Treatment: lubrication, epilation, electrolysis, cryodestruction with double-freeze/thaw technique, radiofrequency or laser (argon, diode, or ruby) ablation, trephination, full-thickness wedge resection, tarsal fracture, or entropion repair; oral azithromycin to reduce recurrence in cases of trachoma

Floppy Eyelid Syndrome

Easily everted upper eyelids

Chronic papillary conjunctivitis caused by lid autoeversion during sleep with resultant mechanical irritation from bed sheets

Associated with obesity, keratoconus, eyelid rubbing, and sleep apnea

Treatment: lubrication, tape/patch/shield lids during sleep; consider surgical correction (upper eyelid lateral tarsal strip, medial and lateral canthal plication, or medial tarsal strip; wedge excision is less effective)

Madarosis

Loss of eyelashes and/or eyebrows resulting from local or systemic disorders

DDx: eyelid neoplasms, chronic blepharitis, trauma, burns, trichotillomania, alopecia, seborrheic dermatitis, chemotherapy agents, malnutrition, lupus, leprosy

Poliosis/Vitiligo

Premature whitening of the eyelashes/eyebrows (poliosis) or skin (vitiligo) as a result of local systemic disorders

Associated with Vogt-Koyanagi-Harada syndrome, sympathetic ophthalmia, Waardenburg syndrome, tuberous sclerosis, radiation, and dermatitis

Eyelid Tumors

Benign Epithelial Tumors

Squamous Papilloma

Keratinized epidermal fronds with fibrovascular cores

Most common benign lesion of eyelid

Associated with papovavirus (HPV) infection

May be sessile or pedunculated

Pathology: papillary configuration, proliferating fibrovascular tissue covered by hyperplastic prickle cell layer of the epidermis, hyperkeratosis and parakeratosis may be present, vacuolated cells containing virus particles may be seen in the upper squamous layer (Fig. 6.28)

Treatment: surgical excision, cryo or laser ablation

Seborrheic Keratosis

Papillomatous proliferation of suprabasalar (prickle) cells

Pigmented keratin crust with greasy, "stuck-on" appearance

Occurs in elderly

Pathology: acanthosis, hyperkeratosis, parakeratosis, and squamous eddies may be present (Fig. 6.29)

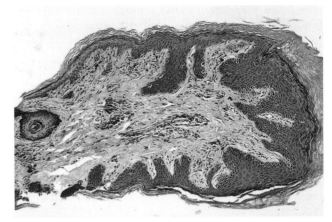

Figure 6.28 Squamous papilloma demonstrating acanthosis and hyperkeratosis. (From Yanoff M, Fine BS. *Ocular Pathology*, 5th ed. St Louis: Mosby; 2002.)

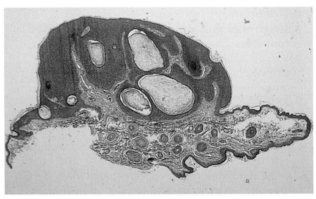

Figure 6.29 Seborrheic keratosis appears as blue lesion above skin surface with blue basaloid cells and keratin cysts. (From Yanoff M, Fine BS. *Ocular Pathology*, 5th ed. St Louis: Mosby; 2002.)

Inverted Follicular Keratosis

Nodular or verrucous lesion

Looks like a cutaneous horn

Inflamed seborrheic keratosis

Pathology: acanthosis, squamous and basal cell proliferation

Cysts

Epithelial-lined chambers filled with debris

Epidermal Inclusion Cyst (Epidermoid Cyst)

Single-lumen, round or oval lesion lined by keratinized, stratified squamous epithelium (epidermis) and filled with cheesy keratin debris

Occurs after a fragment of epidermis is carried into the subepithelium by trauma

Trapped but viable epithelium proliferates and produces keratin

Rupture can cause a foreign body granulomatous reaction

Dermoid Cyst

Lined by keratinized squamous epithelium and dermal appendages such as hair shafts and sebaceous glands

Contains keratin, cilia, and sebum

Often congenital; most common orbital tumor in children

Can be found in eyelid or orbit

Hidrocystoma (Sudoriferous Cyst)

Multilocular, branching lumen that appears empty or contains serous fluid

Lined by a double row of cuboidal epithelium (resembling sweat duct)

Most are eccrine hidrocystoma (can be apocrine if arising from the glands of Moll)

Occur most commonly at eyelid margin or lateral canthus

Sebaceous Gland Tumors

Congenital Sebaceous Gland Hyperplasia

Proliferation of normal sebaceous glands

20% degenerate into basal cell carcinoma

Acquired Sebaceous Gland Hyperplasia

Multiple well-circumscribed yellow nodules

Lobules of mature sebaceous glands around a dilated duct

Muir-Torre Syndrome

Multiple sebaceous neoplasms, keratoacanthomas, and visceral tumors (especially gastrointestinal [GI])

Sweat Gland Tumors

Syringoma

Waxy, yellow nodules on lower lid

Usually occur in young women

Benign proliferation of eccrine ductal structures

Hidrocystoma

Translucent, bluish cyst

Arises from eccrine or apocrine glands

Tumors of Hair Follicle Origin

Trichoepithelioma

Firm, skin-colored nodule

More common in women

Usually occurs on forehead, eyelids, nasolabial fold, and upper lip

Pathology: basaloid cells surrounding a keratin center

Multiple lesions: Brooke tumor (autosomal dominant [AD])

Trichofolliculoma

A keratin-filled dilated cystic hair follicle, surrounded by immature hair follicles

Appears as a small umbilicated nodule usually with central white hairs

Tricholemmoma

Small crusty lesion with rough ulcerated surface

Usually occurs on face

Arises from glycogen-rich clear cells of the outer hair sheath

May resemble basal, squamous, or sebaceous gland carcinoma

Cowden disease (AD): multiple facial tricholemmomas; marker for breast (40%) or thyroid cancer

Pilomatrixoma ("Calcifying Epithelioma of Malherbe")

Solitary, firm, deep nodule with overlying normal, pink, or bluish skin

Freely movable subcutaneous pink-purple nodule

Most common cystic lesion of childhood

In young adult, arises from hair matrix of upper lid or brow

Occurs on the eyelid, face, neck, or arms

Can range from 5-30 mm in diameter

May resemble an epidermal cyst

Associated with myotonic dystrophy and Gardner syndrome

Precancerous Lesions

Actinic Keratosis

Most common precancerous lesion

Related to sun exposure

Occurs in middle-aged individuals

Scaly, white, flat-topped lesion with surrounding erythema

Common on face, eyelid, and scalp

May be single or multiple

12% evolve into squamous cell carcinoma (less aggressive than if it arises de novo); 25% spontaneously resolve

May also evolve into basal cell carcinoma

Pathology: elastotic degeneration in the dermis, overlying hyperkeratosis, focal parakeratosis, clefts in dyskeratotic areas (Fig. 6.30)

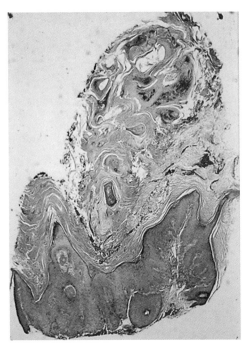

Figure 6.30 Actinic keratosis appears as pink papillomatous lesion with marked hyperkeratosis and acanthosis about skin surface. (From Yanoff M, Fine BS. *Ocular Pathology*, 5th ed. St Louis: Mosby; 2002.)

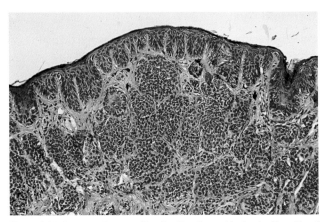

Figure 6.31 Compound nevus with cells at junction and in dermis. (From Yanoff M, Fine BS. *Ocular Pathology*, 5th ed. St Louis: Mosby; 2002.)

Treatment: surgical excision, cryo or freezing with liquid nitrogen

Nevus

Congenital or acquired hamartoma

Can be flat, but is usually elevated and pigmented

Arises from neural crest cells

Pigmentation and size tend to increase during puberty

With time, nevi tend to move deeper, migrating into the dermis

Contains benign-appearing dermal melanocytes

Malignant transformation is rare

Classified by location

Junctional nevus: occurs at epidermal/dermal junction; flat
Greatest malignant potential

Compound nevus:
Both intradermal and junctional components (Fig. 6.31); slightly elevated or papillomatous
Often pigmented
Junctional component gives malignant potential

Intradermal nevus:
Most common
Most benign

Can be papillomatous, dome-shaped, or pedunculated
Slightly pigmented or amelanotic
Hair shafts indicate intradermal variety

Kissing nevus:
Congenital
Involves both upper and lower lids
Secondary to fusion of lids during embryonic development

Spindle cell nevus:
Compound nevus of childhood
Bizarre cellular components
No malignant potential

Giant hairy nevus of the face and scalp:
Congenital; thickened eyelids can cause amblyopia

Nevus of Ota (Oculodermal Melanocytosis)

(See Chapter 5, Pediatrics/Strabismus)

Lentigo Maligna (Melanotic Freckle of Hutchinson)

Acquired cutaneous pigmentation

Often periocular

Occurs in middle-aged or older individuals

Conjunctival pigmentation may be noted

No episcleral pigmentation

Melanoma arises in ~30%

Cutaneous counterpart of primary acquired melanosis (PAM) of the conjunctiva

Xeroderma Pigmentosa (Autosomal Recessive [AR])

Defect in DNA repair (ultraviolet [UV] light endonuclease)

Freckles and scaling at early age

Susceptible to a variety of malignant tumors (basal cell carcinoma, squamous cell carcinoma, malignant melanoma, sarcoma)

3% incidence of skin malignant melanoma

Malignant Epithelial Tumors

Risk factors: increased age, sun exposure, fair skin, previous history of skin cancer, positive family history

Characteristics: irregularity, induration, and altered lid anatomy

Basal Cell Carcinoma (BCC)

Most common malignancy of the eyelid (90%)

40 × more common than squamous cell carcinoma

Develops on sun-exposed skin in elderly patients; smoking is also a risk

Location (in order of frequency): lower lid (50%–60%), medial canthus (20%–30%), upper lid (15%), outer canthus (5%)

Poorest prognosis when found in medial canthus because tumor often extends deeper and can involve lacrimal drainage system

Morbidity and mortality occur from local invasion of skull and CNS

Rarely metastasizes

Pathology: blue basaloid tumor cells arranged in nests and cords (H&E stain); peripheral palisading commonly seen (Fig. 6.32)

Nodular basal cell carcinoma: most common form; firm, raised, pearly, discrete mass, often with telangiectases over tumor margin; if center is ulcerated, called a rodent ulcer

Morpheaform basal cell carcinoma: less common, but much more aggressive; firm, flat lesion with indistinct borders; penetrates into dermis, pagetoid spread can occur; tumor cells may line up in single cell layer ("Indian-file" pattern) (Fig. 6.33)

Treatment: excisional biopsy, wide excision with frozen section, Mohs micrographic surgery, may require supplemental cryotherapy or radiation therapy, exenteration for orbital extension

Squamous Cell Carcinoma (SCC)

Flat, keratinized, ulcerated, erythematous plaque

Can arise de novo or from preexisting actinic keratosis

May spread by direct extension or may metastasize via local lymphatics or hematogenously

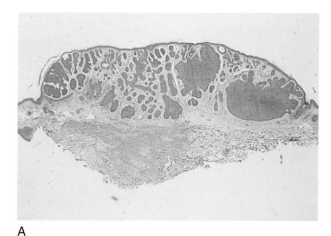

A

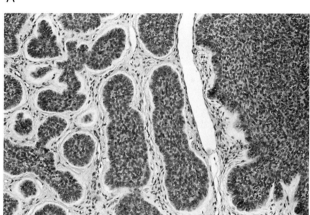

B

Figure 6.32 (A) Basal cell carcinoma appears as blue nests of basal cells proliferating over pale pink desmoplasia (dermal fibroblast proliferation). (B) Basal cell nests with peripheral palisading and mitotic figures. (Courtesy of HG Scheie. From Yanoff M, Fine BS. *Ocular Pathology*, 5th ed. St Louis: Mosby; 2002.)

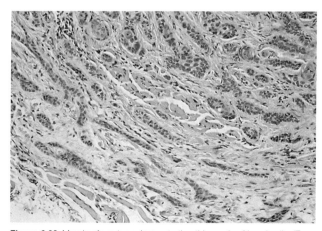

Figure 6.33 Morpheaform type demonstrating thin cords of basal cells. (From Yanoff M, Fine BS. *Ocular Pathology*, 5th ed. St Louis: Mosby; 2002.)

May be associated with HIV and HPV infection

More aggressive than basal cell carcinoma

Usually occurs on lower eyelid

205

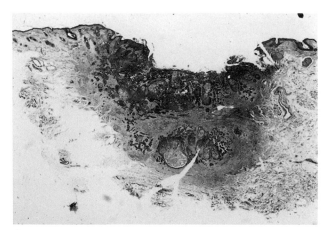

A

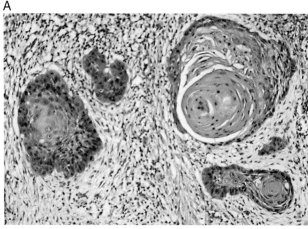

B

Figure 6.34 Squamous cell carcinoma. (A) Pink epithelial cells invading dermis with overlying ulceration. (B) Squamous cells in dermis making keratin. (From Yanoff M, Fine BS. *Ocular Pathology*, 5th ed. St Louis: Mosby; 2002.)

Pathology: pink dyskeratotic cells forming keratin pearls (H&E stain), cordlike infiltrating strands into the dermis containing atypical anaplastic cells (Fig. 6.34)

Treatment: excisional biopsy, wide excision with frozen section, Mohs micrographic surgery, may require supplemental cryotherapy or radiation therapy, exenteration for orbital extension

Keratoacanthoma

Dome-shaped squamous lesion

Rapid onset (4–8 weeks); occurs in elderly

Central keratin-filled crater and elevated rolled edges; clinically resembles basal cell carcinoma

Previously considered a form of pseudoepitheliomatous hyperplasia, now classified as a squamous carcinoma

Spontaneous involution

May cause permanent damage to lid margin and madarosis (loss of lashes)

Pathology: acanthotic, hyperkeratotic, dyskeratotic epithelium and inflammatory cells (Fig. 6.35)

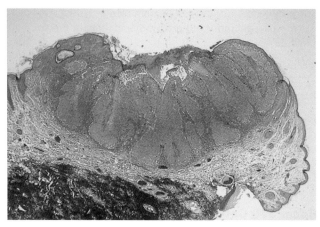

Figure 6.35 Keratoacanthoma appears as cup-shaped lesion with central keratin core above skin surface. (From Yanoff M, Fine BS. *Ocular Pathology*, 5th ed. St Louis: Mosby; 2002.)

Treatment: observation, surgical excision, local steroid injection

Sebaceous Gland Carcinoma

Orange-yellow nodule

2nd most common malignancy of the eyelid (after BCC)

Occurs in the elderly (6th-7th decade of life); higher incidence among Asian populations

Usually arises from meibomian glands; can also arise from glands of Zeis and glands of caruncle

Upper lid more commonly involved (greater number of meibomian glands)

Can masquerade and be misdiagnosed as a recurrent chalazion or chronic blepharitis

Often associated with madarosis

Highly malignant and lethal tumor; regional lymph node and hematogenous metastasis; 5-year mortality rate = 30%

Pathology: lobules of anaplastic cells with foamy, lipid-laden, vacuolated cytoplasm, large hyperchromic nuclei, skip areas and pagetoid invasion (spread of tumor into conjunctival epithelium), positive lipid stains (oil-red-O stain) (Fig. 6.36)

Treatment: wide excision with frozen section and conjunctival map biopsy, exenteration for orbital extension or pagetoid spread, radiotherapy for palliation

Muir-Torre syndrome: multiple sebaceous neoplasms, keratoacanthomas, and visceral tumors (especially GI)

Malignant Melanoma (MM)

< 1% of all eyelid cancers (Fig. 6.37)

Lentigo maligna melanoma (Hutchinson malignant freckle) (10%): occurs in sun-exposed

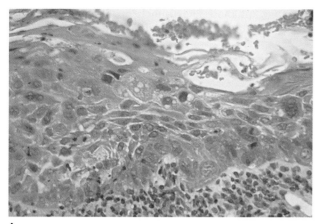

A

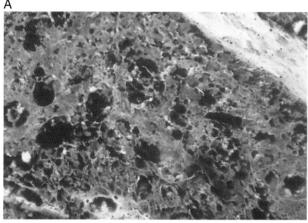

B

Figure 6.36 Sebaceous adenocarcinoma. (A) Large, foamy tumor cells in epidermis demonstrating pagetoid spread. (B) Oil-red-O stains fat in cells. (From Yanoff M, Fine BS, *Ocular Pathology*, 5th ed. St Louis: Mosby; 2002.)

areas of elderly patients; arises from lentigo maligna (see *Precancerous lesions*)
> *Findings:* flat, pigmented macule with irregular borders
> *Pathology:* fascicles of spindle-shaped cells
> 10% metastasize; 5-year survival = 90%

Superficial spreading melanoma (80%): occurs in sun-exposed and nonexposed skin (this form is not directly related to sun exposure) of younger individuals
> Initial horizontal growth phase before invading deeper
> *Findings:* spreading macule with irregular outline, variable pigmentation, invasive phase marked by papules and nodules
> *Pathology:* pagetoid nests in all levels of epidermis
> 5-year survival = 69%

Nodular melanoma (10%):
> Most common type of melanoma in the eyelid
> Usually occurs in 5th decade of life
> More common in men (2:1)
> Always palpable
> More aggressive, with early vertical invasion; 5-year survival = 44%
> 20% of nodular and 50% of superficial spreading arise from nevi

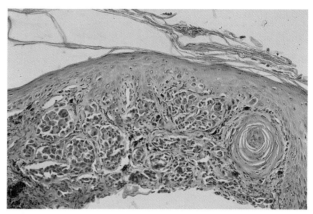

Figure 6.37 Malignant melanoma. (From Yanoff M, Fine BS. *Ocular Pathology*, 5th ed. St Louis: Mosby; 2002.)

Signs of transformation: change in color, change in shape or size, induration, ulceration, bleeding

Treatment: wide surgical excision, lymph node dissection if microscopic evidence of lymphatic or vascular involvement

Prognosis: depends on depth of vertical invasion; <0.75 mm indicates favorable prognosis

Neurogenic Tumors

Neurofibroma

(See Chapter 5, Pediatrics/Strabismus)

Nodular form (fibroma molluscum):
> Usually not associated with neurofibromatosis (NF)

Plexiform form:
> Associated with NF
> Produces S-shaped lid deformity

Pathology: combined proliferation of axons, Schwann cells, and endoneural fibroblasts

Treatment: observation or resection

Neurilemmoma (Schwannoma)

(See *Orbit* section)

Solitary eyelid nodule composed of Schwann cells

Usually located near medial canthus

Usually not associated with NF

Pathology: proliferation of Schwann cells

Treatment: local excision

Merkel Cell Tumor

Rare, vascular, red-blue, sausage-shaped lesion

Rapid growth from Merkel cells (mechanical receptors for touch; amine precursor uptake and decarboxylation [APUD] system)

Usually occurs in upper lid

Occurs in older individuals

Metastasis and death in 30% of patients

Treatment: wide excision with immunohistochemical stains, lymph node dissection, radiation therapy

Vascular Tumors

Lymphangioma

(See Chapter 5, Pediatrics/Strabismus)

Capillary Hemangioma

(See Chapter 5, Pediatrics/Strabismus)

Cavernous Hemangioma

Appears as a port wine stain (nevus flammeus)

Associated with Sturge-Weber syndrome

Grows with the patient; does not involute

Pathology: dilated capillaries without endothelial cell proliferation

Kaposi Sarcoma

Malignant soft tissue sarcoma (solitary or multiple)

More common in immunocompromised patients and those of Mediterranean descent

Various types: epidemic (AIDS related), classic (Mediterranean), endemic (African), and iatrogenic (transplant associated)

May involve orbit

Nontender, violaceous nodules and plaques

May cause lid distortion with edema and entropion

Treatment: complete surgical excision, also responsive to radiotherapy and chemotherapy

Other Lesions

Xanthelasma

Soft, flat or slightly elevated yellow plaques

More common on the medial aspect of the eyelids

Normal serum lipids in 2/3 of patients

Can occur in hyperlipid syndromes such as familial hypercholesterolemia, juvenile xanthogranuloma, histiocytosis X

Associated with **Erdheim-Chester disease (lipoid granulomatosis):** multisystem disease with lipogranuloma formation in the liver, heart, kidneys, lungs, and bones

Findings: proptosis and xanthelasma-like lesions
Pathology: histiocytes and Touton giant cells

Pathology: aggregates of lipid-containing macrophages (foam cells) with surrounding inflammation

Treatment: observation; may recur after excision

Sarcoidosis

(See *Orbit* section)

Slightly elevated, umbilicated papules

Noncaseating granulomas

Amyloidosis

Confluent, yellow, waxy papules

May hemorrhage with minor trauma

Lid lesions are associated with systemic involvement

Pathology: heterogeneous group of substances that stains with Congo red

Necrobiotic Xanthogranuloma

Zonal granuloma with necrobiotic center

Associated with JXG, monoclonal gammopathies, and plasma cell dyscrasias

Pathology: Touton giant cells and xanthoma cells

Mycosis Fungoides

Cutaneous T-cell lymphoma

Pathology: Lutzner cells and Pautrier abscesses

NASOLACRIMAL SYSTEM DISORDERS

Obstructions

Congenital tearing: (See Chapter 5, Pediatrics/Strabismus)
    Must rule out congenital glaucoma; also consider corneal trauma, trichiasis, and superficial foreign body

Acquired tearing:
Etiology: primary idiopathic hypersecretion, ocular surface irritation with reflex tearing, outflow obstruction
Diagnosis:
    DYE DISAPPEARANCE TEST: instill fluorescein in inferior fornix of both eyes, wait 5 minutes, then evaluate for asymmetric clearance of dye from tear meniscus

JONES I TEST: perform dye disappearance test, then attempt to recover fluorescein in inferior nasal meatus with cotton-tipped applicator; abnormal result (no fluorescein) occurs in 33% of normal individuals

JONES II TEST: perform Jones I test, then irrigate saline into nasolacrimal system; dye recovery from nose indicates functional occlusion of nasolacrimal duct; clear saline recovery indicates canalicular occlusion or nonfunctioning lacrimal pump

DACRYOSCINTOGRAM: instillation of technetium 99, physiologic test

DACRYOCYSTOGRAM: injection of Lipiodol (Ethiodol; radiopaque) outlines drainage system

PROBING AND IRRIGATION

Punctal Obstruction

Etiology: senile, cicatrizing (ocular cicatricial pemphigoid, Stevens-Johnson syndrome), trauma, tumor, drug induced

Treatment: dilation, punctoplasty, reapposition of puncta

Canalicular Obstruction

Etiology: trauma, toxic medications (antivirals, strong miotics, epinephrine, chemotherapeutics), infections (HSV, Epstein-Barr virus [EBV], trachoma), dacryolith, inflammation (ocular cicatricial pemphigoid, Stevens-Johnson syndrome), allergy, radiation, tumor, canaliculitis

Treatment:
Repair of canalicular system (in trauma)
Partial obstruction: Crawford tubes, Veirs rods, monocanalicular stents
Obstruction within 8 mm of punctum: conjunctivodacryocystorhinostomy (CDCR) with Jones tubes
Obstruction >8 mm from punctum: dacryocystorhinostomy (DCR) with O'Donoghue tubes

Nasolacrimal Duct Obstruction

Congenital: (See Chapter 5, Pediatrics/Strabismus)

Acquired:
Etiology: involutional stenosis (most common cause, more common in women [2:1], inflammatory infiltrates compress nasolacrimal duct), trauma, chronic sinus disease, nasal polyps, dacryocystitis, granulomatous disease (e.g., sarcoidosis, granulomatosis with polyangiitis)
Treatment: silicone intubation, DCR

Lacrimal Sac Obstruction

Etiology: trauma, acute or chronic dacryocystitis

Treatment: DCR

Infections

Canaliculitis

Infection of canaliculus, usually chronic

Organisms: *Actinomyces israelii* is most common (filamentous gram-positive rod). Also, *Candida albicans, Aspergillus, Nocardia asteroides,* HSV, and varicella-zoster virus (VZV)

More commonly occurs in middle-aged women

Symptoms: tearing, redness, pain, discharge

Findings: erythematous, dilated, tender, pouting punctum; expressible discharge, recurrent conjunctivitis; may have bloody tears

Grating sensation with probing

Often find sulfur granules

Treatment: warm compresses, probing and irrigation with penicillin, canalicular curettage, incision and débridement

Dacryocystitis

Infection of nasolacrimal sac

Organisms: *Staphylococcus, Streptococcus, Pseudomonas, Haemophilus influenzae* (young children), *Klebsiella, Actinomyces, Candida*

Findings:
Acute: edema, erythema, and distention below the medial canthal tendon; may result in mucocele formation, chronic conjunctivitis, or orbital cellulitis
Chronic: distended lacrimal sac, minimal inflammation

Treatment: warm compresses, topical and systemic antibiotics, incision and drainage if abscess present, avoid irrigation and probing during acute infection, DCR after acute inflammation subsides

Dacryoadenitis

Acute or chronic inflammation of lacrimal gland

Etiology:
Acute: infection (*Staphylococcus, Neisseria gonorrhoeae,* mumps, EBV, VZV)
Chronic: inflammation or infection (IOI, sarcoidosis, Mikulicz syndrome, lymphoid lesions, syphilis, tuberculosis [TB])

Symptoms: swelling, redness; may have pain, tearing, discharge with acute infection

Findings: enlarged lacrimal gland; may have tenderness, fever, preauricular lymphadenopathy, globe dystopia, restricted ocular motility

Table 6.7 Differential diagnosis of common disorders

Epithelial Eyelid Lesions
Slow growing:
    Squamous cell papilloma
    Actinic keratosis
    Seborrheic keratosis
    Basal cell carcinoma
    Squamous cell carcinoma
Fast growing:
    Molluscum contagiosum
    Keratoacanthoma
Subepithelial Eyelid Lesions
Cystic
    Cyst of Moll
    Cyst of Zeiss
    Sebaceous cyst
Solid
    Meibomian cyst
    Hordeolum
    Chalazion
    Xanthelasma
    Sebaceous adenocarcinoma
Pseudoproptosis
High myopia (axial myopia)
Contralateral enophthalmos
Shallow orbits (Crouzon, Apert syndrome)
Buphthalmos
Contralateral ptosis
Upper lid retraction
Infantile Proptosis
Capillary hemangioma (most common)
Orbital cellulitis
Dermoid
Encephalocele
Histiocytosis X
Leukemia
Retinoblastoma
Craniofacial disorders
Childhood Proptosis
Orbital cellulitis (most common)
Capillary hemangioma
Dermoid cyst
Inflammatory pseudotumor
Lymphangioma
Metastatic neuroblastoma
Granulocytic sarcoma
Orbital extension of retinoblastoma
Optic nerve glioma
Rhabdomyosarcoma
Lymphoma/leukemia
Meningioma
Neurofibromatosis
Spheno-orbital encephalocele
Optic nerve glioma
Plexiform neurofibroma in the orbit
Adult Proptosis
Thyroid eye disease (most common)
Orbital pseudotumor
Orbital cellulitis/abscess
Mucocele
Granulomatosis with polyangiitis
Sarcoidosis
Optic nerve glioma
Meningioma
Hemangioma
Orbital lymphoma
Metastatic tumor
Orbital cysts
Fibrous histiocytoma
Fibro-osseous tumors
Leukemia
Chloroma
Crouzon disease

Cavernous sinus thrombosis
Orbital varices
Atrioventricular malformations
Acromegaly
Histiocytosis X
Multiple myeloma
Orbital fractures
Pigmented Eyelid Lesions
Nevus
Pigmented basal cell carcinoma
Lentigo maligna (Hutchinson freckle)
Malignant melanoma
Oculodermal melanocytosis (nevus of Ota)
Enlarged Extraocular Muscles on Computed Tomography Scan
Thyroid eye disease (muscle tendons spared)
Orbital pseudotumor (muscle tendons involved)
Metastatic cancer
Lymphoma
Infection
Carotid-cavernous sinus fistula
Acromegaly
Amyloid
Nodular fasciitis
Fibrous histiocytoma
Tenon cyst
Granulomatosis with polyangiitis
Lacrimal Gland Inflammation/Swelling
Mumps
Glandular fever
Suppurative adenitis
Extension of conjunctivitis
Tuberculosis
Sarcoidosis
Malignant lymphoma
Lacrimal gland tumor
Thyroid eye disease
Orbital pseudotumor
Unilateral Periorbital Inflammation
Ruptured dermoid cyst
Rhabdomyosarcoma
Orbital pseudotumor
Leukemia
Eosinophilic granuloma
Infantile cortical hyperostosis
Enophthalmos
Orbital floor fracture
Metastatic tumors with sclerosis (breast carcinoma)
Painless Proptosis
Cavernous hemangioma
Optic nerve tumor
Neurofibroma
Neurilemmoma
Benign lacrimal gland tumors
Rhabdomyosarcoma
Fibrous histiocytoma
Lymphoma
Osteoma
Painful Proptosis
Orbital pseudotumor
Posterior scleritis
Dacryoadenitis
Orbital hemorrhage
Malignant lacrimal gland tumor
Nasopharyngeal carcinoma
Lymphangioma
Orbital abscess
Granulomatosis with polyangiitis
Primary orbital tumors
Hemangioma
Lacrimal gland tumors
Optic nerve meningioma or glioma
Rhabdomyosarcoma

Diagnosis: CT scan; consider culture, laboratory tests (serologies), and biopsy

Treatment: may require systemic antibiotics, incision and drainage, or excision

Tumors of the Lacrimal Sac

Rare; secondary to dacryocystitis

Findings: painless mass located above medial canthal tendon, tearing, may have bloody tears; bleeding with probing

Must be differentiated from dacryocystitis

Dacryocystogram outlines tumor

Squamous papilloma: most common primary lacrimal sac tumor

Squamous cell carcinoma: most common primary malignant lacrimal sac tumor

Lymphoma: second most common primary malignant lacrimal sac tumor

Lacrimal sac can be invaded by other malignant tumors of eyelids and conjunctiva

ORBITAL SURGERY

Evisceration

Removal of intraocular contents, leaving the sclera intact

Indications: blind painful eye, process not involving sclera

Complications: implant extrusion as a result of epithelial downgrowth and poor closure

Enucleation

Removal of entire globe and portion of optic nerve

Implant material: polymethyl methacrylate (PMMA), silicone, hydroxyapatite, dermis fat graft

Integrated implant: painted prosthesis fits into implant via peg

Indications: blind painful eye, intraocular malignancy, after severe trauma to avoid sympathetic ophthalmia

Exenteration

Removal of all orbital contents

Indications: adenoid cystic carcinoma, mucormycosis, orbital extension of sebaceous cell, basal cell, malignant melanoma, and squamous cell carcinomas

Dacryocystorhinostomy (DCR)

Creation of passage between lacrimal sac and nasal cavity

Osteotomy is made by removing the lacrimal sac fossa and superior nasal wall of nasolacrimal duct (NLD) at level of middle turbinate; bony window should measure 15 mm × 15 mm

Indications: focal distal canalicular obstruction and NLDO

Complications: failure resulting from obstruction at common canaliculus or at bony ostomy site

REVIEW QUESTIONS (Answers start on page 418)

1. Which organism is most commonly associated with angular blepharitis?
   a. *Staphylococcus epidermidis*
   b. *Moraxella*
   c. *Staphylococcus aureus*
   d. *Demodex folliculorum*
2. Sequelae of a CN 7 palsy may include all of the following, *except*
   a. filaments
   b. ptosis
   c. decreased vision
   d. dry eye
3. Which procedure is the best treatment option for the repair of a large upper eyelid defect?
   a. Cutler-Beard
   b. Bick
   c. Hughes
   d. Fasanella-Servat
4. The extraocular muscle with the largest arc of contact is the
   a. LR
   b. IO
   c. MR
   d. SO
5. The risk of systemic involvement is highest for an ocular lymphoid tumor in which location?
   a. orbit
   b. eyelid
   c. conjunctiva
   d. bilateral orbit
6. The rectus muscle with the shortest tendon of insertion is the
   a. IR
   b. SR
   c. MR
   d. LR
7. Which of the following bones does *not* make up the medial orbital wall?
   a. lacrimal

b. maxilla
c. sphenoid
d. palatine

8. Which of the following clinical features is *least* commonly associated with a tripod fracture?
   a. restriction of the inferior rectus
   b. flattening of the malar eminence
   c. hypesthesia
   d. displacement of the lateral canthus

9. A carotid-cavernous fistula is commonly differentiated from a dural-sinus fistula by all of the following characteristics, *except*
   a. proptosis
   b. afferent pupillary defect
   c. bruit
   d. CN 6 palsy

10. Basal cell carcinoma is *least* likely to occur at which site?
    a. upper eyelid
    b. medial canthus
    c. lower eyelid
    d. lateral canthus

11. All of the following are sites of attachment of the limbs of the medial canthal tendon, *except*
    a. frontal process of the maxillary bone
    b. anterior lacrimal crest
    c. orbital process of the frontal bone
    d. posterior lacrimal crest

12. Which muscle is most commonly responsible for vertical diplopia after four-lid blepharoplasty?
    a. superior oblique
    b. inferior oblique
    c. superior rectus
    d. inferior rectus

13. Congenital and involutional ptosis can be distinguished by all of the following, *except*
    a. degree of levator function
    b. presence of lid crease
    c. width of palpebral fissure
    d. presence of jaw wink

14. Congenital obstruction of the lacrimal drainage system usually occurs at the
    a. valve of Rosenmüller
    b. common canaliculus
    c. lacrimal sac
    d. valve of Hasner

15. What is the correct order of structures that would be encountered when the upper eyelid is penetrated 14 mm above the lid margin?
    a. preseptal orbicularis muscle, orbital septum, levator aponeurosis, Müller muscle
    b. preseptal orbicularis muscle, orbital septum, levator muscle
    c. pretarsal orbicularis muscle, levator muscle, conjunctiva
    d. pretarsal orbicularis muscle, levator aponeurosis, orbital septum, fat

16. What is the best treatment option for a child who develops recurrent proptosis after upper respiratory infections?
    a. observation
    b. radiation therapy

c. chemotherapy
d. surgery

17. All of the following are features of mucormycosis, *except*
    a. internal ophthalmoplegia
    b. ipsilateral CN 7 palsy
    c. diplopia
    d. involvement of the first branch of the trigeminal nerve

18. All of the following are associated with blepharophimosis, *except*
    a. trisomy 18
    b. ectropion
    c. AR inheritance
    d. wide intercanthal distance

19. Which of the following is the most important test to perform in a patient with a capillary hemangioma?
    a. echocardiogram
    b. hearing test
    c. electrocardiogram
    d. bleeding time

20. For entropion repair, the lateral tarsal strip is sutured
    a. below and anterior to the rim
    b. below and posterior to the rim
    c. above and anterior to the rim
    d. above and posterior to the rim

21. Staged surgery for a patient with severe thyroid eye disease is best done in what order?
    a. decompression, strabismus, lid repair
    b. strabismus, decompression, lid repair
    c. lid repair, decompression, strabismus
    d. decompression, lid repair, strabismus

22. Which of the following best explains why when a ptotic lid is lifted, the contralateral lid falls?
    a. inhibition of Müller muscle
    b. Sherrington's law
    c. relaxation of the frontalis muscle
    d. Hering's law

23. Which study is most helpful in the evaluation of a patient with opsoclonus?
    a. electrocardiogram
    b. MRI
    c. electroretinography
    d. angiogram

24. What is the most appropriate treatment for a benign mixed tumor of the lacrimal gland?
    a. radiation
    b. excision
    c. observation
    d. biopsy

25. What is the most appropriate treatment for a biopsy-positive basal cell carcinoma of the lower eyelid?
    a. cryotherapy to the cancer and margins
    b. local antimetabolite treatment
    c. radiation with 2500 rads to the lesion and margins
    d. excision with frozen section control of the margins

26. Which of the following CT-enhancing lesions has a pathognomonic appearance?
    a. rhabdomyosarcoma
    b. glioma
    c. lymphangioma
    d. meningioma

27. Which of the following factors is *least* likely to contribute to the development of entropion?
    a. preseptal orbicularis override
    b. horizontal lid laxity
    c. posterior lamella foreshortening
    d. capsulopalpebral fascia disinsertion

28. A 24-year-old woman presents after blunt trauma to the left orbit with enophthalmos and restriction of upgaze. Which plain film radiographic view would be most helpful?
    a. Caldwell view
    b. lateral view
    c. Waters view
    d. axial view

29. All of the following may cause enophthalmos, *except*
    a. breast carcinoma
    b. lymphoma
    c. orbital floor fracture
    d. phthisis bulbi

30. All of the following nerves pass through the superior orbital fissure, *except*
    a. CN 3
    b. CN 4
    c. CN V$_2$
    d. CN 6

31. Blepharospasm is associated with
    a. myotonic dystrophy
    b. syphilis
    c. vertebrobasilar insufficiency
    d. Parkinson disease

32. The anatomic boundaries of the superior orbital fissure are
    a. the greater wing of the sphenoid and the zygoma.
    b. the greater and lesser wings of the sphenoid
    c. the lesser wing of the sphenoid and the maxilla
    d. the lesser wing of the sphenoid and the zygoma

33. Which of the following is most likely to exacerbate the symptoms of thyroid eye disease?
    a. alcohol
    b. cigarettes
    c. aspirin
    d. caffeine

34. A 44-year-old woman develops a left lower eyelid ectropion following a severe facial burn. The most appropriate procedure includes
    a. horizontal tightening
    b. vertical shortening
    c. repair of lower eyelid retractors
    d. levator myotomy

35. All of the following are methods of treating spastic entropion, *except*
    a. eyelid taping
    b. botox injection
    c. Wies marginal rotation
    d. Quickert suture

36. The most common complication of a hydroxyapatite orbital implant is
    a. implant migration
    b. infection
    c. orbital hemorrhage
    d. conjunctival erosion

37. Which collagen vascular disease is associated with malignancy?
    a. dermatomyositis
    b. scleroderma
    c. granulomatosis with polyangiitis
    d. systemic lupus erythematosus

38. Oral antibiotics are indicated for
    a. canaliculitis
    b. dacryocystitis
    c. dacryoadenitis
    d. NLD obstruction

39. The levator muscle inserts onto all of the following structures, *except* the
    a. tarsus
    b. lateral orbital tubercle
    c. posterior lacrimal crest
    d. trochlea

40. When performing a DCR, at which level is the ostium created?
    a. superior turbinate
    b. middle turbinate
    c. inferior turbinate
    d. none of the above

41. An adult with a complete NLD obstruction and patent puncta and canaliculi is best treated with which procedure?
    a. silicone stent intubation
    b. Jones tube
    c. dacryocystectomy
    d. dacryocystorhinostomy

42. The most effective procedure for involutional ectropion is
    a. lateral tarsal strip
    b. plication of the orbital septum
    c. shortening of the medial canthal ligament
    d. wedge resection of the tarsus

43. A patient presents with follicular conjunctivitis, and a cluster of umbilicated papules is noted near the eyelashes of the left eye. The most effective treatment for this condition is
    a. acyclovir
    b. antibiotics
    c. cryotherapy
    d. radiation

44. The most common cause of unilateral proptosis in a middle-aged woman is
    a. cavernous hemangioma
    b. thyroid eye disease
    c. dermoid
    d. metastatic breast carcinoma

45. The most common cause of involutional entropion of the lower eyelid is
    a. inflammation.
    b. laxity and retractor disinsertion
    c. orbicularis spasm
    d. posterior lamella scarring

46. An elderly woman with chronic unilateral blepharitis, thickening of the left upper eyelid, and submandibular lymphadenopathy is most likely to have
    a. basal cell carcinoma
    b. keratoacanthoma
    c. molluscum contagiosum
    d. sebaceous gland carcinoma

47. A 56-year-old woman with diabetes presents with pain, swelling, and redness of the left upper eyelid. Orbital involvement is most likely if she also has
    a. headache
    b. discharge
    c. ptosis
    d. pain with eye movement

48. A 72-year-old man has bilateral ptosis and levator function measuring 14 mm OU. The most likely diagnosis is
    a. chronic progressive external ophthalmoplegia
    b. Horner syndrome
    c. levator aponeurotic dehiscence
    d. myasthenia gravis

49. The sensory nerve most likely to be affected by an orbital fracture is
    a. lacrimal
    b. nasociliary
    c. infraorbital
    d. infratrochlear

50. Which of the following findings is most helpful for making the diagnosis in a patient with suspected thyroid eye disease?
    a. abnormal forced ductions
    b. comitant esotropia
    c. presence of ptosis
    d. normal thyroid function tests

51. A patient suddenly develops pain, proptosis, loss of vision, and subconjunctival hemorrhage after a retrobulbar block. The most appropriate action is immediate
    a. administration of IV mannitol
    b. anterior chamber paracentesis
    c. lateral canthotomy
    d. retrobulbar evacuation with a large-bore needle

52. A 60-year-old man with a 1-week history of tearing is found to have a tender, swollen mass in the inferior medial canthal region of the left eye. Which is the most appropriate initial management?
    a. probe the canaliculus
    b. obtain a dacryocystogram
    c. start oral antibiotics
    d. perform a dacryocystorhinostomy

53. Which of the following signs is most helpful in differentiating preseptal cellulitis from orbital cellulitis?
    a. fever
    b. eyelid edema
    c. periorbital tenderness
    d. relative afferent pupillary defect

54. What is the most likely diagnosis in a patient with right upper eyelid retraction and normal thyroid function tests?
    a. idiopathic orbital inflammation
    b. myasthenia gravis
    c. thyroid eye disease
    d. metastatic cancer

55. *Demodex* infection is associated with
    a. angular blepharitis
    b. anterior blepharitis
    c. meibomitis
    d. posterior blepharitis

Please visit the eBook for an interactive version of the review questions. See front cover for activation details.

SUGGESTED READINGS

Basic and Clinical Sciences Course. (2021). *Section 7: Orbit, eyelids and lacrimal system*. San Francisco: AAO.

Black, E. H., & Nesi, F. A. (2012). *Smith and Nesi's ophthalmic plastic and reconstructive surgery* (3rd ed.). New York: Springer.

Chen, W. P., & Kahn, J. A. (2009). *Color atlas of cosmetic oculofacial surgery* (2nd ed.). Philadelphia: Saunders.

Collin, J. R. O. (2006). *Manual of systematic eyelid surgery* (3rd ed.). Philadelphia: Butterworth-Heinemann.

Dutton, J. S. (2011). *Atlas of clinical and surgical orbital anatomy* (2nd ed.). Philadelphia: Saunders.

Dutton, J. S. (2013). *Atlas of oculoplastic and orbital surgery* (2nd ed.). Philadelphia: Lippincott Williams and Wilkins.

Fagien, S. (2007). *Putterman's cosmetic oculoplastic surgery* (4th ed.). Philadelphia: Saunders.

Levine, M. R., & Allen, R. C. (2018). *Manual of oculoplastic surgery* (5th ed.). New York: Springer.

Rootman, J. (2002). *Diseases of the orbit* (2nd ed.). Philadelphia: Lippincott Williams and Wilkins.

Rootman, J. (2013). *Orbital surgery: A conceptual approach* (2nd ed.). Philadelphia: Lippincott Williams and Wilkins.

Smith, B. C., Nesi, F. A., Cantarella, V. H., et al. (1998). *Smith's ophthalmic plastic and reconstructive surgery* (2nd ed.). St. Louis: Mosby.

7

ANATOMY/PHYSIOLOGY
CONJUNCTIVAL DISORDERS
CORNEAL DISORDERS
SCLERAL DISORDERS
SURGERY

ANATOMY/PHYSIOLOGY

Conjunctiva

Mucous membrane composed of nonkeratinized stratified squamous epithelium (2-5 cells thick) with goblet cells (most numerous in tarsal conjunctiva, inferonasal bulbar conjunctiva, and area of plica semilunaris) and underlying vascular stromal tissue (substantia propria) with lymphatics, plasma cells, macrophages, mast cells, lymphocytes

Palpebral conjunctiva: firmly adherent to tarsus, covers inner surface of lids

Forniceal conjunctiva: loose and redundant, combines with fibrous tissue from levator aponeurosis and Müller muscle in upper lid and inferior rectus (IR) sheath and inferior tarsal muscle in lower lid

Bulbar conjunctiva: loosely adherent to globe except at limbus, where it fuses with Tenon's capsule

Plica semilunaris: narrow fold of medial vascular bulbar conjunctiva adjacent to caruncle, contains goblet cells, fat, nonstriated muscle; rudimentary structure analogous to nictitating membrane in certain animals

Caruncle: small fleshy tissue at medial canthus attached to plica semilunaris, intermediate between conjunctiva and skin; 5 mm high, 3 mm wide; contains goblet cells, sebaceous glands, sweat glands, lacrimal tissue, and hairs

Vascular supply: branches of eyelid marginal arcades supply all areas of conjunctiva; posterior and anterior conjunctival arteries (from anterior ciliary arteries) supply forniceal and bulbar, and limbal conjunctiva, respectively

Innervation: via cranial nerve (CN) V_1

Precorneal Tear Film

Thickness = 3.4 μm (2.0–5.5 μm); volume = 7.4 μL (unanesthetized), 2.6 μL (anesthetized)

3 layers (traditional model):
Lipid: outer layer; reduces evaporation; hydrophobic barrier that decreases surface tension and prevents tear overflow; cholesterol and lipids; produced by meibomian (holocrine), Zeis (sebaceous), and Moll (apocrine) glands
Aqueous: middle layer; provides oxygen to epithelium; 98% water, 2% protein, pH = 7.2 (6.5–7.6); osmolarity ~302 mOsm/L (296–308 mOsm/L); produced by lacrimal and accessory lacrimal (exocrine) glands (Krause and Wolfring), basal secretion rate = 3.8 μL/min; turnover rate = 12%-16%/min, controlled by neural feedback loop; lysozyme (antibacterial enzyme) constitutes 30% of total protein in tear film; also, lactoferrin, matrix metalloproteinase 9 (MMP-9), immunoglobulins (IgA, IgG, IgM, IgE, IgD), electrolytes (concentration Na+ similar to serum, K+ is 5–7 × serum, with Cl- regulate osmotic fluid flow from cornea; bicarbonate regulates pH; other electrolytes serve as enzyme cofactors), oxygen, cytokines and growth factors
Mucin: inner layer; reduces surface tension and allows aqueous tear film to be spread evenly; helps structure the tear film; glycoproteins; 3 types: secreted mucins (MUC4 and MUC7) produced by lacrimal gland, gel-forming mucins (MUC5-AC) produced by conjunctival goblet cells (glands of Manz and crypts of Henle, primarily in fornix), and membrane-associated mucins (MUC1 and MUC16) that protect the ocular surface; 2-3 μL/day

Tear film is less discrete, now considered 2-layer uniform gel:
Mucoaqueous combination and overlying lipid layer: apical surface of conjunctiva and corneal epithelium covered with transmembrane mucins (reduce surface friction and barrier function against pathogens) and aqueous

215

(hydration and protection of ocular surface), which act as a combination layer with decreasing concentration of mucus more anteriorly. Glycocalyx (mainly mucin glycoproteins) between tear film and corneal epithelial cells provides tear film stability and corneal wettability

Functions: lubrication of ocular surface, nutrient exchange (especially oxygen), antimicrobial defense, removal of debris, major refractive component

Lacrimal functional unit: lacrimal glands, ocular surface (conjunctiva, cornea, meibomian glands), lids, and sensory and motor nerves connecting these components; maintains healthy ocular surface

Blinking essential for tear film distribution, renewal, and drainage

Cornea (Fig. 7.1)

Average measurements:
Diameter: vertical = 11 mm, horizontal = 12 mm; at birth, horizontal diameter = 9.5-10.5, reaches adult size by age 2
Thickness: central = 550 μm, peripheral = 1.0 mm; typically, inferotemporal paracentral cornea is thinnest; superior paracentral cornea is thickest
Radius of curvature: 7.8 mm anteriorly; 6.2-6.8 mm posteriorly (peripheral cornea is flatter, especially nasal and superior)
Power: anterior surface = +49 D, posterior surface = –6 D, total = 43 D (75% of total power of eye)
Refractive index: 1.376

Epithelium: 40-50 μm thick (10% of corneal thickness); hydrophobic (hydrophilic molecules penetrate poorly)
Smooth refractive surface; protects against infection
Microplicae and microcilli on apical surface coated with glycocalyx
Aerobic metabolism (accounts for 70% of adenosine triphosphate [ATP] production)
Oxygen is obtained via diffusion from the tear film when the eye is open and from the lid vasculature when the eye is closed; also, small amount from the aqueous

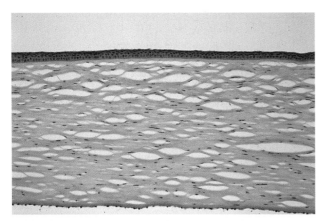

Figure 7.1 Normal cornea. (From Yanoff M, Fine BS. *Ocular Pathology*, 5th ed. St Louis: Mosby; 2002.)

Regenerates from limbal stem cells (turnover = 6–7 days)
Approximately 4-6 cells thick centrally and 7-10 cells thick at limbus
Layers:
   TOP: 3-4 layers of squamous cells (uppermost are apical cells)
   MIDDLE: 1-3 layers of wing cells (flattened polygonal shape)
   DEEP: 1 layer of basal cells
Cells:
   APICAL CELLS: secrete proteins that form the glycocalyx extending from epithelial surface into mucin layer of tear film
   WING CELLS: tightly packed, linked by desmosomes; form protective barrier
   BASAL CELLS: anchor epithelium to stroma by hemidesmosomes; secrete basement membrane
   NERVE CELLS: epithelium contains sensory nerve endings
Pathology:
   CORNEAL EPITHELIAL EDEMA:
      INTRACELLULAR: caused by epithelial hypoxia and nutritional compromise; associated with contact lens (CL) use; fine, frosted-glass appearance (Sattler veil)
      INTERCELLULAR: caused by elevated intraocular pressure (IOP); causes microcystic edema and epithelial bullae
   CORNEAL FILAMENTS: composed of mucus and desquamated epithelial cells; caused by increased mucus production and abnormal epithelial turnover

Basal lamina: scaffold for epithelium; adjacent to Bowman layer; composed of type IV collagen secreted by basal epithelium (use periodic acid-Schiff [PAS] stain)
2 layers: lamina lucida and lamina densa
Basal epithelium is secured by hemidesmosomes; adheres to stroma by anchoring fibrils

Bowman layer (Bowman membrane): 8-15 μm thick; type I and V collagen enmeshed in glycosaminoglycan (GAG) matrix, rich in fibronectin, acellular; formed from secretion from both basal epithelial cells and stromal keratocytes
Not a true basement membrane
Prevents epithelial cell growth factors from reaching stromal keratocytes (which causes corneal haze)
Heals with scarring; does not regenerate

Stroma: 470-500 μm thick centrally, 900 μm peripherally; 90% of corneal thickness, 78% water by weight; collagen in mucopolysaccharide matrix
Collagen lamellae: ~200 sheets (each ~2 μm thick) composed of parallel small-diameter (20-30 nm) fibrils; mainly type I (70%), also types V, VI, VII (anchors epithelium), XII, XIV; type III only in stromal wound healing. Corneal stiffness increases with age from collagen crosslinking
Proteoglycans: glycosylated proteins with at least one GAG (keratan sulfate, chondroitin sulfate, and dermatan sulfate) maintain lamellar spacing, negatively charged, draw in sodium and water (swelling pressure of the stroma)

Cells: keratocytes (2.4 million, denser anteriorly, produce proteoglycans and tropocollagen; in wound repair, tropocollagen is different, resulting in nonparallel collagen fibrils and opacity), Langerhans cells, pigmented melanocytes, lymphocytes, macrophages, histiocytes

Matrix metalloproteinases (MMPs): family of enzymes that break down components of the extracellular matrix; help maintain the normal corneal structure; play a critical role in restructuring the cornea after injury

MMP-1 (collagenase-1): breaks down collagen types I, II, and III

MMP-2 (gelatinase A): breaks down collagen types IV, V, and VII, as well as gelatins and fibronectin

MMP-3 (stomalysin): breaks down proteoglycans and fibronectins

MMP-9 (gelatinase B): breaks down collagen types IV, V, and VII, as well as gelatins and fibronectin.

MMP-1, 2, and 3 are made by the stroma; MMP-9 is made by the epithelium; only MMP-2 is found in healthy cornea, the others are found only after injury

Pathology: during processing, stromal lamellae separate, forming clefts (artifact); if these are absent, suggests corneal edema (lamellae are same thickness, but space between fills with fluid)

Descemet membrane: 3-4 μm (birth) to 10-12 μm (adults) thick; PAS-positive basement membrane

Anchors endothelium to stroma

Type IV collagen secreted by endothelial cells

Layers:

FETAL BANDED LAYER: anterior layer (closer to stroma), striated pattern; organized collagen lamellae (like stroma); no change with age

ADULT NONBANDED LAYER: posterior layer (closer to endothelium), no striations; nonorganized; thickens with age

Regenerates after damage as long as endothelium is intact

Dua layer: posterior 15 μm of stroma may be distinct acellular layer

Pathology:

BREAKS: edges tend to coil or roll into a scroll shape (Haab striae, forceps injury, hydrops) (Fig. 7.2)

EXCRESCENCES: aging change, peripheral = Hassall-Henle warts, central = cornea guttae

FOCAL THICKENING: Fuchs dystrophy, iridocorneal touch, vitreocorneal touch, guttata (Fig. 7.3)

Endothelium: 4-6 μm thick

Monolayer of interdigitating hexagonal cells joined by tight junctions

Transports nutrients into cornea, pumps fluid out of cornea

Rich in mitochondria; metabolizes carbohydrates at 5-6 x the rate of epithelium

Functions:

1. Barrier between stroma and anterior chamber
2. Keeps cornea dehydrated and clear; 1 million cells at birth (~3800 endothelial cells/mm² centrally), young adult central cell count ~3000 cells/mm²; loss of approximately 50% with aging (0.6%/year);

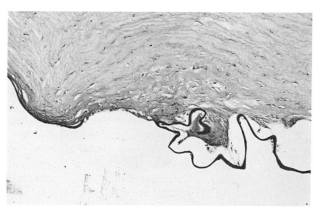

Figure 7.2 Hydrops demonstrating corneal edema (thickening) with breaks in Descemet membrane. (From Yanoff M, Fine BS. *Ocular Pathology*, 5th ed. St Louis: Mosby; 2002.)

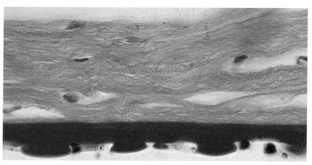

Figure 7.3 Periodic acid-Schiff stain demonstrating guttata as wartlike excrescences of Descemet membrane. (From Yanoff M, Fine BS. *Ocular Pathology*, 5th ed. St Louis: Mosby; 2002.)

adjacent cells stretch to fill gaps (no regeneration), insufficient pump when <500 cells/mm²

Morphology: at least 60% of cells should be hexagonal; less than this represents unhealthy cornea

Pathology:

PLEOMORPHISM: variation in cell shape

POLYMEGATHISM: variation in cell size

Responses to stress (large, unusually shaped cells); surgery, CL wear; certain drugs may cause an osmotic challenge or inhibition of the Na⁺/K⁺ pump, causing stromal edema

Example: diabetes (buildup of sorbitol in endothelial cells with hyperglycemia); CL (inhibits Na⁺/K⁺ pump and cells swell); earliest endothelial change (endothelial bleb response) occurs within minutes of insertion of a thick, soft or rigid CL (resolves rapidly after lens removal or slowly after 30 minutes of lens wear)

SCHWALBE LINE: termination of corneal endothelium (junction between endothelium and trabecular meshwork)

SCHWALBE RING: peripheral termination of Descemet membrane

POSTERIOR EMBRYOTOXIN: thickening and anterior displacement of Schwalbe line

Innervation: via CN V₁

Approximately 70-80 branches of long posterior ciliary nerves enter peripheral cornea after myelin sheath is lost 1-2 mm before limbus

Stains:

Fluorescein: stains epithelial defects; negative staining occurs in areas of epithelial irregularity

PATTERN GIVES CLUE TO ETIOLOGY:

INTERPALPEBRAL: dry eye

HORIZONTAL BAND ACROSS INFERIOR ONE-THIRD OF CORNEA: lagophthalmos/exposure

SUPERIOR PUNCTATE: superior limbic keratoconjunctivitis (SLK), floppy eyelid syndrome

CENTRAL PUNCTATE: focal epithelial keratitis (Thygeson superficial punctate keratitis [SPK], epidemic keratoconjunctivitis [EKC], molluscum)

INFERIOR PUNCTATE: blepharitis

PERILIMBAL (360°): soft CL wear

NEGATIVE STAINING: thickened irregular epithelium (i.e., epithelial basement membrane dystrophy, healing epithelial defect)

Rose bengal: stains tissue deficient of albumin and mucin, including devitalized cells

Lissamine green: devitalized cells of the conjunctiva and cornea, conjunctival intraepithelial neoplasia (CIN); more comfortable than rose bengal

Special techniques:

Pachymetry: measures corneal thickness

Keratometry: measures corneal curvature (only 2 points 3 mm apart in paracentral region)

Topography: measures curvature of entire cornea

Tomography: measures front and back surface of entire cornea

Schirmer test: measures tear production (basal + reflex [without anesthesia]; basal [with anesthesia])

Specular microscopy: measures endothelial cell count and morphology

Confocal microscopy: images corneal layers

Corneal optical coherence tomography (OCT): images corneal layers

Limbus

Corneoscleral junction, not distinct anatomic structure

Area 1-2 mm wide at which cornea and sclera meet; contains corneal epithelial stem cells, episclera, junction of corneoscleral stoma, and aqueous collector channels (see Chapter 10, Anterior Segment)

Sclera

White fibrous layer composed of collagen and elastin, covers posterior 5/6 of globe between cornea and optic nerve. Composed of 3 ill-defined layers: episclera, sclera proper, and lamina fusca

Thickness: 0.6 mm anterior to muscle insertions, 0.3 mm just behind recti insertions, 1.0 mm posteriorly around optic nerve, 0.4-0.5 mm at equator

Most common areas of rupture (blunt trauma): superonasal limbus, circumferential arc parallel to limbus

opposite point of impact, behind recti insertions, equator, and lamina cribrosa

Emissaria: scleral channels, transmit vessels and nerves

Anterior: in front of recti insertions, transmit anterior ciliary arteries

Middle: exit vortex veins, route for extension of choroidal melanoma

Posterior: lamina cribrosa, transmit short and long posterior ciliary vessels and ciliary nerves

Vascular supply: sclera avascular except for intrascleral plexus just behind limbus and episcleral plexus (superficial and deep; involved in episcleritis and scleritis, respectively)

Axenfeld loops: ciliary nerve loops exit sclera behind nasal and temporal limbus, visible when pigmented (small dark spots)

CONJUNCTIVAL DISORDERS

Inflammation

Follicles

Gray-white round elevations with avascular center and vessels at periphery

Well-circumscribed focus of lymphoid hypertrophy (lymphocytes with a germinal center) as a result of reactive hyperplasia

Generally most prominent in inferior fornix (except in trachoma)

Papillae

Small to large elevations with central vascular tuft and pale avascular valleys

Epithelial proliferation, hypertrophy, and infoldings; hyperplasia of vascular stroma with chronic inflammatory cells

Usually upper eyelid

Nonspecific reaction to conjunctival inflammation (edema and leakage of fluid from vessels)

Subepithelial substantia propria of tarsal and limbal conjunctivae contains fibrous tissue septa that interconnect to form polygonal lobules with a central vascular bundle

Giant papillae: >1 mm in diameter

Chemosis

Conjunctival edema; may be caused by allergy or infection, can occur after eyelid surgery, or may be idiopathic

Phlyctenule

Usually unilateral; more common in children and young adults

Etiology: type IV hypersensitivity reaction to *Staphylococci,* coccidioidomycosis, *Candida,* herpes simplex virus (HSV), lymphogranuloma venereum (LGV), tuberculosis (TB)

Findings: round, elevated, focal, sterile infiltrate on bulbar conjunctiva, limbus, or cornea; overlying epithelium breaks down (stains with fluorescein); may have corneal vascularization

Pathology: infiltration of lymphocytes; atypical ulceration; fibrosis

Treatment: topical steroids and antibiotic

Symblepharon

Adhesion between conjunctival surfaces (palpebral and bulbar)

Caused by inflammation, trauma, or surgery

Bilateral in ocular cicatricial pemphigoid and Stevens-Johnson syndrome

Degenerations

Amyloidosis

Yellow-salmon, subepithelial, interpalpebral plaque in primary localized disease

Systemic amyloidosis is not associated with conjunctival amyloid but is associated with amyloid of lid

Pathology: acellular eosinophilic material that stains with Congo red, thioflavin T, metachromatic with crystal violet, apple-green birefringence and dichroism with polarization microscopy

Concretions (Lithiasis)

Small, round, yellow-white deposits in palpebral conjunctiva

May contain calcium

May erode through conjunctiva and abrade ocular surface causing foreign body sensation

Treatment: remove with needle if erodes through conjunctiva

Conjunctivochalasis

Redundant, loose, nonedematous inferior bulbar conjunctiva interposed between globe and lower eyelid

Exact etiology unknown; thought to result from elastoid degeneration and loss of adhesion between conjunctiva and sclera as Tenon capsule thins with age, possible mechanical factor from dry eye or blepharitis (lid rubbing, dry conjunctiva); often coexists or misdiagnosed as dry eye disease; more common in elderly, CL wearers, and patients with autoimmune thyroid disease

Symptoms: tearing (interference with tear meniscus and lacrimal drainage), irritation, foreign body sensation, redness, tearing

Findings: excess folds of inferior bulbar conjunctiva, epiphora; may have conjunctival ulceration, subconjunctival hemorrhage, and signs of dry eye disease

Classification:
  Grade I: no persistent fold
  Grade II: single, small fold
  Grade III: more than two folds and not higher than tear meniscus
  Grade IV: multiple folds and higher than tear meniscus

Treatment: if symptomatic, treat with lubrication; consider topical steroids or surgery (conjunctivoplasty [conjunctival resection] with or without amniotic membrane transplantation, conjunctival fixation to sclera, cautery)

Pingueculum

Small nodule composed of abnormal subepithelial collagen; may calcify

Located at limbus, nasal more common than temporal; does not involve cornea

Caused by actinic (ultraviolet [UV] light) exposure

Pathology: elastoid degeneration (basophilic degeneration of collagen)

Pingueculitis: inflamed pingueculum resulting from dryness and irritation
  Treatment: lubrication, short course of topical steroids

Pterygium

Interpalpebral, wing-shaped, fibrovascular tissue that invades cornea

Associated with actinic exposure

Findings: Stocker line (corneal iron line at head of pterygium); may induce astigmatism with flattening in meridian of pterygium (typically with-the-rule); may decrease vision if crosses visual axis

Pathology: elastoid degeneration with destruction of Bowman layer; may have epithelial dysplasia; in recurrences after excision may have fibrotic response not elastoid degeneration

Treatment: observation or surgical excision
  Up to 50% recurrence rate with primary excision (50% within 4 months, 95% within 1 year)
  Decreased risk of recurrence with amniotic membrane (15%), conjunctival autograft (5%), or mitomycin application at surgery; β-irradiation and thiotepa are no longer used

Deposits

Exogenous

Argyrosis, mascara, adenochrome (topical epinephrine is metabolized to melanin)

Endogenous

Addison disease, Nelson syndrome, alkaptonuria (autosomal recessive [AR], absence of homogentisic acid oxidase)

Biopsy: for cystinosis or oxalosis, fix in 50% alcohol so that crystals do not dissolve; if urate suspected, use absolute alcohol

Conjunctival Telangiectasia

Associated with Louis-Barr syndrome (ataxia telangiectasia), Osler-Weber-Rendu (hereditary telangiectasia), Sturge-Weber syndrome, diabetes, sickle cell disease, Fabry disease, increased orbital pressure (C-C fistula), blood-filled lymphatic tissue, irradiation

Allergy

Type I hypersensitivity reaction: airborne allergens (pollen, mold, dander) crosslink IgE receptors on mast cells, causing degranulation with release of histamine, eosinophil chemotactic factors, platelet-activating factor, major basic protein, and prostaglandin D_2

Symptoms: itching (H_1 receptors), hyperemia (H_2 receptors)

Conjunctival scraping: abundant eosinophils (normally, there are very few)

Treatment: topical antihistamine (emedastine [Emadine], levocabastine [Livostin], cetirizine [Zerviate]), mast cell stabilizer (pemirolast [Alamast], nedocromil [Alocril], lodoxamide [Alomide], cromolyn sodium [Crolom]), antihistamine/mast cell stabilizer combination (azelastine [Optivar], olopatadine [Patanol, Pataday], ketotifen [Zaditor, Alaway], epinastine [Elestat], bepotastine [Bepreve], alcaftadine [Lastacaft]), nonsteroidal anti-inflammatory drug (NSAID; ketorolac [Acular]), steroid, artificial tears, cold compresses

Allergic Conjunctivitis

Allergies affect 20% of the US population

90% of patients with systemic allergies will have ocular symptoms

Most commonly seasonal or perennial allergic conjunctivitis

Associated with allergic rhinitis

Symptoms: itching, tearing, redness

Findings: lid swelling, conjunctival injection, chemosis

Giant Papillary Conjunctivitis

Etiology: allergic reaction to material coating a foreign body (e.g., CL [especially extended wear], exposed suture, ocular prosthesis); true giant papillae also occur in vernal and atopic keratoconjunctivitis

Atopic individuals are at higher risk

Symptoms: itching, tearing, mucus discharge, CL discomfort, then intolerance

Findings: giant papillae (>1.0 mm) on upper palpebral conjunctiva

Treatment: removal of inciting factor (e.g., CL, suture), topical allergy medication; symptoms resolve months before the giant papillae resolve; avoid thimerosal

Atopic Keratoconjunctivitis (AKC)

Atopy: hereditary allergic hypersensitivity (10%–20% of population)

Types I and IV hypersensitivity reactions

Onset usually between ages 30 and 50 years

Clinical diagnosis (atopic skin disease [eczema], hay fever, asthma)

Eczema (atopic dermatitis): 3% of population; AKC in 15%-40% of those with atopic dermatitis

Symptoms: itching, burning, photophobia, tearing, blurred vision

Findings: atopic dermatitis of eyelids (may have blepharitis, madarosis [loss of lashes], punctal ectropion), papillary conjunctivitis (small or medium-sized papillae in inferior fornix); may develop symblepharon, corneal vascularization, and scarring

Associated with keratoconus (10%), subcapsular cataracts (Maltese cross pattern), bilateral HSV keratitis, pellucid marginal degeneration

Pathology: mast cell infiltration of conjunctival epithelium

Treatment: topical allergy medication; consider topical cyclosporine (1%–2%) qid or tacrolimus 0.01% bid, supratarsal steroid injection (0.25–0.50 mL dexamethasone or triamcinolone acetate [Kenalog]), systemic antihistamine

Vernal Keratoconjunctivitis (VKC)

(See Chapter 5, Pediatrics/Strabismus)

Toxic Keratoconjunctivitis

Etiology: direct contact of medication or chemical substance with ocular surface

Findings: conjunctival injection, follicles, papillae, keratitis (SPK, occasionally pseudodendrite)

Superior Limbic Keratoconjunctivitis (SLK)

Recurrent inflammation of superior bulbar and palpebral conjunctiva; unknown etiology

Associated with CL wear and thyroid dysfunction (50%)

Female preponderance (70%), onset usually between ages 30-55 years

Recurrent episodes; lasts 1-10 years, eventually resolves permanently

Bilateral in 70%; symptoms worse than signs

Symptoms: foreign body sensation, burning, photophobia, redness, blurred vision

Findings: conjunctival injection hyperemia, thickening, redundancy of superior bulbar conjunctiva with fine punctate staining (rose bengal), velvety papillary hypertrophy of upper palpebral conjunctiva, micropannus, filamentary keratitis (50%), decreased Schirmer test (25%)

Pathology: thickening and keratinization of superior bulbar conjunctiva with loss of goblet cells

Conjunctival scraping: neutrophils, lymphocytes, plasma cells

Treatment: variety of options, usually requires scarring of superior bulbar conjunctiva
- Steroids of little use
- Pressure patch
- Large-diameter bandage contact lens
- Mechanical scraping of affected area may provide temporary relief
- Topical silver nitrate solution 0.5%-1.0% to produce chemical burn, can retreat for recurrence (never use silver nitrate stick)
- Thermocauterization of upper bulbar conjunctiva
- Recession or resection of upper bulbar conjunctiva

Conjunctivitis Associated With Systemic Diseases

Mucocutaneous disorders: Stevens-Johnson syndrome, ocular cicatricial pemphigoid (OCP), bullous pemphigoid, pemphigus, epidermolysis bullosa, dermatitis herpetiformis, arthropathies (reactive arthritis syndrome, psoriatic arthritis), infections (Parinaud oculoglandular syndrome, Kawasaki disease), granulomatosis with polyangiitis

Infectious Conjunctivitis

May be hyperacute, acute, or chronic; usually viral in adults and bacterial in children

Findings: papillae, follicles, conjunctival injection, chemosis, discharge; may have preauricular lymphadenopathy, lid swelling, membranes, keratitis, corneal infiltrates, anterior chamber (AC) reaction

Subepithelial infiltrates (SEIs): collections of inflammatory cells (mostly lymphocytes) at level of Bowman layer and anterior stroma
- Typically occur 2 weeks after onset of EKC, can last months
- Thought to be immunologic response to viral antigens trapped in stroma
- May cause decreased vision, glare, and photophobia
- DDx: hypoxia (contact lens overwear), infectious keratitis, EKC, Thygeson SPK, hypersensitivity (staph marginal keratitis), medication (postsurgical topical NSAID without concomitant topical steroid), corneal graft rejection, Reis-Bucklers dystrophy, Cogan dystrophy
- **TREATMENT:** topical steroids (SEIs fade but may return if steroids abruptly discontinued) or cyclosporine

Subconjunctival hemorrhages: hemorrhagic conjunctivitis
- **ETIOLOGY:** coxsackie A24, Picorna (enterovirus 70), EKC (adenovirus types 8 and 19)

True membrane: fibrin exudation, inflammatory cells, and invasion by vessels; firmly adherent to epithelium, bleeding occurs when peeled (diphtheria, *Gonococcus*, β-hemolytic *Streptococcus*, Stevens-Johnson syndrome)

Pseudomembrane: less adherent fibrin exudate (HSV, EKC, pharyngoconjunctival fever [PCF], bacterial, chlamydial, VKC, chemical burn, OCP, foreign body, ligneous, Kawasaki disease, graft-versus-host [GVH] disease)

DDx of conjunctivitis with preauricular lymphadenopathy: EKC, HSV, *Gonococcus*, *Chlamydia*, Parinaud oculoglandular syndrome, Newcastle disease

DDx of acute follicular conjunctivitis: EKC, PCF, chlamydial, primary HSV, Epstein-Barr virus (EBV), medicamentosa (antivirals, atropine, Propine, apraclonidine [Iopidine], brimonidine [Alphagan], neomycin), viral lid infections (verruca, molluscum), Newcastle disease, acute hemorrhagic (enteroviral) conjunctivitis

DDx of chronic follicular conjunctivitis (>4 weeks): chlamydial, medicamentosa, viral lid lesion, HSV, psittacosis, Lyme disease, Parinaud oculoglandular syndrome, chronic fiber granuloma (nylon in fornix), type I hypersensitivity (atopic), molluscum, trachoma

Viral

Adenovirus

Most common; double-stranded DNA; primary infection provides lifelong immunity

Initially diffuse epithelial keratitis with normal vision; later, focal epithelial keratitis, coalescence of fine spots that become subepithelial infiltrates

Transmitted by contact; contagious for 12-14 days

Seven subgroups (A–G), >52 serotypes, 1/3 associated with eye infection (majority are group D, some from groups B, C, and E); also cause respiratory (commonly groups B, C, and E) and gastrointestinal (GI; associated with groups A, F, and G) infections

Epidemic keratoconjunctivitis (EKC): types 8, 19 (reclassified as 64), and 37 are most severe, 53, 54, and 56 are less severe; bilateral in 75%-90%
  Findings: preauricular lymphadenopathy, follicular conjunctivitis, lid swelling, watery discharge, pseudo-membrane, subconjunctival hemorrhage, conjunctival scarring (symblepharon), SEIs; rarely, corneal edema, AC reaction, hypopyon; pharyngitis and rhinitis in 50%; can cause corneal ulceration
  Treatment: steroids are useful primarily with a true membrane or vision worse than 20/40 from SEIs, cyclosporine can also be used to treat SEIs; consider topical ganciclovir gel 0.15% (Zirgan) 3-5 times/day for x 1 week, hypochlorous acid 0.015% (Avenova) qid x 4-5 days, or in-office one-time application of povidone-iodine 5% ophthalmic solution for acute adenovirus

COVID-19 (SARS-CoV-2): follicular conjunctivitis; diagnosed with swab of conjunctiva via polymerase chain reaction (PCR) method

Pharyngoconjunctival fever (PCF): types 1, 3 (most common), 4, 5, 6, 7, and 14; young children; spread by respiratory secretions
  Findings: fever, pharyngitis, follicular conjunctivitis; may have punctate keratitis, rarely SEIs

Nonspecific follicular conjunctivitis: types 2-5 (3 and 4 most common), 7, 9-11, 13-18, 20-30, 32, 33, 36, 38, 39, and 42-49

Herpes Viruses

Self-limited follicular conjunctivitis occurs with HSV, varicella-zoster virus (VZV), EBV

Newcastle Disease

Unilateral follicular conjunctivitis, pneumonitis, preauricular lymphadenopathy

Occurs in poultry handlers; self-limited, lasts 1 week

Etiology: RNA virus; causes fatal disease in turkeys and other birds

Measles (Rubeola)

Mild papillary conjunctivitis, epithelial keratitis (associated with vitamin A xerosis), retinopathy (see Chapter 5, Pediatrics/Strabismus)

Rubella (German Measles)

Acquired infection presents with fever, malaise, and maculopapular rash

Conjunctivitis (70%), epithelial keratitis, retinitis with exudative retinal detachment

Optic neuritis may develop after vaccination

Congenital rubella syndrome causes ocular and systemic abnormalities (see Chapter 5, Pediatrics/Strabismus)

Molluscum Contagiosum

Chronic follicular conjunctivitis associated with elevated umbilicated lid lesions

Caused by release of toxic viral products

Treatment: excision of lesions or cryosurgery

Bacterial

Hyperacute (<24 Hours)

Copious purulent discharge, marked conjunctival injection and chemosis
  Neisseria gonorrhoeae: preauricular lymphadenopathy, corneal infiltrates; can penetrate intact corneal epithelium; can perforate within 48 hours

Diagnosis: Gram stain (gram-negative intracellular diplococci)

Treatment: systemic ceftriaxone (1 g intramuscular [IM] if no corneal involvement; 1 g intravenous [IV] or IM qd × 5 days with corneal involvement); topical antibiotic (fluoroquinolone or bacitracin); azithromycin (1 g PO single dose to cover concurrent *Chlamydia* infection)

Acute (Hours to Days)

Purulent discharge, not as severe as hyperacute

Streptococcus pneumoniae, Staphylococcus, Haemophilus influenzae, Pseudomonas

Treatment: topical antibiotic (Polytrim, tobramycin, azithromycin, or fluoroquinolone); add systemic antibiotic for *H. influenzae*

Chronic

Staphylococcus, Moraxella (chronic angular blepharoconjunctivitis), occasionally gram-negative rods

Diagnosis: culture

Treatment: topical antibiotic (Polytrim)

Chlamydial

Inclusion Conjunctivitis (Trachoma Inclusion Conjunctivitis [TRIC])

Chlamydia trachomatis serovars D to K

Chronic follicular conjunctivitis

Associated with urethritis (5%)

Findings: bulbar follicles, subepithelial infiltrates, no membranes

Treatment: doxycycline, also need to treat sexual partners

Trachoma

Bilateral keratoconjunctivitis; leading cause of preventable blindness

Chlamydia trachomatis serovars A to C

Findings (progressive): bilateral infection of upper tarsal and superior bulbar conjunctiva, papillary reaction, conjunctival follicles, repeated infections, conjunctival scarring (Arlt line), tarsal shortening, entropion, trichiasis, corneal abrasion, superior corneal pannus, corneal scarring, cicatrized limbal follicles (Herbert pits)

Classification:
  MacCallan (old):
    STAGE 2 = simple conjunctivitis with immature follicles
    STAGE 2A = mostly follicles
    STAGE 2B = mostly follicles
    STAGE 3 = cicatrizing with trichiasis, entropion, horizontal palpebral conjunctival scar (Arlt line)
    STAGE 4 = inactive with varying degrees of scarring, ptosis, xerosis
  World Health Organization:
    TF = TRACHOMATOUS INFLAMMATION (follicular): >5 follicles larger than 0.5 mm on upper tarsus
    TI = TRACHOMATOUS INFLAMMATION (intense): inflammatory thickening obscuring >50% of large, deep tarsal vessels
    TS = TRACHOMATOUS CICATRIZATION (scarring): visible white lines or sheets of fibrosis (Arlt line)
    TT = TRACHOMATOUS TRICHIASIS: at least one misdirected eyelash
    CO = CORNEAL OPACITY: obscuring at least part of pupil margin, causing vision worse than 20/60

Pathology: epithelial cells contain initial bodies (basophilic intracytoplasmic inclusions of Halberstaedter and Prowazek); Leber cells (macrophages in conjunctival stroma with phagocytosed debris)

Treatment: azithromycin 1 g PO single dose or doxycycline 100 mg bid x 7-10 days, and several months of topical antibiotics (tetracycline) during active disease; management of dry eyes; removal of misdirected lashes

Other Conjunctivitis

Ligneous

(See Chapter 5, Pediatrics/Strabismus)

Parinaud Oculoglandular Syndrome

Monocular granulomatous conjunctivitis, with necrosis and ulceration of follicles; fever, malaise, lymphadenopathy; may have rash

Etiology: cat-scratch disease (*Bartonella henselae,* most common), tularemia, sporotrichosis, TB, syphilis, *Chlamydia, Actinomyces,* EBV, *Rickettsia,* coccidioidomycosis

Pathology: follicles and granulomas

Diagnosis: PCR assay

Reactive Arthritis Syndrome

Formerly Reiter syndrome

Triad of urethritis, arthritis, and conjunctivitis/uveitis; mucopurulent conjunctivitis is the most common ocular finding (30%–50%), uveitis occurs in approximately 10%; may have keratoderma blennorrhagicum

Etiology: non-gonococcal urethritis; *Chlamydia, Shigella,* and *Salmonella* bowel infection; up to 75% HLA-B27 positive

Staphylococcal Disease

Blepharitis, conjunctivitis, keratitis (SPK, marginal infiltrates), phlyctenule

Floppy Eyelid Syndrome

(See Chapter 6, Orbit/Lids/Adnexa)

Autoeversion of eyelids during sleep with mechanical irritation on bedsheets causes papillary reaction on tarsal conjunctiva

Associated with obesity, keratoconus, eyelid rubbing, and sleep apnea

Treatment: lubrication, tape/patch/shield lids during sleep; consider horizontal eyelid tightening

Tumors

Hamartoma: growth arising from tissue normally found at that site (e.g., nevus, neurofibroma, neurilemmoma, schwannoma, glioma, hemangioma, hemangiopericytoma, lymphangioma, trichoepithelioma)

Choristoma: growth arising from tissue not normally found at that site (e.g., dermoid cyst, dermatolipoma, ectopic lacrimal gland)

Congenital Tumors

(See Chapter 5, Pediatrics/Strabismus)

Cystic Tumors

Simple Cyst

Serous

Inclusion Cyst

Clear cyst lined by normal epithelium

Congenital or acquired (after surgery or trauma)

Dislodged epithelium undergoes cavitation within stroma

Lined by nonkeratinized stratified squamous epithelium; contains mucin (goblet cells)

Treatment: complete excision; recurs if not completely excised

Squamous Tumors

Squamous Papilloma

Benign proliferation of conjunctival epithelium, appears as sessile or pedunculated fleshy mass with prominent vascular tufts

Sessile: broad base, usually older patients, often located at limbus

Pedunculated: usually caused by HPV, occurs in children, often located near caruncle; frequently recurs after excision; can regress spontaneously

Pathology: vascular cores covered by acanthotic, nonkeratinized, stratified squamous epithelium (Fig. 7.4)

Treatment:
  Adults: excisional biopsy with cryotherapy to rule out dysplastic or carcinomatous lesion; incomplete excision may result in multiple recurrences
Rare risk of malignant transformation

Conjunctival Intraepithelial Neoplasia (CIN)

Premalignant lesion

Replacement of conjunctival epithelium by atypical dysplastic squamous cells

Usually translucent or gelatinous appearance; <10% exhibit leukoplakia (keratinization)

Carcinoma in situ: total replacement of epithelium by malignant cells; basement membrane (BM) intact; no invasion into substantia propria; characterized by leukoplakia, thickened epithelium, and abnormal vascularization

Usually begins at limbus and spreads onto cornea

Associated with HPV subtypes 16 and 18 (check HIV in young patient) and actinic exposure

Men > women; occurs in older, fair-skinned individuals

Pathology: dysplastic epithelium spreads anterior to Bowman layer, fine vascularity with hairpin configuration (similar to papilloma), anaplastic cells, dyspolarity (Fig. 7.5)

Treatment: wide local excision with cryotherapy; remove involved corneal epithelium (use fluorescein or rose bengal to delimit); excise until margins are clear. Consider topical 5-fluorouracil, topical mitomycin C or interferon alpha-2b (topical or subconjunctival)

Squamous Cell Carcinoma

Malignant cells have broken through epithelial basement membrane

Most common malignant epithelial tumor of conjunctiva; rarely metastasizes

Appearance similar to carcinoma in situ

Associated with ultraviolet radiation, HPV, and smoking; 90% Caucasian, 80% male

Pathology: invasive malignant squamous cells with penetration through basement membrane (Fig. 7.6)

Treatment: wide excision (4 mm margin) with removal of surrounding conjunctiva, episclerectomy and corneal epitheliectomy with 100% alcohol and cryotherapy (reduces recurrence rate from 40% to <10%); consider topical 5-fluorouracil or mitomycin C or interferon alpha-2b (topical or subconjunctival); enucleation for intraocular involvement; exenteration and radiation therapy for intraorbital spread

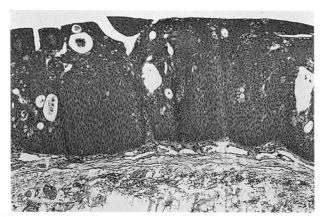

Figure 7.4 Squamous papilloma demonstrating acanthotic epithelium with blood vessels. (From Yanoff M, Fine BS. *Ocular Pathology*, 5th ed. St Louis: Mosby; 2002.)

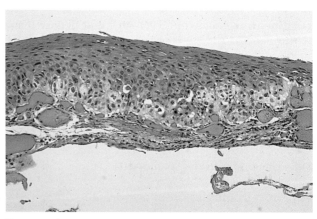

Figure 7.5 Conjunctival intraepithelial neoplasia demonstrating full-thickness atypia and loss of polarity. (From Yanoff M, Fine BS. *Ocular Pathology*, 5th ed. St Louis: Mosby; 2002.)

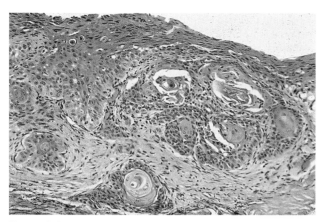

Figure 7.6 Squamous cell carcinoma demonstrating cells in substantia propria forming keratin pearls. (From Yanoff M, Fine BS. *Ocular Pathology*, 5th ed. St Louis: Mosby; 2002.)

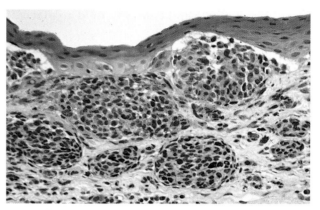

Figure 7.7 Nevus with subepithelial rests of nevus cells. (From Yanoff M, Fine BS. *Ocular Pathology*, 5th ed. St Louis: Mosby; 2002.)

Prognosis: 2%-8% intraocular invasion, 12%-16% intraorbital invasion, metastases rare; up to 8% mortality rate

Mucoepidermoid Carcinoma

Rare, aggressive variant of squamous cell carcinoma with malignant goblet cells

Typically occurs in individuals >60 years old

Very aggressive, can invade globe through sclera

Suspect in cases of recurrent squamous cell carcinoma

Pathology: epidermoid and mucinous components; stains with mucicarmine, Alcian blue, and colloidal iron

Treatment: wide local excision with cryotherapy; high recurrence rate

Melanocytic Tumors

Racial Melanosis

Bilateral, light-brown, flat, perilimbal pigmentation; increased melanin in basal epithelium

Most common in pigmented individuals

No malignant potential

Freckle

Congenital; increased melanin in basal epithelium; normal number of melanocytes

Nevus

Congenital nests of benign nevus cells along basal epithelium and/or substantia propria

Amelanotic in 20%-30%

Freely movable over globe

Epithelial inclusion cysts in 50%

Often enlarges or becomes more pigmented during puberty or pregnancy

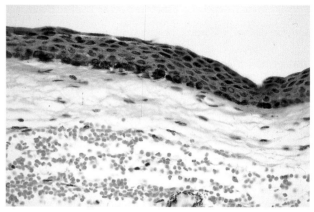

Figure 7.8 Primary acquired melanosis with pigmentation throughout the epithelium. (From Yanoff M, Fine BS. *Ocular Pathology*, 5th ed. St Louis: Mosby; 2002.)

Types (classified by location):

Junctional: nevus cell confined to epithelial/subepithelial junction (anterior to basement membrane); often seen during 1st and 2nd decades of life; appearance similar to primary acquired melanosis (PAM) with atypia

Compound (most common): nevus cells in epithelial and subepithelial locations; cystic or solid epithelial rests are very common; epithelial inclusion cysts common

Subepithelial: nevus cells confined to substantia propria; malignant transformation possible (Fig. 7.7)

Primary Acquired Melanosis (PAM, Acquired Melanosis Oculi)

Unilateral, flat, diffuse, patchy, brown pigmentation; waxes and wanes

Proliferation of intraepithelial melanocytes; no cysts (Fig. 7.8)

Most frequently on bulbar conjunctiva or in fornices but can occur on palpebral (tarsal) conjunctiva

Analogous to lentigo maligna of skin

Occurs in middle-aged to elderly whites

Low risk of malignant transformation, nodular thickening is indication for excisional biopsy

PAM without atypia and PAM with mild atypia: no risk for progression to melanoma

PAM with severe atypia: 13% risk for progression to melanoma

  Greatest risk factor is extent in clock hours

Treatment: observe with photographs; biopsy thickened areas (does not increase risk of metastasis); excisional biopsy with cryotherapy, consider topical interferon alpha-2b or mitomycin C for recurrence; complete excision if malignant

Congenital Ocular Melanosis

(See Chapter 5, Pediatrics/Strabismus)

Secondary Acquired Conjunctival Melanosis

Addison disease, radiation, pregnancy, topical epinephrine

Malignant Melanoma

Rare, variably pigmented, elevated mass most commonly on bulbar conjunctiva

May see feeder vessel

Arises from PAM (70%) or preexisting nevi (20%), or de novo (10%); 2% of ocular malignancies, ~5% of ocular melanomas

Pathology: intraepithelial pagetoid spread; need to bleach specimen to determine amount of atypia (Fig. 7.9), stain with S-100 and HMB-45

Treatment: document with photos; complete excision (no-touch technique) with clear margins, episclerectomy, corneal epitheliectomy with 100% alcohol and cryotherapy (double freeze-thaw); consider adjuvant topical mitomycin C; adjuvant radiotherapy (plaque or proton beam); exenteration now rare

Recurrence may be amelanotic

Prognosis: 25%-45% mortality; 25% risk of metastases (regional lymph nodes and brain); more likely to invade sclera than squamous cell carcinoma (SCC)
If >2 mm thick, increased risk of metastasis and mortality

Involvement of caruncle, fornices, palpebral conjunctiva has worst prognosis

Better prognosis than cutaneous melanoma

Exenteration does not improve survival

Vascular Tumors

Pyogenic Granuloma

Exuberant proliferation of granulation tissue

Vascular mass with smooth convex surface occurring at site of previous surgery (usually strabismus, pterygium, or chalazion excision)

Pathology: loose fibrous stroma containing multiple capillaries and inflammatory cells

Treatment: topical steroids; primary excision, excision with conjunctival graft or cryotherapy

Kaposi Sarcoma

Red mass, often multifocal

Stages 1 and 2: patchy and flat, <3 mm in height, <4 months in duration

Stage 3: more nodular, >3 mm in height, longer duration
  Associated with AIDS (20%)

Pathology: proliferation of capillaries, endothelial cells, and fibroblast-like cells (Fig. 7.10)

Treatment: excision, XRT, paclitaxel (Taxol) (inhibits mitosis)

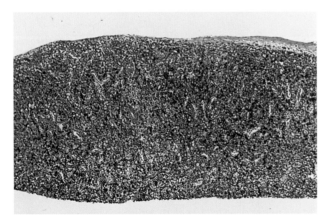

Figure 7.9 Malignant melanoma appears as pigmented tumor with loss of polarity. (From Yanoff M, Fine BS. *Ocular Pathology*, 5th ed. St Louis: Mosby; 2002.)

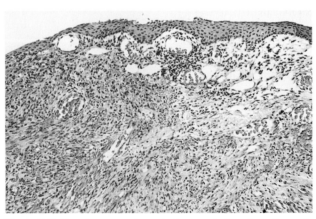

Figure 7.10 Kaposi sarcoma demonstrating neoplastic cells and vascular spaces. (From Yanoff M, Fine BS. *Ocular Pathology*, 5th ed. St Louis: Mosby; 2002.)

Cavernous Hemangioma

Red patch; may bleed

Associated with other ocular hemangiomas or systemic disease

Pathology: endothelial lined canals with red blood cells (RBCs)

Lymphangioma

Cluster of clear cysts; may have areas of hemorrhage

Pathology: dilated lymphatic vessels

Treatment: excision if small

Lymphoid Tumors

(See Chapter 6, Orbit/Lids/Adnexa)

Smooth, flat, fleshy, salmon-colored mass; single or multiple

Occurs in substantia propria; overlying epithelium is smooth; can be bilateral

Most commonly in fornix, may involve orbit

Associated with systemic disease in 20% (but systemic lymphoma rarely presents in conjunctiva)

Spectrum of disease from benign to malignant (non-Hodgkin's; less aggressive mucosa-associated lymphoid tissue [MALT] or more malignant non-MALT); cannot distinguish clinically; requires biopsy with immunohistochemical studies (fresh, unfixed tissue specimen) for diagnosis

Usually middle-aged adults

Requires systemic workup, including computed tomography (CT) scan, bone scan, serum protein electrophoresis (SPEP), medical consultation

DDx: leukemia, metastases

Treatment: low-dose radiation therapy (XRT), surgery, local chemotherapy

Metastatic Tumors

Very rare to conjunctiva

Fleshy yellow-pink mass

Breast, lung, cutaneous melanoma (usually pigmented)

Other Tumors

Fibrous Histiocytoma

Yellow-white mass composed of fibroblasts and histiocytes

Extends from limbus to peripheral cornea

Pathology: storiform pattern

Treatment: local excision

Benign Hereditary Intraepithelial Dyskeratosis (BHID) (Autosomal Dominant [AD])

Mapped to chromosome 4q35

Originally seen in triracial families in Halifax County, North Carolina (Haliwa Indians)

Usually presents in 1st decade of life

Symptoms: itching, burning, photophobia

Findings: bilateral dyskeratotic lesions (plaques with gelatinous base and keratinized surface) involving bulbar conjunctiva near limbus; may have similar plaques on buccal mucosa or oropharynx

Pathology: acanthosis, dyskeratosis, prominent rete pegs; no malignant potential

DDx: Bitot spot, pinugeculum, squamous papilloma, squamous cell carcinoma

Treatment: observe; topical steroids (severe symptoms); excision (diagnostic; lesions recur)

Pseudoepitheliomatous Hyperplasia

Benign proliferation of conjunctiva onto corneal epithelium

Usually occurs away from limbus (in contrast to squamous hyperplasia or carcinoma)

Develops over weeks to months

Findings: raised, whitened hyperkeratotic surface (cannot differentiate clinically from dysplasia)

Pathology: thickened squamous epithelium; occasional mitotic figures; no atypia; no clear demarcation between normal and abnormal cells

Treatment: excision

Caruncle Tumors

Benign

Papilloma (30%), nevus (25%), inclusion cyst, sebaceous hyperplasia, sebaceous adenoma, pyogenic granuloma

Oncocytoma (oxyphilic adenoma): arises from metaplasia of ductal and acinar cells of accessory lacrimal glands; composed of polyhedral cells arranged in nests, cords, or sheets; eosinophilic cytoplasm correlates with abundance of mitochondria; more common in women

Malignant (5%)

SCC, malignant melanoma, sebaceous adenocarcinoma

CORNEAL DISORDERS

Congenital

(See Chapter 5, Pediatrics/Strabismus)

Trauma

Abrasion

Epithelial defect, most commonly traumatic (e.g., fingernail, plant branch)

Increased risk of infection, especially in contact lens wearer

Symptoms: foreign body sensation, pain, tearing, redness, photophobia

Findings: epithelial defect stains with fluorescein, conjunctival injection, ciliary flush; may have mild AC reaction

Treatment: topical antibiotic, consider topical NSAID, cycloplegic, bandage contact lens, or patching for pain control (never patch CL wearer because of increased risk of microbial keratitis)

Foreign Body

May be superficial or deep

Often metal (usually associated with adjacent rust ring), glass, or organic material

Treatment: removal of foreign body, topical antibiotic; old deep inert material may be observed

Laceration

Partial- or full-thickness cut in cornea

Requires surgical repair and topical antibiotic and steroid

Complications include scarring and irregular astigmatism, which, if affect vision, may be treated with rigid C or keratoplasty

Recurrent Erosion

Spontaneous epithelial defect

Associated with epithelial basement membrane dystrophy (EBMD) in 19%-29% or previous corneal trauma (i.e., abrasion) in 45%-64%; also occurs in other corneal dystrophies

Abnormal adhesion of epithelium to Bowman layer allows spontaneous sloughing

Symptoms usually occur in morning upon awakening (epithelium swells 4% overnight, and mechanical force of lids rubbing across corneal surface when open eyes or blink can dislodge epithelium)

Duration of symptoms depends on size of erosion

Findings: epithelial defect (may be partially healed), conjunctival injection; may have mild AC reaction and signs of corneal dystrophy (i.e., anterior basement membrane dystrophy [ABMD] with irregular epithelium, areas of negative stain)

Treatment: lubrication, hypertonic saline (Muro 128 5% ointment qhs × 3–12 months); if recurs, consider bandage contact lens, epithelial débridement, anterior stromal puncture/reinforcement, diamond burr (débride and polish Bowman layer), laser (phototherapeutic keratectomy [PTK] with excimer laser, or micropuncture with Nd:YAG laser [1 mJ, aim just below epithelium]); also, consider treatment with matrix metalloproteinase-9 inhibitors (doxycycline 50 mg PO bid × 2 months and topical steroids tid × 2–3 weeks); débridement for subepithelial scarring

Prognosis: recurrence rates are >25% for medical management, 15%-18% for epithelial débridement, 6% for débridement with diamond burr polishing, rare with PTK

Burns

Tissue destruction resulting from chemical or thermal injury

Acid: denatures and precipitates tissue proteins
Sulfuric (batteries): most common
Sulfurous (bleach): penetrates more easily than other acids
Hydrofluoric (glass polishing/etching): increased penetration
Hydrochloric: severe burn only with high concentration
Acetic: mild burn if concentration <10%
Pathology: superficial coagulative necrosis of conjunctiva and corneal epithelium

Alkali: denatures but does not precipitate proteins, also saponifies fat; therefore penetrates deeply, may perforate; causes most severe injury
Lime (plaster, cement): most common; toxicity increased by retained particulate matter; less penetration
Ammonia (fertilizers), *lye* (drain cleaners): produce most serious injury
Also, *MgOH* (fireworks), *KOH*
Pathology: conjunctival and corneal epithelial loss with corneal clouding and edema; conjunctival and corneal necrosis; ischemia from thrombosis of conjunctival and episcleral vessels

Radiation: thermal burn (similar to acid burn)
UV light (snow blindness, arc-welding): punctate epithelial keratitis 8-12 hours after exposure; completely resolves
Ionizing radiation: superficial keratitis; then stromal disruption from keratocyte damage; corneal drying secondary to keratinization of conjunctiva

Grading systems:
Roper-Hall Classification: based on severity of corneal damage and limbal ischemia
GRADE I: corneal epithelial damage, no ischemia; full recovery
GRADE II: stromal haze but iris details seen, ischemia <1/3 of limbus; good prognosis, some scarring

GRADE III: total corneal epithelial loss, stromal haze, obscuration of iris; ischemia from 1/3-1/2 of limbus; guarded prognosis

GRADE IV: cornea opaque; ischemia >1/2 of limbus; poor prognosis, risk of perforation

McCulley Classification: clinical course classification, helpful for guiding treatment

IMMEDIATE PHASE: emergent intervention

ACUTE PHASE: 0-7 days; monitor reepithelialization, inflammation, intraocular pressure

EARLY REPARATIVE PHASE: 7-21 days; support corneal healing and limit ulceration

LATE REPARATIVE PHASE: 3 weeks to several months; consider surgical interventions to stabilize ocular surface

Treatment:

Immediate phase: copious irrigation (minimum 15 minutes with at least 1 L of fluid) until pH neutralized; remove chemical particulate matter; débride necrotic tissue

Acute and early reparative phases: topical lubrication (preservative-free artificial tears up to q1h and ointment qhs), broad-spectrum antibiotic, and cycloplegic. For grades II-IV, add topical steroids (prednisolone acetate 1% q1–2h during first 10 days then taper [risk of stromalysis], if steroids still necessary after 10–14 days, then change to medroxyprogesterone [Provera 1%]), topical citrate (10% q2h), ascorbate (topical 10% q2h and systemic 2 g PO in divided doses), oral doxycycline 100 mg PO bid (collagenase inhibitor; ethylenediaminetetraacetic acid [EDTA] and acetylcysteine are ineffective); consider bandage contact lens until epithelial defect heals; ocular hypotensive medication for elevated IOP

Late reparative phase: for grades III-IV, surgery may be required, including symblepharon lysis, conjunctival and mucous membrane transplantation, tenoplasty, limbal autograft or keratoepithelioplasty (if epithelium not healed after 3 weeks), punctal occlusion, and tarsorrhaphy; consider cryopreserved amniotic membrane (PROKERA), scleral lenses including the Boston ocular surface prosthesis (PROSE lens), conjunctival flap to treat recurrent or persistent corneal epithelial defects. Later, consider penetrating keratoplasty or keratoprosthesis (poor results; better if performed 1–2 years after injury); may need limbal stem cell transplant

Complications: cataract, glaucoma, uveitis, symblepharon, entropion, xerosis, retrocorneal membrane, neurotrophic keratitis, corneal ulceration, anterior segment ischemia, and neovascularization

Dry Eye Disease

Sporadic or chronic ocular irritation with visual disturbance

Caused by tear film and ocular surface abnormality; usually multifactorial

Tear Film and Ocular Surface Society Dry Eye Workshop (TFOS DEWS) II definition (2017):

Dry eye is a multifactorial disease of the ocular surface characterized by a loss of homeostasis of the tear film, and accompanied by ocular symptoms, in which tear film instability and hyperosmolarity, ocular surface inflammation and damage, and neurosensory abnormalities play etiologic roles

Affects 5%-30% of the population ≥50 years old; female > male

Risk factors: age, Asian race, hormone levels (hormone replacement therapy, androgen deficiency), environmental conditions (low humidity, wind, heat, air-conditioning, pollutants, irritants, allergens), digital screen use, contact lens wear, and diabetes

Aqueous Deficiency

Lacrimal gland dysfunction (aplasia, surgical removal), infiltration (sarcoidosis, thyroid disease, lymphoma, amyloidosis, TB), inflammation (mumps, Sjögren syndrome, radiation), obstruction (Stevens-Johnson syndrome, ocular cicatricial pemphigoid, GVH disease, pemphigus, trachoma, chemical burns), denervation (Riley-Day [familial dysautonomia], Shy-Drager [adult dysautonomia, idiopathic autonomic dysfunction], Möbius syndrome), drugs that decrease lacrimal secretion (antihistamines, diuretics, anticholinergics, psychotropics), androgen deficiency

Keratoconjunctivitis Sicca

Adult women (95%), often associated with Sjögren syndrome

Diagnostic criteria for Sjögren syndrome:

Keratoconjunctivitis sicca (KCS)

Xerostomia (decreased parotid flow rate)

Lymphocytic infiltration on labial salivary gland biopsy

Laboratory evidence of systemic autoimmune disease (positive antinuclear antibody [ANA] titer, rheumatoid factor, or SS-A or SS-B antibody; associated with HLA-B8 [90%])

Symptoms: burning, dryness, foreign body sensation, redness, tearing, fluctuation of vision; worse later in day, with prolonged use of eye, and in dry or windy environments. Can be asymptomatic

Findings: decreased tear meniscus height (<0.2 mm), decreased tear breakup time (<10 seconds), increased mucus, filaments in severe cases, interpalpebral corneal and conjunctival staining with rose bengal/lissamine green or fluorescein, Schirmer test (<10 mm/5 min) or Phenol red thread test (<10 mm/15 seconds), increased tear osmolarity (312 mOsm/L has best sensitivity and specificity as threshold for diagnosis; ≥308 mOsm/L or ≥8 mOsm/L difference between eyes [early disease], ≥316 mOsm/L [moderate disease], ≥336 mOsm/L [severe disease]), increased matrix metalloproteinase-9 level (>40 ng/mL); confocal microscopy shows tortuosity, reflectivity, and beading of corneal nerves

Pathology: lymphocytic infiltration of lacrimal gland

Treatment: stepwise based on level of disease severity

Step 1: education, modification/elimination of

environmental factors and offending agents, lubrication with artificial tears, nutritional supplements (oral fish oils/omega-3 fatty acids: eicosapentaenoic acid [EPA] and docosahexaenoic acid [DHA])

Step 2: nonpreserved lubricating drops, bedtime ointment, Lacrisert, punctal occlusion, humidifier moisture chamber goggles, topical cyclosporine (Cequa, Restasis), topical lifitegrast (Xiidra), short course of topical steroid (Eysuvis), varenicline nasal spray (Tyrvaya), neurostimulation (iTear100)

Step 3: oral secretagogues, autologous serum drops, consider acetylcysteine (Mucomyst), bandage contact lens

Step 4: longer course topical steroid, cryopreserved amniotic membrane (PROKERA), scleral lenses including Boston ocular surface keratoprosthesis (PROSE lens), tarsorrhaphy

Mikulicz syndrome: lacrimal and parotid gland swelling and KCS resulting from sarcoidosis, TB, lymphoma, leukemia

Mucin Deficiency

Goblet cell dysfunction resulting from conjunctival scarring and keratinization (vitamin A deficiency, OCP, Stevens-Johnson syndrome, alkali burns, trachoma, GVH disease); impression cytology measures number of goblet cells

Xerophthalmia

Conjunctival epithelial keratinization caused by vitamin A deficiency

Vitamin A required for conjunctival goblet cell mucin production, corneal stromal metabolism, retinal photoreceptor metabolism, normal iron metabolism, normal growth, resistance to measles

Incidence 5 million new cases/year; affects 20-40 million children worldwide

Usually in developing countries (50% in India); in developed countries, results from lipid malabsorption (short bowel syndrome, chronic liver dysfunction, cystic fibrosis) and poor diet (chronic alcoholism)

WHO Classification:
XN: night blindness
X1A: conjunctival xerosis
X1B: Bitot spot
X2: corneal xerosis
X3A: corneal ulcer (<1/3 cornea)
X3B: corneal ulcer/keratomalacia (≥1/3 cornea)
XS: corneal scarring
XF: xerophthalmic fundus

Findings: night blindness (nyctalopia), conjunctival xerosis (leathery appearance) and Bitot spots (gray, foamy plaques); corneal xerosis with keratomalacia, ulceration, and scarring; xerophthalmic fundus (fine white mottling)

Treatment: vitamin A replacement (i.e., 200,000 IU vitamin A [IM or PO] x 2 days, repeat in 2 months [for children >1 year old and adults])

Stevens-Johnson Syndrome

Young people; 25% recurrence, 10%-33% mortality

Etiology: drugs (sulfa, antibiotics, barbiturates, phenytoin [Dilantin]), infection (herpes, *Mycoplasma*), idiopathic

Findings: acute pseudomembranous conjunctivitis, symblepharon, persistent epithelial defects, dry eye, trichiasis, corneal scarring, vascularization, erosions, and ulcers

Other findings:
Erythema multiforme: cutaneous bullous eruptions (target lesions), crusting, rash involves face, mucosal ulceration and strictures, sore throat, fever, arthralgias
    ERYTHEMA MULTIFORME MINOR: no mucous membrane involvement
    ERYTHEMA MULTIFORME MAJOR: mucous membrane ulceration; 20% mortality from secondary infection

Pathology: occurs at mucocutaneous junction
Early: epithelial thinning with fibrinous exudate and stromal lymphocytic infiltration
Late: patchy epidermalization with keratinization and subepithelial fibrosis

Treatment: topical antibiotic, steroid, lubrication, symblepharon lysis, surgery; consider oral steroids, punctal occlusion, tarsorrhaphy, cryopreserved amniotic membrane (PROKERA), scleral lenses including the Boston ocular surface keratoprosthesis (PROSE lens)

Ocular Cicatricial Pemphigoid

Systemic vesiculobullous disease of mucous membranes resulting in cicatrizing conjunctivitis

Other mucous membrane involvement, including oral (up to 90%), esophageal, tracheal, and genital; skin involved in up to 30% of cases

Usually women (2:1) age >60 years

Etiology: probably autoimmune (immune complexes present in basement membrane zone)

Associated with HLA-DR4, DQw3, and medications (pilocarpine, phospholine iodide, timolol, epinephrine, idoxuridine)

Classification: 2 systems
Foster: based on disease progression
    STAGE I = chronic conjunctivitis with subepithelial fibrosis
    STAGE II = fornix shortening
    STAGE III = symblepharon
    STAGE IV = end-stage
Mondino and Brown: based on degree of fornix shortening
    STAGE I = <25%
    STAGE II = 25%-50%
    STAGE III = 75%
    STAGE IV = end-stage

Findings: symblepharon, ankyloblepharon, fornix shortening, trichiasis, entropion, subconjunctival fibrosis, severe dry eye, corneal ulcers, vascularization, and scarring; oral lesions

Other findings:
Skin: recurrent vesiculobullous lesions of inguinal region and extremities, scarring lesions on scalp and face
Mucous membranes (nose, pharynx, larynx, esophagus): strictures, dysphagia

Pathology: occurs at level of basement membrane (subepithelial bullae); epithelial thinning, loss of goblet cells, keratinization, subepithelial inflammation and fibrosis; IgA in conjunctival basement membrane zone; mostly polys; antigen antibodies are deposited below epidermis
Pemphigus vulgaris: antigen antibodies located within epithelium (intraepithelial acantholysis with epithelial bullae)

Conjunctival scraping: lymphocytes, plasma cells, eosinophils

Treatment: lubrication, immunosuppressive therapy, dapsone, cyclophosphamide, surgery; consider punctal occlusion, tarsorrhaphy, cryopreserved amniotic membrane (PROKERA), scleral lenses including the Boston ocular surface keratoprosthesis (PROSE lens)
Penetrating keratoplasty: poor success rate
Keratoprosthesis: limited success for end-stage disease

Prognosis: remissions and exacerbations

Lipid Deficiency

Meibomian Gland Disease/Dysfunction (MGD; Posterior Blepharitis, Meibomitis, Acne Rosacea)

(See Chapter 6, Orbit/Lids/Adnexa)

~86% of patients with dry eye disease have signs of MGD

Other Factors

Lid abnormalities: increased evaporative loss (lagophthalmos, Bell palsy, ectropion, entropion, thyroid disease); treat with lid taping, tarsorrhaphy, surgical repair of underlying abnormality

Blink related: reading/computer work (reduces blink rate by up to 60%), Parkinson disease, lid malposition (see above)

Aging: reduced basal tear secretion

Environment: wind, low humidity, pollutant, allergens

Iatrogenic: medications (antihistamines, antidepressants, anxiolytics, anticholinergics, β-adrenergic blocking agents, diuretics, retinoids, estrogens), topical anesthetics, preservatives (benzalkonium chloride, thimerosal, polyquad), contact lens wear (approximately 50% of CL wearers have dry eye symptoms), ophthalmic surgery and procedures (most commonly corneal, refractive, and cataract)

Inflammation

Interstitial Keratitis (IK)

Etiology:
Bacteria: syphilis (congenital [90%; most common cause of bilateral IK] or acquired), relapsing fever *(Borrelia)*, TB (unilateral, sectoral), leprosy, LGV
Virus: HSV, EBV, measles, mumps, rubella, influenza, smallpox, vaccinia
Protozoa: leishmaniasis, African sleeping sickness *(Taenia cruzi)*, malaria, onchocerciasis, cysticercosis *(Taenia solium)*
Other causes: sarcoidosis, Hodgkin's disease, Kaposi sarcoma, mycosis fungoides, incontinentia pigmenti, hidradenitis suppurativa, Cogan syndrome (vertigo, tinnitus, hearing loss, IK)
Can be initiated by minor corneal trauma in patients with congenital syphilis

Findings: neovascularization appears as salmon patch, results in hazy corneal scarring, regression of vessels leaves ghost vessels (clear branching pattern within the scar); may develop secondary glaucoma from iris/angle damage

Pathology: diffuse lymphocytic infiltrate with thickened corneal stroma

Treatment: topical steroids

Cogan Syndrome

Ocular inflammation (usually IK) with Meniere-like vestibular dysfunction

Most likely autoimmune

Affects young adults, average age of onset is 29 years

Associated with antecedent upper respiratory illness (50%) and vascular inflammatory disease (10%; aortic insufficiency, aortitis, necrotizing large vessel [Takayasu-like], and polyarteritis nodosa)

Symptoms: pain, redness, photophobia

Findings: SEIs, IK, conjunctivitis, iritis, scleritis, episcleritis

Other findings: sudden onset of Meniere-like symptoms (nausea, emesis, tinnitus, decreased hearing, severe vertigo; may have nystagmus); 80% progress to deafness without systemic steroids

DDx of keratitis with vestibuloauditory symptoms: syphilis, polyarteritis nodosa, granulomatosis with polyangiitis, sarcoidosis, Vogt-Koyanagi-Harada (VKH) syndrome, sympathetic ophthalmia, cerebellopontine angle tumor

Audiogram: most pronounced loss at extreme frequencies, relative sparing of midrange

Treatment: systemic steroids to prevent permanent hearing loss

Thygeson Superficial Punctate Keratopathy

Associated with HLA-DR3; 90% bilateral; spontaneous remissions and exacerbations for years

Symptoms: photophobia, foreign body sensation, burning, tearing

Findings: coarse, punctate, gray-white snowflake opacities in corneal epithelium with faint subepithelial haze; raised center breaks through epithelial surface and stains with fluorescein during acute attack; during remissions, inactive lesions appear flat and do not stain; no associated conjunctivitis or iritis

Treatment: topical steroids (symptomatic relief and rapid resolution of lesions, but may prolong course of disease), therapeutic contact lens, consider cryopreserved amniotic membrane (PROKERA), trifluridine (Viroptic; may help, but idoxuridine does not work and can cause subepithelial scarring), topical cyclosporine (may also be beneficial)

Without treatment symptoms last for 1-2 months, then remission; recurrences can begin 6-8 weeks later

Filamentary Keratitis

Strands composed of mucus and desquamated epithelial cells adherent to cornea at one end

Caused by increased mucus production and abnormal epithelial turnover

Etiology: KCS, SLK, recurrent erosions, bullous keratopathy, prolonged patching, HSV keratitis, neurotrophic keratitis, neuroparalytic keratopathy, ectodermal dysplasia, trauma, atopic dermatitis, adenoviral keratoconjunctivitis, topical medication toxicity (medicamentosa), ptosis

No filaments in OCP because mucus production is diminished in this disorder

Treatment: acetylcysteine (Mucomyst), lubrication, remove filaments, bandage contact lens, treat underlying disorder

Degenerations

Pannus

Peripheral ingrowth of subepithelial fibrovascular tissue, usually superiorly

Inflammatory: destruction of Bowman layer (i.e., trachoma)

Degenerative: Bowman layer remains intact; may contain fatty plaque deposits (i.e., chronic edema)
  Most commonly results from CL wear

White Limbal Girdle of Vogt

Small, white, fleck and needle-like deposits at temporal and nasal limbus

Pathology: subepithelial elastotic degeneration of collagen (sometimes with calcium particles)

Corneal Arcus

Arcus senilis: hazy white peripheral corneal ring with intervening clear zone between limbus

Arcus juvenilis: arcus in persons <40 years old; associated with hyperlipoproteinemia types 2, 3, and 4

Pathology: lipid deposition in stroma

DDx: lecithin cholesterol acyltransferase (LCAT) deficiency, fish eye disease, Tangier disease

Carotid ultrasound: for unilateral arcus senilis (may have stenosis on uninvolved side)

Furrow Degeneration

Thin area peripheral to arcus senilis, more apparent than real; nonprogressive; asymptomatic

Crocodile Shagreen

Mosaic, polygonal, hazy, gray opacities separated by clear zones; "cracked-ice" appearance

Extends to periphery

Anterior crocodile shagreen: occurs at level of Bowman layer

Posterior crocodile shagreen: occurs at level of Descemet membrane

Salzmann Nodular Degeneration

Blue-white elevated nodules; more common in older females

Etiology: chronic inflammation (e.g., old phlyctenulosis, trachoma, IK, staph hypersensitivity)

Pathology: replacement of Bowman layer by hyaline and fibrillar material

Treatment: superficial keratectomy, PTK; may recur after

Polymorphic Amyloid Degeneration

Bilateral, symmetric, small stellate flecks or filaments in deep stroma

Slowly progressive; usually seen in patients >50 years old; asymptomatic

Not associated with systemic amyloid

Spheroidal Degeneration (Labrador Keratopathy, Actinic Keratopathy, Lipid Droplet Degeneration, Bietti Hyaline Degeneration, Keratinoid Degeneration)

Bilateral; male > female

Etiology: combination of genetic predisposition, actinic exposure, and age

Types:
Type 1 (most common): involves peripheral cornea in horizontal meridian; occurs after age 30
Type 2: associated with other corneal pathology; may involve central cornea; occurs earlier in life
Type 3: involves conjunctiva
Usually asymptomatic

Findings: translucent, golden brown, spherical, superficial stromal and conjunctival proteinaceous deposits

Pathology: extracellular basophilic material

Cornea Farinata (AD)

Tiny, dot- and comma-shaped, deep stromal opacities; may contain lipofuscin (degenerative pigment)

Involutional change

Hassall-Henle Bodies

Small, peripheral, wartlike excrescences (guttata) of Descemet membrane (protrude toward AC)

Normal senescent change; rare before age 20 years

Depositions

Band Keratopathy

Interpalpebral band of subepithelial hazy white opacities with ground-glass, Swiss-cheese appearance; begins at limbus

Etiology: uveitis, IK, superficial keratitis, phthisis, sarcoidosis, trauma, intraocular silicone oil, systemic disease (hypercalcemia, vitamin D intoxication, Fanconi syndrome, hypophosphatemia, gout, "milk-alkali" syndrome, myotonic dystrophy, chronic mercury exposure)

Pathology: calcification of epithelial basement membrane, Bowman layer, and anterior stroma, with destruction of Bowman layer; calcium salts are extracellular when process is caused by local ocular disease, calcium salts are intracellular when process is caused by alteration of systemic calcium metabolism

Treatment: chelation with topical disodium EDTA
Gout and hyperuricemia cause brown band from deposition of urate

Lipid Keratopathy

Diffuse or crystalline yellow stromal deposits

Caused by lipid exudation from corneal vascularization

Coat White Ring

Small, discrete, gray-white dots

Follows metallic foreign body

Mucopolysaccharidoses

(See Chapter 5, Pediatrics/Strabismus)

Sphingolipidoses

(See Chapter 5, Pediatrics/Strabismus)

Dyslipoproteinemias

Fish-eye disease (AR): mapped to chromosome 16q22; diffuse corneal clouding, denser in periphery

Hyperlipoproteinemia types 2, 3, and 4: arcus

LCAT deficiency: mapped to chromosome 16; dense arcus and diffuse, fine, gray stromal dots

Tangier disease (AR): high-density lipoprotein (HDL) deficiency, relapsing polyneuropathy, small deep stromal opacities

Hypergammaglobulinemia

Crystals

Cystinosis

(See Chapter 5, Pediatrics/Strabismus)

Ochronosis (Alkaptonuria) (AR)

Mapped to chromosome 3q2

Melanin-like pigment (alkapton; peripheral epithelium and superficial stroma)

Tyrosinemia Type II (Richner-Hanhart Syndrome) (AR)

Mapped to chromosome 16q22

Deposits in epithelium and subepithelial space as a result of tyrosine aminotransferase deficiency

Refractile branching linear opacities, may have dendritic pattern

Triad of painful hyperkeratotic skin lesions (on palms and soles), keratitis, and mental retardation

Wilson Disease (Hepatolenticular Degeneration) (AR)

Increased copper levels as a result of a deficiency in ceruloplasmin

Copper deposition in
Basal ganglia: spasticity, dysarthria, tremor, ataxia
Liver: cirrhosis
Eye: Kayser-Fleischer ring (copper deposition in peripheral Descemet; starts superiorly, then inferiorly, medially, and temporally); sunflower cataract

DDx of Kayser-Fleischer ring: primary biliary cirrhosis, chronic active hepatitis, multiple myeloma, chronic cholestatic jaundice

Treatment: oral tetrathiomolybdate (penicillamine), followed by oral zinc maintenance; Kayser-Fleischer rings resolve with adequate treatment

Chalcosis

Copper (Descemet), results from intraocular foreign body composed of <85% copper

Siderosis

Iron (stroma)

Iron Lines

Caused by stagnation of tears (basal epithelium)

Fleischer ring: base of cone in keratoconus

Stocker line: head of pterygium

Ferry line: adjacent to filtering bleb

Hudson-Stähli line: horizontal at lower 1/3 of cornea; normal aging, nocturnal exposure

Argyrosis

Silver (deep stroma/Descemet)

Chrysiasis

Gold (peripheral deep stroma)

Krukenberg Spindle

Melanin (on endothelium)

Plant Sap

From Dieffenbachia

Cornea Verticillata (Vortex Keratopathy)

Gray to golden-brown phospholipid deposits in whorl pattern (epithelium) resulting from Fabry disease and medications (most commonly amiodarone, chloroquine, indomethacin, ibuprofen, naproxen, tamoxifen, suramin, clofazimine, phenothiazines, and topical netarsudil)

Ulcers

Corneal Melt (Noninfectious Ulcer)

Nonimmune mediated: traumatic, eyelid abnormalities (entropion, ectropion, trichiasis, exposure, lagophthalmos), neurotrophic cornea, acne rosacea, keratomalacia, gold toxicity

Systemic immune mediated: primary KCS, Sjögren syndrome, ocular cicatricial pemphigoid, Stevens-Johnson syndrome, rheumatoid arthritis, systemic lupus erythematosus (SLE), granulomatosis with polyangiitis, polyarteritis nodosa

Localized immune mediated: Mooren ulcer, *Staph* marginal ulcer, vernal keratoconjunctivitis

Peripheral Corneal Ulcers

Mooren Ulcer

Chronic, very painful, progressive ulceration

Typically begins nasally or temporally and spreads circumferentially (up to 360°)

Type II hypersensitivity reaction

Associated with hepatitis C, Crohn disease, and hydradenitis

Symptoms: photophobia, decreased vision (irregular astigmatism)

Findings: undermined leading edge with overhanging margin, absent epithelium in active areas; may have conjunctival injection

Variants:
  USA: unilateral disease of elderly (males = females), usually less aggressive; perforation rare
  Africa: severe bilateral disease in young patients; rapidly progressive with risk of perforation
Diagnosis of exclusion (rule out rheumatologic and autoimmune diseases)

Pathology: adjacent conjunctiva contains increased plasma cells, immunoglobulin, and complement

Treatment: steroids, immunosuppressive agents (methotrexate, cyclosporine), NSAIDs, bandage contact lens, conjunctival recession or resection; may require corneal glue or penetrating or lamellar keratoplasty for perforation

Terrien Marginal Degeneration

Painless, progressive, bilateral, troughlike stromal thinning; starts superiorly

Young to middle-aged men (75%), unknown etiology

Findings: leading edge of lipid, steep central edge, sloping peripheral edge, intact epithelium, superficial vascularization; can progress circumferentially or centrally; induces "against-the-rule" astigmatism; may perforate with mild trauma, rarely spontaneously

Staph Marginal Ulcer

Hypersensitivity reaction

Findings: initial subepithelial infiltrate with peripheral clear zone, progresses to shallow ulcer; adjacent conjunctival injection; blepharitis

Treatment: resolves spontaneously, topical steroids may help; treat blepharitis

Marginal Keratolysis/Peripheral Ulcerative Keratitis (PUK)

Ulceration is typically peripheral and unilateral, can be central and bilateral

Caused by elevated collagenase; melting stops when epithelium heals

Associated with dry eyes (Sjögren) and systemic disease:
Rheumatoid arthritis: painless guttering or acute painful ulceration; also may have scleritis
Granulomatosis with polyangiitis: 60% have ocular involvement, most commonly PUK; also, may have scleritis, conjunctivitis, orbital involvement with proptosis, retinal vasculitis, and anterior ischemic optic neuropathy (AION)
Polyarteritis nodosa: may be presenting feature; also may have pale-yellow, waxy, raised, friable conjunctival vessels, scleritis, conjunctivitis, and retinal vasculitis
SLE: rare manifestation
Scleroderma: also may have KCS and trichiasis
Others: relapsing polychondritis, inflammatory bowel disease, Behçet disease

Diagnosis: blood tests as for scleritis (complete blood count [CBC], erythrocyte sedimentation rate [ESR], ANA, rheumatoid factor [RF], antineutrophil cytoplasmic antibodies [ANCA])

Treatment: lubrication, punctal occlusion, tarsorrhaphy; consider immunosuppressive agents (topical cyclosporine), conjunctival recession or resection; treat underlying disease

Fuchs Superficial Marginal Keratitis

Marginal infiltrates initially, then pseudopterygium with severe corneal thinning underneath

Risk of perforation with surgery or trauma

Microbial Keratitis (Infectious Ulcer)

Bacterial

Most common

Penetration of intact epithelium: *Neisseria, Corynebacterium diphtheriae, Shigella, Haemophilus aegyptius, Listeria monocytogenes*

Through epithelial defect: any organism; most commonly *Staphylococcus, Streptococcus,* and *Pseudomonas*

Risk factors: corneal trauma or surgery, contact lens wear, epithelial ulceration, dry eye, lid abnormalities

Signs of improvement: decrease in infiltrate (density/size), stromal edema, endothelial plaque, AC reaction, hypopyon; and reepithelialization

Treatment:
Empiric: topical fortified antibiotics (vancomycin or ce-fazolin, plus tobramycin alternating q1h) or fluoroquinolone (Besivance, Zymaxid or Vigamox q15min x 2–3 hours, then q1h); consider subconjunctival antibiotic injection (if noncompliant)
If no response to empiric therapy: antibiotic resistance (change regimen based on culture results); fungal, protozoal, or viral process; poor compliance (admit to hospital); anesthetic abuse
Topical cycloplegic
Topical steroid (should be avoided until improvement is noted [usually after 48–72 hours], then dosed at lower frequency than topical antibiotic)
Steroids for Corneal Ulcers Trial (SCUT): evaluated topical moxifloxacin monotherapy or with adjunctive 1% prednisolone phosphate at initial dose of qid after 48 hours of topical antibiotic; no difference in best corrected visual acuity (BCVA) at 3 months, but steroid was safe, no difference in rate of healing, rate of corneal perforation, or rate of worsening of keratitis. At 12 months, patients with non-*Nocardia* species had slightly better visual acuity in steroid group

Complications:
Spread to adjacent structures: sclera *(Pseudomonas),* intraocular (rare in absence of corneal perforation; filamentous fungi may penetrate intact Descemet membrane)
Corneal damage: scarring, neovascularization, endothelial dysfunction (corneal edema), descemetocele, perforation
Synechiae and secondary glaucoma
Cataract

Syphilis

(See Chapter 5, Pediatrics/Strabismus)

Crystalline Keratopathy

Most commonly caused by *Streptococcus viridans,* also *Candida, Staphylococcus epidermidis, Streptococcus pneumoniae, Haemophilus,* and *Enterococcus*

Associated with chronic topical steroid use (after corneal graft)

Branching, cracked-glass appearance without epithelial defect

Treat strep with vancomycin

Herpes Simplex (HSV)

Most common cause of infectious blindness and second-most-common cause of corneal blindness in United States (trauma is first); HSV-1 is more common for ocular infections than HSV-2 (genital)

Often asymptomatic primary infection before age 5 years, 3- to 5-day incubation period

Generally unilateral but can be bilateral (i.e., immunocompromised host)

Seropositivity to HSV is 25% by age 4 years and 100% by age 60 years

Congenital: (see Chapter 5, Pediatrics/Strabismus)

Vesicular blepharitis: primary or secondary HSV; lymphadenopathy does not occur in recurrences; perilimbal involvement is atypical, dendrite uncommon

Acute unilateral follicular conjunctivitis: primary or recurrent HSV; may mimic and often misdiagnosed as EKC; usually punctate epithelial keratitis near limbus, preauricular lymphadenopathy; may develop dendrite and pseudomembrane, may have vesicular skin eruption; bulbar conjunctival ulceration is rare but specific

Primary HSV epithelial keratitis: one or multiple small dendrites, stromal infiltrates; no conjunctivitis; heals in 1-2 weeks with corneal scarring; lid lesions occur (uncommon in recurrences except in children) but without scarring; may have lid margin ulceration (ulcerative blepharitis); associated with decreased corneal sensation and patchy iris atrophy near pupillary margin
> *Cultures:* positive in 75%
> *Pathology:* intranuclear viral inclusions and multinucleated giant cells with Giemsa stain
> *Prognosis:* risk of recurrence is 30% within 2 years; can be induced by many stimuli (stress, sun exposure, hormonal changes, fever, corneal trauma or surgery)

Recurrent HSV: caused by reactivation of latent virus in trigeminal (Gasserian) ganglion; four presentations:
> *Epithelial keratitis:* infectious dendritic ulcer caused by live virus in basal epithelium (Table 7.1)
> > Four lesions:
> > **VESICLES:** clear cystic lesions that coalesce to form dendrite
> > **DENDRITIC ULCER:** branching linear lesion with central trough (stains with fluorescein), swollen heaped-up borders containing active virus (stain with rose bengal or lissamine green), and terminal bulbs (accumulations of vesicular cells); may have stromal edema or infiltrate, iritis (few keratic precipitates [KP]).
> > **GEOGRAPHIC ULCER:** enlarged, nonlinear dendritic ulcer with scalloped borders containing live virus
> > **MARGINAL ULCER:** stromal infiltrate under a limbal dendrite with adjacent limbal injection (no clear

zone as seen in staph marginal keratitis); may have conjunctival dendrite(s)
> > **TREATMENT:** topical antiviral (trifluridine [Viroptic] 9 ×/day, ganciclovir [Zirgan 5 ×/day, or vidarabine [Vira A] or idoxuridine 5 ×/day; use until ulcer heals [1–2 weeks], then taper for 1 week; beware of toxicity from overuse [>2–3 weeks]), cycloplegia, consider débridement and oral antivirals (acyclovir, famciclovir, or valacyclovir)
> > Dendrite usually resolves in 1 week; if still present after 10 days, possible resistance, so switch medication. As the lesion heals, a dendritic shape epitheliopathy persists for several weeks (which should not be treated with antiviral medication)
> > Antiviral toxicity (idoxuridine > vidarabine > trifluridine > acyclovir/ganciclovir): punctate epithelial keratopathy, follicular conjunctivitis, indolent corneal ulceration, preauricular lymphadenopathy with idoxuridine, punctal stenosis
> > Steroids reduce scarring; taper very slowly, critical dose variable (may need steroids for years); potentiate but do not activate live virus
> > Without treatment, 25% of epithelial keratitis resolves in 1 week and 50% resolves in 2 weeks, but increased risk of stromal involvement with scarring, neovascularization, and decreased vision
> *Stromal keratitis* (immune or interstitial keratitis): immunologic reaction caused by recurrent infection in 20%-30% of patients with dendritic ulcer within 5 years. Hallmarks are stromal infiltrate, neovascularization, and scarring
> > **NONNECROTIZING (DISCIFORM) KERATITIS:** inflammatory reaction within endothelium with secondary focal nummular stromal edema as a result of delayed hypersensitivity reaction
> > Localized fine KP, no necrosis; may have iritis, increased IOP (trabeculitis)
> > If severe: diffuse stromal edema, Descemet folds; may have hypopyon, rarely corneal vascularization
> > Culture negative
> > PATHOLOGY: granulomatous reaction, sometimes with retrocorneal membrane
> > TREATMENT: topical steroid (cover with antiviral to prevent epithelial recurrence and antibiotic ointment to prevent secondary bacterial infection); consider topical cyclosporine
> > **NECROTIZING KERATITIS:** rare; antigen–antibody complement-mediated reaction to rapid viral replication in stroma
> > Ulceration with infiltrate and thinning, stromal inflammation, epithelial defect, AC reaction; may perforate, may be difficult to distinguish from bacterial or fungal keratitis
> > TREATMENT: steroid and antiviral; consider cyclosporine or amniotic membrane transplant
> *Endotheliitis:* inflammatory reaction to live virus in the endothelium with varying degrees of isolated stromal edema and stellate KP; can be disciform (round), linear, or diffuse (limbus to limbus); may develop hypopyon, rubeosis, spontaneous hyphema, elevated IOP
> > **TREATMENT:** topical steroid plus oral antiviral; consider oral steroid

Table 7.1	Comparison of herpetic epithelial keratitis	
Lesion	**HSV dendrite**	**VZV pseudodendrite**
Appearance	Delicate, fine, lacy ulcer	Coarse, ropy, elevated, "painted-on" lesion
		Smaller, less branching than HSV dendrite
	Terminal bulbs	Blunt ends (no terminal bulbs)
	Epithelial cells slough	Epithelial cells are swollen and heaped-up
Staining	Base with fluorescein	Poor with fluorescein and rose bengal
	Edges with rose bengal	
Treatment	Do not use steroids	Good response to steroids

HSV, Herpes simplex virus; *VZV*, varicella-zoster virus. Note: Active viral replication in epithelial lesions occurs in both HSV and VZV. Other causes of pseudodendrite: *Acanthamoeba*, tyrosinemia II, epithelial healing ridge

Neurotrophic keratopathy (metaherpetic ulcer): chronic sterile macroulceration as a result of impaired corneal sensation and decreased tear production

Oval-shaped with smooth edges, no staining with rose bengal at edge; no stromal inflammation; may have thinning and scarring

TREATMENT: lubrication; may take months to heal owing to damaged basement membrane, impaired corneal innervation, and abnormal tear film; may require tarsorrhaphy, bandage contact lens, autologous serum drops, amniotic membrane, conjunctival flap

Diagnosis:

Papanicolaou smear: intranuclear inclusion bodies (Lipschütz bodies), Cowdry type A (eosinophilic) intranuclear inclusions

Tzanck prep: multinucleated giant cells with Giemsa stain

Culture: only 60% positive if swab active dendrite

Immunofluorescence: detects HSV antigen

Treatment: depends on lesion (see above); preferred topical antiviral is now ganciclovir (Zirgan); corneal transplant (penetrating keratoplasty [PK]) for visually significant scarring

Herpetic Eye Disease Study (HEDS):

STROMAL DISEASE: treatment with topical steroids and trifluridine (Viroptic) is better than Viroptic alone (prednisolone acetate 8 ×/day and Viroptic qid x 1 week, then 10-week taper; supports immune mediated mechanism for stromal disease); no benefit to concomitant oral acyclovir

IRITIS: acyclovir (400 mg 5 ×/day), in addition to topical Viroptic and steroid, is better than topicals alone

PROPHYLAXIS: acyclovir (400 mg bid x 1 year) decreases by 50% risk of recurrent HSV keratitis

Complications: uveitis, glaucoma, episcleritis, scleritis, secondary bacterial keratitis, corneal scarring and neovascularization, corneal perforation, iris atrophy, punctal stenosis

MAJOR CLINICAL STUDY

Herpetic Eye Disease Study (HEDS)

Objective:

Five trials to evaluate the role of steroids and antiviral medication in the treatment and prevention of ocular HSV disease:

1. Efficacy of oral acyclovir (ACV) in treating stromal keratitis (non-necrotizing [disciform] and necrotizing): 10-week course of ACV 400 mg 5 ×/day or placebo, in addition to topical steroids and trifluridine
2. Efficacy of topical corticosteroids in treating stromal keratitis: 10-week tapering course of prednisolone phosphate or placebo in addition to topical trifluridine (prednisolone acetate 8 ×/day and trifluridine [Viroptic]

qid × 1 week, then gradual taper over 10 weeks)
3. Efficacy of oral ACV in treating iridocyclitis: 10-week course of ACV 400 mg 5 ×/day or placebo, in addition to topical steroids and trifluridine
4. Efficacy of oral ACV in preventing stromal keratitis or iridocyclitis in patients with epithelial keratitis: 3-week course of ACV 400 mg 5 ×/day or placebo, in addition to topical trifluridine
5. Efficacy of oral ACV in preventing recurrent ocular HSV disease: 12-month course of ACV 400 mg bid or placebo and 6-month observation period for patients with a history of ocular HSV within the preceding year
6. Determinants of recurrent HSV keratitis: analyzed the placebo group from the acyclovir prevention trial

Results:

1. Oral ACV, in addition to topical steroids and trifluridine (Viroptic), for the treatment of stromal keratitis did not improve the number of treatment failures, time to resolution of keratitis, or 6-month BCVA
2. Topical corticosteroids reduced the risk of persistent or progressive stromal keratitis by 68% and shortened the duration of keratitis
3. Trial was stopped because of slow recruitment. Treatment failure occurred in 50% of the ACV group versus 68% of the placebo group
4. Oral ACV did not reduce the risk of stromal keratitis or iridocyclitis development in patients with epithelial keratitis. Stromal keratitis or iridocyclitis developed in 11% of patients in the ACV group vs. 10% in the placebo group, and such an occurrence was more common in those with a previous history of stromal keratitis or iritis (23% vs. 9% without previous history)
5. Oral ACV reduced the risk of recurrent ocular disease during the treatment period (19% vs. 32%), especially in the stromal keratitis subset (14% vs. 28%). Recurrence of nonocular HSV disease was also lower in the treated group (19% vs. 36%). No rebound in the rate of disease was seen during the 6-month observation period after treatment
6. In the placebo group of the previous trial, 18% developed epithelial keratitis, and 18% developed stromal keratitis. Previous epithelial keratitis did not significantly affect the subsequent risk of epithelial keratitis; previous stromal keratitis significantly increased the subsequent risk of stromal keratitis (10 ×)

Conclusions:

1. Oral ACV, in addition to topical steroid and trifluridine (Viroptic), is not useful for the treatment of stromal keratitis
2. Topical corticosteroids are beneficial for the treatment of stromal keratitis
3. Results were not statistically significant but suggest a possible benefit of oral ACV for the treatment of iridocyclitis
4. In patients with epithelial keratitis, a 3-week course of oral ACV has no apparent benefit in preventing

stromal disease or iridocyclitis

5. Oral ACV prophylaxis significantly reduces the risk of recurrent ocular and orofacial HSV disease, especially in patients with previous stromal keratitis

6. In patients with ocular HSV disease in the previous year, a history of epithelial keratitis is not a risk factor for recurrent epithelial keratitis, but a history of stromal keratitis increases the risk of subsequent stromal keratitis, and this risk is strongly associated with the number of previous episodes

Herpes Zoster Ophthalmicus (HZO)

Herpes zoster involvement of first branch of trigeminal nerve CN 5 (V_1)

Acute, painful, unilateral dermatomal vesicular eruption (obeys midline) with prodrome; new lesions occur for ~1 week with resolution in 2-6 weeks

May occur without rash (zoster sine herpete)

After chickenpox, 20% to 30% risk of developing varicella-zoster (shingles); increased incidence and severity with age >60 years, up to 50% at age 85 years; 10%-25% have HZO, and 50% of these have ocular involvement if untreated

Most common single dermatome is CN 5: ophthalmic (V_1) > maxillary (V_2) > mandibular (V_3)

3 branches of ophthalmic division: frontal nerve > nasociliary nerve > lacrimal nerve

Hutchinson sign: skin lesion on tip or side of nose (nasociliary nerve) is a strong indication of ocular involvement

Symptoms: 2- to 3-day prodrome (fever, malaise, headache, paresthesia)

Findings:
Lid: vesicles, cicatricial changes (ectropion, entropion, madarosis, ptosis), trichiasis, lagophthalmos, blepharitis
Conjunctiva: follicular conjunctivitis, vesicles, pseudo-membranes, symblepharon
Cornea: keratitis (65%) (see Table 7.1)
   PUNCTATE EPITHELIAL: precursor to pseudodendrite; viral replication with epithelial destruction
   PSEUDODENDRITIC: blunt ends, no terminal bulbs, no ulceration, minimal staining; self-limited (appears within a few days of rash, resolves in 4–6 days)
   INFLAMMATORY ULCERATION: immune response; often peripheral; may lead to perforation
   MUCUS PLAQUES: can occur at any time, even months or years later; vary in size, shape, and location daily; sharply demarcated gray-white lesion on epithelial surface; mild fluorescein staining, vivid rose bengal staining; interference with normal mucus–epithelial interaction, no active virus replication; associated with decreased corneal sensation, stromal keratitis, anterior segment inflammation, increased intraocular pressure, and cataracts
   STROMAL: occurs in 50% with epithelial disease within first 1-3 weeks; nummular subepithelial infiltrates

and disciform keratitis beneath initial keratitis; immune response (may develop ring)
   ENDOTHELIITIS: occurs in 10% with epithelial disease; keratouveitis with focal stromal edema, KP, anterior chamber cells and flare; viral infection or immune response
   INTERSTITIAL: corneal vascularization and scarring
   NEUROTROPHIC: occurs in 20%; caused by decreased corneal sensation; leads to ulceration, stromal scarring, pannus, exposure keratopathy (as a result of lid abnormalities)
   EXPOSURE KERATOPATHY: caused by lid scarring, lagophthalmos, and neurotrophic cornea may develop severe dry eye with ulceration and scarring
Episcleritis/scleritis: limbal vasculitis, sclerokeratitis, scleral atrophy, posterior scleritis
Iris: segmental atrophy as a result of vasculitis with ischemia and necrosis; Argyll-Robertson pupil (ciliary ganglion involvement)
Uveitis: can occur months later; may have elevated IOP, 45% develop glaucoma; may develop cataract
Retina: central retinal artery occlusion, acute retinal necrosis (ARN); progressive outer retinal necrosis (PORN) in patients with AIDS
Optic nerve: ischemic optic neuropathy
CN palsies: CN 3, 4, or 6 palsy occurs in 25%; self-limited; may involve pupil; may have orbital apex syndrome (optic neuropathy, ophthalmoplegia, and anesthesia) from vasculitis
Syndromes:
   RAMSAY HUNT SYNDROME: CN 5 and 7 involvement with facial paralysis
   ZOSTER SINE HERPETE: zoster-type dermatomal pain without rash

Diagnosis: characteristic skin lesions, Tzanck prep, serology (IgG antibodies), culture, ELISA

Prevention: vaccination in patients ≥50 years old (safety and efficacy demonstrated in Shingles Prevention Study); Zostavax reduces incidence (51%), severity and duration of zoster; reduces incidence of pain (61%) and postherpetic neuralgia (67%), but efficacy decreases with increasing age and may need to be readministered after 10 years. Newer recombinant Shingrix vaccine more effective (97% in patients 50–69 years old, >91% in patients >69 years old; 89% against HZO)

Treatment:
Oral antiviral within 72 hours of rash: acyclovir (800 mg 5 ×/day), famciclovir (Famvir, 500 mg tid), or valacyclovir (Valtrex, 1000 mg tid) × 7 days; IV acyclovir × 10-14 days if immunocompromised
   Reduces time course (formation of new lesions, healing of lesions, period of viral shedding) and risk and severity of ocular involvement. Famvir and Valtrex reduce risk, duration, and severity of postherpetic neuralgia
   Despite treatment, 25% develop chronic or recurrent HZO within 5 years; overall recurrence rate as high as 51%

Oral steroid: prednisone 60 mg qd × 1 week, then 30 mg
qd × 1 week, then 15 mg qd × 1 week
Reduces time course, duration and severity of acute
pain, and incidence of postherpetic neuralgia
For intraocular and ocular surface involvement: topical steroid (may require indefinitely to prevent recurrence),
cycloplegic, and antibiotic; may require IOP control
and treatment of ocular complications; consider low-
dose suppressive therapy with valacyclovir ([Valtrex]
500 mg PO qd) or acyclovir ([Zovirax] 400 mg PO bid)
to reduce risk of HZO recurrence
For postherpetic neuralgia: capsaicin cream (Zostrix;
depletes substance P), cimetidine, tricyclic antidepressants (amitriptyline, desipramine), carbamazepine (Tegretol), gabapentin (Neurontin), pregaba-
lin (Lyrica), lidocaine (Lidoderm patch), opioids,
Benadryl; consider nerve block, Botox map injections

Complications: occur in 50%; most common is
postherpetic neuralgia
Postherpetic neuralgia (PHN): neuropathic pain syndrome
that persists or occurs after resolution of rash; risk factors include age >60 years, severity of prodromal and
acute pain, severity of rash, and HZO. Occurs in 10%
of all patients with zoster, 10%-20% with HZO; 50%
resolve within 1 month, 80% within 1 year
Meningoencephalitis and myelitis: rare; occurs 7-10 days
after rash with fever, headache, cranial nerve palsies,
hallucinations, altered sensorium; most common in
patients with cranial zoster, dissemination, or immunocompromised (may be fatal in AIDS)
Granulomatous arteritis: contralateral hemiplegia weeks
to months after acute disease; involves middle cerebral
artery; 65% are >60 years old; 25% mortality

Chickenpox

Findings: papillary conjunctivitis, "pock" lesions on bulbar
conjunctiva and at limbus, keratitis (dendritic, disciform,
interstitial)

Fungi

Types:
Molds (filamentous): form hyphae
SEPTATE: most common cause of fungal keratitis; most
common in southern/southwestern United States
Fusarium (F. solani is most virulent), *Aspergillus,
Curvularia, Paecilomyces, Penicillium, Phialophora*
NONSEPTATE: *Mucor* (rare cause of keratitis)
Yeast: Candida (most common cause of mycotic ocular
infections in northern United States), *Cryptococcus*
(associated with endogenous endophthalmitis; rarely
keratitis)
Dimorphic fungi: grow as yeast or mold
Histoplasma, Blastomyces, Coccidioides

Risk factors:
Molds: corneal injury especially from tree branch or vegetable material, soft CL wear
Yeast: therapeutic soft CL wear, topical steroid use, nonhealing epithelial defect, decreased host resistance

Findings: satellite infiltrates, feathery edges, endothelial
plaque; can penetrate Descemet membrane

Treatment: topical antifungal (natamycin 5%
[filamentous], clotrimazole *[Aspergillus]*, amphotericin B
0.15% [yeast], flucytosine 1%, ketoconazole 2%, miconazole
1%, voriconazole 1%, itraconazole 1%, fluconazole 0.5%);
cycloplegic
Topical natamycin is better than voriconazole for filamentous fungal ulcers, particularly *Fusarium* (Mycotic Ulcer
Treatment Trail [MUTT] I conclusion)
No benefit of adding oral voriconazole to topical antifungal for severe filamentous fungal ulcers, but consider
for *Fusarium* (MUTT II conclusion)
Corneal epithelium is significant barrier to natamycin
penetration
Topical steroids contraindicated

Acanthamoeba

Exists as trophozoite or cyst; 22 species

Initially misdiagnosed as HSV in 90%

Risk factors: cleaning soft CL with homemade saline
solution; swimming or hot tubbing while wearing CL

Prevention: heat disinfectant (75°C)

Findings: epithelial cysts (can look like EKC with
subepithelial infiltrates and punctate keratopathy), perineural
infiltrate (enlarged corneal nerves, decreased corneal
sensation, pain [perineuritis]), ring-shaped infiltrate, corneal
edema, pseudodendrite, iritis, hypopyon (30%–40%), scleritis;
may perforate

Diagnosis: calcofluor white, Giemsa stain, culture
(nonnutrient agar with *Escherichia coli* overlay; can grow on
blood or chocolate agar but not as well), confocal microscopy

Pathology: oval amoebic double-walled cysts in stroma

Treatment: débridement if infection limited to epithelium
(may be curative), combination of topical agents
Antibacterial: neomycin or paromomycin (Humatin)
1% q2 hours initially
Antifungal: miconazole 1% or clotrimazole 1% q1 hour
initially, and oral voriconazole, ketoconazole or itra-
conazole
Antiparasitic: polyhexamethylene biguanide (PHMB;
Baquacil; swimming pool cleaner) 0.02%-0.06% or
chlorhexidine 0.02%, and propamidine isethionate
(Brolene) 0.1% or hexamidine (Desomedine) 0.1%
q1 hour initially
Steroid: controversial
Recurrence after penetrating keratoplasty in 30%

Microsporidia

Obligate intracellular spore-forming parasite *(Encephalitozoon
hellem, Encephalitozoon cuniculi)*

Keratitis in HIV-positive patients

Symptoms: blurred vision, photophobia, foreign body sensation

Findings: diffuse punctate epithelial erosions and intraepithelial opacities; may have sinusitis

Diagnosis: epithelial cells with cytoplasmic inclusions on Giemsa stain

Treatment: topical fumagillin (10 mg/mL) up to q2h or voriconazole 1% q2h x 2 weeks, then taper slowly for 1 month

Onchocerciasis

(See Chapter 8, Uveitis)

Leprosy

(See Chapter 8, Uveitis)

Epstein-Barr virus (EBV)

Findings: multifocal stromal keratitis; may rarely have episcleritis, follicular conjunctivitis, uveitis, optic neuritis

Diagnosis:
Antibodies: viral capsid antigen IgM and IgG and early antigen-diffuse (EA-D) peak at 6-12 weeks; viral capsid antigen (VCA)-IgM and Epstein-Barr nuclear antigen (EBNA) are detectable for life; heterophile antibodies (IgM that reacts to horse and sheep blood cells) peak at 2-3 weeks and last 1 year (Monospot test)
Lymphocytosis: occurs in 70%; peaks at 2-3 weeks
Liver enzymes: elevated

Ectasias

Keratoconus

Bilateral in 90%; onset often in childhood/early adolescence

Associations:
Systemic conditions: atopy (eye rubbing), Down syndrome, connective tissue disease (Ehlers-Danlos syndrome, Brittle cornea syndrome, Marfan syndrome, osteogenesis imperfecta)
Ocular conditions: aniridia, retinitis pigmentosa, VKC, Leber congenital amaurosis, ectopia lentis, floppy eyelid syndrome, congenital hereditary endothelial dystrophy (CHED), posterior polymorphous dystrophy (PPCD)

Findings: in early keratoconus, slit lamp exam is normal. In more advanced disease, findings include inferior corneal protrusion, stromal thinning at cone apex (apical thinning), apical scarring, Fleischer ring (epithelial iron deposition at base of cone), Vogt striae (fine deep striae anterior to Descemet membrane; disappear with external pressure), prominent corneal nerves, oil-droplet reflex (Charleaux sign; with red reflex on ophthalmoscopy), scissors reflex on retinoscopy, Munson sign (angulation of lower lid on downgaze as a result of corneal protrusion), Rizzuti sign

(conical reflection of light from temporal light source on nasal iris); may develop hydrops
Hydrops: acute corneal edema and clouding as a result of break in Descemet membrane; painful or painless; decreased IOP; heals over 6-10 weeks; scarring and corneal flattening can occur, occasionally with stromal neovascularization

Pathology: breaks in Bowman layer, stromal folds, superficial scarring, stromal thinning; Descemet is normal unless hydrops has occurred (breaks with curled edges covered by adjacent endothelial cells and new Descemet)

DDx: contact lens-induced corneal warpage, pellucid marginal degeneration, keratoglobus, EBMD

Diagnosis: corneal topography (irregular astigmatism, central or inferior steepening), keratometry (steep readings, irregular mires), tomography (corneal thinning), epithelial mapping with OCT or high-resolution ultrasound (ArcScan), corneal biomechanics (Corvis, ocular response analyzer [ORA]), genetic testing (Avagen)

Treatment: CL (rigid, piggyback, scleral, hybrid) for visual improvement; rigid CL will not stop progression of disease. Corneal collagen crosslinking (to stop progression), Intacs; penetrating keratoplasty for advanced cases; supportive for hydrops (topical steroids, cycloplegic, bandage contact lens)

Posterior Keratoconus

(See Chapter 5, Pediatrics/Strabismus)

Keratoglobus

Rare, sporadic, globular corneal deformity

Associated with connective tissue disorders, Leber congenital amaurosis

Findings: bilateral corneal thinning, maximal in midperiphery at base of protrusion

Treatment: CL (rigid), penetrating keratoplasty

Pellucid Marginal Degeneration

Onset age 20-40 years; no sex predilection; more common in Europeans and Japanese

Findings: bilateral, inferior corneal thinning with protrusion above thinnest area; no vascularization; acute hydrops rare

Pathology: resembles keratoconus

Diagnosis: corneal topography (irregular, against-the-rule astigmatism with inferior annular/claw/lazy-c pattern of steepening)

Treatment: contact lenses for visual improvement; corneal collagen crosslinking to stop progression. If severe, a large penetrating keratoplasty may be required

Dystrophies

Inherited genetic disorders (usually defective enzyme or structural protein)

AD except macular, gelatinous drop-like, and CHED, which are AR; and Lisch epithelial and X-linked endothelial corneal dystrophies, which are X-linked dominant

Many dystrophies have a mutation of the TGFB1 (also known as BIGH3) gene on chromosome 5; these dystrophies tend to be AD and include granular, lattice type 1 and variants, Reis-Bucklers, and Thiel-Behnke; central cloudy and Fuchs endothelial corneal dystrophies are of unknown etiology (some may be AD), and epithelial basement membrane dystrophy is mostly degenerative

Onset by age 20 years, except epithelial basement membrane dystrophy (ages 30–40), pre-Descemet (ages 30–40), and Fuchs (ages 40–50)

Not associated with systemic diseases, except Schnyder (associated with hyperlipoproteinemia), and lattice type 2 (not considered a corneal dystrophy; Meretoja syndrome associated with systemic amyloidosis)

Affect central cornea only, except Meesmann, macular, fleck, congenital stromal corneal dystrophy (CSCD), and CHED, which extend to limbus

The classification of corneal dystrophies has traditionally been anatomic according to the corneal layer most affected (anterior, stromal, and endothelial). This was changed in 2008 by the International Committee for Classification of Corneal Dystrophies (IC3D), which divided the major corneal dystrophies into four categories: epithelial and subepithelial dystrophies, Bowman layer dystrophies, stromal dystrophies, and Descemet membrane and endothelial dystrophies. In 2015, the IC3D revised the classification to reflect the involvement of cellular layers (excluding Bowman layer and Descemet membrane): epithelial and subepithelial dystrophies, epithelial-stromal (TGFB1) dystrophies, stromal dystrophies, and endothelial dystrophies.

Epithelial and Subepithelial Dystrophies

EBMD; Cogan Microcystic Epithelial Dystrophy; Map-Dot-Fingerprint Dystrophy; ABMD (Majority Degenerative; AD in Isolated Familial Cases)

Most common anterior corneal dystrophy

Usually bilateral, can be asymmetric; primarily affects middle-aged women

Symptoms more common in those >30 years old

Symptoms: usually asymptomatic; may have pain, redness, tearing, irritation (recurrent epithelial erosions), or decreased vision (subepithelial scarring)

Findings: irregular and often loose epithelium with characteristic appearance (map, dot, fingerprint):

Map lines: subepithelial connective tissue

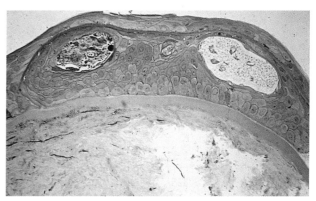

Figure 7.11 Anterior basement membrane dystrophy demonstrating cysts and aberrant production of basement membrane material in the epithelium. (From Yanoff M, Fine BS. *Ocular Pathology*, 5th ed. St Louis: Mosby; 2002.)

Microcysts: white, putty-like dots (degenerated epithelial cells trapped in abnormal epithelium)

Fingerprints: parallel lines of basement membrane separating tongues of reduplicated epithelium

May develop recurrent erosions (10% with the dystrophy get erosions, 50% with erosions have the dystrophy) or decreased vision or monocular diplopia from subepithelial scarring (irregular astigmatism)

Pathology: epithelial reduplication with excess subepithelial and intraepithelial production of basement membrane material and collagen (caused by poor epithelial adhesion to BM) (Fig. 7.11)

Treatment: none unless symptomatic. For erosions, treat with lubrication, hypertonic saline (Muro 128 5% ointment qhs × 3–12 months); if recurs, consider bandage contact lens, epithelial débridement, anterior stromal puncture/reinforcement, diamond burr (débride and polish Bowman layer), laser (PTK with excimer laser, or micropuncture with Nd:YAG laser [1 mJ, aim just below epithelium]); also, consider treatment with MMP-9 inhibitors (doxycycline 50 mg PO bid × 2 months and topical steroids tid × 2–3 weeks); débridement for subepithelial scarring

Epithelial Recurrent Erosion Dystrophies (EREDs) (AD)

Onset early childhood

3 variants: Franceschetti corneal dystrophy (FRCD), dystrophia smolandiensis (DS), dystrophia helsinglandica (DH)

Symptoms: decreased vision, photophobia, tearing

Findings: recurrent epithelial erosions lasting 1-7 days; less frequent and severe by age 30-40 years, but develop central subepithelial opacity, fibrosis, and keloid-like elevated scar

Pathology: destruction and absence of Bowman layer with connective tissue pannus (FRCD); keloid-like deposit of amyloid (stains with Congo red) (DS)

Subepithelial Mucinous Corneal Dystrophy (SMCD) (AD)

Onset in 1st decade of life

Symptoms: pain, photophobia, tearing from epithelial erosions; decreased vision in adolescence

Findings: recurrent corneal erosions, diffuse subepithelial opacities and haze

Pathology: subepithelial deposits of fine fibrillar substance

Meesmann Corneal Dystrophy (MECD) (AD)

Mapped to chromosomes 12q13 *(KRT3)* and 17q12 *(KRT12)* (Stocker-Holt variant)

Appears early in life

Minimal symptoms; may have mildly reduced vision, photophobia

Stocker-Holt variant more severe

Findings: tiny epithelial vesicles, most numerous interpalpebrally, extend to limbus, may have epithelial erosions

Pathology: epithelial cells contain PAS-positive material (peculiar substance); thickened epithelial basement membrane (Fig. 7.12)

No treatment

Lisch Epithelial Corneal Dystrophy (LECD; Band-Shaped or Whorled Microcystic Dystrophy of the Corneal Epithelium) (X-Linked Dominant)

Mapped to chromosome Xp22.3

Onset in childhood, slowly progressive

Symptoms: asymptomatic or blurred vision

Findings: various patterns of gray opacities (whorl, radial, band, flame, feather, or club-shaped)

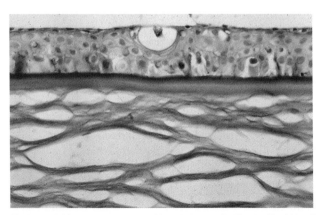

Figure 7.12 Meesmann dystrophy with periodic acid-Schiff stain. (From Yanoff M, Fine BS. *Ocular Pathology*, 5th ed. St Louis: Mosby; 2002.)

Pathology: vacuolated cells containing glycogen

Gelatinous Drop-Like Corneal Dystrophy (GDLD) (AR)

Mapped to chromosome 1p32 *(TACSTD2;* formerly *M1S1)*

Rare; onset in 1st-2nd decade of life, more common in Japanese; not associated with systemic amyloidosis

Symptoms: decreased vision, pain, photophobia, tearing

Findings: progressive central, mulberry-like, subepithelial deposits and stromal opacity; recurs after treatment (keratectomy and keratoplasty)

Pathology: absence of Bowman layer; amyloid (subepithelial and stromal)

Epithelial-Stromal (TGFB1) Dystrophies

Reis-Bucklers Corneal Dystrophy (Corneal Dystrophy of Bowman Layer Type I [CDB1]) (AD)

Mapped to chromosome 5q31 *(TGFB1)*

Onset in childhood

Symptoms: pain (recurrent epithelial erosions), decreased vision

Findings: irregular, diffuse, geographic gray-white opacities at Bowman layer and stroma, begin centrally with clear interruptions, then more confluent extending to limbus and deeper stroma; epithelial erosions, corneal scarring

Pathology: absence of Bowman layer and replacement by granular highly reflective irregular deposits extending into stroma; stain with Masson trichrome

Treatment: PTK, penetrating keratoplasty (recurrence in the corneal transplant is common)

Thiel-Behnke Corneal Dystrophy (TBCD; Corneal Dystrophy of Bowman Layer Type II [CDB2]; Honeycomb-Shaped Corneal Dystrophy; Curly Fibers Corneal Dystrophy; Waardenburg-Jonkers Corneal Dystrophy) (AD)

Mapped to chromosomes 5q31 *(TGFB1)*

Onset in early childhood

Less visual loss and does not recur in graft as early and extensively (compared with Reis-Bucklers [CDB type I])

Symptoms: pain (recurrent epithelial erosions), gradual decreased vision

Findings: flecks and irregular scattered opacities at Bowman layer progress to reticular or honeycomb pattern; epithelial erosions, corneal scarring

Pathology: Bowman layer is replaced by fibrocellular material in a pathognomonic wavy "sawtooth" pattern; curly fibers on electron microscopy

Lattice Corneal Dystrophy Type I (LCD1; Biber-Haab-Dimmer Corneal Dystrophy) and Variants (AD)

Mapped to chromosome 5q31 *(TGFB1)*

Classic form of lattice dystrophy: onset in 1st decade of life; starts centrally, spares periphery, no systemic amyloid

Four variants (present later in life): type IIIA (5th-7th decade of life, epithelial erosions, thicker lattice lines extending to limbus), type I/IIIA (thinner lattice lines), type IV (7th-9th decade of life, smaller lattice lines in deep stroma, no epithelial erosions), and polymorphic amyloidosis (no lattice lines)

Meretoja syndrome (Finnish familial amyloidosis; formerly Lattice corneal dystrophy type II [LCD2; Gelsolin type]) (AD): not a true corneal dystrophy. Mapped to chromosome 9q34 *(GSN)*; Finnish descent; systemic amyloidosis syndrome (facial mask; dry, lax skin; blepharochalasis, dermatochalasis; pendulous ears; cranial and peripheral nerve palsies); corneal lattice lines more peripheral and moves centrally

Symptoms: pain (recurrent epithelial erosions), decreased vision by 4th decade of life

Findings: branching refractile lines in anterior stroma (best seen in retroillumination), central subepithelial white dots, subepithelial diffuse haze with ground-glass appearance, peripheral cornea typically clear (depends on type); eventually epithelial erosions with scarring

Pathology: amyloid deposits, stain with Congo red, thioflavin T, metachromatic with crystal violet, apple-green birefringence and dichroism with polarization microscopy (Fig. 7.13)

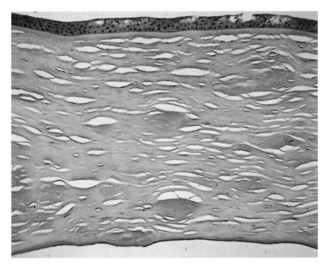

Figure 7.13 Deposits in lattice dystrophy. (From Yanoff M, Fine BS. *Ocular Pathology*, 5th ed. St Louis: Mosby; 2002.)

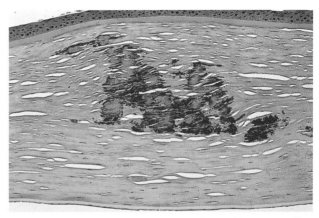

Figure 7.14 Deposits in granular dystrophy stain red with trichrome. (From Yanoff M, Fine BS. *Ocular Pathology*, 5th ed. St Louis: Mosby; 2002.)

Treatment: PTK, penetrating keratoplasty (recurrence more likely than in macular or granular, but less likely than in Reis-Bucklers)

Granular Corneal Dystrophy Type I (GCD1; Groenouw Corneal Dystrophy Type I) (AD)

Most common stromal dystrophy

Mapped to chromosome 5q31 *(TGFB1)*

Deposits present in 1st decade of life, can remain asymptomatic for decades

Symptoms: glare, photophobia, decreased vision; pain (recurrent epithelial erosions)

Findings: discrete focal, white, granular deposits with breadcrumb or snowflake appearance in central anterior stroma, intervening clear areas; epithelial erosions

Pathology: hyaline deposits (from deep epithelium to Descemet membrane), stain with Masson trichrome (Fig 7.14)

Treatment: PTK, penetrating keratoplasty

Granular Corneal Dystrophy Type II (GCD2; Avellino Dystrophy; Combined Granular-Lattice Dystrophy) (AD)

Mapped to chromosome 5q31 *(TGFB1)*; later identified in family from Avellino, Italy

Onset usually in teens or early adulthood, may occur in 1st decade of life; slowly progressive

Findings: white dots with small spokes, discoid or ring-shaped patches, spiky deposits (star, icicle, spider-shaped), and short lines or dashes (rarely cross); dots and rings appear early in anterior stroma, dashes occur later in deeper stroma; stromal haze; may get erosions

Pathology: hyaline and amyloid deposits from basal epithelium to deep stroma; stain with Masson trichrome and Congo red

Mnemonic: **M**arilyn **M**onroe **A**lways **G**ets **H**er **M**en in **LA** **C**ounty

Refers to name of dystrophy, substance deposited in cornea, special stain (for the three classic "stromal" dystrophies):

Macular, **M**ucopolysaccharide, **A**lcian blue
Granular, **H**yaline, **M**asson trichrome
Lattice, **A**myloid, **C**ongo red

Stromal Dystrophies

Macular Corneal Dystrophy (MCD; Groenouw Corneal Dystrophy Type II) (AR)

Mapped to chromosome 16q22 *(CHST6)*; error in synthesis of keratan sulfate

3 variants (type I, type IA, type II) based on immunoreactivity of keratan sulfate in cornea and serum

Most severe but less common than granular or lattice dystrophies

Deposits present in 1st decade of life

Symptoms: severe decreased vision in 2nd-3rd decade of life

Findings: gray-white stromal flecklike opacities at all levels extending to periphery with diffuse haze (no intervening clear spaces), develop central corneal thinning and guttata; epithelial erosions rare

Pathology: mucopolysaccharide (glycosaminoglycan) deposits, stain with Alcian blue and colloidal iron (Fig. 7.15)

Treatment: PTK, penetrating keratoplasty

Schnyder corneal dystrophy (SCD; Schnyder crystalline corneal dystrophy) (AD)

Mapped to chromosome 1p36 *(UBIAD1)*

Onset usually 2nd-3rd decade

Slowly progressive, rarely reduces vision enough to require corneal transplantation

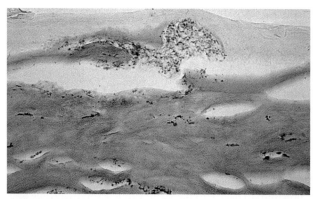

Figure 7.15 Deposits in macular dystrophy stain with Alcian blue. (From Yanoff M, Fine BS. *Ocular Pathology*, 5th ed. St Louis: Mosby; 2002.)

Symptoms: decreased vision, glare

Findings: age dependent, only 50% have corneal crystals (may be unilateral, rarely regress, occur late)

≤23 years old: ringlike central corneal opacity, comma-shaped subepithelial crystals
23-38 years old: arcus lipoides
>38 years old: diffuse midperipheral stromal haze
May have hyperlipoproteinemia (type IIa, III, or IV)

Pathology: cholesterol and neutral fat deposits, stain with oil-red-O and Sudan black

Can recur in graft

Congenital Stromal Corneal Dystrophy (CSCD)

(See Chapter 5, Pediatrics/Strabismus)

Fleck Corneal Dystrophy (FCD; Francois-Neetens Corneal Dystrophy) (AD)

Mapped to chromosome 2q34 *(PIKFYVE;* previously known as *PIP5K3)*

Congenital, nonprogressive may be asymmetric or unilateral

Vision usually not affected

Findings: discrete, flat, gray-white, dandruff-like speck and ring-shaped opacities, scattered throughout stroma extending to periphery; may have decreased corneal sensation

Associated with limbal dermoid, keratoconus, central cloudy dystrophy of Francois, punctate cortical lens changes, pseudoxanthoma elasticum, atopy

Pathology: glycosaminoglycan and lipid deposits, stain with Alcian blue and colloidal iron (GAGs), Sudan black and oil-red-O (lipid)

Posterior Amorphous Corneal Dystrophy (PACD) (AD)

Mapped to chromosome 12q21.33 *(KERA, LUM, DCN,* and *EPYC)*

Early in life, minimally progressive or nonprogressive

Vision mildly affected

Findings: diffuse gray-white sheetlike stromal opacities concentrated in posterior stroma, mostly centrally but extends to periphery

Associated with corneal thinning (as thin as 380 μm), corneal flattening (<41 D), hyperopia, prominent Schwalbe line, fine iris processes, pupillary remnants, iridocorneal adhesions, corectopia, pseudopolycoria; no association with glaucoma

Central Cloudy Dystrophy of FRANCOIS (CCDF)

Unknown inheritance (may be AD); may be posterior crocodile shagreen (corneal degeneration)

Nonprogressive, asymptomatic; onset in 1st decade of life

Findings: multiple, nebulous, polygonal gray areas separated by cracklike intervening clear zones (indistinguishable from posterior crocodile shagreen); most dense centrally and posteriorly, fade anteriorly and peripherally

Pre-Descemet Corneal Dystrophy (PDCD; Deep Filiform Dystrophy) (AD)

Onset in 4th-7th decade of life; several subgroups: isolated (hereditary or degenerative), subtype (punctiform and polychromatic; AD), and associated with X-linked ichthyosis (mapped to chromosome Xp22.31 [STS])

Usually asymptomatic

Findings: central, annular, or diffuse fine, gray deep stromal polymorphic opacities

Pathology: lipid deposits in posterior stromal keratocytes

Endothelial Dystrophies

Fuchs Endothelial Corneal Dystrophy (FECD) (Unknown, AD)

Early onset (mapped to chromosome 1p34.3-32 [FECD1]) or late onset (mapped to chromosomes 13pter-q12.13 [FECD2], 18q21 [FECD3], 20p13-12 [FECD4], 5q33.1-35.2 [FECD5], 10p11.2 [FECD6], 9p24.1-22.1 [FECD7], and 15q25 [FECD8])

Variable expressivity and incomplete penetrance, may be sporadic; most commonly inheritance unknown

Onset usually in 4th decade of life or after, early variant onset in 1st decade; female > male (approximately 3:1); progressive

Symptoms: blurred vision (initially, only in morning; later, all day); may have pain, photophobia, tearing (ruptured bullae)

Findings: cornea guttata starts centrally, may spread peripherally (stage 1); endothelial decompensation, stromal edema, Descemet folds, endothelial beaten metal appearance with or without pigment dusting (stage 2); epithelial bullae, bullous keratopathy (stage 3); subepithelial fibrosis, scarring, and peripheral superficial vascularization (pannus) (stage 4)

Pathology: hyaline excrescences (guttae) on thickened Descemet membrane, atrophic endothelium with areas of cell dropout, endothelial cell polymegathism and pleomorphism

Treatment: hypertonic ointment, consider topical steroid for mild edema; contact lens or conjunctival flap (Gunderson) for comfort; may require Descemet stripping endothelial keratoplasty (DSEK) or penetrating keratoplasty

Posterior Polymorphous Corneal Dystrophy (PPCD) (AD)

3 types: PPCD1 mapped to chromosome 20p11.2-q11.2; PPCD2 mapped to chromosome 1p34.3-32.3 (COL8A2); PPCD3 mapped to chromosome 10p11.22 (ZEB1)

Minimally or nonprogressive, often asymmetric; occurs early in life

Vision usually normal

Endothelium behaves like epithelium, forming multiple layers with occasional migration of cells into angle causing glaucoma (15%)

Findings: isolated grouped vesicles, geographically shaped discrete gray lesions, broad bands with scalloped and flaky material (railroad tracks) at level of Descemet membrane and endothelium; corneal steepening (>48 D in most PPCD3); may develop stromal edema, corectopia, peripheral iridocorneal adhesions (25%), and increased intraocular pressure (15%)

Pathology: irregular excrescences at level of Descemet membrane surrounded by gray opacification, thickened Descemet membrane, abnormal endothelial cells (resemble epithelial cells; contain keratin, microvilli, desmosomes) with blebs, discontinuities, reduplication

DDx: Haab striae in congenital glaucoma, iridocorneal endothelial (ICE) syndrome

Treatment: penetrating keratoplasty for endothelial decompensation, can recur in graft

Congenital Hereditary Endothelial Dystrophy (CHED)

(See Chapter 5, Pediatrics/Strabismus)

X-Linked Endothelial Corneal Dystrophy (XECD)

(See Chapter 5, Pediatrics/Strabismus)

Miscellaneous

Cornea Guttata

Associated with aging and with corneal endothelial dystrophy

Beaten metal appearance

Most never develop corneal edema

Pathology: thickened Descemet with localized excrescences of collagen; variable endothelial size and shape and reduced number on specular microscopy

Delle(n)

Focal thinning(s) from dehydration as a result of adjacent area of elevation (i.e., pingueculum, pterygium, filtering bleb)

Treatment: lubrication; punctal occlusion to raise tear film; may require removal of inciting lesion

Descemetocele

Extreme focal thinning of cornea in which only Descemet membrane remains

Caused by corneal melt (see Corneal melt section)

High risk of perforation

Bullous Keratopathy

Corneal edema with epithelial bullae, thickened stroma, but no guttata

Caused by loss or dysfunction of endothelial cells

May develop fibrovascular pannus

Etiology: aphakia, pseudophakia (rigid AC IOL), vitreocorneal touch, iridocorneal touch, sequela of severe or chronic keratitis

Pathology: blister-like elevations of corneal epithelium, damaged hemidesmosomes

DDx of corneal edema: aphakic bullous keratopathy (ABK), PBK, inflammation, infection, Fuchs endothelial dystrophy, PPCD, CHED, hydrops, acute angle-closure glaucoma, congenital glaucoma, graft failure, contact lens overwear, hypotony, birth trauma, ICE syndrome, anterior segment ischemia, toxicity (amantadine, chlorhexidine), Brown-McLean syndrome
> *Brown-McLean Syndrome:* peripheral corneal decompensation in aphakic patients, central cornea clear
>> **ETIOLOGY:** uncertain, possibly mechanical irritation from floppy peripheral iris

Neurotrophic Keratitis

Corneal degeneration caused by impaired corneal innervation (damage to CN 5 or branches)

Etiology: most commonly herpes simplex, varicella-zoster, trigeminal neuralgia surgery, acoustic neuroma, diabetes, topical medication toxicity (*beware*: topical anesthetic abuse), corneal injury (burn, contact lens abuse, ocular surgery); also, cerebrovascular accident, tumor, aneurysm, trauma, multiple sclerosis, Riley-Day syndrome, leprosy

Findings: conjunctival injection, corneal edema, nonhealing epithelial defects, ulceration, scarring, risk of infection and perforation; may have AC reaction
> *Mackie classification:*
>> **STAGE 1** = corneal staining
>> **STAGE 2** = nonhealing corneal epithelial defects
>> **STAGE 3** = corneal stromal melting

Diagnosis: decreased corneal sensation, or sectoral or complete anesthesia (test with cotton-tipped applicator or Cochet-Bonnet esthesiometer)

Treatment: lubrication, recombinant human nerve growth factor (rhNGF; cenegermin [Oxervate] q4h × 8 weeks); consider prophylactic antibiotic, bandage CL, punctal plugs, autologous serum drops, tarsorrhaphy, cryopreserved amniotic membrane (PROKERA), scleral lenses including the Boston ocular surface keratoprosthesis (PROSE lens); corneal neurotization surgery for severe disease

Familial Dysautonomia (Riley-Day Syndrome)

(See Chapter 5, Pediatrics/Strabismus)

Exposure Keratopathy

Desiccation of corneal epithelium resulting from CN 7 lesion (failure to close eyelids)

Findings: epithelial defects; may develop infection, melt, perforation

Treatment: lubrication, moisture chamber goggles, lid taping at bedtime; consider tarsorrhaphy, lid weights

Contact Lens–Related Problems

SPK: mechanical or chemical (solutions)

3 and 9 o'clock staining: results from poor wetting of peripheral cornea; refit lens

Abrasion: increased risk of infection in CL wearers
> *Treatment:* topical antibiotics, never patch

Infiltrates: hypoxia, antigenic reaction to preservatives in CL solutions, infection
> *Treatment:* stop CL wear, topical antibiotics

Edema: epithelial microcystic edema as a result of altered metabolism; associated with extended wear CL
> *Treatment:* decrease wear time; switch to daily wear lenses

Giant papillary conjunctivitis (GPC): sensitivity to CL material, deposits on CL, or mechanical irritation
> *Treatment:* stop CL wear, topical allergy medication

Superior limbic keratoconjunctivitis (SLK): may be a result of hypersensitivity or toxic reaction to thimerosal
> *Treatment:* resolves with discontinuation of lens wear

Neovascularization: superficial, deep, sectoral, or 360°; results from chronic hypoxia
> *Treatment:* refit lens with increased oxygen transmission; stop lens wear if significant vascularization

Corneal warpage: irregular astigmatism related to lens material (hard > rigid gas-permeable [RGP] > soft), fit, and length of time of wear; not associated with corneal edema. Usually asymptomatic; may have contact lens intolerance, blurred vision with glasses, loss of best spectacle-corrected visual acuity, or change in refraction (especially axis of astigmatism); corneal topography is abnormal (irregular astigmatism)
> *Treatment:* discontinue lens wear; repeat refraction and corneal topography until stable

Corneal Transplant Failure

Early (primary): poor tissue or surgery

Late: allograft rejection (delayed onset [at least 2 weeks]); homograft reaction

Risk factors: young age, stromal vascularization, previous graft failure, after chemical burns, inflammatory disease

Symptoms: decreased vision, redness, pain, irritation

Findings:
Epithelial rejection line: "battle" line of host-versus-donor epithelium; occurs in 10%, often precedes more destructive rejection events
Endothelial rejection: anterior chamber reaction, KP, graft edema, Khodadoust rejection line (moves across cornea destroying endothelium, resulting in stromal edema)
Other findings: subepithelial infiltrates, new KP, increased IOP (trabeculitis from AC reaction)

Treatment:
Endothelial rejection: IV steroids (methylprednisone 500 mg; reduces risk of subsequent rejection episodes [33% vs. 67% for oral steroids]), topical steroids (40% reversal rate alone), oral steroids
Epithelial rejection or stromal infiltrates with no graft swelling: treat with topical therapy alone

Prognosis: graft survival rate for treating endothelial rejections with a single pulse of IV steroids is 90% when presents within 1 week and 67% when presents later than 1 week (probably caused by irreversible damage to endothelial cells despite reversal of rejection)

Epithelial Downgrowth

Can occur following almost any intraocular surgery; increased risk with complicated surgery associated with hemorrhage, inflammation, vitreous loss, or incarcerated tissue

Surface epithelium grows through wound into eye, covering anterior segment structures

Appears as advancing line on corneal endothelium

Epithelium can cover the endothelium (leading to edema) and the angle (resulting in glaucoma); contact inhibition by healthy endothelium may inhibit this

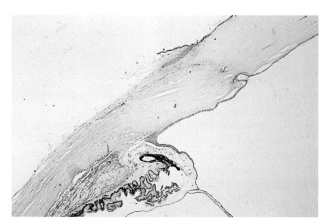

Figure 7.16 Epithelial downgrowth with epithelium present on corneal endothelium, angle, and iris, and into vitreous. (From Yanoff M, Fine BS. *Ocular Pathology*, 5th ed. St Louis: Mosby; 2002.)

Pathology: multilayered nonkeratinized squamous epithelium; PAS stains conjunctival goblet cells (differentiates between corneal and conjunctival epithelium) (Fig. 7.16)

DDx of retrocorneal membrane: mesodermal dysgenesis, ICE syndrome, trauma, posterior polymorphous dystrophy, disciform keratitis (HSV or VZV), alkali burn

Diagnosis: argon laser application to surface of iris produces white burn if iris involved; helps delineate extent of epithelial membrane

Treatment: excision of epithelial membrane and involved tissue with cryotherapy to remaining corneal membrane; high-power laser ablation of entire membrane may occasionally work; complete excision is difficult

Prognosis: poor, often develop secondary glaucoma

Fibrous Ingrowth

Fibrous proliferation through wound into AC

Less progressive and destructive than epithelial downgrowth

Fibroblasts originate from episclera or corneal stroma

Limbal Stem Cell Deficiency

Dysfunction or destruction of limbal stem cells causes loss of their barrier function and replacement of the corneal epithelium with conjunctival epithelial cells. Range of severity depending on extent of limbal involvement; may be stationary, progressive, diffuse, or sectoral

Etiology: autoimmune (Stevens-Johnson syndrome, ocular cicatricial pemphigoid, graft-versus-host disease), trauma (chemical injury, thermal injury, multiple ocular surgeries, cryotherapy, radiation, CL overwear), toxicity (preservative, mitomycin C, 5-fluorouracil), infection (extensive corneal/ocular surface infection [i.e., herpes, trachoma]), inflammation (atopic keratoconjunctivitis, vernal keratoconjunctivitis, neurotrophic keratopathy, bullous keratopathy), congenital (aniridia, epidermal dysplasia, xeroderma pigmentosum, dominantly inherited keratitis, multiple endocrine deficiencies, Turner syndrome, dyskeratosis congenita, lacrimo-auriculo-dento-digital [LADD] syndrome), and ocular surface tumors

Symptoms: asymptomatic or may have decreased vision, photophobia, pain, foreign body sensation, redness, tearing, blepharospasm

Findings: conjunctivalization of cornea, irregular corneal epithelium (ranging from mild fluorescein stippling to streaming/vortex-like pattern from area of limbal damage), flattening/loss of palisades of Vogt, epithelial haze, epithelial defects; may develop recurrent erosions, corneal ulceration, melt, perforation, vascularization, pannus, stromal scarring, and calcification; may have decreased visual acuity, conjunctival hyperemia, and other signs depending on etiology

Pathology: Bowman layer destruction, fibrous tissue ingrowth

Diagnosis: impression cytology (presence of goblet cells on cornea demonstrates conjunctivalization of corneal epithelium; goblet cells absent in 1/3 of cases); immunohistochemical staining (most specific are presence of conjunctival cytokeratin markers [CK7 and CK13] and absence of corneal marker [CK12]); confocal microscopy (loss of limbal architecture and palisades of Vogt, altered limbal and corneal epithelial cell morphology, decreased cell density, and decreased thickness; subepithelial vascularization and fibrosis); corneal epithelium takes up fluorescein

Treatment: treat underlying condition; optimize ocular surface (topical lubrication and steroids, may require autologous serum drops, punctal occlusion, bandage contact lens, cryopreserved amniotic membrane [PROKERA], scleral lenses including the Boston ocular surface prosthesis [PROSE lens], partial tarsorrhaphy); limbal stem cell transplant (autograft from fellow eye if unilateral [low risk of LSCD in donor eye if graft size <4–6 clock hours] or keratolimbal allograft if bilateral), cultivated limbal epithelial transplantation, or cultivated oral mucosal epithelial transplantation; poor candidate for penetrating keratoplasty unless performed after successful limbal transplant; consider keratoprosthesis; risk of recurrent conjunctivalization

Graft-Versus-Host Disease (GVHD)

Mild to severe immune-mediated disease in transplant recipients

Life-threatening complication of allogeneic hematopoietic cell transplantation (HCT; most common), solid organ transplantation containing lymphoid tissue, and transfusions of unirradiated blood. 2 types:

Acute GVHD: syndrome of dermatitis, hepatitis, and enteritis occurring within first 100 days

Chronic GVHD: syndrome affecting same organs as acute GVHD and also mouth, lungs, neuromuscular system, and genitourinary tract occurring after day 100 (with or without prior acute GVHD)

Depending on human leukocyte antigen (HLA) matching and donor relationship, up to 20%-90% develop acute GVHD, and 33%-64% develop chronic GVHD

Acute GVHD is the main risk factor for chronic GVHD

Findings:
Acute GVHD: hemorrhagic cicatricial conjunctivitis, pseudomembranes, symblepharon, punctate keratitis, KCS, lagophthalmos, entropion, microvascular retinopathy (4%–10%)
Chronic GVHD: KCS, punctate keratitis, optic neuropathy (2%; thought to be caused by cyclosporine, resolves with discontinuation)

Other findings:
Acute GVHD: maculopapular rash (pruritic or painful), weight loss, diarrhea, intestinal bleeding, abdominal pain, ileus
Chronic GVHD: maculopapular rash (palms and soles, spreading to face and trunk; may develop bullae and vesicles), sclerodermatoid or lichenoid skin changes (may cause contractures), atrophy and lesions of oral mucosa, jaundice, myositis, arthritis, hematuria, vaginitis, penile dysfunction

Diagnosis: skin, liver, intestinal biopsy

Treatment:
Prevention: standard primary prophylaxis of acute GVHD in allogeneic HCT is systemic cyclosporine or tacrolimus × 6 months and short course of methotrexate; before unrelated-donor HCT, treat with antithymocyte globulin
Acute GVHD (grade II-IV): continue immunosuppressive prophylactic agent and add high-dose methylprednisolone; may also require antithymocyte globulin, sirolimus, mycophenolate mofetil, daclizumab, anti-interleukin-2 receptor; may require secondary therapy with other agents
Chronic GVHD: primary therapy includes systemic prednisone, tacrolimus, cyclosporine, sirolimus, and thalidomide; may require secondary therapy with other agents

Prognosis: depends on type and severity as well as response to treatment
Acute GVHD (stage II or higher): up to 75% mortality in patients with no response to treatment or progression; 20%-25% mortality in patients with complete response
Chronic GVHD: overall survival is 42%

Iridocorneal Endothelial (ICE) Syndrome

(See Chapter 10, Anterior Segment)

Multiple Endocrine Neoplasia (MEN)

MEN 1 (Werner syndrome): mapped to chromosome 11
Neoplasias of pituitary, parathyroid, and islet cells of pancreas
Findings: visual field defects from pituitary tumors

MEN 2a (Sipple syndrome) (AD): mapped to chromosome 10
Medullary thyroid carcinoma, pheochromocytoma, parathyroid adenomas
Findings: prominent corneal nerves
Pathology: thickened conjunctival nerves contain numerous Schwann cells and partially myelinated axons; thickened corneal nerves result from an increased number of axons per nerve fiber bundle
Diagnosis: elevated calcitonin and vanillylmandelic acid

MEN 2b (Sipple-Gorlin syndrome) (AD): mapped to chromosome 10
Medullary thyroid carcinoma, pheochromocytoma, mucosal and GI neuromas, marfanoid habitus
Eye findings: prominent corneal nerves, conjunctival neu-

roma (87%), eyelid neuroma (80%), dry eye (67%), prominent perilimbal blood vessels (40%)

DDx of prominent corneal nerves: leprosy, *Acanthamoeba*, Down syndrome, neurofibromatosis, keratoconus, congenital glaucoma, Refsum disease, Fuchs corneal endothelial dystrophy, failed corneal graft, KCS, trauma, advanced age, ichthyosis, posterior polymorphous dystrophy

Tumors

Corneal Intraepithelial Neoplasia (CIN)

(See Conjunctiva section)

Squamous Cell Carcinoma (SCC)

(See Conjunctiva section)

SCLERAL DISORDERS

Episcleritis

Inflammation of episclera

Self-limited, usually young adults

Bilateral = 33%; recurrent = 67%

Associated with VZV, rheumatoid arthritis (RA), gout

Signs: sectoral (70%) or diffuse (30%) injection with mild or no discomfort; may have nodule (20%), chemosis, AC reaction

Pathology: nongranulomatous vascular dilatation, perivascular lymphocytic infiltration; diffuse or nodular (similar to rheumatoid scleritis but limited to episclera); palisade of epithelioid cells bordering central fibrinoid necrosis

Diagnosis: blanches with topical 2.5% phenylephrine; if lasts for >3 weeks, perform systemic workup

Treatment: topical vasoconstrictor (Naphcon A), mild topical steroid (fluorometholone [FML], loteprednol [Alrex, Lotemax]); consider oral NSAID

Scleritis

Inflammation of sclera

More common in females; onset age of 30-60 years

Bilateral in >50%

Etiology: 40% associated with systemic disease; 50%-60% for necrotizing scleritis

Collagen vascular diseases (RA [20% of all cases of scleritis; only 3% of patients with RA develop scleritis; 75% of RA-related scleritis is bilateral], SLE, polyarteritis nodosa), vascular disease (granulomatosis with poly-

angiitis, giant cell arteritis, Takayasu disease), relapsing polychondritis, sarcoidosis, ankylosing spondylitis, reactive arthritis syndrome, Crohn disease, ulcerative colitis, infections (HSV, VZV, *Pseudomonas, Nocardia, Actinomyces*, mycobacteria, fungi *[Fusarium, Aspergillus]*, gram-positive cocci), gout, rosacea

Classification:

Anterior: 98%

DIFFUSE (40%): most benign; widespread involvement

PATHOLOGY: sclera thickened, diffuse nongranulomatous inflammation with macrophages, lymphocytes, and plasma cells; perivascular distribution

NODULAR (44%): focal involvement; nodule is immobile; up to 10% progress to necrotizing, rule out infectious cause

PATHOLOGY: zonal necrotizing granuloma, fibrinoid necrosis, chronic inflammation, fusiform thickening, immune complex deposition with complement activation; once collagen has been destroyed, inflammation recedes, uvea herniates into defect

NECROTIZING (14%): associated with life-threatening autoimmune disease (5-year mortality rate = 25%; has improved with biologic therapy); more common in older patients, female > male

WITH INFLAMMATION (granulomatous, vasoocclusive, postsurgical): focal or diffuse, progressive, pain and redness; vascular sludging and occlusion; underlying blue uveal tissue may be visible giving redness a "violaceous" hue; 40% lose vision; 60% have ocular complications: anterior uveitis, sclerosing keratitis, cataract, glaucoma, peripheral corneal melt, scleral thinning

WITHOUT (OVERT) INFLAMMATION (scleromalacia perforans): minimal symptoms, minimal injection; scleral thinning, marked ischemia; seldom perforate; females with severe rheumatoid arthritis; 8-year mortality rate = 21%

Posterior: 2%; posterior to ora serrata; usually unilateral and very painful, mild or no pain in 30%-40%; often decreased vision

Usually no associated systemic disorder

80% have anterior scleritis

FINDINGS: thickened and inflamed posterior sclera, choroidal detachment and folds, amelanotic fundus mass, optic nerve edema; may have vitritis, macular edema, limitation of motility, ptosis, proptosis, exudative retinal detachment (RD), elevated IOP (forward shift of lens-iris diaphragm as a result of anterior rotation of ciliary body)

Mnemonic: **POST SCLER** (**P**roptosis, **O**phthalmoplegia, **S**welling of disc, **T**hickening of sclera and T-sign, **S**ubretinal exudates, **C**horoidal folds, **E**xudative RD, **R**ing choroidal detachment)

B-SCAN ULTRASOUND: pocket of fluid in Tenon space (sclerotenonitis), T-sign (when adjacent to optic nerve shadow), thickened sclera

FLUORESCEIN ANGIOGRAPHY (FA): early patchy hypofluorescence, late staining, disc leakage

OCT: delineate scleral involvement and fundus changes

CT SCAN: thickening of posterior sclera with contiguous involvement of orbital fat (T-sign)

DDX: choroidal tumor, orbital pseudotumor (idiopathic orbital inflammation [IOI]), uveal effusion syndrome, VKH, thyroid eye disease, orbital tumors

Symptoms: pain, redness, photophobia

Findings: diffuse or sectoral area of deep injection (violaceous hue), tender to touch, chemosis, scleral edema; may have scleral nodule, scleral thinning, AC reaction (33%), keratitis (acute stromal keratitis, sclerosing keratitis, marginal keratolysis); chorioretinal folds and serous RD in posterior scleritis

Diagnosis: does not blanch with topical phenylephrine
  Lab tests: CBC, ESR, RF, ANA, ANCA, Venereal Disease Research Laboratory (VDRL), fluorescent treponemal antibody absorption (FTA-ABS), uric acid, blood urea nitrogen (BUN), purified protein derivative (PPD), chest X-ray (CXR)
  ANCA: positive in granulomatosis with polyangiitis; also polyarteritis nodosa, Churg-Strauss, and crescentic glomerulonephritis
    2 types:
      C-ANCA (cytoplasmic; positive in granulomatosis with polyangiitis)
      P-ANCA (perinuclear; positive in polyarteritis nodosa [PAN])
  Anterior segment fluorescein angiogram: may detect nonperfusion and vaso-obliteration

Treatment: oral NSAID, consider oral steroids or immunosuppressive agents; treat underlying disorder; topical steroids are not effective; sub-Tenon steroid injection is contraindicated; may require patch graft for perforation

Complications: keratitis, cataract, uveitis, glaucoma

Granulomatosis With Polyangiitis

Formerly Wegener granulomatosis

Systemic disease of necrotizing vasculitis and granulomatous inflammation involving sinuses, respiratory system, kidneys, and orbit

Males > females

Findings (60%): nasolacrimal duct obstruction, proptosis, painful ophthalmoplegia, conjunctivitis, chemosis, KCS, episcleritis, necrotizing scleritis (most common type of ocular involvement), keratitis, cotton-wool spots, arterial narrowing, venous tortuosity, choroidal thickening, cystoid macular edema (CME), central retinal artery occlusion (CRAO), optic nerve involvement

Other findings: upper respiratory tract (hemoptysis), renal failure (major cause of death), hemorrhagic dermatitis, cerebral vasculitis, weight loss, peripheral neuropathy, fever, arthralgia, saddle nose (destruction of nasal bones)

Diagnosis: C-ANCA positive in 67%

Treatment: systemic steroids and immunosuppressives (cyclophosphamide)

Complications: fatal if untreated

Takayasu Disease

Narrowing of large branches of aorta

Diminished pulsations in upper extremities

Decreased blood pressure in upper extremities, increased blood pressure in lower extremities

Findings: scleritis, amaurosis fugax, ocular ischemia, AION

Polyarteritis Nodosa

Systemic vasculitis affecting medium-size and small arteries

Males > females

Findings: necrotizing sclerokeratitis, vascular occlusions, ischemic optic neuropathy, rarely aneurysms of retinal vessels

Other findings: kidneys (nephritic or nephrotic syndrome, hypertension, renal failure), heart (myocardial infarction, angina, pericarditis), intestines (pain, infarction), arthritis, peripheral neuropathy

Relapsing Polychondritis

Multisystem disorder characterized by recurrent episodes of inflammation in cartilaginous tissues throughout body

Findings (60%): episcleritis, scleritis, iritis, conjunctivitis, KCS, exudative RD, optic neuritis, proptosis, CN 6 palsies

Other findings: migratory polyarthritis, fever, diffuse inflammation of cartilage (nose, ear, trachea, larynx)

Treatment: topical or systemic steroids; dapsone

Discoloration

Blue sclera: sclera appears blue owing to thinning and visualization of underlying uvea
  DDx: Ehlers-Danlos, Hurler, Turner, and Marfan syndromes; osteogenesis imperfecta, scleromalacia perforans, congenital staphyloma, high myopia, buphthalmos
    Mnemonic: **HOPES B** (**H**igh myopia, **O**steogenesis imperfecta, **P**seudoxanthoma elasticum, **E**hlers-Danlos syndrome, **S**cleritis, **B**uphthalmos)

Scleral icterus: yellow sclera caused by hyperbilirubinemia

Ochronosis (alkaptonuria) (AR): homogentisic acid oxidase deficiency
  Homogentisic acid accumulates, metabolized into melanin-like compound with brown pigmentation of cartilage (ear, nose, heart valves) and sclera; excreted in urine (dark)
  Findings: triangular pigment deposits anterior to rectus muscle insertions, pinhead-size peripheral corneal stromal deposits, pigmentation of tarsus and lids

Cogan senile scleral plaque: blue-gray hyalinization of sclera anterior to horizontal rectus muscle insertions

SURGERY

Penetrating Keratoplasty (PK; PKP)

Full-thickness corneal graft/transplant

Most common indications: bullous keratopathy (pseudophakic, aphakic), keratoconus, graft failure, corneal scar; Peter anomaly (children)

Success rate: 90% of grafts are clear at 1 year (>90% for keratoconus; 65% for HSV)

Complications: rejection (20%), failure, glaucoma, suprachoroidal or expulsive hemorrhage, endophthalmitis, recurrence of pathology

Collaborative Corneal Transplant Treatment Study (CCTS): ABO blood type incompatibility is a possible risk factor for rejection
   HLA matching is not cost-effective or advantageous
   High-risk status: vascularization of cornea in 2 quadrants, history of previous graft rejection, glaucoma, extensive PAS, traumatic or hereditary ocular surface disorders

Donor screening:
   Contraindications for donor corneas: septicemia, lymphoma or leukemia, systemic malignancy with ocular metastasis, anterior segment tumors (choroidal melanoma is not a contraindication), Creutzfeldt-Jakob disease, rabies, subacute sclerosing panencephalitis, progressive multifocal leukoencephalopathy (PML), HIV, hepatitis B and C (neither HIV nor hepatitis C has ever been transmitted)

Tissue preservation:
   4°C moist chamber: use within 48 hours
   M-K medium (McCarey-Kaufman): TC-199 medium with dextran (5% concentration) and gentamicin stored at 4°C; use within 48 hours
   Chondroitin sulfate: acts as antioxidant and membrane growth factor
   K-Sol (Kaufman): chondroitin sulfate in TC-199 at 4°C; discontinued
   Corneal storage media (CSM): from Minnesota Lions Eye Bank researchers plus mercaptoethanol (antioxidant) and chondroitin sulfate; discontinued with introduction of Dexsol and Optisol
   Dexsol: minimal essential medium with chondroitin sulfate and dextran 1% (osmotic agent to keep cornea thin)
   Optisol: hybrid of K-sol, Dexsol, and CSM, plus vitamins, amino acids, and antioxidants; amphotericin B can also be added; as effective as Dexsol but keeps cornea thinner
   Many media contain pH indicators that change color with a change in pH (i.e., microbial contamination)

Lamellar Keratoplasty (Anterior Lamellar Keratoplasty [ALK], Deep Anterior Lamellar Keratoplasty [DALK])

Partial or full-thickness stromal graft composed of epithelium, Bowman layer, and stroma. ALK involves a stromal dissection, whereas DALK entails replacement of stromal tissue down to the level of Descemet membrane. DALK is safer, has increased wound strength, and has less chance of rejection. The dissection can be performed manually, with an air bubble or viscoelastic; intraoperative OCT can be helpful (OCT-guided DALK)

Indications: stromal pathology (scar, dystrophy) and keratoconus (DALK)

Contraindications: corneal endothelial dysfunction

Complications: graft rejection, suture-related complications, and interface opacification can occur with both procedures; intraoperative Descemet membrane tear or perforation can occur with DALK requiring conversion to penetrating keratoplasty.

Endothelial Keratoplasty (EK; Deep Lamellar EK [DLEK], Descemet Stripping EK [DSEK], Descemet Stripping and Automated Endothelial Keratoplasty [DSAEK], Descemet Membrane EK [DMEK], Descemet Membrane and Automated Endothelial Keratoplasty [DMAEK])

Techniques have evolved from DLEK to DSEK, DMEK, and DMAEK, making the procedure faster and safer with better visual outcomes. DSAEK involves manually stripping the endothelium and replacing with donor lenticule composed of endothelium, Descemet membrane, and thin layer of stroma prepared with a microkeratome. DMEK (requires peripheral iridotomy/iridectomy) and DMAEK (lenticule has peripheral ring of stroma) have faster recovery, better vision, and lower rejection rate

Indications: corneal edema resulting from Fuchs dystrophy and bullous keratopathy

Complications: endothelial rejection, lenticule separation or displacement requiring rebubble (SF6 gas)

Keratophakia (No Longer Performed)

Donor lenticule is placed between the cornea and a microkeratome-created lamellar section to correct aphakia

Contraindications: thinned corneas, infants, glaucoma

Keratomileusis (No Longer Performed)

Lamellar section is removed, frozen, shaped on a cryolathe, then replaced in stromal bed to correct myopia or hyperopia. Donor lenticule can be used instead (Fig. 7.17)

Contraindications: glaucoma

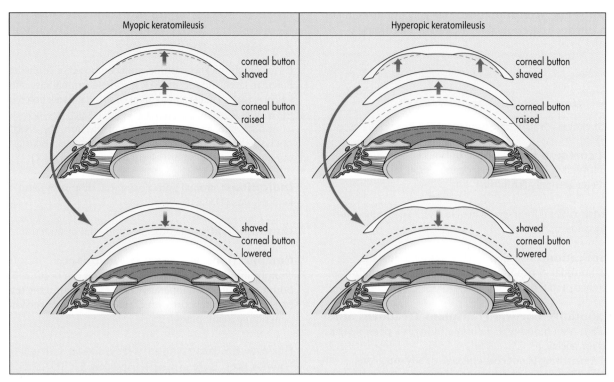

Figure 7.17 Keratomileusis. In a myopic keratomileusis, a corneal button is raised using a microkeratome, and it is reshaped using a cryolathe *(upper part)*. When the button is replaced, the central cornea is flattened *(lower part)*. (From Chang SW, Azar DT. Automated and manual lamellar surgical procedures and epikeratoplasty. In: Yanoff M, Duker JS, eds. *Ophthalmology*. London: Mosby; 1999.)

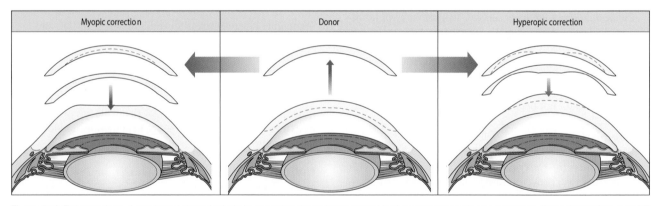

Figure 7.18 Epikeratoplasty. A preshaped donor lenticule is sutured to the recipient stromal bed to correct myopia and hyperopia. (From Chang SW, Azar DT. Automated and manual lamellar surgical procedures and epikeratoplasty. In: Yanoff M, Duker JS, eds. *Ophthalmology*. London: Mosby; 1999.)

Epikeratophakia (Epikeratoplasty) (No Longer Performed)

Epithelium is removed and a lathed donor lenticule is placed to correct myopia or hyperopia (Fig. 7.18)

Can be performed in children; reversible

Contraindications: blepharitis, dry eye, lagophthalmos

Pathology: 2 Bowman layers (donor lenticule and patient)

Astigmatic keratotomy (AK)

Procedure in which 99% depth arcuate or straight incisions typically placed at the 7 or 8 mm optical zone (OZ) to correct astigmatism

Various nomograms exist (i.e., Lindstrom ARC-T)

Do not make arcuate incisions >90° (decreased efficacy, increased instability)

When combined with RK, crossed incisions created wound gape and instability

Limbal/corneal relaxing incisions are performed at 10-12 mm OZ, usually at time of cataract surgery, with preset diamond knife (500-600 μm depth)

Radial Keratotomy (RK) (Rarely Performed)

Deep radial corneal incisions to correct low to moderate myopia

Effect dependent on number of incisions, depth of incisions, size of OZ, patient age

Number of incisions: the greater the number of incisions, the greater the effect; never use >8 incisions (additional incisions have limited effect and cause greater destabilization of the cornea)

Incision depth: the deeper the incision, the greater the effect; diamond knife is set at 100% of thinnest pachymetry measurement (usually paracentral inferotemporal region; temporal < inferior < nasal < superior)

Optical zone: the smaller the diameter of the OZ (the longer the incision), the greater the effect; do not make OZ <3 mm (visual aberrations [starburst])

Patient age: the older the patient, the greater the effect

Patient sex: greater effect in males than in females

Technique: American (downhill cut [toward limbus], safer but shallower) versus Russian (uphill cut [toward central cornea], deeper but risk of invading OZ); combined technique with special knife gives deep cut with safety

Complications: undercorrection or overcorrection, perforation, infection, scarring, irregular astigmatism, progressive hyperopia (in Prospective Evaluation of Radial Keratotomy [PERK] study, 43% had ≥1.00 D of hyperopia after 10 years), glare/starburst, fluctuating vision

Results: 85% achieved 20/40 or better vision after initial procedure; 96% achieved 20/40 or better after enhancement, 85% achieved 20/25 or better after enhancement

Photorefractive Keratectomy (PRK)

Laser ablation of corneal surface to correct myopia, hyperopia, and astigmatism

Excimer (excited dimer) laser: argon-fluoride (wavelength = 193 nm; far ultraviolet), energy = 64 eV

Functions as a "cold" laser (breaks molecular bonds to ablate tissue; no thermal damage)

Each pulse removes ~0.25 μm of corneal tissue

Depth of ablation is related to diameter of OZ and amount of intended correction

Munnerlyn equation: depth = (refractive error/3) × OZ^2
   Example: 12 μm for 6 mm OZ and 1 D of myopia

Advantages of PRK: precise removal of tissue, minimal adjacent tissue damage

Disadvantages of PRK: involves visual axis, risk of haze/scarring, regression, requires removal of epithelium

Contraindications: collagen vascular, autoimmune, or immunodeficiency disorders; pregnancy; corneal ectasia; keloid formation; isotretinoin (Accutane), amiodarone, sumatriptan (Imitrex)

Cautions: unstable refraction (change of >0.5 D/year), systemic diseases that affect wound healing (diabetes, atopy, connective tissue diseases, immunocompromised

status), herpes keratitis (HSV or VZV), ocular inflammation (keratitis, acne rosacea, pannus that extends into visual axis)

Complications: undercorrection or overcorrection, haze/scarring, delayed reepithelialization, sterile infiltrates, infection, decentered ablation, central island, irregular astigmatism, keratectasia, regression, glare/halos, dry eye, glaucoma, or cataract (from steroids)

Corneal haze: risk and severity increase with deeper ablations and postoperative UV radiation exposure; results in decreased vision with regression of effect. Mitomycin C (MMC) used intraoperatively can reduce risk of haze. Oral vitamin C 1000 mg/day x 1 week before surgery and 2 weeks postoperatively, and avoidance of UV exposure may also help prevent haze

Treatment of complications:

Enhancements: it is recommended to wait at least 3 months or until the refraction and corneal topography are stable before performing an enhancement for overcorrection or undercorrection

Haze: treat with topical steroids; consider application of MMC 0.02% x 2 minutes along with scar débridement with either a diamond burr or a superficial excimer laser treatment (PTK). Once the haze is reduced, the refraction can change dramatically, so do not treat residual refractive error at time of haze removal

Irregular astigmatism: scleral lens, topography-guided retreatment

Laser In Situ Keratomileusis (LASIK)

Combination of keratomileusis and excimer laser ablation to correct myopia, hyperopia, and astigmatism

Corneal flap created with mechanical or laser microkeratome and excimer laser ablation performed on underlying stromal bed

Advantages of LASIK: more rapid healing, less discomfort, less risk of haze, less postoperative medications

Disadvantages of LASIK: flap complications, interface complications

Complications:

Intraoperative: flap creation complication (buttonhole, incomplete, or irregular flap, free cap) epithelial abrasion or sloughing, programming error, decentered ablation

Immediate postoperative: diffuse lamellar keratitis (DLK; sands of Sahara), epithelial ingrowth, flap dislocation, flap striae, central island, irregular astigmatism, dry eye, undercorrection or overcorrection, night vision problems (glare, halos)

Delayed postoperative: late DLK, pressure-induced stromal keratopathy (PISK), late flap slip or flap laceration, undercorrection or overcorrection, keratectasia, dry eye, photophobia (from laser keratome, 1–3 weeks to 3 months postop, treat with topical steroids)

Treatment of complications:

Buttonhole (increased risk with steep corneas), *incomplete or irregular flap:* replace flap, do not perform ablation;

when cornea stabilizes, either cut a new flap or perform surface ablation (PRK/PTK)

Free cap (increased risk with flat corneas): place free cap in moisture chamber epithelial side down, perform ablation, then replace cap and let dry

Epithelial slough or corneal abrasion: increased risk with certain microkeratomes and in eyes with epithelial BM dystrophy; increases risk of developing DLK and epithelial ingrowth. Treat with bandage contact lens and close follow-up. If large defect occurs in first eye, consider postponing treatment of second eye

Flap striae or flap dislocation: replace flap and stretch; consider use of epithelial débridement, hypotonic saline or sterile water, ironing with a warm spatula, or suturing (interrupted radials or antitorque)

DLK: inflammation within flap interface; etiology often unknown; increased risk with epithelial defect. Late DLK may result from epithelial defect and cornea ulcer

CLASSIFICATION:

STAGE 1: peripheral inflammatory cells (usually postop day 1–2)

STAGE 2: inflammatory cells migrate centrally (usually postop day 3–4)

STAGE 3: more central inflammatory cells with scarring

STAGE 4: stomal melting and scarring

TREATMENT: frequent topical steroids for stages 1 and 2 flap lifting and interface irrigation for stages 3 and 4; consider a short pulse of oral steroids for stages 2-4

Central toxic keratopathy: noninflammatory central corneal opacity and hyperopic shift; appears on postop day 3-5, usually preceded by DLK. No treatment. Spontaneously resolves in 2-18 months. May also occur after PRK

Interface fluid syndrome (IFS; pressure-innduced stromal keratitis [PISK]): steroid-induced elevated intraocular pressure causes pocket of aqueous fluid accumulation within flap interface with stromal opacification; produces myopic shift, increased corneal thickness, inaccurately low intraocular pressure measurement. Can look like DLK. Stop steroids; initiate IOP-lowering drops

Epithelial ingrowth: nests of epithelium growing under the flap; active areas of ingrowth detected with fluorescein staining of adjacent flap edge; more common in eyes with epithelial BM dystrophy and after enhancements. Ingrowth that is progressive or affects the vision is treated with flap lifting and débridement of the stromal bed and flap undersurface. Consider radial sutures or glue to help seal the flap edge; if ingrowth recurs, consider Nd:YAG laser treatment

Irregular ablation (decentered, irregular astigmatism): requires custom or topo-guided retreatment

Corneal ectasia (keratectasia): often occurs with treatment of eyes with a preexisting ectasia (keratoconus, forme fruste keratoconus, pellucid marginal degeneration) or excessive depth of ablation in normal corneas (residual stromal depth <250 μm) can result in progressive myopic astigmatism and corneal ectasia; can also occur without risk factors. Treat with corneal collagen cross-linking to halt progression. A scleral lens or RGP contact lens can help with visual improvement, but will not stop progression. Consider Intacs to improve the shape of the cornea, or penetrating keratoplasty for severe cases where the visual axis has developed significant scarring

Dry eye: can worsen postoperatively if untreated before surgery; can also occur in patients without preexisting dry eye. Superior hinged flap may cause greater dryness than is caused by nasal hinged flap. Treat with frequent lubrication; consider punctal occlusion and topical cyclosporine, lifitegrast, or steroids

Glare/halos: often caused by residual refractive error. The role of scotopic pupil size as a contributing factor is controversial (may have been a risk with older laser ablations, but is not a risk factor with modern laser ablations). Treatment options include pharmacologic miosis (Alphagan-P or pilocarpine) or retreatment with larger optical zone or blend zone

Infectious keratitis: uncommon but serious complication; most common organisms are Gram-positive cocci and atypical *Mycobacteria*. Suspected infection requires lifting flap and culturing; treat with fortified topical antibiotics (vancomycin and amikacin); may require flap amputation

Laser-Assisted Epithelial Keratomileusis (LASEK)

Variation of PRK; epithelial flap is created with alcohol, excimer laser is applied, and epithelial flap is replaced

Advantages of LASEK: may have less risk of haze than PRK

Disadvantages of LASEK: slower visual recovery than with PRK

Complications: same as with PRK: undercorrection or overcorrection, haze/scarring, delayed reepithelialization, infection, decentered ablation, central island, irregular astigmatism, regression, glare/halos, dry eye, stromal incursion (with mechanical flap device)

Risk of haze can be reduced with oral vitamin C and avoidance of UV exposure

Small Incision Lenticule Extraction (SMILE)

Intrastromal corneal lenticule cut by femtosecond laser is removed through a small incision to correct myopia, astigmatism, and hyperopia

Requires careful dissection and removal of lenticule to prevent retained fragment

Advantages of SMILE: eliminates large incision and flap complications of LASIK

Disadvantages of SMILE: lenticule complications

Complications: undercorrection or overcorrection, glare/halos, incomplete lenticule extraction (irregular astigmatism), decentered treatment, incision tear, pocket perforation, haze, inflammation, infection, keratectasia

Phototherapeutic Keratectomy (PTK)

Use of excimer laser to ablate corneal pathology limited to anterior 1/3 of cornea

Indications: superficial scars, dystrophies, irregularities, residual band keratopathy, recurrent erosions

Can use confocal microscopy to determine depth of pathology

Complications: recurrence of pathology, reactivation of HSV, induced hyperopia or irregular astigmatism

Intracorneal Inlays

A thin, contact lens-like implant placed in the central optical zone beneath a corneal flap or within a corneal pocket to correct myopia, hyperopia, astigmatism, or presbyopia without removing corneal tissue

Presbyopic implants are inserted in the patient's nondominant eye to improve near vision. Strategies for presbyopia correction: implant thickness and shape alter the corneal curvature, implant has power, or implant acts as a pinhole (KAMRA Inlay)

Advantages: reversible, adjustable, no removal of tissue

Complications: undercorrection or overcorrection, irregular astigmatism, glare, halos, flap striae, epithelial ingrowth, DLK, corneal deposits/haze, infection, implant decentration or extrusion

Intrastromal Corneal Ring Segments (Intacs)

Ring segment implants placed into peripheral corneal channels outside the visual axis to correct low to moderate myopia. Implants flatten the cornea without cutting or removing tissue from the central optical zone. Also used to reshape corneas with keratoconus or post-LASIK ectasia (Fig. 7.19). Rarely performed for treatment of myopia

Advantages: reversible, adjustable, spares visual axis, no removal of tissue

Complications: undercorrection or overcorrection, irregular astigmatism, glare, halos, infection, implant decentration or extrusion, stromal deposits

Conductive Keratoplasty (CK) (Rarely Performed)

A contact probe directly delivers radiofrequency (thermal) energy to the peripheral cornea in a ring pattern to steepen the central cornea and correct low to moderate hyperopia.

Advantages: spares visual axis, no removal of tissue

Complications: undercorrection or overcorrection, irregular astigmatism, regression

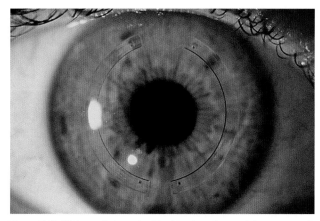

Figure 7.19 Slit-lamp photograph of the intrastromal corneal ring segments in position in patient's cornea. (Courtesy of Mr. Thomas Loarie. From Friedman NJ, Husain SE, Kohnen T, et al. Investigational refractive procedures. In: Yanoff M, Duker JS, eds. *Ophthalmology*. London: Mosby; 1999.)

REVIEW QUESTIONS (Answers start on page 420)

1. Which is the *least* desirable method for corneal graft storage?
   a. moist chamber at 4°C
   b. glycerin
   c. Optisol
   d. cryopreservation
2. Presently in the United States, phlyctenule is most commonly associated with
   a. HSV
   b. TB
   c. *Staphylococcus*
   d. fungus
3. Which blood test is most helpful in the evaluation of a patient with Schnyder corneal dystrophy?
   a. calcium
   b. uric acid
   c. immunoglobulins
   d. cholesterol
4. Which disease has never been transmitted by a corneal graft?
   a. CMV
   b. Creutzfeldt-Jakob
   c. rabies
   d. *Cryptococcus*
5. Which corneal dystrophy does *not* recur in a corneal graft?
   a. granular
   b. macular
   c. lattice
   d. posterior polymorphous
6. A conjunctival map biopsy is typically used for which malignancy?
   a. squamous cell carcinoma
   b. basal cell carcinoma
   c. sebaceous gland carcinoma
   d. malignant melanoma

7. All of the following may cause follicular conjunctivitis, *except*
   a. *Chlamydia*
   b. *Neisseria*
   c. Iopidine
   d. EKC

8. Which of the following tests is *least* helpful in determining the etiology of enlarged corneal nerves?
   a. electrocardiogram
   b. calcitonin
   c. urinary vanillylmandelic acid
   d. acid-fast stain

9. Corneal filaments are *least* likely to be present in which condition?
   a. KCS
   b. Thygeson SPK
   c. SLK
   d. medicamentosa

10. Which of the following is *not* an appropriate treatment for SLK?
    a. bandage contact lens
    b. conjunctival resection
    c. silver nitrate stick
    d. conjunctival cautery

11. In what level of the cornea does a Kayser-Fleischer ring occur?
    a. epithelium
    b. Bowman layer
    c. stroma
    d. Descemet membrane

12. Cornea verticillata–like changes are associated with all of the following, *except*
    a. indomethacin
    b. haloperidol
    c. chloroquine
    d. amiodarone

13. The *least* common location for a nevus is
    a. bulbar conjunctiva
    b. palpebral conjunctiva
    c. caruncle
    d. lid skin

14. All of the following ions move across the corneal endothelium by both active transport and passive diffusion, *except*
    a. Cl⁻
    b. K⁺
    c. Na⁺
    d. H⁺

15. Which organism is associated with crystalline keratopathy?
    a. *S. aureus*
    b. *H. influenzae*
    c. *Enterococcus*
    d. *S. viridans*

16. Which of the following conditions is associated with the best 5-year prognosis for a corneal graft?
    a. PBK
    b. Fuchs dystrophy
    c. ABK
    d. HSV

17. The best strategy for loosening a tight contact lens is to
    a. increase the diameter
    b. increase the curvature
    c. decrease the diameter
    d. decrease the curvature

18. The type of contact lens that causes the *least* endothelial pleomorphism is
    a. soft daily wear
    b. soft extended wear
    c. rigid gas permeable
    d. hard/polymethylmethacrylate

19. Which of the following conditions is associated with the *worst* prognosis for a corneal graft?
    a. PBK
    b. Fuchs dystrophy
    c. Reis-Bucklers dystrophy
    d. keratoglobus

20. Which is *not* a treatment of acute hydrops?
    a. steroid
    b. homatropine
    c. bandage contact lens
    d. corneal transplant

21. Which organism *cannot* penetrate intact corneal epithelium?
    a. *C. diphtheriae*
    b. *N. gonorrhoeae*
    c. *P. aeruginosa*
    d. *H. aegyptius*

22. Which of the following medications would be the best choice in the treatment of microsporidial keratoconjunctivitis?
    a. fumagillin
    b. chloramphenicol
    c. galardin
    d. paromomycin

23. All of the following agents are used in the treatment of *Acanthamoeba* keratitis, *except*
    a. paromomycin
    b. natamycin
    c. chlorhexidine
    d. miconazole

24. Goblet cells are *least* abundant in which location?
    a. tarsal conjunctiva
    b. plica
    c. bulbar conjunctiva
    d. limbus

25. Thygeson SPK is best treated with topical
    a. cyclosporine
    b. idoxuridine
    c. loteprednol
    d. trifluridine

26. EKC is typically contagious for how many days?
    a. 5 days
    b. 7 days
    c. 10 days
    d. 14 days

27. A shield ulcer is associated with
    a. AKC
    b. SLK
    c. VKC
    d. GPC

28. Which of the following is most likely to be associated with melanoma of the uvea?
    a. dysplastic nevus syndrome
    b. melanosis oculi
    c. nevus of Ota
    d. secondary acquired melanosis

29. Which of the following is *not* associated with *N. gonorrhoeae* conjunctivitis?
    a. pseudomembrane
    b. preauricular lymphadenopathy
    c. purulent discharge
    d. corneal ulcer

30. Even spreading of the tear film depends most on which factor?
    a. lipid
    b. aqueous
    c. mucin
    d. epithelium

31. A neurotrophic ulcer should *not* be treated with
    a. tarsorrhaphy
    b. antiviral
    c. antibiotic
    d. bandage contact lens

32. Which layer of the cornea can regenerate?
    a. Bowman layer
    b. stroma
    c. Descemet membrane
    d. endothelium

33. The most appropriate treatment for a patient with scleromalacia is
    a. topical steroid
    b. sub-Tenon steroid injection
    c. oral NSAID
    d. oral immunosuppressive agent

34. The HEDS recommendation for treating stromal (disciform) keratitis is
    a. topical steroid alone
    b. topical steroid and topical antiviral
    c. topical steroid and oral antiviral
    d. topical steroid, topical antiviral, and oral antiviral

35. Feathery edges and a satellite infiltrate are most characteristic of a corneal ulcer caused by
    a. *Pseudomonas*
    b. *Acanthamoeba*
    c. *Microsporidia*
    d. *Fusarium*

36. PTK would be most appropriate for treating which of the following corneal disorders?
    a. superficial granular dystrophy
    b. anterior stromal neovascularization
    c. mid-stromal herpes scar
    d. Fuchs dystrophy

37. A 62-year-old woman with KCS is most likely to demonstrate corneal staining in which location?
    a. superior 1/3
    b. middle 1/3 (interpalpebral)
    c. inferior 1/3
    d. diffuse over entire cornea

38. Which of the following findings is most commonly associated with SLK?
    a. filaments
    b. giant papillae
    c. pseudomembrane
    d. follicles

39. Which lab test is most helpful to obtain in a 38-year-old man with herpes zoster ophthalmicus?
    a. ANCA
    b. Lyme titer
    c. CXR
    d. HIV test

40. A patient with conjunctival intraepithelial neoplasia is most likely to have
    a. CMV
    b. EBV
    c. HSV
    d. HPV

41. Which of the following disorders is most likely to be found in a patient suffering from sleep apnea?
    a. iritis
    b. interstitial keratitis
    c. follicular conjunctivitis
    d. trichiasis

42. A patient with GVH disease is most likely to have which eye finding?
    a. scleritis
    b. symblepharon
    c. optic neuropathy
    d. iritis

43. Topical corticosteroids should *not* be used in a patient with which form of herpes simplex keratitis?
    a. epithelial
    b. endothelial
    c. disciform stromal
    d. necrotizing stromal

44. What is the most appropriate management for a patient who reports recurrent foreign body sensation when waking up but does not have a discrete epithelial defect on exam?
    a. epithelial debridement
    b. lubrication
    c. anterior stromal puncture
    d. phototherapeutic keratectomy

45. A 24-year-old woman reports a painful, red left eye and blurry vision after sleeping with her CL in for several days. Examination shows a corneal ulcer with edema and a hypopyon. The most likely diagnosis is
    a. HSV
    b. *Candida*
    c. *Acanthamoeba*
    d. *P. aeruginosa*

46. The best test to measure basal tear secretion is
    a. dye disappearance test
    b. Jones I test
    c. Schirmer test with anesthesia
    d. tear film breakup time

47. Adenoviral membranous conjunctivitis is most likely to cause which of the following?
    a. symblepharon
    b. corneal perforation
    c. irregular astigmatism
    d. corneal neovascularization

48. After a corneal alkali burn, which of the following signs is associated with the *worst* prognosis?
    a. conjunctival chemosis
    b. complete corneal epithelial defect
    c. corneal edema
    d. complete limbal blanching

49. The most likely cause of a corneal keratometry measurement 2.5 D steeper inferiorly than superiorly at the 3 mm zone is
    a. pterygium
    b. Mooren ulcer
    c. keratoconus
    d. Terrien marginal degeneration

50. The nasociliary branch of the trigeminal nerve innervates the tip of the nose and the
    a. frontal sinus
    b. lacrimal gland
    c. upper eyelid
    d. cornea

51. The most common complication of pterygium surgery is
    a. dellen
    b. scleral melt
    c. pyogenic granuloma
    d. recurrence

52. The refractive effect of Intacs is titrated by the
    a. number of ring segments inserted
    b. optical zone of the ring segments
    c. thickness of the ring segments
    d. curvature of the ring segments

53. At the 4-week postop exam of a patient who underwent uncomplicated PRK for moderate myopia, the manifest refraction is –0.25 D OD and –1.25 D OS. Slit-lamp exam shows moderate anterior stromal haze OS. How would you manage this patient?
    a. add topical antibiotic
    b. increase topical steroids
    c. place bandage contact lens
    d. perform PRK enhancement with MMC

54. A buttonhole flap is most likely to occur with a microkeratome if the patient has
    a. axial length >26 mm
    b. corneal pachymetry <520 μm
    c. keratometry >47 D
    d. white-to-white >12.5 mm

55. The best surgical option for a patient with Fuchs dystrophy, corneal edema, and a visually significant cataract is
    a. phacoemulsification and IOL
    b. phacoemulsification, IOL, and penetrating keratoplasty
    c. phacoemulsification, penetrating keratoplasty, and CL
    d. phacoemulsification, IOL, and endothelial keratoplasty

56. A large epithelial defect occurs during LASIK flap creation. This patient is most at risk for
    a. flap dislocation
    b. diffuse lamellar keratitis
    c. epithelial ingrowth
    d. irregular astigmatism

57. The Kamra inlay improves near vision by which of the following methods?
    a. containing add power on implant
    b. pinhole effect
    c. increasing corneal curvature
    d. decreasing corneal curvature

58. Which type of CL is most likely to cause giant papillary conjunctivitis?
    a. polymethylmethacrylate
    b. rigid gas permeable
    c. soft daily wear
    d. soft extended wear

59. Which method of astigmatism correction provides the best visual acuity after cataract surgery in a patient with keratoconus?
    a. rigid contact lens
    b. toric iol
    c. limbal relaxing incisions
    d. LASIK

60. According to the Munnerlyn equation, the depth of an excimer laser corneal ablation is most dependent on the
    a. degree of myopia
    b. degree of astigmatism
    c. size of the blend zone
    d. diameter of the optical zone

Please visit the eBook for an interactive version of the review questions. See front cover for activation details.

SUGGESTED READINGS

Arffa, R. C. (1998). *Grayson's diseases of the cornea* (4th ed.). St. Louis: Mosby.

Basic and Clinical Sciences Course. (2021). *Section 8: External disease and cornea.* San Francisco: AAO.

Brightbill, F. S., McDonnell, P. J., McGhee, C. N. J., et al. (2008). *Corneal surgery theory, technique and tissue* (4th ed.). St. Louis: Mosby.

Foster, C. S., Azar, D. T., & Dohlman, C. H. (2005). *Smolin and Thoft's the cornea: Scientific foundations and clinical practice* (4th ed.). Philadelphia: Lippincott Williams & Wilkins.

Kaufman, H. E., Barron, B. A., & McDonald, M. B. (1997). *The cornea* (2nd ed.). Philadelphia: Butterworth-Heinemann.

Krachmer, J. H., & Palay, D. A. (2013). *Cornea color atlas* (3rd ed.). Philadelphia: Saunders.

Mannis, M. J., & Holland, E. J. (2016). *Cornea* (4th ed.). Philadelphia: Elsevier.

8

Uveitis

ANATOMY/PHYSIOLOGY

Uvea

Vascular layer of eye: iris, ciliary body, choroid

Attached to sclera at scleral spur, vortex veins at exit sites, and optic nerve (results in dome-shaped appearance of choroidal detachment)

Iris (see Chapter 10, Anterior Segment)

Ciliary body (See Chapter 9, Glaucoma)

Choroid (See Chapter 11, Posterior Segment)

PATHOPHYSIOLOGY

Inflammatory reaction:
Acute: chemical mediators (histamine, serotonin, kinins, plasmin, complement, leukotrienes, prostaglandins)
Chronic: cellular infiltrates
  NONGRANULOMATOUS: lymphocytes, plasma cells
  GRANULOMATOUS: epithelioid and giant cells (Langhans, foreign body, Touton)
    3 PATTERNS: diffuse (e.g., Vogt-Koyanagi-Harada [VKH] syndrome), discrete (e.g., sarcoidosis), zonal (e.g., lens-induced)

Soluble retinal antigen (S-Ag):
Protein (arrestin) found in human rod photoreceptor outer segments and pineal gland

Most potent uveitic antigen; induces experimental autoimmune uveitis (EAU; type 4 hypersensitivity reaction), best animal model of human uveitis
EAU: intradermal injection of S-Ag in rats and rabbits produces panuveitis; removal of thymus prevents EAU (supports T-cell–mediated basis of inflammatory response)
Human diseases that resemble EAU: VKH, sympathetic ophthalmia, birdshot chorioretinopathy; lymphocytes from these patients develop an in vitro proliferative response to retinal S-Ag, suggesting an autoimmune basis for these diseases

CLASSIFICATION

Pathology: nongranulomatous (lymphocyte and plasma cell infiltrates), granulomatous (epithelioid and giant cell infiltrates)

Etiology: infectious (20%), noninfectious (80%; immune response, malignancy, trauma, chemical, idiopathic)

Location: anterior uveitis (70%–80%; iritis, iridocyclitis), intermediate uveitis (15%; vitritis), posterior uveitis (13%; retinitis, choroiditis, chorioretinitis), panuveitis (18%; involvement of all uveal layers: iris, ciliary body, choroid). Keratouveitis is corneal inflammation with secondary involvement of anterior chamber (AC); sclerouveitis is scleral inflammation with involvement of uveal tract

Course: acute, recurrent (episodes separated by ≥3 months without treatment), chronic

ANTERIOR UVEITIS

Inflammation of iris (iritis) and ciliary body (cyclitis); exudation of white blood cells and protein into AC secondary to breakdown of the blood–aqueous barrier and increased vascular permeability, may have minimal spill-over into retrolental space

Most common cause of anterior uveitis in adults is idiopathic (50%), followed by HLA-B27–associated uveitis; must rule out infection, malignancy, medication, trauma

Most common cause of acute, noninfectious, hypopyon iritis is HLA-B27–associated iritis

Etiology:

Children: juvenile idiopathic arthritis (JIA), ankylosing spondylitis, psoriatic arthritis, tubulointerstitial nephritis and uveitis syndrome, Fuchs heterochromic iridocyclitis, familial juvenile systemic granulomatosis (Blau syndrome), sarcoidosis, postviral, herpes simplex virus (HSV), trauma, Kawasaki disease, retinoblastoma
50% have posterior component (toxoplasmosis in 50% with posterior component)

Young adults: HLA-B27 associated, sarcoidosis, HSV, syphilis, Fuchs, Behçet disease, tubulointerstitial nephritis and uveitis syndrome, spillover from intermediate or posterior uveitis

Older adults: idiopathic, sarcoidosis, HSV, varicella-zoster virus (VZV), masquerade syndromes (peripheral retinal detachment [RD; Schwartz-Matsuo syndrome], intraocular foreign body, malignancies [large cell lymphoma, malignant melanoma])

Classification:

Nongranulomatous:

ACUTE: idiopathic, HLA-B27 associated (8% of general population; associated with acute, recurrent uveitis [40%–50% are HLA-B27 positive]; alternating involvement of both eyes [~75%]; up to 90% develop seronegative spondyloarthropathy: ankylosing spondylitis, reactive arthritis syndrome, psoriatic arthritis, inflammatory bowel disease, Whipple disease), Behçet disease, glaucomatocyclitic crisis (Posner-Schlossman syndrome), HSV, VZV, Kawasaki disease, Lyme disease, cytomegalovirus (CMV), Ebola (convalescent phase; anterior, posterior, or panuveitis), traumatic, postoperative, other autoimmune diseases (lupus, relapsing polychondritis, granulomatosis with polyangiitis, tubulointerstitial nephritis and uveitis syndrome), drugs (rifabutin, cidofovir, sulfonamides, bisphosphonates, diethylcarbamazine, metipranolol, systemic moxifloxacin, oral contraceptives, immune checkpoint inhibitors)

CHRONIC (duration >6 weeks): JIA, Fuchs heterochromic iridocyclitis, HSV, VZV

Granulomatous:

INFECTIOUS: syphilis, tuberculosis (TB), leprosy, brucellosis, toxoplasmosis, *Propionibacterium acnes*, fungal (*Cryptococcus, Aspergillus*), HIV

IMMUNE-MEDIATED: sarcoidosis, VKH syndrome, sympathetic ophthalmia, lens-induced (phacoanaphylactic/phacoantigenic), multiple sclerosis (MS)

Symptoms: pain, photophobia, blurred vision, redness, floaters, photopsias

Findings: conjunctival and episcleral injection, ciliary injection (circumcorneal flush from branches of anterior ciliary arteries), miosis (iris sphincter spasm), AC reaction; may have hypopyon, keratic precipitates, iris nodules, dilated iris vessels (occasionally, rubeosis), synechiae (posterior [iris adhesions to lens; seclusiopupillae is a complete adhesion that can result in iris bombe] or anterior [iris adhesions to cornea and angle]), altered intraocular pressure (low from ciliary body [CB] shutdown [chronic uveitis can cause CB atrophy or detachment resulting in hypotony and eventual phthisis], or high from trabeculitis, trabecular meshwork clogging from inflammatory cells, pupillary block, peripheral anterior synechiae, steroid response) (Fig. 8.1)

Keratic precipitates (KP): aggregates of white blood cells on corneal endothelium; typically located inferiorly and centrally (Fig. 8.2)

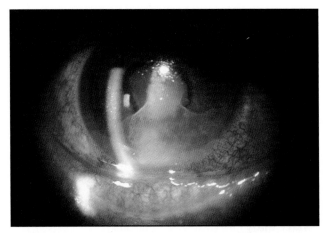

Figure 8.1 Severe idiopathic anterior uveitis with fibrinoid reaction. (From Hooper PL. Idiopathic and other anterior uveitis. In: Yanoff M, Duker JS, eds. *Ophthalmology*. London: Mosby; 1999.)

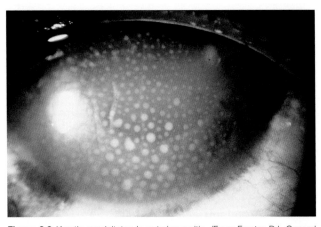

Figure 8.2 Keratic precipitates in anterior uveitis. (From Forster DJ. General approach to the uveitis patient and treatment strategies. In: Yanoff M, Duker JS, eds. *Ophthalmology*. London: Mosby; 1999.)

May occur with any intraocular inflammation, most commonly with uveitis

May be white or pigmented, small or large, nongranulomatous (fine) or granulomatous (mutton fat), diffuse or focal

NONGRANULOMATOUS: composed of lymphocytes and polymorphonuclear leukocytes (PMNs)

GRANULOMATOUS: composed of macrophages, lymphocytes, epithelioid cells, and multinucleated giant cells

DDX OF DIFFUSE KP: Fuchs heterochromic iridocyclitis, sarcoidosis, syphilis, keratouveitis, toxoplasmosis (rarely)

Iris nodules:

KOEPPE: located at pupil margin; occur in granulomatous and nongranulomatous uveitis

BUSACCA: located on anterior iris surface; occur only in granulomatous uveitis (Fig. 8.3)

BERLIN: located in AC angle; occur in granulomatous uveitis

DDx of hypopyon: HLA-B27 associated, infection (keratitis, endophthalmitis), foreign body, JIA, Behçet disease, VKH syndrome, malignancy (leukemia, lymphoma, retinoblastoma), toxic (rifabutin)

DDx of uveitic glaucoma: HSV, VZV, Posner-Schlossman syndrome, Fuchs heterochromic iridocyclitis, sarcoidosis; rarely toxoplasmosis, syphilis, sympathetic ophthalmia

DDx of retinal vasculitis:

Primarily arteritis: systemic lupus erythematosus, polyarteritis nodosa, syphilis, HSV/VZV (acute retinal necrosis [ARN]/progressive outer retinal necrosis [PORN]), Churg-Strauss syndrome, Susac disease

Primarily phlebitis: sarcoidosis, MS, Behçet disease, birdshot chorioretinopathy, HIV, Eales disease

Arteritis and phlebitis: toxoplasmosis, relapsing polychondritis, granulomatosis with polyangiitis, Crohn disease, frosted branch angiitis

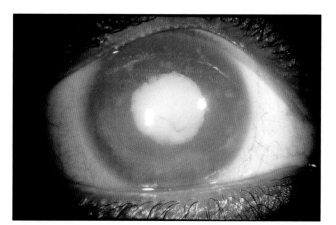

Figure 8.3 Chronic granulomatous uveitis demonstrating Busacca nodules. (From Forster DJ. General approach to the uveitis patient and treatment strategies. In: Yanoff M, Duker JS, eds. *Ophthalmology*. London: Mosby; 1999.)

Diagnosis: tailor workup according to examination and history; purpose of testing is to eliminate a diagnosis, rule out systemic infections (i.e., syphilis, TB), and confirm suspected diagnosis

No testing: first episode of mild, unilateral, nongranulomatous anterior uveitis not associated with systemic symptoms or signs suggestive of an underlying etiology (usually idiopathic), or if diagnosis known

Test: uveitis is moderate or severe, bilateral, recurrent, granulomatous, involves posterior segment, or associated with systemic symptoms or signs suggestive of an underlying etiology

Retest: consider when initial test results do not match clinical suspicion, and if uveitis changes (becomes more severe, bilateral, diffuse, or new symptoms or signs appear)

Minimum: complete blood count (CBC) with differential, erythrocyte sedimentation rate (ESR), Venereal Disease Research Laboratory (VDRL) and fluorescent treponemal antibody absorption (FTA-ABS), QuantiFERON-TB Gold

Expanded: granulomatous, positive review of systems, or posterior involvement: angiotensin-converting enzyme (ACE), antinuclear antibody (ANA), antineutrophil cytoplasmic antibodies (ANCA), QuantiFERON-TB Gold, chest X-ray (CXR) or chest computed tomography (CT); consider HSV and VZV titers, enzyme-linked immunosorbent assay (ELISA) for Lyme immunoglobulin M (IgM) and immunoglobulin G (IgG) in endemic areas, human leukocyte antigen (HLA) typing (25% with HLA-B27 develop sacroiliac disease, so obtain sacroiliac X-ray), urinalysis and urine beta-2 microglobulin (tubulointerstitial nephritis and uveitis syndrome), urethral cultures (reactive arthritis syndrome), HIV Ab test; for endophthalmitis, culture by tap to determine organism

Targeted approach:

RECURRENT UVEITIS, WITH BACK STIFFNESS UPON AWAKENING: rule out ankylosing spondylitis

HLA-B27

Lumbosacral spine imaging (CT)

GRANULOMATOUS UVEITIS: rule out TB and sarcoidosis

CXR

Upper-body gallium scan

ACE elevated in 60% with sarcoidosis; also in Gaucher disease, miliary TB, silicosis; check to make sure not on an ACE-inhibitor

Lysozyme

Serum calcium

Liver function tests and bilirubin

QuantiFERON-TB Gold

CHILD WITH RECURRENT OR CHRONIC IRIDOCYCLITIS: rule out JIA (usually ANA-positive, rheumatoid factor [RF]-negative)

ANA

RF

HLA-B27

RETINAL VASCULITIS, RECURRENT APHTHOUS ULCERS, PRETIBIAL SKIN LESIONS: rule out Behçet disease

Skin lesion biopsy

HLA-B51 and HLA-B5

PARS PLANITIS AND EPISODIC PARESTHESIAS: rule out
multiple sclerosis (MS)
Brain magnetic resonance imaging (MRI)
Lumbar puncture (LP)
**RETINOCHOROIDITIS ADJACENT TO PIGMENTED
CHORIORETINAL SCAR:** rule out toxoplasmosis
Toxoplasma IgM and IgG titers
RETINAL VASCULITIS AND SINUSITIS: rule out
granulomatosis with polyangiitis
ANCA
CXR
Sinus films
Urinalysis
RECURRENT UVEITIS AND DIARRHEA: rule out
inflammatory bowel disease (IBD)
Gastrointestinal (GI) consult
Endoscopy with biopsy
CHOROIDITIS, EXUDATIVE RD, EPISODIC TINNITUS:
rule out Harada disease/VKH syndrome
Fluorescein angiography (FA)
LP
Brain MRI
Audiometry
ELDERLY WITH VITRITIS: rule out intraocular
lymphoma or infection
Vitreal biopsy for culture or cytology
**UNILATERAL IRIDOCYCLITIS, FINE WHITE KP,
LIGHTER IRIS IN AFFECTED EYE:** rule out Fuchs
heterochromic iridocyclitis
Intraocular pressure (IOP)
Gonioscopy (fine-angle vessels)

Complications: iris atrophy, band keratopathy, synechiae
(anterior and posterior), cataract, glaucoma, cystoid macular
edema, retinal detachment, retinal vasculitis, optic neuritis,
neovascularization, cyclitic membranes, hypotony, phthisis

Treatment: topical steroids, cycloplegic; may require
systemic steroids, immunomodulatory therapy (IMT; i.e.,
antimetabolites, T-cell inhibitors, alkylating agents, biologic
agents), antibiotics; use safest, most potent agent
Goal: prevent ocular damage and vision loss; treat until
no cells (*exception:* JIA can have trace cell)
Poor response to steroids: Fuchs, syphilis, toxoplasmosis,
keratouveitis, Lyme disease, chronic postoperative
endophthalmitis, ARN, CMV

Prognosis: depends on location; 35% have visual
impairment or blindness, usually caused by cystoid macular
edema (CME), cataract, and glaucoma
Risk of 25% decrease in visual acuity: 1%-4% for anterior
uveitis, 66% for intermediate uveitis, 43% for posterior
uveitis, 40% for panuveitis

Seronegative Spondyloarthropathies

Group of conditions with the following features:
radiographic sacroiliitis (with or without spondylitis),
asymmetric peripheral arthritis without rheumatoid nodules,
negative RF and ANA, HLA-B27 association, variable
mucocutaneous lesions, and anterior uveitis

Ankylosing Spondylitis

90% HLA-B27-positive; typically young men

Symptoms: lower back pain and stiffness with inactivity
(upon awakening in morning, long car rides)

Findings: anterior uveitis (30%; recurrent in 40%),
episcleritis, scleritis

Other findings: arthritis (sacroiliac and peripheral joints),
heart (aortic insufficiency, heart block), colitis (10%), lungs
(restricted chest expansion, apical fibrosis)

Sacroiliac X-ray: sclerosis and narrowing of joint space;
ligamentous ossification can occur

Reactive Arthritis Syndrome

Formerly Reiter syndrome; inflammatory arthritis following
GI or genitourinary infection; 1%-3% with nonspecific
urethritis develop episode of arthritis

Triad of urethritis, arthritis, and conjunctivitis; majority do
not present with classic triad

50%-75% HLA-B27; 2nd-3rd decade of life; mainly males
(10% females)

Thought to be aberrant autoimmune response to infection:
*Chlamydia, Ureaplasma, Yersinia, Campylobacter, Shigella,
Salmonella*; rare case after bacillus Calmette-Guerin (BCG)
treatment for bladder cancer

Criteria (≥2 features plus skeletal involvement): sausage-
shaped finger, toe or heel pain; asymmetric oligoarthritis
(usually knees, ankles, sacroiliac joints, lumbar spine);
conjunctivitis or iritis; acute diarrhea or cervicitis (within 4
weeks of onset of arthritis); urethritis or genital ulcers

Findings: mucopurulent conjunctivitis (30%), keratitis,
acute anterior uveitis

Other findings: tendonitis (30%; plantar fasciitis, Achilles
tendinitis), keratoderma blennorrhagicum (20%; scaling
skin lesion on feet and hands; similar to pustular psoriasis),
circinate balanitis (scaling, erythematous rash on distal
penis), prostatitis, cystitis, mouth ulcers, geographic tongue,
erythema nodosum, heart (carditis, aortic, conduction and
valvular abnormalities), nails (onycholysis, subungual
keratosis, pits)

Complications: recurrent arthritis (15%–50%), chronic
arthritis or sacroiliitis, ankylosing spondylitis, urethral
stricture, aortic root necrosis, cataracts, CME

Psoriatic Arthritis

Associated with HLA-B17 and HLA-B27

Uveitis in 25% (usually bilateral and chronic), associated with sacroiliitis, rarely in psoriasis without arthritis

Findings: conjunctivitis, dry eyes, anterior uveitis

Other findings: arthritis (hands, feet, sacroiliac joints [20%]), psoriatic skin and nail changes

Inflammatory Bowel Disease (IBD)

Uveitis, usually bilateral with posterior component; occurs in ulcerative colitis (up to 12%) and Crohn disease (2.4%)

Findings: conjunctivitis, keratoconjunctivitis sicca, episcleritis, scleritis, anterior uveitis, orbital cellulitis, vasculitis, optic neuritis

Other findings: arthritis (20% have sacroiliitis; 60% with sacroiliitis are HLA-B27–positive), erythema nodosum, pyoderma gangrenosum, hepatitis, sclerosing cholangitis

Behçet Disease

Triad of recurrent hypopyon iritis, aphthous stomatitis, and genital ulcers; also arthritis, thromboembolism, and central nervous system (CNS) problems

Anterior uveitis is usually bilateral with posterior involvement, hallmark is occlusive retinal vasculitis (see Posterior Uveitis below)

Fuchs Heterochromic Iridocyclitis (Fuchs Uveitis Syndrome)

Unilateral (90%), anterior uveitis; young adults

Associated with CMV, rubella, and ocular toxoplasmosis

Symptoms: blurred vision

Findings: diffuse small white stellate KP, minimal AC reaction, no posterior synechiae, iris heterochromia (diffuse atrophy of stroma, loss of iris crypts; involved iris is usually lighter; 15% bilateral), fine-angle vessels (may bleed during gonioscopy, cataract surgery, or paracentesis) (Fig. 8.4)

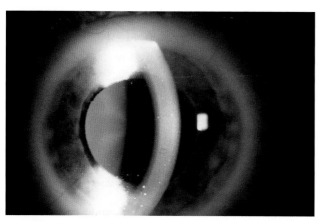

Figure 8.4 Fuchs uveitis. (From Hooper PL. Idiopathic and other anterior uveitis. In: Yanoff M, Duker JS, eds. *Ophthalmology*. London: Mosby; 1999.)

DDx of iris heterochromia: trauma (intraocular metallic foreign body), inflammation, congenital Horner syndrome, iris melanoma, Waardenburg syndrome (iris heterochromia, telecanthus, white forelock, congenital deafness), Parry-Romberg syndrome (iris heterochromia, Horner syndrome, ocular motor palsies, nystagmus, facial hemiatrophy), glaucomatocyclitic crisis, medication (topical prostaglandin analogues [Xalatan, Lumigan, Travatan]), nevus of Ota

Pathology: plasma cells in ciliary body

Complications: glaucoma (up to 60%), cataract (posterior subcapsular cataract [PSC]; up to 90%)

Treatment: poor response to steroids

Juvenile Idiopathic Arthritis (JIA; formerly juvenile rheumatoid arthritis [JRA])

(See Chapter 5, Pediatrics/Strabismus)

Kawasaki Disease

(See Chapter 5, Pediatrics/Strabismus)

Tubulointerstitial Nephritis and Uveitis Syndrome (TINU)

Acute nongranulomatous anterior uveitis, usually bilateral; may have intermediate, posterior, or panuveitis; usually young females in 2nd-4th decades of life

Unknown etiology; associated with HLA-DQA1, DQB1, and DRB1; some cases may be hypersensitivity reaction to medications (antibiotics, nonsteroidal anti-inflammatory drugs [NSAIDs])

Criteria: abnormal serum creatinine or decreased creatinine clearance, abnormal urinalysis (increased β_2-microglobulin, proteinuria, eosinophils, pyuria or hematuria, white cell casts, and normoglycemic glycosuria), and systemic illness (fever, weight loss, anorexia, fatigue, arthralgias, myalgias; may have abnormal liver function, eosinophilia, and elevated ESR)

Pathology: interstitial edema and fibrosis with mononuclear inflammatory cells; eosinophils can be present

Treatment: oral steroids to prevent renal failure, may require IMT

Posner-Schlossman Syndrome (Glaucomatocyclitic Crisis)

Recurrent, unilateral, anterior uveitis and increased IOP; episodes self-limited (hours to days)

Associated with HLA-Bw54; CMV may be causative agent

Symptoms: unilateral pain

Findings: mild AC reaction, few or no KP, elevated IOP, mid-dilated pupil, no synechiae

Treatment: may require topical glaucoma medications to control IOP, steroids to control inflammation

Phacoanaphylactic Endophthalmitis (Phacoantigenic Uveitis)

Immune complex disease (type 3 hypersensitivity reaction) when normal tolerance to lens protein is lost

Previous rupture of lens capsule in same or fellow eye, followed by latent period; with re-exposure to lens protein during surgery, zonal granulomatous uveitis occurs

Associated with trauma (80%)

May develop severe granulomatous uveitis with hypotony, secondary open-angle glaucoma

Pathology: zonal pattern (PMNs infiltrate central lens material; epithelioid histiocytes and mononuclear cells around nidus)

Treatment: remove lens

Infections

Herpes Simplex Virus (HSV) and Varicella Zoster Virus (VZV)

Acute or chronic, recurrent iritis, especially VZV (up to 40%); may also have corneal involvement

Findings: KP (granulomatous, nongranulomatous, or stellate) underlying areas of dendritic or stromal keratitis or endotheliitis, elevated intraocular pressure common; may have skin lesions, iris atrophy (patchy or sectoral), corneal scarring, decreased corneal sensation, neurotrophic keratitis

Treatment: topical steroid and cycloplegic; consider topical antiviral (prophylactically or for keratitis) and systemic antiviral acutely and for long-term prevention (HSV: acyclovir 400 mg PO bid or valacyclovir 500 mg PO qd. VZV: acyclovir 800 mg PO bid or valacyclovir 1 g PO qd)

Epstein-Barr Virus (EBV)

Bilateral granulomatous anterior uveitis occurs in acquired infection (mononucleosis); may also have other anterior segment and posterior segment involvement (see Posterior Uveitis below)

Cytomegalovirus (CMV)

Unilateral, chronic, recurrent anterior uveitis in immune-competent individuals

Findings: mimics Fuchs heterochromic iridocyclitis or Posner-Schlossman syndrome with small KP, elevated IOP, sectoral iris atrophy; may have corneal edema

and endotheliitis; severe hemorrhagic retinitis in immunocompromised patients (see Posterior Uveitis below)

Treatment: systemic antivirals (valganciclovir), topical and intravitreal ganciclovir

Lyme Disease

Caused by infection with *Borrelia burgdorferi* (spirochete); transmitted by infected tick (*Ixodes scapularis* and *Ixodes pacificus*)

Ocular involvement is usually bilateral

Affected organ systems: skin, CNS, cardiovascular, musculoskeletal

3 stages:
Stage 1 (local disease; within 4 weeks in 70%): erythema chronicum migrans ("bull's-eye" macular rash at tick bite), fever, malaise, fatigue, myalgias, arthralgias
Stage 2 (disseminated disease; 1–4 months): hematogenous spread causes rash, arthritis (up to 80%; commonly knee), carditis, neurologic manifestations (up to 40%; meningitis, encephalitis, radiculitis, Bell palsy)
Stage 3 (persistent disease; >5 months): arthritis (chronic associated with HLA-DR4 and HLA-DR2), acrodermatitis chronica atrophicans (blue–red lesion on extremities, can develop fibrosis and nodules), neurologic changes (neuropsychiatric disease, radiculopathy, chronic fatigue, peripheral neuropathy, memory loss)

Findings:
Stage 1: follicular conjunctivitis (most common; 11%), episcleritis
Stage 2 and 3: uveitis (most common in stage 2), often chronic granulomatous iridocyclitis with posterior synechiae and vitreous cells, intermediate or posterior uveitis, choroiditis (peripheral multifocal with small round punched-out lesions and vitritis), retinal vasculitis, branch retinal vein occlusion (BRVO), exudative RD, neuroretinitis, papillitis, optic neuritis, optic atrophy, cranial nerve palsies (cranial nerve [CN] VII most common), papilledema (with meningitis); keratitis (most common in stage 3; bilateral nummular stromal infiltrates, may develop edema and neovascularization), episcleritis

Diagnosis: antibody testing (ELISA for IgM and IgG)

Treatment: systemic antibiotics (oral amoxicillin, doxycycline, or cefuroxime; or intravenous [IV] ceftriaxone); topical steroid and cycloplegic for uveitis, topical steroid for keratitis (immune reaction in cornea)

Syphilis

Caused by infection with *Treponema pallidum* (spirochete)

Findings: chronic or recurrent nongranulomatous or granulomatous anterior uveitis; may also have interstitial keratitis, dilated iris vascular tufts (iris roseola), vitritis, chorioretinitis, papillitis, and mucocutaneous manifestations (see Panuveitis below)

Tuberculosis

Rarely caused by direct ocular infection of *Mycobacterium tuberculosis,* usually an immune response to organism

Findings: chronic granulomatous iritis; may also have conjunctival nodules, phlyctenules, interstitial keratitis, scleritis, iris nodules, vitritis, choroiditis (see Panuveitis below)

INTERMEDIATE UVEITIS

Etiology: idiopathic (pars planitis), MS (5%–25% have periphlebitis and intermediate uveitis), sarcoidosis, Lyme disease, peripheral toxocariasis, syphilis, TB, human T-lymphotropic virus type 1 (HTLV-1)

Pars Planitis

Most common type of intermediate uveitis (85%–90%)

Male = female, usually aged 5-40 years; 80% bilateral, often asymmetric

25% of uveitis in children

Up to 15% develop MS

Etiology: unknown; diagnosis of exclusion

Symptoms: floaters, blurred vision

Findings: light flare with a few KP, anterior vitritis, snowballs (white vitreous cellular aggregates near ora serrata; may coalesce to form peripheral fibrovascular accumulation [snowbank] over inferior pars plana and vitreous base), CB detachment, retrolental membrane, peripheral retinal periphlebitis, hyperemic disc, no chorioretinitis, no synechiae (Fig. 8.5)

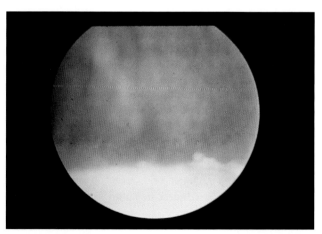

Figure 8.5 Inferior pars plana snowbank with attached snowballs. (From Zimmerman PL. Pars planitis and other intermediate uveitis. In: Yanoff M, Duker JS, eds. *Ophthalmology*. London: Mosby; 1999.)

Pathology:
> *Snowballs:* epithelioid cells and multinucleated giant cells
> *Snowbank:* preretinal membrane of fibroglial and vascular elements
> *Peripheral retinal veins:* often have perivascular cuff of lymphocytes

DDx: sarcoidosis, toxoplasmosis, toxocariasis, syphilis, Lyme disease, MS, HTLV-1
> *Multiple sclerosis:* intermediate uveitis can occur (up to 30% of patients with MS develop uveitis, associated with HLA-DR15; usually intermediate); bilateral (up to 95%), milder than idiopathic cases; may present with band keratopathy, mild AC reaction, vitreous cells, periphlebitis in a young patient; can also have cataract (PSC), epiretinal membrane, CME
> *HTLV-1:* retrovirus endemic in Japan, Caribbean, Central and South America; infects CD4+ T cells; causes adult T-cell leukemia/lymphoma, HTLV-1–associated myelopathy/tropical spastic paralysis, and uveitis. Uveitis is most commonly intermediate (75%) with anterior uveitis (20%), vitritis (60%), retinal vasculitis (60%), exudative retinal lesions (25%), optic disc involvement (20%), CME; recurrence in 50%. Also associated with interstitial keratitis, dry eye, retinal degeneration, optic neuropathy

Complications: cataract (up to 60%), glaucoma (10%), cyclitic membrane, retinal NV, vitreous hemorrhage, tractional or rhegmatogenous RD (up to 10%), CME (50%), band keratopathy

Treatment (main indication is CME with reduced vision): periocular and oral steroids; consider IMT, intravitreal anti–vascular endothelial growth factor (VEGF) agents, vitrectomy; areas of retinal ischemia and neovascularization (NV) can be treated with laser photocoagulation or cryotherapy (rarely used, may cause more inflammation)

Prognosis: 10% self-limited, 30% smoldering with remissions and exacerbations, 60% chronic, 75% maintain vision ≥20/40 after 10 years

POSTERIOR UVEITIS

Most common cause of posterior uveitis in adults is toxoplasmosis (followed by retinal vasculitis)

Signs: vitreous cells, membranes, opacities, inflammatory exudates ("snowballs"), vasculitis (opacification around vessels [sheathing: whole vessel, cuffing: segment of vessel]), hemorrhages, exudates (candlewax drippings), retinitis (edema or necrosis, causes whitening), pigmentary changes (caused by retinal pigment epithelium [RPE] inflammation), choroiditis (focal, multifocal, or diffuse), choroidal infiltrates (creamy yellow lesions), choroidal detachment, retinal detachment (exudative, tractional, or rhegmatogenous), preretinal/subretinal fibrosis

DDx of vitritis:

Panuveitis: idiopathic, sarcoidosis, TB, syphilis, VKH, sympathetic ophthalmia, Behçet disease, Ebola

Postsurgical/trauma: Irvine-Gass syndrome

Endophthalmitis: infection, sterile

Choroiditis: acute posterior multifocal placoid pigment epitheliopathy (APMPPE), serpiginous choroiditis, birdshot chorioretinopathy, multifocal choroiditis, punctate inner chorioretinopathy, *Toxocara*, presumed ocular histoplasmosis syndrome [POHS]

Retinitis: ARN, CMV, toxoplasmosis, candidiasis, cysticercosis, onchocerciasis

Vasculitis: Eales disease

Other infections: nematodes, Whipple disease, EBV, Lyme disease

Other: amyloidosis, ocular ischemia, masquerade syndromes, spillover from anterior uveitis

Intermediate uveitis: pars planitis, MS, IBD, TINU

Diagnosis: consider vitrectomy or chorioretinal biopsy if unresponsive to treatment or suspected infection or malignancy

Complications: neovascularization (retinal or choroidal), CME, optic nerve swelling and atrophy

CME: common cause of vision loss in pars planitis, birdshot chorioretinopathy, retinal vasculitis, and any iridocyclitis (especially chronic, recurrent cases)

Indications for IMT: vision-threatening inflammation, inflammations unresponsive to maximum steroid therapy, steroid contraindicated, not tolerated, or dependent; Behçet disease, sympathetic ophthalmia, VKH, pars planitis, Eales disease, retinal vasculitis, serpiginous choroiditis, ocular cicatricial pemphigoid (OCP), necrotizing scleritis

Collagen Vascular Diseases

Systemic Lupus Erythematosus (SLE)

Multisystem autoimmune connective tissue disease

Usually females, childbearing age; more common in African Americans and Hispanics

Autoantibodies: antinuclear antibodies (ANA; high false-positive rate if no signs or symptoms), antibodies to DNA (anti-ssDNA, anti-dsDNA), antibodies to cytoplasmic components (anti-Sm, anti-Ro, anti-La), and antiphospholipid antibodies

Findings: ocular involvement in 50%; lids (discoid lupus), Sjögren syndrome, scleritis, cranial nerve palsies, optic neuropathy, retinal and choroidal vasculopathy (cotton-wool spots, hemorrhages, vascular occlusions, exudative RD, choroidal infarction, neovascularization); rarely uveitis

Other findings: skin lesions (70%–80%; malar rash, discoid lupus, photosensitivity, mucosal lesions), arthritis (80%–85%), renal disease (50%–75%), Raynaud phenomenon (30%–50%), neurologic (35%); may have heart, lung, and liver involvement

Treatment: systemic steroids, IMT, hydroxychloroquine; may require anticoagulation; panretinal photocoagulation, intravitreal anti-VEGF agents, vitrectomy

Polyarteritis Nodosa (PAN)

Systemic vasculitis with focal, necrotizing inflammation of small and medium-size arteries

5th-7th decades of life, male > female (3:1)

Associated with hepatitis B

Findings: hypertensive retinopathy, retinal artery occlusions, choroidal infarction, retinal vasculitis, exudative RD, cranial nerve palsies, amaurosis fugax, homonymous hemianopia, Horner syndrome, optic atrophy, scleritis, peripheral ulcerative keratitis

Other findings: fever, weight loss, fatigue, arthralgia, peripheral neuropathy, skin lesions (subcutaneous nodules, purpura, Raynaud phenomenon), kidney involvement (secondary hypertension), small bowel ischemia/infarction, coronary arteritis, pericarditis

Treatment: 90% 5-year mortality if untreated; systemic steroids and IMT increase survival to 80%

Granulomatosis With Polyangiitis (GPA)

Formerly Wegener granulomatosis

Multisystem autoimmune disease; triad of necrotizing granulomatous vasculitis of respiratory tract, focal segmental glomerulonephritis, and necrotizing vasculitis of small vessels

Organ involvement: paranasal sinus > lungs > kidneys

Findings: ocular or orbital (usually from sinus extension) involvement in up to 50%; orbital cellulitis, dacryocystitis, orbital pseudotumor, scleritis (40%), peripheral ulcerative keratitis, uveitis (10%; unilateral or bilateral anterior, intermediate, or posterior), retinitis (20%; cotton-wool spots, hemorrhages, vascular occlusions, retinal vasculitis)

Other findings: sinusitis (bloody nasal discharge), pulmonary changes, arthritis; may have skin lesions (purpura, ulcers, subcutaneous nodules) and neurologic changes (mononeuritis multiplex, cranial neuropathies, seizures, stroke symptoms, cerebral vasculitis with possible neovascularization, vitreous hemorrhage, and neovascular glaucoma)

Diagnosis: tissue biopsy, CXR, lab tests (ESR, C-reactive protein [CRP], ANCA [c-ANCA, p-ANCA, PR3-ANCA, MPO-ANCA], urinalysis [proteinuria, hematuria])

Treatment: 80% 1-year mortality if untreated, vision loss in up to 40%; oral steroids and IMT (cyclophosphamide, rituximab) increase survival to 93%

Susac Syndrome

SICRET syndrome (small infarctions of cochlear, retinal, and encephalic tissue)

Rare; triad of encephalopathy, hearing loss, and branch retinal artery occlusion (BRAO)

Age range 16-58 years old, usually young females

MRI: multifocal supratentorial white matter lesions; may involve corpus callosum

Audiometry: sensorineural hearing loss

Treatment: controversial, includes high-dose IV steroids, IMT, anticoagulation

Infections

Rubella

(See Chapter 5, Pediatrics/Strabismus)

Measles

(See Chapter 5, Pediatrics/Strabismus)

Toxoplasmosis

(See Chapter 5, Pediatrics/Strabismus)

Toxocariasis

(See Chapter 5, Pediatrics/Strabismus)

Presumed Ocular Histoplasmosis Syndrome (POHS)

Caused by infection with *Histoplasma capsulatum,* a dimorphic fungus (mold in soil, yeast in animals and birds) endemic in Mississippi and Ohio River valleys; rare in Europe; rare among African Americans

Age of onset commonly 20-45 years; male = female; 90% with ocular signs have positive skin reaction (>5 mm) to intracutaneous 1:100 histoplasmin (test usually not used because it may incite macular disease)

Macular involvement associated with HLA-B7, HLA-DRw2

Primary infection from inhalation of spores, usually asymptomatic or have self-limited flu-like illness; hematogenous spread to spleen, liver, and choroid

Primary choroidal infection causes granulomatous, clinically unapparent inflammation that resolves into a small, atrophic scar that can disrupt Bruch membrane, choriocapillaris, and RPE

Findings: triad of peripapillary atrophy, multiple punched-out chorioretinal scars ("histo spots," may enlarge, >20% develop new spots), and maculopathy. No anterior or posterior segment cell; may have linear equatorial streaks; may develop choroidal neovascularization (CNV; different

from that in AMD in that vessels penetrate Bruch membrane and extend over RPE; a second layer of RPE forms [basal side up] and attempts to encircle the CNV) (see Fig. 11.51)

Risk of CNV: 1% if no signs of POHS in fellow eye, 5% if no histo spots in macula and 15% (within 5 years) if histo spots in macula

CXR: calcifications

Treatment: intravitreal anti-VEGF agents, intravitreal steroids, and other therapies for CNV (see Chapter 11, Posterior Segment)

Cytomegalovirus (CMV)

Progressive hemorrhagic necrotizing retinitis involving all retinal layers

Occurs in immunocompromised individuals and congenital CMV

Before highly active antiretroviral therapy (HAART) therapy, 30% of patients with HIV/AIDS with CD4 count <50 cells/mm³; modern antiretroviral drugs have reduced risk by 80%

40% bilateral at presentation

Symptoms: often asymptomatic; may have floaters, scotoma

Findings: well-circumscribed necrotizing retinitis (3 variants), mild AC and vitreous reaction

Fulminant: "pizza-pie" fundus with thick, yellow–white areas of edema, necrosis, hemorrhage, vascular sheathing, Kyrieleis plaques; usually in posterior pole (Fig. 8.6)

ZONE 1: 1-disc diameter surrounding the disc and 2-disc diameter around the fovea: immediately sight threatening

ZONE 2: anterior to zone 1 and posterior to vortex vein ampullae

ZONE 3: peripheral to zone 2

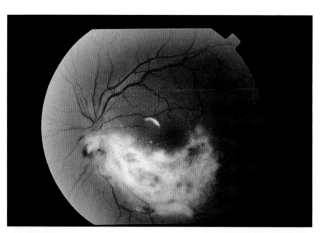

Figure 8.6 Cytomegalovirus retinitis. (From Hudson HL, Boyer DS, Martin DF, et al. Viral posterior uveitis. In: Yanoff M, Duker JS, eds. *Ophthalmology.* London: Mosby; 1999.)

Indolent: "brushfire" appearance with granular, yellow–white advancing edge and peripheral atrophic "burned-out" region; minimal hemorrhage, edema, vascular sheathing; usually in periphery

Perivascular: similar to "frosted-branch" angiitis

Other findings (congenital CMV infection): fever, pneumonitis, hepatosplenomegaly, thrombocytopenia, anemia. Approximately 10%-20% have retinitis, may have RD (up to 1/3), cataract, optic atrophy

Pathology: infected retinal cells are markedly enlarged, then necrotic, finally atrophic; large owl's eye intranuclear inclusions

Complications: rhegmatogenous RD (up to 30%)

Treatment: antiviral therapy (induction during first 2 weeks); intravitreal injections for sight-threatening lesions

Ganciclovir (Cytovene): virostatic
TOXICITY: myelosuppression with neutropenia and thrombocytopenia (5%–10% of patients)
INDUCTION: 5 mg/kg IV bid × 2-4 weeks
MAINTENANCE: 5-10 mg/kg IV qd
INTRAVITREAL INJECTION: 2 mg/0.1 mL 2-3 times a week × 2-3 weeks

Foscarnet: virostatic
TOXICITY: renal, seizures, anemia
INDUCTION: 90 mg/kg IV bid or 60 mg/kg IV tid × 2 weeks
MAINTENANCE: 90-120 mg/kg IV qd
INTRAVITREAL INJECTION: 2.4 mg/0.1 mL 2-3 times a week × 2-3 weeks, then 1-2 times a week

Cidofovir (Vistide): longer half-life
TOXICITY: renal, anterior uveitis (50%), hypotony
INDUCTION: 3-5 mg/kg IV once a week × 2 weeks
MAINTENANCE: 3-5 mg/kg IV once every 2 weeks
Administered through peripheral line (central line required for ganciclovir and foscarnet)
INTRAVITREAL INJECTION: 165-330 μg once a week × 3 weeks, then every 2 weeks
Associated with lowering of IOP (~2 mm Hg), 20%-50% develop iritis (~5 days after last infusion)

Probenecid and hydration with each dose to reduce renal toxicity and decrease iritis
Median time to progression = 120 days

Ganciclovir implant (Vitrasert): median time to progression = 194 days (vs. 72 days with IV ganciclovir and 15 days with no treatment); lasts ~8 months

Oral valganciclovir: L-valyl ester of ganciclovir (prodrug), 60% bioavailability, fatty foods increase bioavailability, reaches peak concentration after 2 hours
INDUCTION: 900 mg bid × 3 weeks
MAINTENANCE: 900 mg qd

Surgery: vitrectomy with long-acting tamponade for rhegmatogenous retinal detachment (RRD)

Acute Retinal Necrosis (ARN)

Acute self-limited confluent peripheral necrotizing retinitis resulting from infection with VZV, HSV, or rarely, CMV or EBV

Usually occurs in healthy (immunocompetent) individuals, mostly in 5th-7th decades of life

36% bilateral (BARN), especially if immunocompromised

Association with HLA-DQw7, HLA-Bw62, and HLA-DR4 in American Caucasians and HLA-Aw33, HLA-B44, and HLA-DRw6 in Japanese

Symptoms: acute decreased vision, ocular/periocular pain, pain on eye movement, redness, photophobia, floaters

Findings: diffuse episcleral injection, anterior uveitis with granulomatous KP, posterior synechiae, elevated intraocular pressure, vitreous cells/haze; within 2 weeks develop triad of vitritis, multifocal peripheral retinitis ("thumbprint" nummular creamy infiltrates posterior to equator with isolated peripheral patches of necrotizing retinitis that becomes confluent; sawtooth demarcation line between necrotic and healthy retina), and generalized obliterative retinal arteritis with peripheral vasoocclusion (Fig. 8.7); multiple retinal breaks and proliferative vitreoretinopathy cause traction RDs (75%); may have optic nerve edema and relative afferent pupillary defect (RAPD); within 2 months, retinitis gradually resolves and necrotic retina sloughs, leaving coarse salt-and-pepper pigmentation

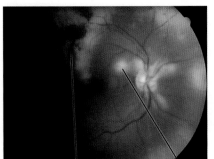
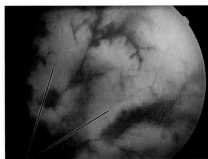

intraretinal hemorrhages   retinal necrosis

Figure 8.7 Acute retinal necrosis. (From Kaiser PK, Friedman NJ, Pineda R II. *Massachusetts Eye and Ear Infirmary Illustrated Manual of Ophthalmology*, 2nd ed. Philadelphia: WB Saunders; 2004.)

Pathology: necrosis occurs from virally induced cytolysis, arteriolar and choriocapillaris occlusion; necrotic cells slough into vitreous, leaving large areas devoid of retina

FA: focal areas of choroidal hypoperfusion early; late staining

Treatment: treatment needs to be individualized
Systemic antiviral agents (tapered slowly over months following resolution of the acute herpetic phase):
INDUCTION: acyclovir 10 mg/kg IV q8h × 10-14 days, valacyclovir 2 g PO tid, ganciclovir 500 mg IV q12h, or valganciclovir 900 mg PO bid × 3 weeks
MAINTENANCE: acyclovir 800 mg PO 5 ×/day, famciclovir 500 mg PO tid, valacyclovir 1 g PO tid, or valganciclovir 450 mg PO bid × 3-4 months
Intravitreal injections (for sight-threatening retinitis): ganciclovir (2 mg/0.1 mL) foscarnet (1.2–2.4 mg/0.1 mL)
Systemic steroids: prednisone (1 mg/kg/day PO × up to 6–8 weeks), initiated 24-48 hours after the start of antiviral therapy or once regression of retinal necrosis has been demonstrated

Prognosis: watch fellow eye closely (usually develops ARN within 6 weeks); antiviral agents reduce risk by 50%; 65%-90% develop RRD (usually within 3 months)

Progressive Outer Retinal Necrosis (PORN)

Variant of ARN in immunosuppressed patients (usually AIDS); painless, with minimal intraocular inflammation

Often have history of cutaneous zoster

74% unilateral at presentation, 70% become bilateral

Findings: multiple discrete peripheral or central areas of retinal opacification/infiltrates (deep with very rapid progression), "cracked mud" appearance after resolution; vasculitis is not prominent (Fig. 8.8)

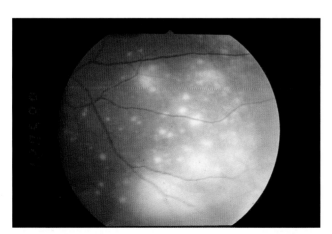

Figure 8.8 Progressive outer retinal necrosis, early stage. (From Hudson HL, Boyer DS, Martin DF, et al. Viral posterior uveitis. In: Yanoff M, Duker JS, eds. *Ophthalmology*. London: Mosby; 1999.)

Treatment: systemic and intraocular antiviral with foscarnet and ganciclovir; poor response to antivirals

Prognosis: 67% have no light perception (NLP) within 4 weeks; RD in 70%

Nonnecrotizing Herpetic Retinitis

Typically during convalescence from acute VZV infection

Usually bilateral, acute retinochoroiditis with hemorrhages in children; chronic choroiditis or retinal vasculitis in adults

Treatment: systemic antiviral; poor response to systemic steroids/IMT

Epstein-Barr Virus (EBV)

Ocular involvement from congenital (usually cataract) or more commonly from acquired infection (mononucleosis)

Associated with Burkitt lymphoma, nasopharyngeal carcinoma, and Hodgkin disease

Findings: follicular conjunctivitis, Parinaud oculoglandular syndrome, episcleritis, stromal keratitis, dacryadenitis, anterior uveitis (bilateral granulomatous); may have cranial nerve palsies, vitritis, retinitis, multifocal choroiditis and panuveitis (MCP), CME, subretinal fibrosis, CNV, ARN, optic disc edema, optic neuritis

Treatment: usually self-limited; topical steroid and cycloplegic for anterior uveitis, systemic steroid for posterior uveitis, systemic antiviral for necrotizing retinitis

Candidiasis

Yeast-like form (blastoconidia), or pseudohyphae or elongated branching structures (pseudomycelia)

Occurs in debilitated patients on hyperalimentation and in IV drug abusers

Most cases occur without positive blood cultures or ongoing fungemia

~10% with candidemia develop endophthalmitis

Findings: anterior uveitis, retinal hemorrhages, perivascular sheathing, chorioretinitis with fluffy white lesions ("puff balls"; may be joined by opaque vitreous stands ["string of pearls"]), vitreous abscess; may have subretinal abscess

DDx of pale subretinal mass: metastasis, amelanotic melanoma, choroidal osteoma, old subretinal hemorrhage, granuloma

Culture: blood agar or Sabouraud glucose (large, creamy-white colonies)

Treatment: IV amphotericin B

Prognosis: 70% mortality within 1 year

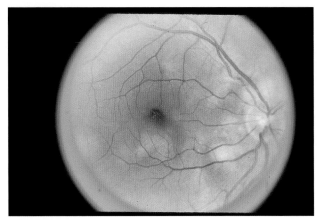

Figure 8.9 Multiple choroidal lesions in *Pneumocystis* choroiditis. (From Cowan CL. Sarcoidosis. In: Yanoff M, Duker JS, eds. *Ophthalmology*. London: Mosby; 1999.)

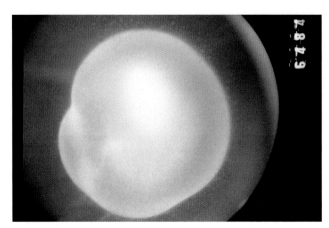

Figure 8.10 Cysticercus in the eye. (From Cowan CL. Sarcoidosis. In: Yanoff M, Duker JS, eds. *Ophthalmology*. London: Mosby; 1999.)

Pneumocystis Choroiditis

Caused by infection with *Pneumocystis carinii*

Choroiditis with multifocal orange nummular lesions; lesions contain cysts of P. carinii (Fig. 8.9)

Associated with use of inhaled pentamidine (which is prophylaxis for pulmonary *Pneumocystis* only)

Cysticercosis

Caused by infection with *Cysticercus cellulosae* (larval stage of pork tapeworm *Taenia solium* or *Taenia saginata*), endemic in Mexico, Africa, Southeast Asia, Eastern Europe, Central and South America, India

Humans are definitive host, and pigs are intermediate host; acquired by ingestion (fecal-oral or undercooked infected pork)

Adult worm lives in small intestine, larvae penetrate gut mucosa, hematogenous spread to eye

Usually occurs in patients aged 10-30 years

Ocular involvement can be eye, orbit, or adnexa; most commonly subretinal or in vitreous (up to 46%)

Findings: mass lesion, exudative RD, intravitreal cyst (globular, translucent, with undulating head [scolex]), eyelid or subconjunctival nodule; larval death causes panuveitis (Fig. 8.10)

Other findings: may have intracerebral calcification, hydrocephalus with CNS involvement

Treatment: vitrectomy required for posterior segment disease; laser photocoagulation can produce severe inflammation; systemic anthelmintics and steroids for extraocular disease

Leprosy

Caused by infection with *Mycobacterium leprae*

5–15 million infected; 250,000 blind

Findings:
Lids: lagophthalmos, madarosis, blepharochalasis, nodules, trichiasis, entropion, ectropion, reduced blinking
Lacrimal: acute and chronic dacryocystitis
Cornea: anesthesia, exposure keratopathy, band keratopathy, corneal leproma, interstitial keratitis, thickened nerves, superficial stromal keratitis
Sclera: episcleritis, scleritis, staphyloma, nodules
Iris: miosis, iritis, synechiae, seclusiopupillae, atrophy, iris pearls, leproma
Ciliary body: loss of accommodation, hypotony, phthisis
Fundus: peripheral choroidal lesions, retinal vasculitis

Complications: cataract, glaucoma

Diffuse Unilateral Subacute Neuroretinitis (DUSN)

Caused by infection with dog hookworm (*Ancylostoma caninum*; 400–1000 μm long) or raccoon nematode (*Baylisascaris procyonis*; 1500–2000 μm long) in subretinal space

Occurs in patients aged 11-65 years (mean age = 14 years)

Causes recurrent focal, multifocal, or diffuse inflammation of retina, RPE, and optic nerve with unilateral decreased vision; rare reports of bilateral disease

Findings: deep, gray–white retinal lesions, optic disc edema, vitritis; may have exudative RD and visible subretinal worm; late findings include retinal vascular narrowing, diffuse RPE pigmentary changes, optic atrophy; results in unilateral "wipe-out" syndrome

Electroretinogram (ERG): decreased

Treatment: laser photocoagulation of nematode if visible or systemic anthelmintics (thiabendazole 22 mg/kg PO bid × 2–4 days and albendazole 200 mg PO bid × 30 days)

Cat-Scratch Disease

Caused by infection with *Bartonella henselae* (gram-negative rod; formerly *Rochalimaea henselae*)

Transmitted by scratch, lick, bite of cats (usually kittens)

Seasonal pattern (fall and winter), most prevalent in southern US, California, and Hawaii

Findings (5%–10%): Parinaud oculoglandular syndrome, retinal/choroidal granulomas (50–300 μm), neuroretinitis (1%–2%; acute vision loss, optic disc edema, and macular star; may have mild iritis and vitritis; usually resolves within 2–3 months); may have vascular occlusions, exudative RD, epiretinal membrane (ERM), optic disc edema, orbital abscess

Other findings: skin lesion (papule, vesicle, pustule) 3-10 days after injury, flu-like symptoms and local adenopathy 1-2 weeks later; may have encephalopathy, aseptic meningitis, osteomyelitis, pneumonia, pleural effusions, pericardial effusions, hepatosplenomegaly

Diagnosis: serum antibody testing (IgG or IgM), skin testing, polymerase chain reaction (PCR)

Treatment: oral antibiotics (doxycycline 100 mg bid and rifampin 300 mg bid × 4–6 weeks)

Leptospirosis

Caused by infection with *Leptospira interrogans* (spirochete)

Acquired from exposure to contaminated soil or water from urine of infected animal

Biphasic: initial/leptospiremic phase (after 2- to 4-week incubation) and second/immune phase

Findings: fever, chills, headache, vomiting, diarrhea, myalgias in initial phase; **Weil disease** (10%; severe septicemia with liver and kidney involvement, fatal in up to 30%); meningitis, myelitis, cranial nerve palsies, uveitis (up to 40%; mild anterior uveitis to severe panuveitis with retinal vasculitis) in second phase

Diagnosis: ELISA for IgM

Treatment: systemic antibiotics (penicillin G 1.5 million units IV qid or doxycycline 100 mg PO bid × 1 week)

Nocardiosis

Caused by infection with *Nocardia asteroides* (gram-positive rod that acts like fungus)

Found in soil, acquired by ingestion or inhalation

Causes pneumonia and abscesses, rarely ocular involvement (any part of eye)

Findings: mild anterior uveitis to severe panuveitis with choroidal or subretinal abscesses, keratitis, necrotizing scleritis

Treatment: systemic antibiotics (Bactrim)

West Nile Virus

RNA virus transmitted from birds by mosquito; endemic in Europe, Australia, Asia, Africa

Occurs between July and December, peak in late summer

80% subclinical, 20% febrile illness

Diabetes associated with increased risk of eye involvement and death

Findings: conjunctivitis, nongranulomatous anterior uveitis, vitritis, multifocal chorioretinitis (flat, deep, white–yellow lesions [200–1000 μm] with pigmentation and atrophy), intraretinal hemorrhages, optic disc edema, optic atrophy, retinal vascular sheathing and occlusions, CN VI palsy, nystagmus; may develop CNV, foveal scar, ischemic maculopathy, vitreous hemorrhage (VH), traction RD

Other findings: myalgia, arthralgia, headache, lymphadenopathy, maculopapular rash; may develop meningitis, encephalitis

FA: hypofluorescence and late staining of active lesions, early hyperfluorescence and late staining of old lesions; lesions may have central blockage from pigment and peripheral hyperfluorescence from atrophy

Indocyanine green (ICG): hypocyanescent spots (more numerous than on fundus exam)

Treatment: supportive; topical steroid for anterior uveitis

Dengue Fever

Caused by infection with dengue virus (4 types); transmitted by *Aedes aegypti* mosquito, endemic in tropics/subtropics

Infection causes fever, headache, myalgia, thrombocytopenia (purpuric rash, other bleeding)

Findings: subconjunctival hemorrhages, maculopathy (10%; foveolitis with acute decreased vision, central scotoma)

Zika Virus (ZIKV)

Transmitted by mosquito (commonly *A. aegypti*)

Congenital Zika syndrome: causes severe abnormalities, no uveitis (see Chapter 5, Pediatrics/Strabismus)

Acquired infection: often presents with minimal or no symptoms; may have fever, headache, rash, myalgia, arthralgia; ocular findings include conjunctivitis, anterior uveitis, posterior uveitis with chorioretinal lesions, unilateral acute maculopathy

Coronavirus 2019 (COVID-19)

Infection with SARS-CoV-2, an enveloped, single-stranded RNA coronavirus, leading to COVID-19 disease

Findings: follicular conjunctivitis, keratoconjunctivitis, episcleritis, uveitis, retinitis, vasculitis, cotton wool spots, retinal hemorrhages, optic neuritis, neuromyelitis optica spectrum disorder

Labs: SARS-CoV-2 PCR test

Ebola Virus Disease (EVD)

Life-threatening viral hemorrhagic fever caused by *Ebolavirus*, a group of 5 RNA viruses endemic in West Africa; transmitted by direct contact with infected blood/body fluids

Uveitis is common; 40% of survivors have severe visual loss/blindness

Findings: conjunctivitis, subconjunctival hemorrhage, and uveitis (anterior, posterior, and panuveitis) that can be blinding in convalescent stage of EVD as a result of posterior synechiae, cataract, epiretinal membrane, macular edema, multifocal retinal lesions, macular scarring, optic disc swelling; may also have episcleritis, interstitial keratitis, optic neuropathy

Other findings: high fever, abdominal pain, diarrhea, vomiting, headache, weakness, fatigue, bruising, arthralgia, myalgia, back pain

Labs: *Ebolavirus* antibody test

Treatment: supportive; systemic steroids and experimental antiviral therapy; topical steroid and cycloplegic for uveitis

Onchocerciasis (River Blindness)

Caused by infection with *Onchocerca volvulus*, endemic in sub-Saharan Africa and parts of Central and South America

Larvae mature in humans, forming adult worms that live in fibrous, subcutaneous nodules (usually in joints); female worms (100 cm long, live for up to 20 years) and male worms (5 cm long, live for much shorter time) reproduce sexually, females give birth to ~2000 microfilariae/day; microfilariae (300 μm long, live for 1–2 years) migrate all over body by direct invasion and hematogenous spread, prefer skin and eyes; live microfilariae induce little or no inflammation; death of organism causes severe granulomatous inflammation and scarring

Transmitted by black fly: breeds along fast-moving streams; bites infected host and acquires microfilariae, which mature into infectious larvae; transmits larvae to humans with bite;

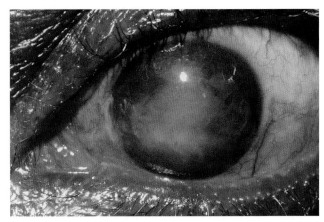

Figure 8.11 Sclerosing keratitis as a result of onchocerciasis. (Courtesy of Professor HR Taylor. From Cowan CL. Sarcoidosis. In: Yanoff M, Duker JS, eds. *Ophthalmology*. London: Mosby; 1999.)

≥25 million infected, with ~300,000 blind and 800,000 visually impaired

Ocular involvement by direct invasion of cornea from conjunctiva (second-leading cause of corneal blindness in world (trachoma is first), invasion of sclera, and possibly hematogenous spread

Findings: live microfilariae in AC and in cornea, anterior uveitis, stromal punctate keratitis (from dead microfilariae), sclerosing keratitis, scleritis, chorioretinitis, optic neuritis and atrophy; may develop cataract, peripheral anterior synechia, and glaucoma (Fig. 8.11)

Other findings: pruritus, pigmentary changes (leopard-skin appearance), chronic inflammation, scarring, maculopapular rash, subcutaneous nodules

Diagnosis: skin snip (place piece of skin in tissue media, 20–100 microfilariae emerge)

Treatment: ivermectin (kills microfilariae) and doxycycline (helps eliminate adult worms)

Ophthalmomyiasis

Results from direct ocular invasion by fly larvae (maggots) that invade AC, posterior segment, or subretinal space

Subretinal invasion: larvae travel through fundus, leaving crisscrossing tracks of atrophied RPE; death of organism causes ocular inflammation

Whipple Disease

Caused by infection with *Tropheryma whipplei* (gram-positive bacillus; *Actinomycetes* family)

Rare multisystem disease; most common in middle-aged males

Associated with HLA-B27, HLA-DRB1, and HLA-DQB1

Intraocular involvement in <5%

Findings: uveitis (bilateral panuveitis and retinal vasculitis), multifocal chorioretinitis; may develop retinal vascular occlusions, retinal hemorrhages, optic disc edema and optic atrophy; may have cranial nerve palsies, nystagmus, ophthalmoplegia

Other findings: malabsorption (75%; diarrhea, steatorrhea), weight loss, fever, abdominal pain, migratory arthritis (80%), sacroiliitis, heart (pericarditis, endocarditis, cardiomyopathy, valvular disease), CNS (ataxia, seizures, dementia, coma)

Pathology: periodic acid-Schiff (PAS)-positive bacillus in macrophages within lamina propria of "clubbed" (abnormal) microvilli on duodenal biopsy, PCR for *T. whipplei* on vitreous biopsy

Treatment: ceftriaxone or penicillin (PCN) × 2 weeks, then Bactrim × 12 months; shorter courses lead to relapses (30%); can be fatal if untreated

Propionibacterium acnes

Gram-positive rod; anaerobic

May become sequestered in capsular bag following cataract surgery

Findings: delayed onset, chronic granulomatous uveitis, often with fibrin or hypopyon; white plaque on posterior capsule is characteristic

Treatment: intravitreal antibiotics (vancomycin, cephalosporins; resistant to aminoglycosides) but usually requires partial or total removal of capsular bag with/without intraocular lens (IOL) removal/exchange with intravitreal injection of antibiotics

Inflammations (Table 8.1)

White Dot Syndromes

Group of inflammatory chorioretinopathies of unknown etiology; common features include multiple, well-circumscribed, white–yellow lesions, often with a viral prodrome, and usually affecting females younger than 50 years old. Distinguished by lesion appearance, natural history, and imaging modalities

Table 8.1 White dot syndromes

	APMPPE	MEWDS	Serpiginous	Birdshot	MCP	PIC	SFU	ARPE	AZOOR
Age	20–50	10–50	20–60	30–70	10–70	20–40	10–35	16–40	15–65
Sex	F = M	F > M (3:1)	F = M	F > M	F > M (3:1)	F (90%)	F (>95%)	F = M	F > M (3:1)
Laterality	Bilateral	Unilateral	Bilateral, asymmetric	Bilateral	Bilateral	Bilateral	Bilateral, asymmetric	Unilateral (75%)	Bilateral (76%)
Association	HLA-B7 and DR2 Viral prodrome, cerebral vasculitis	Viral prodrome (50%)	HLA-B7 Rule out TB	HLA-A29	None	None	None	None	Autoimmune disease (28%)
Onset	Acute	Acute	Variable	Insidious	Insidious	Acute	Insidious	Acute	Insidious
Course	Self-limited	Self-limited	Chronic, recurrent	Chronic, recurrent	Chronic, recurrent	Self-limited	Chronic, recurrent	Self-limited	Chronic, recurrent (31%)
Vitritis	Mild	Mild	Mild	Chronic, moderate	Chronic, moderate	None	Chronic, moderate	Mild or none	Mild or none
Lesions	1–2 disc areas, yellow–white placoid lesions; geographic hyper- or hypopigmented scars	100–200 μm, soft, white–orange, transient dots; no scarring	Geographic scars, active yellow–gray edges, centrifugal extension	50–150 μm, ovoid, cream-colored spots; indistinct margins; yellow scars without pigmentation	50–200 μm gray–white to yellow lesions; mixture of old scars and new spots	100–200 μm, yellow or gray spots; punched-out scars	50–500 μm, white–yellow lesions; scars, subretinal fibrosis	100–200 μm, hyperpigmented lesions with yellow–white halos	Minimal changes early, late pigmentation and perivenous sheathing
Macula	Rare CNV	Granularity Rare CNV	Subretinal scars 25% CNV	CME Rare (6%) CNV	CME 33% CNV	Atrophic scars 70% CNV	CME CNV	None	Rare CME
Prognosis	Good	Excellent	Poor	Fair	Fair	Good, unless macula CNV	Poor	Excellent	Poor
Treatment	None, Steroids for CNS involvement	None	Steroids, IMT Anti-VEGF for CNV	Steroids, IMT	Steroids, IMT Anti-VEGF for CNV	None, Steroids, IMT Anti-VEGF for CNV	Steroids, IMT	None	Steroids, IMT

Acute Posterior Multifocal Placoid Pigment Epitheliopathy (APMPPE)

Occurs in healthy adults aged 20-50 years; female = male; bilateral

Acute, self-limited; may be nonspecific choroidal hypersensitivity reaction

Association with HLA-B7 and HLA-DR2; also cerebral vasculitis, erythema nodosum, GPA, PAN, scleritis, episcleritis, sarcoidosis, ulcerative colitis, and infections (group A streptococcus, adenovirus type 5, TB, Lyme disease, mumps, and hepatitis B vaccination)

Flu-like prodrome (50%)

Symptoms: acute, usually bilateral, decreased vision with central/paracentral scotomas (fellow eye involved within days to weeks), may be preceded by photopsias

Findings: multiple, flat, yellow–white placoid lesions (1–2 disc areas) at level of RPE or choriocapillaris (possibly a result of choroidal hypoperfusion) scattered in posterior pole; lesions fade over 2-6 weeks, leaving geographically shaped RPE changes (hypopigmentation and hyperpigmentation); may have mild vitritis, minimal or no AC reaction; rarely retinal vasculitis, retinal vascular occlusions, CME, exudative RD, optic disc edema, CNV (Fig. 8.12)

Other findings: thyroiditis, erythema nodosum, cerebral vasculitis, regional enteritis

FA: initial blockage with late hyperfluorescent staining; window defects in old cases (Figs. 8.13 and 8.14)

ICG: early and late hypocyanescence of placoid lesions; hypocyanescence larger than actual lesions; generally improve over time

Fundus autofluorescence (FAF): hypoautofluoresence of acute lesions with hyperautofluorescent halo; older lesions are hypoautoflourescent

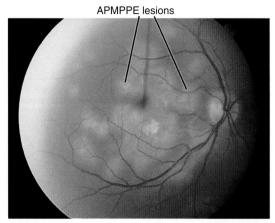

APMPPE lesions

Figure 8.12 Acute posterior multifocal placoid pigment epitheliopathy demonstrating multiple posterior pole lesions. (From Kaiser PK, Friedman NJ, Pineda R II. *Massachusetts Eye and Ear Infirmary Illustrated Manual of Ophthalmology*, 2nd ed. Philadelphia: WB Saunders; 2004.)

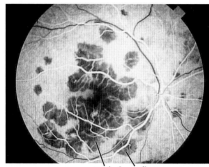

early hypofluorescence

Figure 8.13 Fluorescein angiogram of same patient as shown in Fig. 8.12 demonstrating early hypofluorescence of the lesions. (From Kaiser PK, Friedman NJ, Pineda R II. *Massachusetts Eye and Ear Infirmary Illustrated Manual of Ophthalmology*, 2nd ed. Philadelphia: WB Saunders; 2004.)

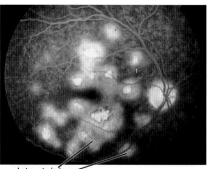

late staining

Figure 8.14 Fluorescein angiogram of same patient as shown in Fig. 8.13 demonstrating late staining of the lesions. (From Kaiser PK, Friedman NJ, Pineda R II. *Massachusetts Eye and Ear Infirmary Illustrated Manual of Ophthalmology*, 2nd ed. Philadelphia: WB Saunders; 2004.)

Optical coherence tomography (OCT): hyperreflectivity in outer plexiform layer; focal areas of discontinuous outer segment ellipsoid zone, relatively healthy photoreceptor layers; OCTA shows choriocapillaris nonperfusion

Treatment: none; steroids for CNS involvement

Prognosis: vision recovers in most patients to ≥20/40 within 6 months; rarely recurs

Multiple Evanescent White Dot Syndrome (MEWDS)

Occurs in 2nd-5th decades of life; female > male (3:1); moderate myopia; unilateral (rare cases of bilateral)

Viral prodrome (33%)

Symptoms: decreased vision, central/paracentral scotomas, photopsias

Findings: granular macular pigmentary appearance (pathognomonic) with small (100-200 μm) white-orange transient spots at level of RPE or deep retina, mainly perifoveal also in midperiphery and periphery; may have vitreous cells, positive RAPD, mild optic disc swelling (Fig. 8.15)

Visual field (VF): enlarged blind spot, generalized depression, paracentral or peripheral scotomas

FA: early hyperfluorescence in wreath-like configuration around fovea; late staining of lesions and optic nerve (Fig. 8.16)

ICG: hypocyanescent spots (more numerous than on fundus exam)

FAF: hyperautofluorescent spots (correspond to lesions on fundus exam)

OCT: abnormal reflectivity of photoreceptor ellipsoid zone

ERG: reduced a wave (involvement of RPE and outer retina) and early receptor potential amplitudes

Treatment: none, observation

Prognosis: vision recovers over 2-10 weeks but may be permanently decreased as a result of pigmentary changes in

fovea; photopsias and enlarged blind spot may last months; recurs in 10%-15% in same or fellow eye

Serpiginous Choroiditis (Geographic or Helicoid Choroidopathy)

Occurs in adults aged 20-60 years; female = male; bilateral, asymmetric

Chronic, progressive, indolent disease of unknown etiology; thought to be immune-mediated occlusive vasculitis

Must distinguish from TB, which can cause similar pattern of inflammation

Symptoms: painless decreased vision with paracentral scotomas

Findings: helicoid or geographic (map-like) pattern of scars with active edges (yellow–gray, edematous) at level of RPE, usually peripapillary and extend to posterior pole; active areas become atrophic over weeks to months; new lesions occur contiguously or elsewhere (often in snake-like/ serpiginous pattern); may have mild AC reaction, vitritis, vascular sheathing, RPE detachment, neovascularization of the disc (NVD); may develop subretinal fibrosis and CNV at border of old scar (up to 25%) (Fig. 8.17)

VF: absolute scotomas (correspond to atrophic scars)

FA: early hypofluorescence with late staining of active borders

ICG: hypocyanescence and late staining of lesions

FAF: hyperautofluorescent active lesions and hypoautofluorescent inactive areas

OCT: outer retinal swelling with hyperreflectivity in acute lesions with loss of outer retinal details, loss of photoreceptors in old lesions

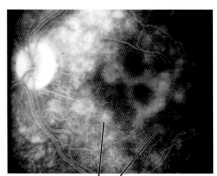

Figure 8.15 Multiple evanescent white dot syndrome demonstrating faint white spots. (From Kaiser PK, Friedman NJ, Pineda R II. *Massachusetts Eye and Ear Infirmary Illustrated Manual of Ophthalmology*, 2nd ed. Philadelphia: WB Saunders; 2004.)

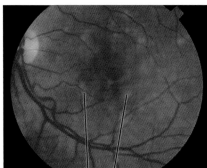

Figure 8.16 Same patient as shown in Fig. 8.15 demonstrating early fluorescein angiogram appearance. (From Kaiser PK, Friedman NJ, Pineda R II. *Massachusetts Eye and Ear Infirmary Illustrated Manual of Ophthalmology*, 2nd ed. Philadelphia: WB Saunders; 2004.)

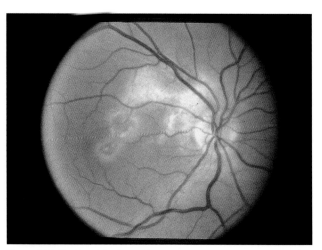

Figure 8.17 Fundus view of the right eye of a 57-year-old woman with early serpiginous choroiditis. (From Moorthy RS, Jampol LM. Posterior uveitis of unknown cause. In: Yanoff M, Duker JS, eds. *Ophthalmology*. London: Mosby; 1999.)

ERG: normal

Treatment: oral, periocular, and intravitreal steroids, IMT

Prognosis: poor, up to 38% have vision ≤20/200; commonly recurs months to years later

Ampiginous Chorioretinitis

Also known as *relentless placoid chorioretinitis*; often with viral prodrome; etiology unknown

Findings: deep, creamy, amoeba-shaped lesions like APMPPE but progressive like serpiginous that start centrally and extend peripherally; become more pigmented during convalescence

FA: early hypofluorescence

FAF: mixed hypofluorescence; convalescent lesions are hypofluorescent

OCT: loss of outer retina and RPE

Birdshot Chorioretinopathy (Vitiliginous Chorioretinitis)

Occurs in adults aged 30-70 years; female > male; usually bilateral

Associated with HLA-A29 (sensitivity 96%, specificity 93%)

Symptoms: blurred vision, nyctalopia, decreased color vision, peripheral visual field loss, floaters (may be out of proportion to visual acuity)

Findings: deep, multifocal, ovoid, cream-colored hypopigmented choroidal lesions (50–150 μm; at level of choroid and RPE) scattered throughout fundus, mainly in nasal and radial distribution from optic nerve following underlying choroidal vessels (similar to birdshot from a shotgun); may have mild AC reaction, vitritis, retinal vasculitis, optic disc edema, CME; may develop optic atrophy, epiretinal membrane, and rarely CNV (6%) (Fig. 8.18)

FA: early hypofluorescence or silence, mild late staining; leakage from disc, vessels, CME

ICG: hypocyanescent lesions (more numerous than on fundus exam); may resolve with treatment

FAF: hypoautofluorescent lesions (more numerous than on fundus exam)

OCT: macular edema; patchy or diffuse photoreceptors loss with loss of ellipsoid zone

ERG: abnormal photoreceptor response, reduced b wave

Treatment: oral and/or local steroids, IMT

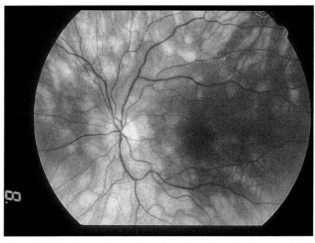

Figure 8.18 Birdshot retinochoroidopathy. (From Moorthy RS, Jampol LM. Posterior uveitis of unknown cause. In: Yanoff M, Duker JS, eds. *Ophthalmology*. London: Mosby; 1999.)

Prognosis: stabilizes over several years; ~20% have vision ≤20/200, with IMT vision stabilizes or improves in up to 90%

Multifocal Choroiditis and Panuveitis (MCP)

Onset between age 10-70 years (median age 45); usually myopic women; female > male (3:1)

May be spectrum of disease, including punctate inner choroiditis (PIC) and subretinal fibrosis and uveitis syndrome (SFU; see below)

Viral etiology (HSV, EBV) has been implicated

Symptoms: decreased vision, floaters, photopsias, enlarged blind spot

Findings: multiple, discrete, gray–white to yellow lesions (50–200 μm) at level of choroid or RPE; vitreous and AC reaction; chronic lesions become atrophic with punched-out margins, variable amounts of pigmentation and occasionally fibrosis; may develop CNV (33%; most common cause of vision loss), CME, ERM (Fig. 8.19)

FA: acute lesions block or fill early and stain late; older lesions behave like window defects with early hyperfluorescence and late fading

ICG: hypocyanescent lesions (more numerous than on fundus exam)

FAF: old lesions are hypoautofluorescent, active lesions are hyperautofluorescent; may have numerous smaller hypoautofluorescent spots in macula and peripapillary area than on fundus exam

OCT: outer retinal swelling, sub-RPE deposits with disruption of overlying outer segment ellipsoid zone

ERG: extinguished responses

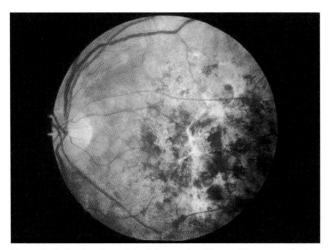

Figure 8.19 Fundus view of the left eye of a 50-year-old woman who has progressive subretinal fibrosis and uveitis syndrome. (From Moorthy RS, Jampol LM. Posterior uveitis of unknown cause. In: Yanoff M, Duker JS, eds. *Ophthalmology*. London: Mosby; 1999.)

Treatment: oral and periocular steroids, IMT; reduces risk of complications (CNV, CME, ERM) by 83% and risk of vision loss to ≤20/200 by 92%, anti-VEGF for CNV

Prognosis: 75% have vision loss in at least one eye

Punctate Inner Choroidopathy (PIC)

Occurs in healthy myopic women aged 20-40 years (10% males)

Symptoms: acute scotomas, photopsias, metamorphopsia

Findings: small (100-200 μm) yellow or gray inner choroidal lesions, rarely extend to midperiphery; resolve over weeks to form atrophic scars that may enlarge and become pigmented; new lesions do not appear; no AC reaction or vitritis; may have exudative RD, CNV (up to 70%) (Fig. 8.20)

VF: enlarged blind spot (40%)

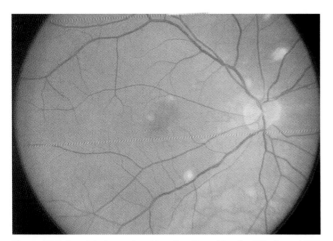

Figure 8.20 Punctate inner choroidopathy. (From Moorthy RS, Jampol LM. Posterior uveitis of unknown cause. In: Yanoff M, Duker JS, eds. *Ophthalmology*. London: Mosby; 1999.)

FA: acute lesions block or hyperfluorescent early and stain late

ICG: hypocyanescent lesions (correspond to lesions on fundus exam)

FAF: similar to MCP (see above)

OCT: similar to MCP (see above)

ERG: normal

Treatment: steroids, IMT, anti-VEGF for CNV

Prognosis: good, unless CNV involving fovea

Subretinal Fibrosis and Uveitis Syndrome (SFU)

Very rare bilateral chronic panuveitis

Occurs in healthy myopic women aged 10-35 years (<5% males); bilateral, asymmetric

May be autoimmune reaction to RPE

Symptoms: acute vision loss, scotomas, photopsias, metamorphopsia

Findings: small (50- 500 μm) white–yellow RPE lesions in posterior pole and midperiphery; fade, become atrophic, or enlarge and coalesce into white subretinal fibrosis over weeks to months; AC reaction, mild to moderate vitritis; may have exudative RD, CME, CNV

Pathology: lymphocytic granulomatous infiltration of choroid, retinal gliosis, subretinal fibrosis

FA: areas of hyper and hypofluorescence early; late staining

OCT: retinal edema, subretinal fluid, subretinal fibrosis

ERG and electro-oculogram (EOG): reduced

Treatment: steroids, IMT

Prognosis: poor; commonly recurs

Acute Retinal Pigment Epitheliitis (ARPE; Krill Disease)

Rare, self-limited disorder of RPE

Occurs in healthy adults aged 16-40 years; male = female, unilateral (75%)

Symptoms: acute decreased vision, metamorphopsia, central scotoma

Findings: clusters of hyperpigmented spots (300–400 μm) in macula surrounded by yellow–white halos; with resolution, the spots lighten or darken, but halos remain; no vitritis (Fig. 8.21)

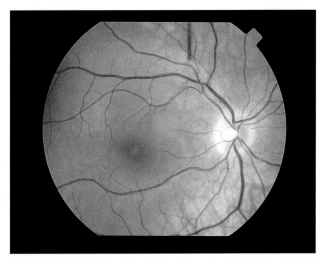

Figure 8.21 Retinal pigment epitheliitis. (From Moorthy RS, Jampol LM. Posterior uveitis of unknown cause. In: Yanoff M, Duker JS, eds. *Ophthalmology*. London: Mosby; 1999.)

DDx: central serous chorioretinopathy, acute macular neuroretinopathy (wedge-shaped or cloverleaf dark-red perifoveal dots; paracentral scotoma; normal ERG)

VF: central scotoma

FA: blockage of spots with halos of hyperfluorescence; late staining

ICG: early patchy hypercyanescence; late hypercyanescence of halos

FAF: normal autofluorescence or hypoautofluorescent spots (correspond to lesions on fundus exam)

OCT: disruption of ellipsoid zone and RPE inner band

ERG: normal

EOG: abnormal

Treatment: none

Prognosis: resolves completely in 6-12 weeks

Acute Zonal Occult Outer Retinopathy (AZOOR)

Occurs in adults aged 16-65 years; female > male (3:1), usually myopic women; starts unilateral, becomes bilateral (75%)

Associated with autoimmune disease (28%)

Symptoms: acute VF loss, photopsias, and scotomas

Findings: minimal changes initially; retinal degeneration/pigmentary changes late, often peripapillary; mild vitritis (50%), decreased vision acuity (20/40 range)

DDx: MEWDS, acute macular neuroretinopathy, multifocal choroiditis, punctate inner choroiditis, ocular histoplasmosis syndrome, acute idiopathic blind spot enlargement syndrome, cancer-associated retinopathy, retinitis pigmentosa

VF: paracentral scotomas, enlarged blind spot

FA: normal in early disease, hyperfluorescent window defects in late disease

ICG: hypocyanescent atrophic areas, late leakage in subacute areas

FAF: central hypoautofluorescence, peripheral hyperautofluorescence at lesion border

OCT: loss of ellipsoid zone and photoreceptor segments

ERG: reduced rod and cone

Treatment: steroids, IMT

Prognosis: recurs in 31%; scotomas stabilize in 75%, improve in 25%; 68% have vision in 20/40 range, 18% legally blind

Autoimmune Retinopathy (AIR)

Rare immune-mediated disease against retinal proteins; antiretinal antibodies (most commonly to recoverin [photoreceptor calcium-binding protein])

2 categories: paraneoplastic (cancer-associated retinopathy [CAR; usually small cell lung cancer] and melanoma-associated retinopathy [MAR]) and nonparaneoplastic (50% have autoimmune disease)

Diagnosis of exclusion, rule out malignancy

Symptoms: vision loss, scotomas, photopsias, nyctalopia, dyschromatopsia

Findings: develop pigmentary changes, vascular attenuation, diffuse atrophy of retina and optic nerve; rare or no vitreous cells

VF: scotoma

ERG: depressed cone response in CAR; normal photoreceptor response, reduced b wave in MAR

Prognosis: vision usually poor but variable

Frosted-Branch Angiitis

Retinal perivasculitis originally found in healthy children

Findings: white spots along retinal arterioles (Fig. 8.22)

DDx: CMV retinitis, toxoplasmosis (Kyrieleis plaques), dermatomyositis

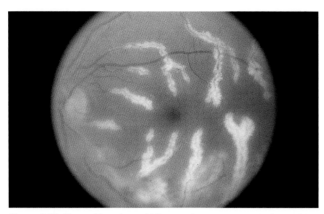

Figure 8.22 "Frosted-branch angiitis" secondary to cytomegalovirus retinitis. (From Hudson HL, Boyer DS, Martin DF, et al. Viral posterior uveitis. In: Yanoff M, Duker JS, eds. *Ophthalmology*. London: Mosby; 1999.)

Idiopathic Uveal Effusion Syndrome

Occurs in healthy, middle-aged males

Chronic, recurrent disorder

Symptoms: blurred vision, metamorphopsia, scotomas

Findings: exudative retinal, choroidal, and ciliary body detachments; mild vitritis, RPE changes (leopard spots), conjunctival injection; key finding is shifting subretinal fluid

B-scan ultrasound: thickened sclera, exudative RD, choroidal detachments

FA: no discrete leakage

Treatment: steroids and IMT not effective; consider scleral resection in nanophthalmic eyes, or quadrantic partial-thickness scleral windows

ENDOPHTHALMITIS

Inflammation involving one or more coats of the eye and adjacent ocular cavities

Etiology: infectious or sterile; must rule out infection

Symptoms: pain, decreased vision

Findings: lid edema, chemosis, AC reaction, hypopyon (pink hypopyon = *Serratia*), vitritis. Endogenous cases may have fever, positive cultures (blood, urine, sputum), chorioretinitis, retinal/choroidal abscesses, vascular sheathing, hemorrhages, Roth spots

Classification: postoperative (70%), traumatic (20%), endogenous (2%–15%)

   Acute postoperative (<6 weeks after surgery; 90% in 1st week):

RISK FACTORS: blepharitis, wound leak, iris prolapse, vitreous loss, contaminated IOL, diabetes, chronic alcoholism

ORGANISMS: 94% gram-positive bacteria (*Staphylococcus epidermidis* [70%], *Staphylococcus aureus* [10%], *Streptococci* [11%]), 6% gram-negative (most commonly *Pseudomonas*)

INCIDENCE:

   Extracapsular extraction (ECCE) or intracapsular cataract extraction (ICCE) (with or without IOL): 0.072%

   Secondary IOL: 0.3%

   Pars plana vitrectomy (PPV): 0.51%

   Penetrating keratoplasty (PK): 0.11%

   Glaucoma filter: 0.061% (early bleb-associated endophthalmitis [BAE; within 1 month]: *S. epidermidis*; late-onset BAE [after 1 month]: *Streptococcus* 31%, *Staphylococcus* up to 22%, and gram-negatives [*Haemophilus influenzae* 23%, *Enterococcus* 7%, *Pseudomonas* 7%])

PREVENTION:

   TREAT BLEPHARITIS: 85% of responsible organisms (*S. epidermidis* and *S. aureus*) are found on lids; hot compresses, lid hygiene, Polysporin ointment × 1 week preop; add doxycycline 100 mg bid × 1 week for acne rosacea or seborrheic dermatitis

   STERILIZE OPERATIVE FIELD: 5% povidone-iodine (Betadine); preoperative topical antibiotics (fluoroquinolone)

   AVOID INOCULATION: drape eyelashes

   ANTIBIOTICS: intracameral (injection or in irrigating solution); topical preop for 1-3 days and postop for 7-10 days; consider subconjunctival antibiotics with broken posterior capsule or vitreous loss

Delayed postoperative (>6 weeks after surgery): *P. acnes* (anaerobic gram-positive rod), coagulase-negative *Staphylococci*, and fungi (*Aspergillus*, *Candida*)

Traumatic:

RISK FACTORS: retained intraocular foreign body, delayed surgery (>24 hours), rural setting (soil contamination), and disruption of the crystalline lens

CULTURE POSITIVE IN 25%: *Bacillus* (30%), *S. epidermidis* (25%), *Streptococci* (13%), *S. aureus* (8%), *Pseudomonas*, *Clostridium*; fungi less common but suspect in vegetable matter injuries (i.e., tree branch), usually *Candida, Aspergillus, Fusarium, Paecilomyces*

INCIDENCE: 2%-7% after penetrating trauma

   Poor visual outcome

PREVENTION: prophylaxis with combination of systemic (IV [vancomycin and ceftazidime] and/or oral [levofloxacin]), intraocular, subconjunctival, and topical antibiotics depending on risk

Endogenous: hematogenous spread; up to 90% have extraocular focus (pneumonia, endocarditis, urinary tract infection, sinusitis, osteomyelitis, meningitis, tooth or liver abscess)

RISK FACTORS: immunosuppression, indwelling venous catheters, intravenous drug abuse (IVDA), following intra-abdominal surgery

ORGANISMS: most commonly fungi (*Candida* [most common], *Aspergillus*, *Coccidioides*; less commonly *Histoplasma*, *Cryptococcus*, *Blastomyces*), some bacteria (usually gram-positives: *Streptococcus*, *S. aureus*, *Bacillus*, *Nocardia*; gram-negatives: *Neisseria meningitidis*, *H. influenzae*, *Escherichia coli*, *Klebsiella*)

Up to 37% of patients with untreated *Candida* septicemia develop endophthalmitis (decreases to 3% with antifungal treatment)

Sterile: culture negative

DDx: uveitis, sterile inflammation (usually from prolonged intraoperative manipulations, especially involving vitreous; retained lens material; rebound inflammation after sudden decrease in postoperative steroids; or toxic anterior segment syndrome [TASS; acute postoperative AC reaction and corneal edema caused by contaminants from surgical instruments, intraocular solutions, or IOL implant]), blebitis (infection of filtering bleb), intraocular foreign body, intraocular tumor, sympathetic ophthalmia, anterior segment ischemia (from carotid artery disease [ocular ischemic syndrome] or following muscle surgery [usually on three or more rectus muscles in same eye at the same surgery])

Treatment: rule out infection (AC and vitreous taps for culture, stain, PCR evaluation; culture blood and body fluids in endogenous cases)

Intravitreal antibiotics/antifungals: vancomycin 1 mg/0.1 mL, ceftazidime 2.25 mg/0.1 mL or amikacin 0.4 mg/0.1 mL; consider intravitreal dexamethasone 0.4 mg/0.1 mL; amphotericin B (5–10 µg/0.1 mL) or voriconazole (100 µg/0.1 mL) if endogenous fungal or delayed onset with presumed fungal etiology (do not use long-acting steroids)

Systemic antibiotics/antifungals: in severe cases, most traumatic cases, and endogenous bacterial cases; vancomycin 1 g IV q12h or cefazolin 1 g IV q8h; ceftazidime 1 g IV q12h; fluconazole or voriconazole (200 mg PO bid × 2–4 weeks) for endogenous candidiasis; amphotericin B (0.25–1.0 mg/kg IV divided equally q6h) for disseminated fungal infection

Subconjunctival antibiotics and steroid: vancomycin 25 mg, ceftazidime 100 mg or gentamicin 20 mg, dexamethasone 12-24 mg

Topical fortified antibiotics/antifungals: vancomycin 25-50 mg/mL, ceftazidime 50 mg/mL q1h; amphotericin B (1.0–2.5 mg/mL q1h) or natamycin (50 mg/mL q1h)

Topical steroids and cycloplegics

Delayed postoperative endophthalmitis: partial or total capsulectomy, PPV, or IOL removal or exchange

Endogenous endophthalmitis: systemic treatment of underlying infection

MAJOR CLINICAL STUDY

Endophthalmitis Vitrectomy Study (EVS)

Objective: To evaluate the treatment of acute (<6 weeks) postoperative (cataract or secondary IOL surgery) endophthalmitis with immediate vitrectomy versus "tap and inject," and whether IV antibiotics (ceftazidime and amikacin) are necessary

Methods: Patients with clinical evidence of acute (<6 weeks) postoperative (cataract or secondary IOL surgery) endophthalmitis and visual acuity of light perception (LP) or better and sufficient clarity to see at least some part of the iris were randomly assigned to emergent AC and vitreous taps alone or with vitrectomy and with injection of intravitreal antibiotics (0.4 mg amikacin and 1.0 mg vancomycin). Patients were also given subconjunctival injections of antibiotics (25 mg vancomycin, 100 mg ceftazidime, and steroid [6 mg dexamethasone phosphate]), topical fortified antibiotics (50 mg/mL vancomycin and 20 mg/mL amikacin) and steroid (prednisolone acetate), and oral steroid (prednisone 30 mg bid × 5–10 days). Patients were also randomly assigned to receive systemic IV antibiotics (2 g ceftazidime IV q8h and 7.5 mg/kg amikacin IV, followed by 6 mg/kg q12h) or no systemic antibiotics. Intravitreal steroids were not used

Results

420 patients enrolled

On average, signs and symptoms occurred 6 days after surgery (75% presented within 2 weeks of surgery)

Positive cultures in 69%; gram-positive bacteria in 94% (70% coagulase-negative *Staphylococcus*, 10% *S. aureus*, 9% *Streptococci* species)

IV antibiotics were of no benefit

Immediate vitrectomy had significant benefits only when patients presented with LP vision or worse

Conclusions

For endophthalmitis after cataract or secondary IOL surgery, perform emergent treatment with AC tap and injection of intravitreal antibiotics when vision is better than LP

Vitrectomy should be reserved for patients presenting with light perception vision or worse

IV antibiotics do not improve the outcome

PANUVEITIS

Sarcoidosis

Multisystem granulomatous disease characterized by noncaseating granulomas; unknown etiology

Females > males; more common among African Americans (20:1)

Systemic disease: acute or chronic (>2 years)

Ocular disease: 30% unilateral, 70% bilateral; 40% acute, 60% chronic; 67% uveitis (usually anterior), 20% posterior segment involvement

Findings (25%–30%): anterior uveitis (2 forms: acute granulomatous [responds well to corticosteroids] and chronic recurrent [difficult to control with corticosteroids]), KP, iris nodules, peripheral anterior synechiae, lacrimal gland infiltration (25%; painless bilateral enlargement, may cause dacryoadenitis, keratoconjunctivitis sicca), eyelid and orbit granulomas, conjunctival nodules, nummular corneal infiltrates, episcleritis and scleritis with nodules, intermediate uveitis, vitritis (snowballs and linear strands ["strings of pearls"]), choroiditis with yellow or white nodules, retinal periphlebitis, retinal granulomas along venules (candlewax drippings), CME, retinal macroaneurysms, retinal vein occlusions, retinal NV, vitreous hemorrhage, optic nerve granulomas, optic disc edema; may develop secondary cataracts, glaucoma, and band keratopathy; papilledema or optic neuropathy in neurosarcoidosis (with or without uveitis)

Other findings: pulmonary (90%; hilar adenopathy [most common], diffuse fibrosis), constitutional (40%; malaise, fever, weight loss), skin (15%; erythema nodosum, subcutaneous nodules), lymphadenopathy (20%), arthralgias, hepatosplenomegaly, peripheral neuropathy, parotid gland infiltration, cardiac and CNS involvement, hypercalcemia

2 types of acute sarcoidosis: often with anterior uveitis and spontaneous remission within 2 years
    Löfgren syndrome: hilar lymphadenopathy, erythema nodosum, anterior uveitis, fever, arthralgia
    Heerfordt syndrome (uveoparotid fever): fever, parotid gland enlargement, anterior uveitis, facial nerve palsy
Mikulicz syndrome (lacrimal, parotid, and salivary gland swelling, sicca syndrome) also caused by sarcoidosis (as well as by TB, lymphoma/leukemia)

Pathology: noncaseating granulomas (caseating granulomas occur in TB) with Langhans multinucleated giant cells (Fig. 8.23)

Diagnosis:

    Lab tests (not diagnostic or specific): ACE (elevated in any diffuse granulomatous disease affecting the lung; may be artificially low with ACE-inhibitor medication), serum lysozyme (more sensitive than ACE, but less specific); consider calcium levels (serum and urine) and liver function tests for widespread involvement
    Chest X-ray or chest CT: hilar adenopathy (Fig. 8.24)
    Gallium scan: look for parotid, lacrimal, or pulmonary involvement
    Biopsy: skin lesion, conjunctival nodule, lymph node, salivary or lacrimal gland, lung, liver; if elevated ACE and positive CXR, 60%-70% of blind conjunctival biopsies will be positive

Treatment: topical, periocular, and systemic steroids, IMT

Prognosis: morbidity mainly from pulmonary involvement; ~5% mortality, up to 10% in neurosarcoidosis;

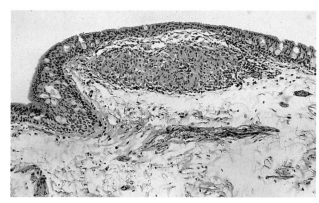

Figure 8.23 Sarcoidosis demonstrating conjunctival granuloma with giant cells surrounded by lymphocytes and plasma cells. (From Yanoff M, Fine BS. *Ocular Pathology*, 5th ed. St Louis: Mosby; 2002.)

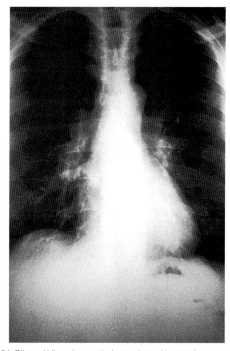

Figure 8.24 Bilateral hilar adenopathy in a patient without pulmonary symptoms. (From Cowan CL. Sarcoidosis. In: Yanoff M, Duker JS, eds. *Ophthalmology*. London: Mosby; 1999.)

vision loss associated with chronic intermediate or posterior uveitis, glaucoma, and delayed treatment (>1 year)

Familial Juvenile Systemic Granulomatosis (Blau Syndrome)

(See Chapter 5, Pediatrics/Strabismus)

Behçet Disease

Chronic recurrent multisystem condition characterized by relapsing inflammation and occlusive vasculitis; may predominantly affect 1 organ system (ocular, neurologic, intestinal, vascular)

Triad of oral ulcers, genital ulcers, and inflammatory eye disease (panuveitis)

Usually occurs in 3rd-4th decades of life; males = females (may be more severe in males); more common in Asians and Middle Easterners

Associated with HLA-B5 (subtypes Bw51 and B52; ocular) and HLA-B12 (mucocutaneous)

Findings (70%): recurrent, explosive episodes of nongranulomatous, necrotizing inflammation with occlusive vasculitis. Uveitis (posterior more common than anterior); can present with nongranulomatous anterior uveitis (80% bilateral; may have transient hypopyon); occasionally, conjunctivitis, episcleritis, or keratitis can occur; posterior involvement is sight-threatening with recurrent vascular occlusions, retinal hemorrhages, exudates, vascular sheathing, CME, vitritis, retinal NV, traction RD, ischemic optic neuropathy and atrophy (25%); may develop posterior synechiae, glaucoma, and cataract (Fig. 8.25)

Other findings: oral (aphthous) ulcers (painful, recurrent, round, white, discrete borders; 2–15 mm; last 7–10 days, heal without scarring), genital ulcers (similar to oral but deeper, larger, heal with scarring), skin lesions (erythema nodosum, acne-like lesions, folliculitis), arthritis (50%; knee,

elbow, wrist, ankle), vasculitis (25%; thrombophlebitis, large vessel occlusion, aneurysms, varices, pulmonary arteritis), cardiac (50%; endocarditis, myocarditis, pericarditis, endomyocardial fibrosis, coronary arteritis), GI (abdominal pain, diarrhea, constipation, ulcers), CNS involvement (25%; meningoencephalitis, strokes, palsies, papilledema, cognitive impairment)

Mnemonic: **ORAL UPSET (O**cclusive periphlebitis, **R**etinitis, **A**nterior uveitis, **L**eakage from retinal vessels, **U**lceration [oral, genital], **P**ustules after skin puncture [pathergy test], **S**cratching leaves lines [dermatographia], **E**rythema nodosum, **T**hrombophlebitis)

Pathology: obliterative vasculitis with activation of both cellular and humoral limbs of immune system; circulating immune complexes in >50%

Diagnosis:

Clinical: (Box 8.1)

Positive skin pathergy test (Behcetin skin test): intradermal puncture produces pustule formation within minutes (occurs in 40%; not pathognomonic of Behçet disease)

Box 8.1 Criteria for Behçet disease

Major criteria

1. Oral aphthous ulcers
2. Genital ulcers
3. Skin lesions (erythema nodosum, acneiform pustules, folliculitis)
4. Ocular disease (75%): nongranulomatous iridocyclitis with sterile hypopyon, necrotizing retinal vasculitis (may cause vascular occlusion), posterior synechiae, glaucoma (pupillary block, uveitic), cataract, traction retinal detachment (TRD)

Minor criteria

1. Arthritis (50%)
2. Gastrointestinal lesions
3. Epididymitis
4. Occlusive vascular lesions of major vessels (vena cava)
5. Migratory thrombophlebitis (33%)
6. Central nervous system involvement (25%; neuro-Behçet; meningoencephalitis, involvement of brain stem, spinal cord, peripheral nerves)
7. Pulmonary artery aneurysm (pathognomonic chest X-ray finding)
8. Interstitial lung changes

Treatment: systemic steroids, IMT (especially tumor necrosis factor [TNF] inhibitors infliximab or adalimumab)

Prognosis: up to 25% have vision <20/200 (usually from CME, occlusive retinal vasculitis, optic atrophy, glaucoma); up to 10% mortality

Vogt-Koyanagi-Harada Syndrome (VKH)

Uveoencephalitis: bilateral diffuse chronic granulomatous panuveitis, exudative RD, optic disc edema, meningeal irritation, skin pigmentary changes, and auditory disturbance

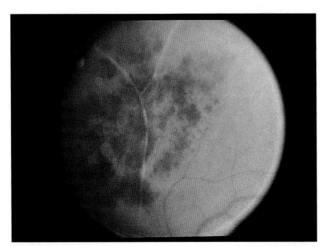

Figure 8.25 Fundus view of a patient who has Behçet disease. (From Yanoff M, Fine BS. *Ocular Pathology*, 5th ed. St Louis: Mosby; 2002.)

Harada disease if only eye findings

Associated with HLA-DR1, HLA-DR4, and HLA-Dw53

Presumed autoimmune process against melanocytes

Occurs in adults aged 30-50 years; more common in Asians, Native Americans, Hispanics, Middle Easterners; female > male

Symptoms: blurred vision, pain, redness, photophobia, stiff neck, headache, deafness, tinnitus, vertigo

Findings: bilateral diffuse granulomatous anterior uveitis, vitritis, exudative RDs (shallow, cloverleaf pattern around posterior pole, may coalesce and form large RDs), exudative choroiditis, CB detachment, altered IOP (increased or decreased), CME, optic disc hyperemia and edema, poliosis; later develop perilimbal vitiligo (Sugiura sign; up to 85% Japanese patients), Dalen-Fuchs nodules (yellow–white retinal spots), sunset-glow fundus (RPE disturbance with focal areas of atrophy and hyperpigmentation causing orange–red discoloration)

Other findings: temporary deafness, tinnitus, vertigo, meningeal irritation, skin lesions (30%; alopecia, vitiligo, poliosis)

Clinical stages:
Prodromal: flu-like symptoms, including headache, nausea, meningismus, fever, tinnitus, dysacousia, photophobia, skin hypersensitivity; rarely have neurologic signs (cranial neuropathies, hemiparesis, aphasia, transverse myelitis, seizures)
Acute uveitic (1–2 days later): diffuse granulomatous inflammation with bilateral blurred vision, pain, redness, exudative RDs (similar to sympathetic ophthalmia)
Convalescent (several weeks later): nongranulomatous inflammation and loss of melanocytes with resorption of exudative RDs and choroidal depigmentation; sunset-glow fundus, Dalen-Fuchs nodules, peripheral nummular chorioretinal scars, perilimbal vitiligo, skin and hair changes (vitiligo, alopecia, poliosis)
Chronic recurrent: granulomatous anterior uveitis with KP, posterior synechiae, iris nodules, iris atrophy; recurrent posterior inflammation uncommon; develop cataracts (50%), glaucoma (33%), CNV (15%), subretinal fibrosis

Pathology: inflammation of choriocapillaris and retina; Dalen-Fuchs nodules (epithelioid cells between Bruch membrane and RPE) (Fig. 8.26)

DDx: sympathetic ophthalmia, posterior scleritis, syphilis, lupus choroiditis, hypotony, uveal effusion syndrome, APMPPE, TB, sarcoidosis, primary intraocular lymphoma

Diagnosis:
LP: cerebrospinal fluid (CSF) pleocytosis (>80%; can last up to 8 weeks)

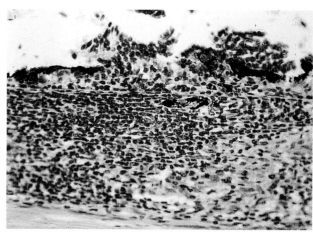

Figure 8.26 Vogt-Koyanagi-Harada (VKH) syndrome demonstrating granulomatous inflammation in choroid extending into choriocapillaris and through retinal pigment epithelium (RPE). (From Yanoff M, Fine BS. *Ocular Pathology*, 5th ed. St Louis: Mosby; 2002.)

FA: multiple focal hyperfluorescent areas of subretinal leakage ("1000 points of light"), pooling in exudative RDs, disc leakage; window defects in late stages of disease
FAF: granular hyperautofluorescence corresponding to areas of inflammation
OCT: grossly thickened choroid; monitor exudative RDs, CME, CNV

Treatment: steroids (6–12 months) and IMT (significantly reduce risk of CNV and subretinal fibrosis)

Prognosis: up to 70% retain vision ≥20/40

Sympathetic Ophthalmia (SO)

Rare, bilateral granulomatous panuveitis following penetrating trauma to an eye (exciting eye)

Fellow eye (sympathizing eye) develops uveitis after a latent period; chronic with exacerbations

Results from immune sensitization to melanin or melanin-associated proteins in uveal tissues; T-cell–mediated (delayed hypersensitivity reaction); latency of 10 days to 50 years after injury, 80% within 3 months, 90% within 1 year

Incidence: 0.5% of penetrating injuries; 0.01% of intraocular surgery (usually vitreoretinal)

Associated with HLA-A11, HLA-DR4, HLA-DRw53, and HLA-DQw3

Findings: Koeppe nodules, mutton fat KP, posterior synechiae, altered intraocular pressure (increased or decreased), vitritis, retinal edema, Dalen-Fuchs nodules, exudative RD; may develop cataract, CME, CNV, optic atrophy (Fig. 8.27)

Other findings: may rarely have hearing loss, alopecia, poliosis, vitiligo, CSF pleocytosis (similar to VKH)

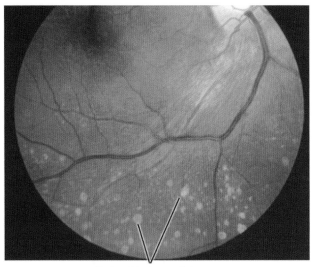

Dalen-Fuchs nodules

Figure 8.27 Dalen-Fuchs nodules in a patient with sympathetic ophthalmia. (From Kaiser PK, Friedman NJ, Pineda R II. *Massachusetts Eye and Ear Infirmary Illustrated Manual of Ophthalmology*, 2nd ed. Philadelphia: WB Saunders; 2004.)

Pathology: diffuse lymphocytic infiltration of choroid with ill-defined, patchy accumulations of epithelioid (giant) cells that contain phagocytosed uveal pigment; inflammation can extend into optic nerve, causing granulomatous optic neuritis; Dalen-Fuchs nodules (epithelioid giant cells between Bruch membrane and RPE that appear as small, round, yellow depigmented spots in peripheral retina [also seen in VKH, sarcoidosis, TB]); no involvement of choriocapillaris (Figs. 8.28 and 8.29)

B-scan ultrasound: choroidal thickening

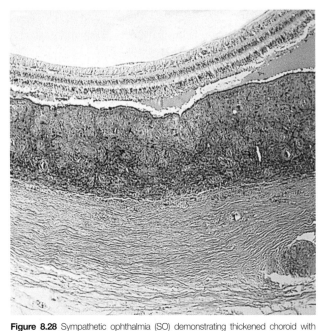

Figure 8.28 Sympathetic ophthalmia (SO) demonstrating thickened choroid with epithelioid cells and lymphocytes; the choriocapillaris is spared. (From Yanoff M, Fine BS. *Ocular Pathology*, 5th ed. St Louis: Mosby; 2002.)

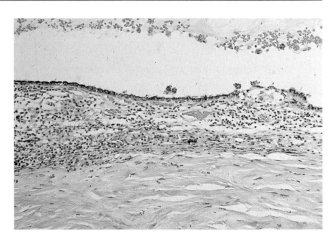

Figure 8.29 High magnification of a Dalen-Fuchs nodule between retinal pigment epithelium (RPE) and Bruch membrane. (From Yanoff M, Fine BS. *Ocular Pathology*, 5th ed. St Louis: Mosby; 2002.)

FA: multiple hyperfluorescent sites of leakage

OCT: intraretinal edema, exudative RD

Treatment: systemic and local steroids, IMT; consider enucleation of injured eye within 2 weeks if NLP vision to prevent SO, but once inflammation has started in fellow eye, removal of exciting eye is controversial

Prognosis: many patients retain good vision in sympathizing eye with prompt treatment; 60% have 20/40 vision, but up to 25% have vision ≤20/200

Syphilis

Panuveitis ("great mimic," great masquerader) resulting from infection with spirochete *Treponema pallidum*

Acquired:
  Findings (secondary and tertiary): panuveitis (10%), iris papules and gummata (yellow–red nodules, also in choroid), chorioretinitis (salt-and-pepper changes), retinitis, retinal vasculitis, exudative RD, neuroretinitis, optic neuritis, optic atrophy, Argyll-Robertson pupil, ocular motor nerve palsies, ectopia lentis, interstitial keratitis (Fig. 8.30)
  Other findings:
    PRIMARY (after 3-week incubation): chancre (painless lesion at inoculation site)
    SECONDARY (6–8 weeks later): rash (maculopapular; especially palms and soles), lymphadenopathy, condylomata
    TERTIARY (>1 year later; 1/3 of untreated): benign tertiary syphilis (gummata on skin, mucous membranes), cardiovascular syphilis (aortic aneurysm), neurosyphilis (CNS, ocular)
  Diagnosis: serology (nontreponemal tests [VDRL or rapid plasma reagin] and treponemal tests [FTA-ABS or microhemagglutination assay for *Treponema pallidum* antibodies, ELISA, PCR); must rule out neurosyphilis with LP

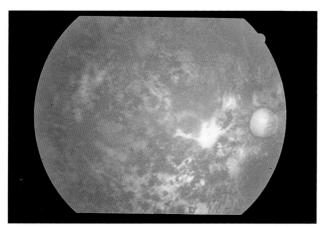

Figure 8.30 Extensive chorioretinal damage with hyperplasia of retinal pigment epithelium as a result of syphilis. (From Dugel PU. Syphilitic uveitis. In: Yanoff M, Duker JS, eds. *Ophthalmology*. London: Mosby; 1999.)

FALSE-POSITIVE VDRL: rheumatoid arthritis, anticardiolipin antibody, SLE, leprosy, hepatitis, mononucleosis, HIV, Lyme disease, leptospirosis, rheumatic fever, malaria, pregnancy, and certain drugs

Treatment: as for neurosyphilis

Penicillin G 18-24 million units/day IV × 10-14 days, followed by penicillin G 2.4 million units/week intramuscularly (IM) × 3 weeks

In penicillin-allergic patients: doxycycline, erythromycin

Congenital:

Findings (at birth or decades later): interstitial keratitis (up to 50%, usually girls; new vessels meet in center of cornea [salmon patch], then atrophy [ghost vessels]), anterior uveitis, ectopia lentis, Argyll-Robertson pupil, cataract, glaucoma, optic neuritis and atrophy, chorioretinitis (salt-and-pepper fundus), retinal vasculitis

Other findings:

EARLY (≤2 years old): death (in utero or perinatal), inflammation of internal organs (hepatosplenomegaly), rhinitis, osteochondritis, desquamative skin rash, pneumonia, anemia, low birth weight

LATE (≥3 years old): dental abnormalities (Hutchinson teeth [peg-shaped], mulberry molars), facial deformities (saddle nose, frontal bossing), saber shins, tabes dorsalis, deafness (CN VIII), skin fissures (rhagades; especially corners of mouth and nose), neurosyphilis

Hutchinson triad: interstitial keratitis, deafness, Hutchinson teeth

Tuberculosis (TB)

Caused by infection with *Mycobacterium tuberculosis*; usually from aerosolized droplets

Lesions common in lungs and choroid (highly oxygenated)

90% systemic infection from reactivation in immunocompromised patient, may develop **miliary TB** (widespread hematogenous dissemination)

Pulmonary (80%), extrapulmonary (20%); usually asymptomatic

Symptoms (10%): fever, night sweats, weight loss

Findings (active infection or immune reaction): lupus vulgaris on eyelids, phlyctenule, primary conjunctival TB, interstitial keratitis, scleritis, lacrimal gland involvement, orbital periostitis, iris nodules, granulomatous uveitis (anterior, posterior, panuveitis) most commonly disseminated choroiditis with multiple yellow lesions (tubercles, 0.5–3 mm), but can be single large choroidal mass (tuberculoma, 4–14 mm) or multifocal choroiditis serpiginous pattern; may have exudative RD, vitreous opacities, CME, CNV, subretinal abscess, retinal perivasculitis with retinal and vitreous hemorrhage, periphlebitis with venous occlusion and NV, optic neuritis, cranial nerve palsies (often caused by basal meningitis), secondary glaucoma and cataract

Diagnosis: definitive diagnosis requires identification of organism in body fluid or tissue biopsy; presumptive (most cases) based on history, exam, purified protein derivative (PPD) tuberculin skin test, QuantiFERON-TB Gold, chest radiograph

FA: early hypofluorescence with late leakage of active lesions; blockage and late staining of old lesions

ICG: hypocyanescence of lesions (more numerous than on fundus exam)

Treatment: systemic antitubercular therapy, including isoniazid, rifampin, ethambutol, pyrazinamide (induction with all 4 drugs × 2 months, then continuation with 2 drugs × 4–7 months); systemic steroids may cause flare-up; ethambutol and isoniazid can cause toxic optic neuropathy

MASQUERADE SYNDROMES

Conditions that present as uveitis, may be neoplastic or nonneoplastic: malignancies (primary vitreoretinal lymphoma [most common], systemic lymphoma, leukemia, benign reactive uveal lymphoid hyperplasia, retinoblastoma, malignant melanoma, metastases, juvenile xanthogranuloma [JXG], bilateral diffuse uveal melanocytic proliferation [BDUMP]), intraocular foreign body, ocular ischemic syndrome, retinitis pigmentosa, multiple sclerosis, chronic peripheral rhegmatogenous RD (Schwartz-Matsuo syndrome [photoreceptor outer segments in AC and increased IOP])

(See Chapter 11, Posterior Segment)

Primary Vitreoretinal Lymphoma (PVRL)

Rare type of primary CNS lymphoma

98% non-Hodgkin B-cell lymphoma, 2% T-cell

Usually occurs in 6th-7th decades of life; male = female

90% of PVRL develop CNS involvement; 25% with CNS lymphoma develop intraocular involvement

Symptoms: decreased vision, floaters

Findings: bilateral AC and vitreous cells, retinal hemorrhage and exudates, creamy subretinal infiltrates, exudative RD, multifocal chorioretinal scars, vasculitis (may appear similar to ARN, toxoplasmosis, "frosted-branch" angiitis, retinal artery occlusion)

Other findings: hemiparesis, seizures, cranial nerve palsies, behavioral changes

Diagnosis: cytology and flow cytometry (aqueous and vitreous) to identifying biomarkers such as CD20+ or monoclonal kappa or lambda B-cell populations; interleukin (IL)-10:IL-6 ratio >1 is highly suggestive; consider retinal biopsy if vitreous biopsy not diagnostic; MRI/CT scan neuroimaging to assess CNS involvement

Treatment: intravitreal chemotherapy (methotrexate, rituximab), external beam radiation; systemic and intrathecal chemotherapy for CNS disease

Prognosis: high-grade malignancy with poor prognosis (median survival ~60 months), 60% 5-year survival; high risk of recurrence and CNS involvement

Leukemia

Retina is most common ocular tissue affected clinically

Choroid is most common ocular tissue affected histopathologically

Findings: AC reaction, iris heterochromia, Roth spots, retinal hemorrhages, cotton-wool spots, peripheral NV, exudative RDs, vascular dilation and tortuosity, optic nerve infiltration; may have exudative RD, hypopyon, pseudohypopyon, hyphema, iris heterochromia

Diagnosis: bone marrow, peripheral blood smear, aqueous cytology
   FA with exudative retinal detachment: multiple areas of hyperfluorescence (similar to VKH)

Malignant Melanoma

Inflammation in 5% of uveal melanoma (anterior, posterior, or panuveitis; episcleritis); usually epithelioid or mixed-cell choroidal melanomas

Necrotic tumor may seed tumor cells into the vitreous and anterior segment, causing an inflammatory response

Findings: AC reaction, iris heterochromia, vitreous hemorrhage; may have brown pseudohypopyon (melanin-laden macrophages) and melanomalytic glaucoma

Diagnosis: FA, B-scan ultrasound (low internal reflectivity)

Metastatic Tumors (Mets)

Intraocular malignancy in adults usually metastases

Usually to choroid and iris, most commonly lung and breast cancer

Rare to retina, most commonly cutaneous melanoma, lung, GI, breast

Findings:
   Choroidal mets: vitritis, choroidal lesions (usually bilateral, multifocal), exudative RD, CME
   Iris mets: AC reaction, iris nodules, iris NV, increased IOP
   Retinal mets: lesions (brown in melanoma, white–yellow in others), perivascular sheathing

Retinoblastoma (RB)

Inflammation in up to 3%; usually diffuse infiltrating RB in children aged 4-6 years

Findings: may have chemosis, pseudohypopyon (white), vitreous cells

Diagnosis:
   AC tap: lactate dehydrogenase (LDH) levels, cytology
   B-scan ultrasound: lack of calcifications

Juvenile Xanthogranuloma (JXG)

Histiocytic disorder in young children involving skin, may affect eyes and other organs

Findings: small fleshy iris tumors, AC reaction, spontaneous hyphema

Diagnosis: skin lesions, iris biopsy (foamy histiocytes and Touton giant cells)

Multiple Sclerosis (MS)

Findings: periphlebitis, intermediate uveitis, optic neuritis

Diagnosis: neurologic examination, head MRI

Intraocular Foreign Body (IOFB)

Retained foreign body, especially organic IOFB, may cause chronic inflammation; IOFB seen in 17%-40% of penetrating ocular injuries; age 20-40 years most common

Findings: signs of ocular trauma, hyphema, corneoscleral laceration, lens disruption, visible FB, iris heterochromia, vitritis, choroidal hemorrhage, retinal detachment, proliferative vitreoretinopathy (PVR), endophthalmitis

Diagnosis: X-ray, B-scan ultrasound, orbital CT scan; MRI is contraindicated if metallic IOFB being considered

Treatment: surgical removal; tetanus immunization history should be obtained, and tetanus toxoid or tetanus immune globulin should be administered if necessary; endophthalmitis prophylaxis with antibiotics:

Systemic: vancomycin 1 g IV q12h or cefazolin 1 g IV q8h; ceftazidime 1 g IV q12h; continue with a course of oral clindamycin 300 mg tid, amikacin 240 mg tid, or moxifloxacin 400 mg PO qd × 10-15 days

Intravitreal (at time of surgery): vancomycin 1 mg/0.1 mL, ceftazidime 2.25 mg/0.1 mL, or amikacin 0.4 mg/0.1 mL; consider amphotericin B (5–10 µg/0.1 mL) or voriconazole (100 µg/0.1 mL) if organic IOFB

Topical (fortified antibiotics/antifungals): vancomycin 25-50 mg/mL, ceftazidime 50 mg/mL q1h

Prognosis: sympathetic ophthalmia in up to 2% of cases

Ocular Ischemic Syndrome

Hypoperfusion of eye, usually from carotid artery obstruction; most commonly males ≥65 years old

Causes intraocular inflammation with decreased vision and pain

Findings: corneal edema, AC reaction (flare > cells), rarely vitreous cells; may have neovascularization (iris, angle, retina, or disc), altered IOP (increased or decreased), cataract, optic disc edema, retinal hemorrhages, dilated/tortuous retinal venules and narrowed arterioles

Diagnosis: FA (delayed filling, diffuse leakage, capillary nonperfusion), carotid Doppler ultrasound (ipsilateral stenosis >90%)

Treatment: topical steroids and cycloplegic for inflammation, panretinal photocoagulation, consider intravitreal anti-VEGF agents; carotid endarterectomy

Prognosis: poor for vision; 40% 5-year mortality

Retinitis Pigmentosa

Findings: vitreous cells, pigmentary retinopathy with vascular attenuation and optic nerve pallor; may develop CME

Diagnosis: ERG, EOG, VF

DDX OF UVEITIS AND ASSOCIATED SIGNS

Band keratopathy: JIA, sarcoidosis, MS

Hyphema: Fuchs heterochromic iridocyclitis, trauma, JXG, VZV

Vitreous hemorrhage: VKH, POHS

Iris nodules: TB, syphilis, sarcoidosis, leprosy, sympathetic ophthalmia, VKH, multiple sclerosis, Fuchs heterochromic iridocyclitis

Iris atrophy: herpetic (diffuse or sectoral), Fuchs heterochromic iridocyclitis (diffuse), traumatic (focal, usually surgical)

Bell palsy (bilateral): Lyme disease, sarcoidosis

Genitourinary involvement: reactive arthritis syndrome, gonococcal disease, Behçet disease

Jaundice: leptospirosis, IBD, CMV, schistosomiasis

Liver enlargement: toxocariasis, toxoplasmosis, CMV

CNS involvement: TB, VKH, congenital toxoplasmosis, congenital CMV, Behçet disease, large cell lymphoma

Skin rash: secondary syphilis, sarcoidosis, Behçet disease, psoriasis, reactive arthritis syndrome, VKH, POHS

Erythema nodosum: sarcoidosis, TB, IBD, POHS, Behçet disease, APMPPE

Oral ulcers: Behçet disease, reactive arthritis syndrome, HSV, IBD, OCP, Stevens-Johnson syndrome (SJS), SLE

Genital ulcers: syphilis, reactive arthritis syndrome, Behçet disease, OCP, SLE

Pulmonary involvement: TB, sarcoidosis, Churg-Strauss syndrome, *Toxocara*, aspergillosis, coccidioidomycosis, POHS, granulomatosis with polyangiitis

SURGERY AND UVEITIS

Usually wait at least 3 months for cataract surgery, 6 months for corneal transplant

JIA: no IOL; can develop cyclitic membranes and CB detachments; consider lensectomy with partial vitrectomy

Pars planitis: increased risk of complications, higher risk for CME; vitreous opacities may limit vision; therefore, consider lensectomy with pars plana vitrectomy

Fuchs heterochromic iridocyclitis: cataract surgery is safe; increased risk of transient postoperative hyphema

REVIEW QUESTIONS *(Answers start on page 422)*

1. The most effective antibiotic for the treatment of *P. acnes* endophthalmitis is
   a. amikacin
   b. gentamicin
   c. vancomycin
   d. ceftazidime

2. For the diagnosis of granulomatous inflammation, which cell type must be present?
   a. Langhans cell
   b. lymphocyte
   c. Touton giant cell
   d. epithelioid histiocyte

3. All of the following are true concerning sarcoidosis, *except*
   a. Touton giant cells are common
   b. lymphocytes surround the granuloma
   c. histiocytes are abundant
   d. necrosis is rare

4. Which of the following is *not* characteristic of Fuchs heterochromic iridocyclitis?
   a. iris neovascularization
   b. cataract
   c. posterior synechiae
   d. vitreous opacities

5. The most common organism causing endophthalmitis following cataract surgery is
   a. *S. pneumoniae*
   b. *H. influenzae*
   c. *S. aureus*
   d. *S. epidermidis*

6. MEWDS can be differentiated from APMPPE by
   a. age of onset
   b. female predilection
   c. paracentral scotomas
   d. viral prodrome

7. All of the following disorders are correctly paired with their HLA associations, *except*
   a. presumed ocular histoplasmosis syndrome, B9
   b. Behçet disease, B51
   c. birdshot chorioretinopathy, A29
   d. reactive arthritis syndrome, B27

8. Decreased vision in a patient with intermediate uveitis is most likely a result of
   a. cataract
   b. macular edema
   c. papillitis
   d. glaucoma

9. A 71-year-old woman with a 6-month history of fatigue, anorexia, and 10-pound weight loss is found to have left-sided weakness, visual acuity of 20/80 OD and 20/60 OS, and vitreous cells. The most helpful workup is
   a. LP and vitrectomy
   b. ESR and temporal artery biopsy
   c. CBC and lymph node biopsy
   d. PPD and chest X-ray

10. The most common organisms causing endophthalmitis following trauma are
    a. *Enterococcus* species and *S. aureus*
    b. *Bacillus* species and *S. epidermidis*
    c. *Pseudomonas* species and *S. aureus*
    d. *S. aureus* and *S. epidermidis*

11. All of the following are features common to both sympathetic ophthalmia and VKH syndrome, *except*
    a. exudative retinal detachments
    b. Dalen-Fuchs nodules
    c. pathology localized to choroid
    d. vitritis

12. Which disorder is more common in males?
    a. MEWDS
    b. uveal effusion syndrome
    c. APMPPE
    d. birdshot chorioretinopathy

13. EVS findings include all of the following, *except*
    a. vitrectomy was beneficial only in patients with LP vision
    b. intravitreal corticosteroids were helpful
    c. IV antibiotics were not helpful
    d. the most common organism was *S. epidermidis*

14. Which of the following is *not* characteristic of MEWDS?
    a. enlargement of the blind spot
    b. bilaterality
    c. flu-like illness
    d. female preponderance

15. The most common cause of posterior uveitis is
    a. sarcoidosis
    b. syphilis
    c. CMV
    d. toxoplasmosis

16. All of the following are causes of HLA-B27–associated uveitis, *except*
    a. ankylosing spondylitis
    b. ulcerative colitis
    c. Crohn disease
    d. psoriasis

17. Which of the following is *not* part of the classic triad of findings in reactive arthritis syndrome?
    a. iritis
    b. arthritis
    c. conjunctivitis
    d. urethritis

18. Phacoantigenic endophthalmitis is characterized by which pattern of granulomatous inflammation?
    a. zonal
    b. diffuse
    c. discrete
    d. necrotizing

19. A 35-year-old man with decreased vision OD is found to have optic disc edema and a macular star. The causative organism most likely is
    a. *Onchocerca volvulus*
    b. *Bartonella henselae*
    c. *Treponema pallidum*
    d. *Borrelia burgdorferi*

20. A person living in which area of the United States would be most likely to develop POHS?
    a. Southwest
    b. Northwest
    c. Midwest
    d. Southeast

21. All of the following are true of birdshot chorioretinopathy, *except*
    a. more common in males
    b. usually bilateral
    c. CME is common
    d. associated with HLA-A29

22. Which of the following is *least* commonly associated with *T. pallidum* infection?
    a. interstitial keratitis
    b. chorioretinitis
    c. ectopialentis
    d. glaucoma

23. The HLA association for intermediate uveitis with multiple sclerosis is
    a. B8
    b. B51
    c. DR4
    d. DR15

24. Retinal S antigen is found in
    a. ganglion cells
    b. retinal pigment epithelium
    c. photoreceptors
    d. Mueller cells

25. Features of Harada disease include all of the following, *except*
    a. vitritis
    b. deafness
    c. exudative retinal detachments
    d. Dalen-Fuchs nodules

26. Larva cause all of the following infections, *except*
    a. cysticercosis
    b. diffuse unilateral subacute neuroretinitis
    c. onchocerciasis
    d. cat-scratch disease

27. Which of the following signs of intermediate uveitis is most associated with multiple sclerosis?
    a. subretinal neovascularization
    b. snowbank
    c. periphlebitis
    d. CME

28. CSF abnormalities are associated with all of the following disorders, *except*
    a. VKH syndrome
    b. ocular sarcoidosis
    c. APMPPE
    d. pars planitis

29. All of the following can present as uveitis, *except*
    a. retinoblastoma
    b. choroidal hemangioma
    c. leukemia
    d. juvenile xanthogranuloma

30. Which of the following is *not* associated with inflammatory bowel disease?
    a. conjunctivitis
    b. episcleritis
    c. interstitial keratitis
    d. iritis

31. Anterior vitreous cells are *least* likely to be found in
    a. retinitis pigmentosa
    b. CMV
    c. serpiginous choroiditis
    d. chronic cyclitis

32. GI disorders associated with uveitis include all of the following, *except*
    a. ulcerative colitis
    b. Whipple disease
    c. diverticulitis
    d. Crohn disease

33. All of the following may occur in ocular sarcoidosis, *except*
    a. optic disc nodules
    b. pars planitis
    c. cranial nerve palsies
    d. low serum gamma globulin

34. The choroid is the primary location of the pathologic process in
    a. toxoplasmosis
    b. CMV
    c. Coats disease
    d. VKH syndrome

35. Which of the following is *least* likely to be found in a patient with sympathetic ophthalmia?
    a. onset after a latent period of 40 years
    b. granulomatous nodules in the retina
    c. history of evisceration of the traumatized eye
    d. iris nodules in the sympathizing eye

36. Band keratopathy is *least* likely to occur in a patient with
    a. sarcoidosis
    b. JIA
    c. Behçet disease
    d. multiple sclerosis

37. A patient with APMPPE is most likely to have
    a. unilateral involvement
    b. enlarged blind spot
    c. viral prodrome
    d. CNV

38. A patient with a mild AC reaction, increased intraocular pressure, and iris heterochromia is most likely to also exhibit which other finding?
    a. anisocoria
    b. ptosis
    c. posterior synechiae
    d. fine vessels in the angle

39. Which of the following cell types is found in both granulomatous and nongranulomatous KP?
    a. epithelioid cells
    b. giant cells
    c. lymphocytes
    d. macrophages

40. All of the following are masquerade syndromes, *except*
    a. vitreous hemorrhage
    b. retinal detachment
    c. intraocular foreign body
    d. multiple sclerosis

41. A false-positive VDRL test is *least* likely to occur in a patient with
    a. granulomatosis with polyangiitis
    b. lupus
    c. rheumatoid arthritis
    d. anticardiolipin antibody

42. A 54-year-old man with chronic recurrent uveitis OS controlled with topical steroids has developed a visually significant cataract. What is the most appropriate treatment?
    a. do not delay cataract surgery and treat with oral steroids
    b. do not delay cataract surgery and treat with oral cyclosporine
    c. delay cataract surgery for 6 weeks and treat with oral cyclosporine
    d. delay cataract surgery until the eye has been quiet for at least 3 months

43. All of the following are risk factors for traumatic endophthalmitis, *except*
    a. delayed surgery
    b. disruption of the lens
    c. retained intraocular foreign body
    d. double penetrating injury

44. A pseudophakic patient develops granulomatous inflammation 8 months after cataract surgery, and a white plaque is present on the posterior capsule. The organism most likely to be causing this condition is
    a. *A. fumigatus*
    b. *C. albicans*
    c. *P. acnes*
    d. *B. cereus*

45. A 28-year-old woman acutely develops reduced vision, pain, redness, and floaters OS. Exam shows a mild iritis with granulomatous KP and discrete patches of peripheral necrotizing retinitis. The most appropriate management is to begin treatment with systemic
    a. acyclovir
    b. foscarnet
    c. ranibizumab
    d. vancomycin

46. CNV is most likely to occur in
    a. acute zonal occult outer retinopathy
    b. birdshot chorioretinopathy
    c. serpiginous choroiditis
    d. punctate inner choroiditis

47. A 30-year-old man with photophobia for a week is found to have 2+ AC cells and flare OU. Initial treatment should be with
    a. topical nonsteroidal anti-inflammatory
    b. topical steroid and cycloplegic
    c. sub-Tenon steroid injection
    d. oral nonsteroidal anti-inflammatory

48. Which of the following tests should be obtained before starting oral steroids for a patient with chronic noninfectious uveitis?
    a. chest X-ray, albumin, and electrolytes
    b. blood pressure, electrolytes, fasting blood glucose
    c. liver enzymes, CBC, and urinalysis
    d. CBC, creatinine, and albumin

49. Which systemic antibiotic is *not* used for endophthalmitis?
    a. ceftazidime
    b. levofloxacin
    c. tobramycin
    d. vancomycin

50. Which white dot syndrome has the best visual prognosis?
    a. acute retinal pigment epitheliitis
    b. acute posterior multifocal placoid pigment epitheliopathy
    c. multifocal choroiditis and panuveitis
    d. subretinal fibrosis and uveitis syndrome

51. The neoplastic condition that most commonly masquerades as uveitis is
    a. leukemia
    b. primary vitreoretinal lymphoma
    c. malignant melanoma
    d. metastases

52. Iris nodule biopsy shows foamy histiocytes. The most likely diagnosis is
    a. sarcoidosis
    b. sympathetic ophthalmia
    c. tuberculosis
    d. juvenile xanthogranuloma

53. The most common cause of endogenous endophthalmitis is
    a. fungi
    b. gram-positive bacteria
    c. gram-negative bacteria
    d. parasite

54. Maculopathy with foveolitis is associated with which viral infection?
    a. Zika
    b. Ebola
    c. West Nile
    d. Dengue

55. Necrotizing scleritis is caused by
    a. *Candidiasis*
    b. *Cysticercosis*
    c. *Leptospirosis*
    d. *Nocardiosis*

Please visit the eBook for an interactive version of the review questions. See front cover for activation details.

SUGGESTED READINGS

Basic and Clinical Sciences Course. (2021). *Section 9: Intraocular inflammation and uveitis*. San Francisco: AAO.

Foster, C. S., & Vitale, A. T. (2013). *Diagnosis and treatment of uveitis* (2nd ed.). New Delhi: Jaypee Brothers Medical Publishers.

Jones, N. P. (2012). *Uveitis* (2nd ed.). London: JP Medical Ltd.

Michelson, J. B. (1992). *Color atlas of uveitis* (2nd ed.). St. Louis: Mosby.

Nussenblatt, R. B., & Whitcup, S. M. (2010). *Uveitis: Fundamentals and clinical practice* (4th ed.). Philadelphia: Mosby.

Glaucoma

ANATOMY/PHYSIOLOGY
TESTING
PATHOLOGY
DISORDERS
TREATMENT

ANATOMY/PHYSIOLOGY

Ciliary Body (CB)

Central portion of uvea, bridges anterior and posterior segments, 6–7 mm wide, located between the scleral spur and ora serrata; gives rise to iris; composed of the pars plicata (anterior 2 mm with ciliary processes) and the pars plana (posterior 4 mm, flat)

Pars plicata consists of:

Ciliary muscle: longitudinal fibers (insert into scleral spur and affect outflow facility), circular fibers (anterior inner fibers oriented parallel to limbus and affect accommodation), and radial fibers (connect longitudinal and circular fibers). Innervation via short ciliary nerves from parasympathetic fibers of cranial nerve (CN) 3 (97% travel to ciliary muscle, 3% travel to iris sphincter), stimulation causes contraction; sympathetic fibers relax muscle

Ciliary vessels: major arterial circle of the iris (in CB near iris root) formed by anastomosis of branches of anterior and long posterior ciliary arteries; drainage through vortex veins and some via intrascleral and episcleral plexus

Ciliary processes: 70 finger-like projections composed of pigmented and nonpigmented epithelial cell bilayer, capillaries, and stroma

Functions:

Suspends and alters shape of lens: zonular fibers that originate between the ciliary processes of the pars plicata, attach to the crystalline lens, and suspend it. Helmholtz theory of accommodation explains the changes in lens shape and thus refractive power with contraction and relaxation of the ciliary muscle. Contraction of the longitudinal fibers pulls the lens forward, shallowing the anterior chamber (AC). Contraction of the circular fibers relaxes the zonules, making the lens more spherical, with greater focusing power. Relaxation of circular fibers (or cycloplegia)

tightens the zonules, stretching the lens and making it thinner, with less focusing power.

Produces aqueous humor: production of aqueous is primarily by active secretion from nonpigmented ciliary epithelium (also passive by diffusion and ultrafiltration); both an Na^+/K^+ pump and carbonic anhydrase are involved. β-blockers act through adenylcyclase to inhibit the Na^+/K^+ pump; glucose enters by passive diffusion.

Rate = 2–3 µL/min (decreases to 1 µL/min at night), AC volume = 220 µL, posterior chamber volume = 60 µL (AC volume turnover is approximately 1%/min). Rate measured by fluorophotometry (direct optical measurement of decreasing fluorescein concentration) or tonography (indirect calculation from outflow measurement). Diurnal production of aqueous (may be related to cortisol levels) decreases with sleep (45%), age (2%/decade; counterbalanced by the decreased outflow with age), inflammation, surgery, trauma, and drugs

AQUEOUS COMPOSITION: slightly hypertonic and acidic (pH 7.5–7.6) compared with plasma; 15 × more ascorbate (vitamin C) than plasma; lower protein (0.02% vs. 7% in plasma, mostly albumin and transferrin); lower calcium and phosphorus (50% of the level in plasma); lower glucose (50%–70% of the plasma level; increased levels in diabetics result in increased levels in lens, causing refractive changes and cataract progression); chloride and bicarbonate vary (from 25% above or below plasma levels); sodium, potassium, magnesium, iron, zinc, and copper levels similar to those in plasma. Other components include glutathione, urea, enzymes, growth factors, oxygen, and carbon dioxide

FUNCTIONS OF AQUEOUS: maintains intraocular pressure (IOP), provides metabolic substrates (glucose, oxygen, electrolytes) to the cornea and lens, removes metabolic waste (lactate, pyruvate, carbon dioxide), prevents oxidative stress and ultraviolet (UV) damage (oxidation-reduction enzymes, antioxidant properties of ascorbate)

Affects aqueous outflow: contraction of ciliary muscle longitudinal fibers causes traction on the trabecular meshwork (TM), increasing outflow, also contributes to uveoscleral outflow

Synthesizes acid mucopolysaccharide component of vitreous: occurs in nonpigmented epithelial cells of pars plana and enters vitreous body at its base

Maintains blood–aqueous barrier: composed of tight junctions of nonpigmented ciliary epithelium, iris vasculature, and inner wall endothelium of Schlemm canal, which prevents proteins from entering aqueous

Within the ciliary processes, plasma enters from thin fenestrated endothelium of capillary core → passes through stroma → 2 layers of epithelium with apposing apical surfaces (which forms the ciliary epithelial bilayer):

PIGMENTED EPITHELIUM: outer layer, faces ciliary stroma, continuous with the retinal pigment epithelium (RPE; basal lamina continuous with Bruch membrane), solutes can move between cells (leaky epithelium)

NONPIGMENTED EPITHELIUM: inner layer, faces aqueous humor, equivalent to the sensory retina (basal lamina continuous with inner limiting membrane [ILM]), site of active secretion, tight junctions between cells

Both layers have basal basement membranes with their apices facing each other. During passage from the bloodstream to the posterior chamber, a molecule must pass through capillary basement membrane, pigmented epithelium basement membrane, pigmented epithelium, nonpigmented epithelium, nonpigmented epithelium basement membrane

Cryodestruction and inflammation cause loss of barrier function (tight junctions open), resulting in flare (proteins in aqueous); atropine reduces flare by closing tight junctions

Outflow Pathways

Trabecular meshwork (traditional pathway): pressure dependent; represents major aqueous drainage system; uveoscleral meshwork → corneoscleral meshwork → juxtacanalicular connective tissue → Schlemm canal → collector channels → aqueous veins → episcleral and conjunctival veins → anterior ciliary and superior ophthalmic veins → cavernous sinus

The pore size of the meshwork decreases toward Schlemm canal:

Uveal meshwork: collagenous core surrounded by endothelial cells; pore size up to 70 μm; linked to ciliary muscle

Corneoscleral meshwork: sheet-like beams insert into scleral spur; pore size up to 30 μm

Juxtacanalicular meshwork: links corneoscleral trabeculae with Schlemm endothelium; pore size up to 10 μm; site of greatest aqueous outflow resistance

Canal of Schlemm is lined by a single layer of endothelial cells (mesothelial cells) and connects to the venous system by 30 collector channels

Uveoscleral outflow (15%–20% of total outflow): pressure independent; aqueous passes through face of ciliary body in the angle, enters the ciliary muscle and suprachoroidal space, and is drained by veins in the ciliary body, choroid, and sclera

Cyclodialysis cleft increases aqueous outflow through the uveoscleral pathway (without reducing aqueous production); cycloplegics and prostaglandin analogues increase uveoscleral outflow; miotics decrease uveoscleral outflow and increase TM outflow

Angle Structures

Visible only by gonioscopy because of total internal reflection at the air–cornea interface (Fig. 9.1)

Mnemonic: **I C**an't **S**ee **T**his **S**tuff (**I**ris, **C**iliary body, **S**cleral spur, **T**rabecular meshwork, **S**chwalbe line)

Schwalbe line: peripheral/posterior termination of Descemet membrane, which corresponds to apex of corneal light wedge (optical cross section of the cornea with narrow slit beam reveals two linear reflections, one from external and one from internal corneal surfaces, which meet at Schwalbe line)

Trabecular meshwork (TM): anterior nonpigmented portion appears as a clear white band; posterior pigmented portion has variable pigmentation (usually darkest inferiorly). Increased pigmentation of TM occurs with pseudoexfoliation syndrome (Sampaolesi line), pigment dispersion syndrome, uveitis, melanoma, trauma, surgery, hyphema, darkly pigmented individuals, and increasing age. Mnemonic: **PIGMENT** (**P**seudoexfoliation and **P**igment dispersion syndrome, **I**ritis, **G**laucoma [after angle closure], **M**elanosis, **E**ndocrine [diabetes, Addison disease], **N**evus, **T**rauma)

Schlemm canal: circular channel like lymphatic vessel, usually not visible or only faintly visible as a light-gray band at the level of posterior TM; elevated venous pressure or pressure from the edge of the gonioscopy lens may cause blood to reflux, making Schlemm canal visible as a faint red band

DDx of blood in Schlemm canal: elevated episcleral venous pressure, oculodermal melanocytosis (nevus of Ota), neurofibromatosis, congenital ectropion uveae, hypotony, secondary to gonioscopy

Scleral spur (SS): narrow white band that corresponds to the site of insertion of longitudinal fibers of ciliary muscle to sclera

Ciliary body (CB): pigmented band that represents the anterior face of the ciliary body; iris processes may be seen

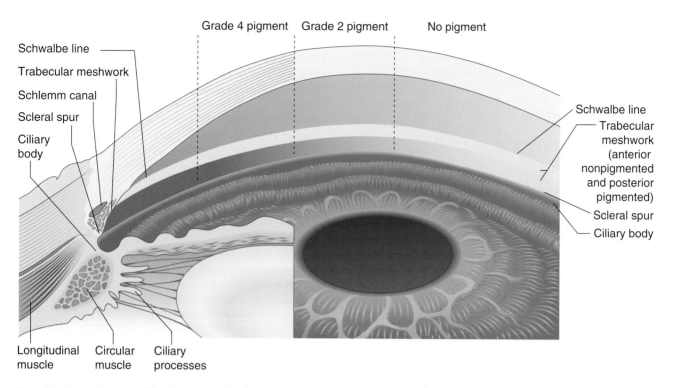

Figure 9.1 Composite drawing of the microscopic and gonioscopic anatomy. (From Becker B, Shaffer RN. *Diagnosis and Therapy of the Glaucomas*. St Louis: Mosby; 1965.)

as lacy projections crossing this band but not the scleral spur (occur in 33% of population)

Angle Abnormalities

Peripheral anterior synechia (PAS): any pigmented structure that crosses scleral spur

Etiology: angle closure, uveitis, neovascularization, flat anterior chamber, iridocorneal endothelial (ICE) syndrome, ciliary body tumors, mesodermal dysgenesis

Normal vessels: radial iris vessels, portions of arterial circle of CB, and rarely, vertical vessels deep in CB; do not branch or cross the scleral spur; present in 7% of patients with blue irides and 10% with brown

Abnormal vessels: fine, often branch, no orientation, cross-scleral spur
  DDx: neovascularization (rubeosis iridis), iris neoplasm, Fuchs heterochromic iridocyclitis (sparse, faint, and delicate; bleed easily on decompression of AC)

Angle recession: tear between longitudinal and circular fibers of the ciliary muscle. Because longitudinal fibers are still attached to the scleral spur, miotics still work, but because they decrease uveoscleral outflow, IOP may actually increase. Breaks in posterior TM result in scarring and a nonfunctional TM; aqueous drains primarily through uveoscleral outflow; 60%–90% of patients with traumatic hyphemas have angle recession; 5% of eyes with angle recession will develop glaucoma

Gonioscopic findings: widened CB band, increased visibility of scleral spur, torn iris processes, sclera visible through disrupted ciliary body tissue, marked variation in CB width in different quadrants of same eye

Cyclodialysis cleft: separation of ciliary body from scleral spur; often from trauma. Results in direct communication between AC and suprachoroidal space, causing hypotony; spontaneous closure may occur (unlikely after 6 weeks) with marked IOP rise; shortly thereafter, the TM should begin to function normally again
  Gonioscopic findings: cleft at junction of scleral spur and CB band
  Treatment: cycloplegic to relax ciliary body in an attempt to close cleft (avoid pilocarpine, which may open the cleft through ciliary muscle traction); laser (argon induces inflammation to close the cleft; spot size = 50–100 μm, duration = 0.1–0.2 s; power = 0.5–1.0 watts to uvea and 1–3 watts to sclera); cryotherapy, suture CB to sclera (direct cyclopexy); intravitreal air bubble for a superior cleft; neodymium:yttrium aluminium garnet (Nd:YAG) laser can be used to open a closed cleft

Iridodialysis: tear/disinsertion of iris root. If large or symptomatic, consider surgical repair with mattress sutures

Optic Nerve (Fig. 9.2)

Approximately 1.2 million axons; cell bodies of ganglion cells are located in the ganglion cell layer. Optic nerve (ON)

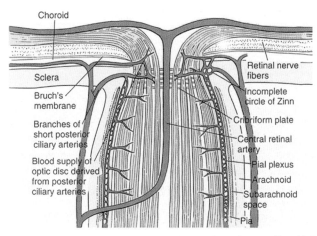

Figure 9.2 Vascular supply and anatomy of the anterior optic nerve. (From Hart WM Jr. In: Podos SM, Yanoff M, eds. *Textbook of Ophthalmology*, vol 6. London: Mosby; 1994.)

head is oval structure (optic disc), variable size (average 1.76 mm horizontal and 1.92 mm vertical) with central depression (cup)

4 layers of ON head based on blood supply:

Nerve fiber: supplied by branches of central retinal artery

Prelaminar: supplied by capillaries of the short posterior ciliary arteries

Laminar (lamina cribrosa): supplied by dense plexus from short posterior ciliary arteries

Retrolaminar: supplied by both ciliary (via recurrent pial vessels) and retinal (via centripetal branches from pial region) circulations

Optic nerve blood flow is influenced by mean blood pressure, IOP, blood viscosity, blood vessel caliber, and blood vessel length

TESTING

Intraocular Pressure

Goldmann equation: $IOP = F/C + EVP$ relates 3 factors important in determination of IOP

F = rate of aqueous formation = $2-3\,\mu L/min$

C = facility of outflow = $0.28\,\mu L/min/mmHg$; <0.20 is abnormal; decreases with age, increases with medication; measured by tonography

EVP = episcleral venous pressure = $8-12$ mmHg; increases with venous obstruction or atrioventivular (AV) shunt: measured by manometry

IOP = $8-21$ mmHg is considered normal; average = 16 $+/-2.5$ mmHg; distribution is not Gaussian and is skewed to higher IOPs

IOP is influenced by age (may increase with age), genetics, race (higher in African Americans), season (higher in winter, lower in summer), blood pressure, obesity, exercise (lower after exercise), Valsalva, time of day (diurnal variation [2–6 mm/day]; peak in morning), posture (higher when lying down vs. sitting up), various hormones, and drugs. Also ocular factors: refractive error (higher in myopes) and eyelid closure

Tonometry

IOP measurement can be performed with a variety of devices (tonometers)

Indentation:

Schiøtz tonometer: known weight indents cornea and displaces a volume of fluid within the eye; amount of indentation estimates pressure; falsely low readings occur with a very elastic eye (low scleral rigidity as with high myopia, buphthalmos, retinal detachment, treatment with cholinesterase inhibitors, thyroid disease, and previous ocular surgery) or a compressible intraocular gas (e.g., SF_6 and C_3F_8); falsely high readings occur with scleral rigidity and hyperopia

Applanation: based on the Imbert-Fick principle: $P = F/A$ (for an ideal thin-walled sphere, pressure inside sphere equals force necessary to flatten its surface divided by the area of flattening). The eye is not an ideal sphere: the cornea resists flattening, and capillary action of the tear meniscus pulls the tonometer to the eye. However, these 2 forces cancel each other when the applanated diameter is 3.06 mm

Goldmann tonometer: biprism attached to a spring; fluorescein semicircles align when area applanated has a diameter = 3.06 mm; error can occur with squeezing, Valsalva, vertical gaze, irregular or edematous cornea, corneal thickness (thick corneas overestimate IOP [~5 mm Hg per 70 μm], and thin corneas underestimate IOP [~5 mm Hg per 70 μm]), amount of fluorescein, external pressure on or restriction of globe, and astigmatism >1.5 D (must align red mark on tip with axis of MINUS cylinder)

Perkins tonometer: portable form of Goldmann device

Mackay-Marg tonometer: applanates small area; good for corneal scars and edema. Examples of this style tonometer include the tonopen and the pneumotonometer

TONOPEN: probe indents cornea, and microprocessor calculates IOP and reliability

PNEUMOTONOMETER: central sensing device is controlled by air pressure

Noncontact:

Air puff tonometer: noncontact device; time required for air jet to flatten cornea is proportional to IOP; varies with cardiac cycle

Gonioscopy

Classification systems:

Scheie:

GRADE I = wide open (CB visible)

GRADE II = SS visible; CB not visible

GRADE III = only anterior TM visible

GRADE IV = closed angle (TM not visible)

Schaffer: opposite of Scheie (Grade 0 is closed; Grade IV is wide open) (Fig. 9.3)

GRADE I = 10% open

Grade II = 20% open

GRADE III = 30% open

GRADE IV = 40% open

Spaeth: most descriptive; 4 elements

FIRST ELEMENT: level of iris insertion (capital letter A–E)

A = Anterior to TM

B = Behind Schwalbe line or at TM

C = at SS

D = Deep angle, CB visible

E = Extremely deep, large CB band

Perform indention gonioscopy: if true insertion is more posterior, place original impression in parentheses followed by true insertion location

SECOND ELEMENT: number that denotes the iridocorneal angle width in degrees from 5 to 45

THIRD ELEMENT: peripheral iris configuration (lowercase letter *r, s,* or *q*)

r = regular (flat)

s = steep (convex)

q = queer (concave)

FOURTH ELEMENT: pigmentation of posterior TM (graded from 0 [none] to 4 [maximal])

Example: (A)B15 r, 1 + (appositionally closed 15° angle that opens to TM with indentation, regular iris configuration, and mildly pigmented posterior TM)

Types of lenses:

Koeppe lens: direct view

Goldmann 3-mirror lens: requires coupling solution (Goniosol)

Zeiss, Posner, and Sussman 4- or 6-mirror lenses: can perform indentation gonioscopy to determine whether angle closure is appositional or synechial

Grading system of shallow/flat anterior chamber:

Grade I: contact between cornea and peripheral iris

Grade II: contact between cornea and iris up to pupil (consider reforming AC with BSS or viscoelastic)

Grade III: contact between cornea and crystalline lens (surgical emergency)

Visual Fields

Perimetry measures the "island of vision" or topographic representation of differential light sensitivity. Peak = fovea; depression = blind spot; extent = 60° nasally, 60° superiorly, 70–75° inferiorly, and 100–110° temporally

Central field test points only within a 30° radius of fixation

Types:

(Fig. 9.4)

Kinetic: uses a moving stimulus of constant intensity to produce an isopter or points of equal sensitivity (horizontal cross section of the hill of vision)

Static: uses a fixed stimulus with constant or variable intensity to produce a profile (vertical cross section of the hill of vision)

Goldmann (kinetic and static):

Test distance: 0.33 m

Test object size: I–V (each increment doubles the diameter [quadruples the area] of test object; III4e test object will have 2 × the diameter and 4 × the area of II4e)

Light filters: 1–4 (increments of 5db), a–e (increments of 1db)

Humphrey (static):

Test distance = 0.33 m; background illumination = 31.5 apostilbs (asb); stimulus size = III; stimulus

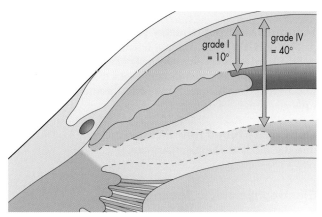

Figure 9.3 Shaffer's angle-grading system. (From Fran M, Smith J, Doyle W. Clinical examination of glaucoma. In: Yanoff M, Duker JS, eds: *Ophthalmology,* 2nd ed, St Louis, 2004, Mosby.)

Kinetic (isopter) perimetry

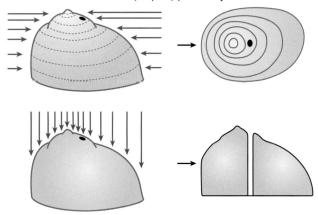

Static (profile) perimetry

Figure 9.4 Kinetic and static perimetry. (From Bajandas FJ, Kline LB. *Neuro-Ophthalmology Review Manual,* 3rd ed. Thorofare, NJ: Slack; 2004.)

duration = 0.2 s; various programs (i.e., central 30°, 24°, 10°, neuro fields, ptosis fields, etc.)

Reliability indices:

FIXATION LOSS: patient responds when a target is displayed in blind spot. There is also a gaze-tracking printout at the bottom of the page that shows the deviation of fixation during each stimulus presentation

FALSE POSITIVE: patient responds when there is no stimulus (nervous or trigger-happy; causes white areas)

FALSE NEGATIVE: patient fails to respond to a superthreshold stimulus at a location that was previously responded to (indicates loss of attention or fatigue; causes cloverleaf pattern)

Global indices:

MEAN DEVIATION (MD): average departure of each test point from the age-adjusted normal value. This represents the overall deviation (mean elevation or depression) of the visual field (VF) from the normal reference field

PATTERN STANDARD DEVIATION (PSD): standard deviation of the differences between the threshold and expected values for each test point. This represents the change in shape of the field from the expected shape for a normal field

SHORT-TERM FLUCTUATION (SF): variability in responses when the same 10 points are retested; measure of consistency

CORRECTED PATTERN STANDARD DEVIATION (CPSD): PSD adjusted for patient reliability (correcting for SF)

Patient vision ≤20/80 will cause a scotoma to appear larger and deeper

Pupil <3 mm will cause reduction in total deviation

Tangent screen (usually kinetic): test distance is 1 m, test object may vary in size and color; tests only central field. Magnifies scotoma and is of low cost; however, poor reproducibility and lack of standardization

VF defect: a scotoma is an area of partial or complete blindness

Corresponds to a defect on Humphrey testing that is at least 3° wide and 6 decibels (dB) deep; also 1 point that is depressed >10 dB or at least 2 points that are depressed at least 5 dB

Typical localized glaucomatous scotomas: (Fig. 9.5)

PARACENTRAL: within central 10°

ARCUATE (Bjerrum): isolated, nasal step of Rönne and Seidel (connected to blind spot)

TEMPORAL WEDGE: temporal to blind spot

Glaucomatous scotomas do not respect the vertical meridian (vs. neurologic VF defects, which do)

VF should correlate with ON appearance; otherwise, consider refractive error, level of vision, media opacities, pupil size, and other causes of VF defects (tilted ON head, ON head drusen, retinal lesions, etc.)

Optic Nerve Head (ONH) Analyzers

Various digital and video cameras that capture ONH image; computer then calculates cup area in an attempt to objectively quantify ONH appearance (Table 9.1)

Confocal scanning laser ophthalmoscopy (CSLO; Heidelberg retinal tomograph [HRT]; TopSS): low-power laser produces digital three-dimensional (3D) picture of ON head by integrating coronal scans of increasing tissue depth; indirectly measures nerve fiber layer (NFL) thickness (Figs. 9.6 and 9.7)

Optical coherence tomography (OCT): measures optical backscattering of light to produce high-resolution, cross-sectional image of the NFL (Fig. 9.8)

Scanning laser polarimetry (SLP; nerve fiber analyzer, GDx): uses a confocal scanning laser ophthalmoscope with an integrated polarimeter to detect changes in light polarization from axons to measure the NFL thickness; quantitative analysis of NFL thickness to detect early glaucomatous damage (Fig. 9.9)

Optic nerve blood flow measurement: color Doppler imaging and laser Doppler flowmetry (Fig. 9.10)

Electrophysiologic Testing

Pattern electroretinogram (pERG), visual evoked response (VEP): may detect pre-perimetric glaucomatous visual function loss in glaucoma suspects

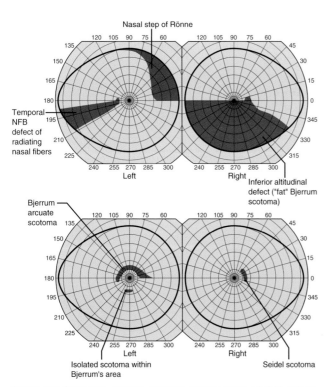

Figure 9.5 Composite diagram depicting different types of field defects. (From Bajandas FJ, Kline LB. *Neuro-Ophthalmology Review Manual*, 3rd ed. Thorofare, NJ: Slack; 2004.)

Table 9.1 Summary of techniques for retinal nerve fiber layer analysis

Technique	Equipment needed	Governing principles	Advantages	Disadvantages
Ophthalmoscopy	Direct ophthalmoscope or slit lamp and 78 D or 90 D lens Red-free light	Nerve fiber layer visibility is enhanced with short-wavelength light	Easy to perform using readily available equipment	May be difficult without clear media Nerve fiber layer not easily seen in lightly pigmented fundi
Red-free, high-contrast fundus photography	Fundus camera with red-free filter High contrast black-and-white film and paper	Nerve fiber layer visibility is enhanced with short-wavelength light	Nerve fiber layer defects may be easy to detect	Requires skilled photographer Requires dilated pupil Limitations of ophthalmoscopy apply
Retinal contour analysis	Scanning laser ophthalmoscope that can perform tomographic topography	Three-dimensional construction of retinal surface can measure retinal height above a reference plane—height is related to thickness of nerve fiber layer	Easy to perform through undilated pupil No discomfort to patient Can image through most media opacities unless very dense	Equipment is expensive Height measurements depend upon location of reference plane Retinal thickness may not be true indirect measure of thickness of nerve fiber layer
Optical coherence tomography	Optical coherence tomography unit	Uses reflected and backscattered light to create images of various retinal layers (analogous to the use of sound waves in ultrasonography)	Can differentiate layers within the retina, including the nerve fiber layer, with a 10 μm resolution Correlates with known histology	Equipment is expensive Requires dilated pupil Resolution may not be high enough to detect small changes
Scanning laser polarimetry	Scanning laser polarimeter	Birefringent properties of the nerve fiber layer cause a measurable phase shift of an incident polarized light proportional to the tissue thickness	Easy to perform through undilated pupil No discomfort to patient Can image through most media opacities, unless very dense Resolution limited to size of a pixel (possibly as small as 1 μm) Reproducibility 5–8 μm	Equipment is expensive Measurements not correlated histologically in humans Requires compensation for other polarizing media (e.g., cornea)

From Chopin NT. Retinal nerve fiber layer analysis. In: Yanoff M, Duker JS, eds. Ophthalmology. *London: Mosby; 1999.*

PATHOLOGY

Glaucoma

Dropout of ganglion cells, replacement of NFL with dense gliotic tissue and some glial cell nuclei; partial preservation of inner nuclear layer with loss of Müller and amacrine cells (normal 8–9 cells high; in glaucoma, 4–5 cells high); earliest histologic changes occur at level of lamina cribrosa; advanced cases may show backward bowing of lamina or "beanpot" appearance (Figs. 9.11 and 9.12)

Schnabel Cavernous Optic Atrophy

Histologic finding in eyes with increased IOP or atherosclerosis and normal IOP; hyaluronic acid infiltration of nerve (originally thought to be from vitreous; may be from in situ production); also occurs in eyes with ischemic optic neuropathy

Pathology: atrophy of neural elements with cystic spaces containing hyaluronic acid (mucopolysaccharides), which stains with colloidal iron and Alcian blue (Fig. 9.13)

Gliosis of the Optic Nerve

With optic atrophy, glial cells replace nerve cells and assume a random distribution throughout the ON

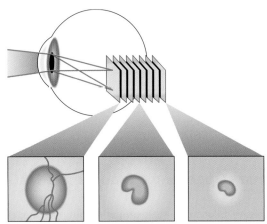

Figure 9.6 Confocal scanning laser ophthalmoscopy. (Adapted from Schuman JS, Noeker RJ. Imaging of the optic nerve head and nerve fiber layer in glaucoma. *Ophthalmol Clin North Am.* 1995;8:259–279.)

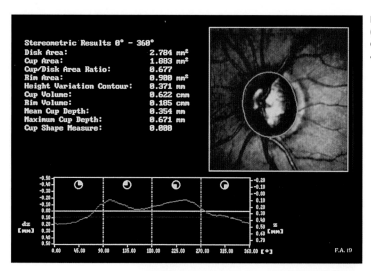

Figure 9.7 Confocal scanning laser ophthalmoscopy printed report. (From Zangwill L, de Souza K, Weinrob RN. Confocal scanning laser ophthalmoscopy to detect glaucomatous optic neuropathy. In: Shuman JS, ed. *Imaging in Glaucoma*. Thorofare, NJ: Slack; 1997.)

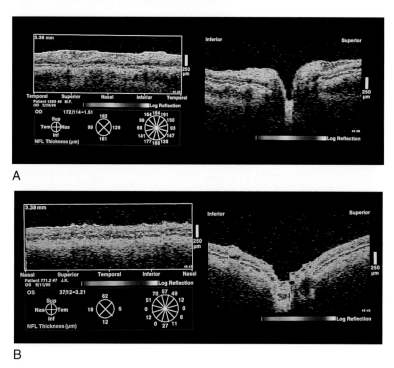

Figure 9.8 Optical coherence tomography. (From Pedut-Kloizman TP, Schuman JS. Disc analysis. In: Yanoff M, Duker JS, eds. *Ophthalmology*. London: Mosby; 1999.)

DISORDERS

Childhood Glaucoma

(See Chapter 5, Pediatrics/Strabismus)

Primary Open-Angle Glaucoma (POAG)

Progressive, bilateral, optic neuropathy with open angles, typical pattern of nerve fiber bundle VF loss, and increased intraocular pressure (IOP >21 mm Hg) not caused by another systemic or local disease

Epidemiology: second-leading cause of blindness in US; most common form of glaucoma (60%–70%); 7% of population has ocular hypertension; 3% of population in Baltimore Eye Study had glaucomatous VF defects. If damage in one eye, untreated fellow eye has 29% risk over 5 years. Steroid responders have 31% risk of developing glaucoma within 5 years

Genetics: juvenile-onset POAG has been mapped to chromosome 1q21-q31 (*GLC1A, MYOC/TIGR*). Adult POAG has been mapped to chromosomes 2qcen-q13 (*GLC1B*), 2p15-p16 (*GLC1H*), 3q21-q24 (*GLC1C*), 8q23 (*GLC1D*), 10p14 (*GLC1E, OPTN* [optineurin]). A mutation in the *OPTN* gene accounts for ~17% of POAG. Congenital glaucoma mapped to chromosome 2p21 (*GLC3A*) and chromosome 1p36 (*GLC3B*).

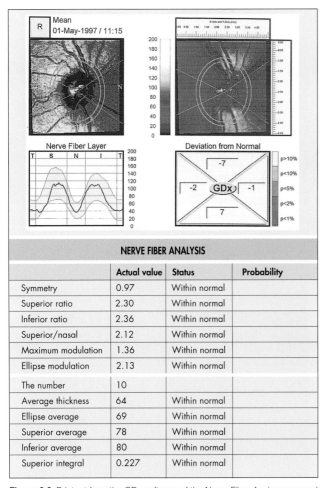

NERVE FIBER ANALYSIS			
	Actual value	Status	Probability
Symmetry	0.97	Within normal	
Superior ratio	2.30	Within normal	
Inferior ratio	2.36	Within normal	
Superior/nasal	2.12	Within normal	
Maximum modulation	1.36	Within normal	
Ellipse modulation	2.13	Within normal	
The number	10		
Average thickness	64	Within normal	
Ellipse average	69	Within normal	
Superior average	78	Within normal	
Inferior average	80	Within normal	
Superior integral	0.227	Within normal	

Figure 9.9 Printout from the GDx software of the Nerve Fiber Analyzer; normal eye. (From Chopin NT. Retinal nerve fiber layer analysis. In: Yanoff M, Duker JS, eds. *Ophthalmology*. London: Mosby; 1999.)

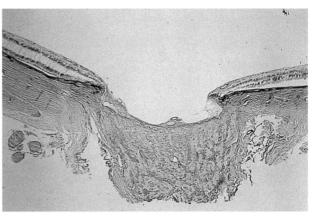

Figure 9.11 Primary open-angle glaucoma demonstrating cupping of the optic nerve head. (From Yanoff M, Fine BS. *Ocular Pathology*, 5th ed. St Louis: Mosby; 2002.)

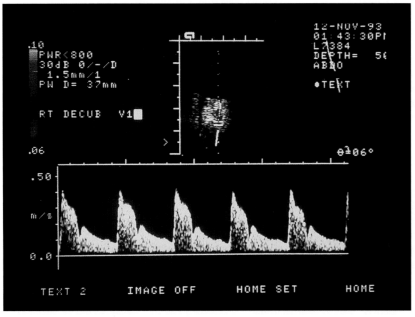

Figure 9.10 Color Doppler imaging of the ophthalmic artery. (From O'Brien C, Harris A. Optic nerve blood flow measurement. In: Yanoff M, Duker JS, eds. *Ophthalmology*. London: Mosby; 1999.)

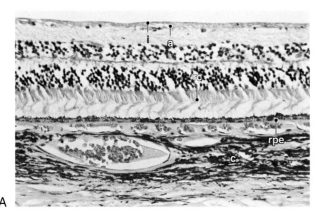
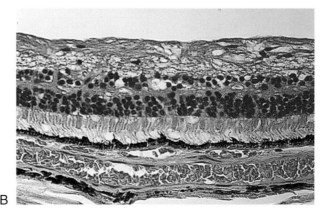

Figure 9.12 Primary open-angle glaucoma demonstrating atrophy of the inner retinal layers: (A) low power, (B) higher magnification. (From Yanoff M, Fine BS. *Ocular Pathology,* 5th ed. St Louis: Mosby; 2002.)

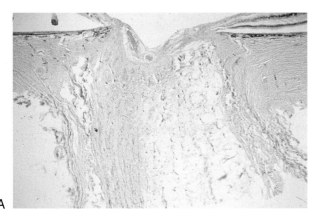
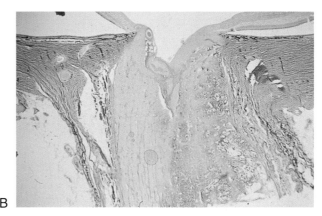

Figure 9.13 Schnabel cavernous optic atrophy demonstrating cystic spaces in optic nerve parenchyma. (A) Hematoxylin and eosin stain. (B) Colloidal iron stain. (From Yanoff M, Fine BS. *Ocular Pathology,* 5th ed. St Louis: Mosby; 2002.)

Risk factors: increased IOP, increased cup-to-disc (C/D) ratio, thinner central corneal thickness (less than approximately 550 μm), positive family history (6 × increase in first-degree relatives), age (increased in patients >60 years old; 15% of those >80 years old have glaucoma), race (3–6 × increase in African Americans vs. Caucasians; POAG also occurs earlier, is 6 × more likely to cause blindness, and is the leading cause of blindness in African Americans), low ocular perfusion pressure; other possible risk factors include diabetes mellitus (DM), myopia, hypertension, migraines; nocturnal hypotension and use of oral antihypertensive drugs are independent risk factors for glaucoma progression

Pathogenesis: unknown

Theories of ON damage:

> *Mechanical:* resistance to outflow, trabecular meshwork dysfunction, difference between IOP and cerebrospinal fluid (CSF) pressure
>
> *Vascular:* poor ON perfusion (low ocular perfusion pressure, nocturnal hypotension [mean arterial blood pressure 10 mm Hg lower than during daytime]); ischemia occurs with systemic hypotension; possible contribution of vasospasm; increased IOP reduces blood flow to ON

> *Fluctuation:* large diurnal fluctuations in IOP
>
> *Neurogenic:* other pathways leading to ganglion cell necrosis or apoptosis, such as excitotoxicity (glutamate), neurotrophin starvation, autoimmunity, abnormal glial-neuronal interactions (tumor necrosis factor [TNF]), defects in endogenous protective mechanisms (heat shock proteins)

Findings: increased IOP, large C/D ratio (especially vertical elongation of optic cup; notching of rim; asymmetry of C/D ratio), NFL loss (evaluate with red-free light), disc splinter hemorrhage (Drance hemorrhage; often followed by notching in region of hemorrhage), bayonetting of vessels at optic cup, characteristic VF defects; may have beta-zone peripapillary atrophy (atrophy of RPE and choriocapillaris between optic disc and alpha-zone)

> With ON damage, loss of yellow–blue color axis occurs first
> Combined sensitivity of tonometry and disc exam = 67%

Visual fields: sensitivity (percent of diseased properly identified) = 85%; specificity (% of normals properly identified) = 85%. Risk of initial field loss is 1%–2%/year for ocular hypertensive patients, risk of field loss increases with increasing IOP

Secondary Open-Angle Glaucoma

Mechanism/Etiology:

Clogging of TM: red blood cells (RBCs; hyphema, sickle cell, ghost cells), macrophages (hemolytic, phacolytic, melanocytic, melanomalytic), neoplastic cells (malignant tumors, neurofibromatosis, juvenile xanthogranuloma), pigment (pigmentary glaucoma, pseudoexfoliation, chronic uveitis, malignant melanoma), lens protein (lens-particle glaucoma), photoreceptor outer segments (Schwartz-Matsuo syndrome), zonular fragments (α-chymotrypsin induced), viscoelastic

Toxic/medication: steroid induced, siderosis, chalcosis

Inflammation: uveitis, uveitis–glaucoma–hyphema (UGH) syndrome, interstitial keratitis (IK)

Increased episcleral venous pressure: orbital mass, thyroid eye disease, arteriovenous fistulas, orbital varices, superior vena cava syndrome, Sturge-Weber syndrome, idiopathic

Trauma: angle recession, chemical injury, hemorrhage, postoperative

Hyphema

27% risk of glaucoma if hyphema >50% of AC volume; 52% risk with total hyphema

Surgical intervention for uncontrolled IOP, corneal blood staining, prolonged presence of large hyphema (>5–10 days), rebleed, 8-ball hyphema (see Chapter 10, Anterior Segment)

Sickle Cell

Sickled cells are rigid; therefore, even small hyphemas can obstruct TM and raise IOP; acetazolamide (Diamox) contraindicated (increases ascorbic acid in AC, causing greater sickling, also causes hemoconcentration and systemic acidosis, both of which favor sickling)

Ghost Cells

Weeks to months after vitreous hemorrhage, degenerated RBCs pass through hyaloid face. These khaki-colored, spherical cells are less pliable than RBCs and do not pass through TM; layer of cells forms a pseudohypopyon

Lytic Glaucomas

Macrophages laden with various materials

Hemolytic: hemosiderin-laden macrophages deposit in TM

Phacolytic: denatured lens proteins escape from hypermature or morgagnian cataract; with intact lens capsule; proteins and macrophages that have ingested lens material clog the outflow tract; appears as milky substance in AC; requires surgical removal of lens. Reduce the inflammation preoperatively with topical steroid, cycloplegic, and ocular hypotensive medications

Melanomalytic: melanin from malignant melanoma is engulfed by macrophages, which clog TM

Melanocytomalytic: melanin from necrotic melanocytoma

Tumor Cells

Deposition of tumor cells, inflammatory cells, and cellular debris; also macrophages laden with melanin from melanomas, direct infiltration of TM, or neovascularization with subsequent intraocular hemorrhage or neovascular glaucoma (NVG); 45% of anterior uveal melanomas and 15% of choroidal melanomas are associated with glaucoma. Retinoblastoma causes glaucoma in 25%–50% from NVG, pupillary block, or tumor material; also lymphoma

Pigmentary Glaucoma (PG) (Autosomal Dominant [AD])

Mapped to chromosome 7q35-q36 *(GLC1F)*

Typically young myopic males; up to 50% of patients with pigment dispersion syndrome (PDS) develop glaucoma

Mechanism: reverse pupillary block bows iris against zonules, and iris movement results in pigment liberation; pigment obstructs TM

Findings: halos and blurry vision with IOP spikes (pigment may be released with exercise); Krukenberg spindle (melanin phagocytized by corneal endothelium); heavy TM pigmentation; iridodonesis; iris transillumination defects (radial midperipheral spoke-like appearance); associated with lattice degeneration (20%) and retinal detachment (5%) (Fig. 9.14)

Treatment: miotics minimize iris-zonule touch; very good response to laser trabeculoplasty; laser peripheral iridotomy may help reduce posterior bowing of iris

Pseudoexfoliation Glaucoma (PXG)

Mapped to chromosome 15q24 *(LOXL1)*

High incidence (up to 50%) of secondary open-angle glaucoma in patients with pseudoexfoliation syndrome (PXS); more common among Scandinavians. Amyloid-like substance deposits in eye and clogs TM, also found in other organs (Fig. 9.15)

Findings: iridopathy (blood–aqueous barrier defect, pseudouveitis, iris rigidity, posterior synechiae, poor pupillary dilation), keratopathy (reduced endothelial cell count, endothelial decompensation, corneal endothelial proliferation over trabecular meshwork), Sampaolesi line (scalloped band of pigmentation anterior to Schwalbe line), weak zonules (phacodonesis, risk of lens dislocation during cataract surgery, and angle closure from anterior movement of lens), lens capsule (white fibrillar material)

Treatment: very good response to laser trabeculoplasty. PXS usually presents with higher initial IOP and is more difficult to control with medical treatment alone versus POAG

Lens-Particle Glaucoma

Lens material in setting of violated capsule blocks TM following trauma or cataract surgery. Greater inflammation than with phacolytic; PAS, posterior synechiae, and inflammatory membranes are common; IOP can be very high

Treatment: cycloplegics, steroids (careful, because steroids slow absorption of lens material), and ocular hypotensive medications

Schwartz-Matsuo Syndrome

High IOP associated with chronic rhegmatogenous retinal detachment (RD; usually shallow and anterior involving ora serrata or nonpigmented epithelium of CB). Photoreceptor outer segments migrate transvitreally into aqueous and block TM; outflow obstruction is also caused by pigment released from RPE and glycosaminoglycans released from photoreceptors. Usually resolves after repair of RD

Alpha-Chymotrypsin Induced

Zonular fragments accumulate in TM after intracapsular cataract extraction (ICCE) with enzymatic zonulysis. Alpha-chymotrypsin itself does not cause damage

Corticosteroid Induced

Risk factors include open-angle glaucoma, family history of glaucoma, increasing age, diabetes, and high myopia. Topical steroids have greater pressure-raising effects than do systemic steroids:

> In response to topical dexamethasone 0.1% qid for 6 weeks, 65% had IOP rise of <5 mm Hg, 30% had a rise of 5–14 mm Hg, and 5% had a rise of at least 15 mm Hg Fluorometholone, rimexolone (Vexol), and loteprednol (Lotemax, Eysuvis, Alrex) are less likely to increase IOP

Siderosis (Iron) or Chalcosis (Copper)

TM toxicity and scarring from intraocular foreign body

Uveitic

Inflammation of the ciliary body (cyclitis) often decreases aqueous production; however, aqueous outflow may also be acutely impaired by trabeculitis and inflammatory cells causing TM obstruction. Chronic inflammation may cause PAS

JIA-associated uveitis: glaucoma occurs in about 20% of cases

Glaucomatocyclitic crisis (Posner-Schlossman syndrome): episodic trabeculitis (mononuclear cells in TM) with high IOP for hours to weeks; minimal inflammatory signs; prolonged use of steroid is not recommended. Association with herpes virus

Fuchs heterochromic iridocyclitis: up to 60% develop high IOP (glaucoma occurs more commonly in patients with bilateral disease and spontaneous hyphema); may persist after resolution of uveitis; do not develop PAS. Association with rubella, herpes, and toxoplasmosis

Phacoantigenic uveitis (phacoanaphylactic endophthalmitis): type 3 hypersensitivity reaction to lens material following trauma or surgery, causing zonal granulomatous reaction after latent period

Uveitis–glaucoma–hyphema (UGH) syndrome: nongranulomatous inflammation; IOL physically irritates iris and ciliary body

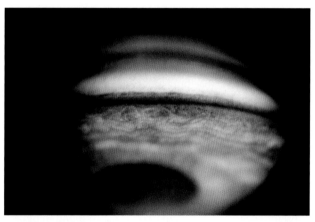

Figure 9.14 Gonioscopic view of pigmentary glaucoma. (From Ball SF. Pigmentary glaucoma. In: Yanoff M, Duker JS, eds. *Ophthalmology*. London: Mosby; 1999.)

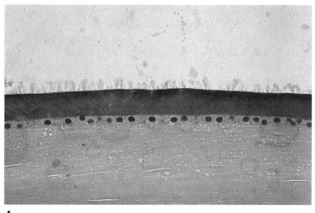

A

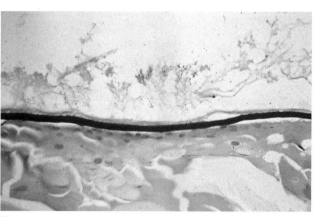

B

Figure 9.15 Pseudoexfoliative syndrome demonstrating exfoliative material on lens capsule. (From Samuelson TW, Shah G. Pseudoexfoliative glaucoma. In: Yanoff M, Duker JS, eds. *Ophthalmology*. London: Mosby; 1999.)

Traumatic

Angle recession: glaucoma develops in 10% of cases with >180° of involvement as a result of scarring of the angle and TM

Chemical burn: can damage trabecular meshwork or uveal circulation, or cause shrinkage of scleral collagen

After vitrectomy: most common complication is glaucoma; caused by intraocular gas, hyphema, ghost cells, uveitis, silicone oil

After corneal transplant: distortion of TM

Elevated Episcleral Venous Pressure

Causes resistance to aqueous outflow

Etiology: carotid-cavernous sinus fistula, cavernous sinus thrombosis, Sturge-Weber syndrome, neurofibromatosis, orbital mass (tumor, varices), thyroid eye disease (false elevation of IOP can be caused by inferior rectus [IR] fibrosis with increased resistance in upgaze), superior vena cava obstruction, mediastinal tumors and syndromes, scleral buckle, idiopathic. May see blood in Schlemm canal

Primary Angle-Closure Glaucoma

Definitions:
Primary angle-closure suspect (PACS): appositional contact of TM and iris considered possible from narrow angles on gonioscopy
Primary angle-closure (PAC): PACS with increased IOP and/or signs of intermittent TM obstruction (PAS, glaukomflecken, excessive TM pigment deposition) without glaucomatous optic neuropathy
Primary angle-closure glaucoma (PACG): PAC with glaucomatous optic neuropathy, classified as acute, subacute/intermittent, or chronic

Mechanism: peripheral iris obstructing TM
Pupillary block (most common): iridolenticular touch causes resistance of aqueous flow from posterior to anterior chamber, causing increased posterior pressure. When the pupil is mid-dilated (i.e., stress, low ambient light levels, sympathomimetic or anticholinergic medications), the elevated posterior chamber pressure causes peripheral iris tissue to bow anteriorly and occlude the TM 360°
Lens-induced iridotrabecular contact: lens size relatively too large for size of globe causes iridocorneal angle narrowing and intermittent/chronic iridotrabecular contact; chronic microtrauma produces PAS and/or decreased aqueous outflow as a result of TM dysfunction, resulting in increased IOP
Plateau iris syndrome: form of primary angle closure without pupillary block (see below)

Epidemiology: acute form is most common in Eskimos and Asians, followed by Caucasians, then African Americans;

highest risk is between 55–65 years old; more common in women (2–4 ×) only among Caucasians. Chronic form is more common in African Americans than Asians, who have a higher risk than Caucasians. 5% of population >60 years of age have occludable angles, 0.5% of these individuals develop angle closure; usually bilateral (75% risk in untreated fellow eye within 5 years)

Genetics: hereditary component, gene associations mapped to chromosomes 1p21 *(COL11A1)*, 3q27 *(ABCC5)*, 7 *(EPDR1)*, 8q11.23 *(PCMTD1-ST18)*, 9 *(DPM2-FAM102A)*, 9p24.2 *(GLIS3)*, 10 *(CHAT)*, 11p15.1 *(PLEKHA7)*, 14q22.1 *(FERMT2)*, 17 *(COL1A1)*, 21 *(COL18A1)*

Anatomic features predisposing to angle closure: small anterior segment (hyperopia, nanophthalmos, microcornea, microphthalmos); hereditary narrow angle; anterior iris insertion (Eskimos, Asians, and African Americans); shallow AC (AC diameter <2.5 mm and especially <2.1 mm; large lens, plateau iris configuration, loose or dislocated lens); short axial length (AL)

Acute Angle Closure

Symptoms: blurred vision, colored halos around lights, pain, redness, nausea and vomiting, headache

Findings: high IOP (40–80 mm Hg), corneal epithelial edema, conjunctival injection, mid-dilated sluggish pupil, shallow anterior chamber, mild AC cell and flare, closed angle (perform indentation gonioscopy to differentiate between appositional and synechial angle closure; glycerin can be used to clear corneal edema; evaluate angle in other eye), may have ON head swelling and hyperemia; with rapid rise in IOP, may see arterial pulsations (retinal ischemia can occur)

Sequelae of ischemia: segmental iris atrophy (focal iris stroma necrosis), dilated irregular pupil (sphincter and dilator necrosis), glaukomflecken (focal anterior lens opacities resulting from epithelial necrosis), retinal vascular occlusion, anterior ischemic optic neuropathy, optic atrophy

Late findings: decreased vision, PAS, chronic corneal edema

Provocative tests: prone test, darkroom test, prone darkroom test, pharmacologic pupillary dilation; positive if IOP rises >8 mm Hg

Thymoxamine test: α-adrenergic antagonist used to distinguish angle closure from glaucoma with narrow angles; thymoxamine blocks iris dilator muscle producing miosis; however, it does not affect trabecular meshwork and normally does not decrease IOP; therefore, decrease in IOP suggests miosis has removed iris from the outflow channel reversing angle closure

Treatment of acute angle-closure glaucoma: peripheral iridotomy or iridectomy (PI; definitive treatment); compression gonioscopy (may force aqueous through block and open angle); pilocarpine (may not be effective at IOP

>40 mm Hg because of sphincter ischemia; may also cause lens–iris diaphragm to move forward, worsening pupillary block); reduce IOP with β-blocker, α_2-agonist, topical or oral carbonic anhydrase inhibitor (CAI), or hyperosmotic agent (isosorbide, glycerin [contraindicated in diabetics], or intravenous [IV] mannitol [risk of cardiovascular adverse effects]); topical steroids for inflammation; laser PI in fellow eye (75% chance of attack in untreated fellow eye; pilocarpine lowers risk to 40% but may lead to chronic angle closure)

If attack of angle closure is broken medically, consider waiting a few days before performing laser PI because corneal edema, iridocorneal touch, and iris congestion make the procedure more difficult

Persistently increased IOP following laser PI may be a result of PAS, incomplete iridotomy, underlying open-angle glaucoma, or secondary angle closure

Consider cataract extraction; goniosynechiolysis for PAS

Subacute/Intermittent Angle Closure

Ratio of nonacute to acute presentations is 2:1; may be asymptomatic or have similar presentation as acute angle closure but less severe and occurs over days to weeks; often complain of headaches, episodes resolve spontaneously, especially by entering a well-lit area (induces miosis); IOP may be normal; glaukomflecken, PAS, and increased TM pigment deposition are evidence of previous attack. Treat with laser PI

Chronic Angle Closure

Gradual closure of angle by apposition or development of PAS leads to slow rise in IOP; variable IOP, but less than with acute angle closure. Often asymptomatic; cornea usually clear because of gradual rise in IOP, but can have extensive VF loss

Plateau Iris

Configuration: angle anatomy resulting in deep central AC and shallow peripheral AC

Syndrome: angle closure in an eye with plateau iris configuration; usually occurs in 4th–5th decades of life and in individuals with less hyperopia than typical angle-closure patient

Findings: may present with acute or chronic angle closure; anteriorly positioned ciliary processes force the peripheral iris more anteriorly than normal; deep chamber centrally; flat iris contour with sharp drop-off peripherally; with dilation, peripheral iris folds into the angle and occludes TM; with compression gonioscopy, angle is more difficult to open and does not open as widely as in primary angle closure

Treatment: laser peripheral iridotomy, laser iridoplasty, and miotics; plateau iris appearance remains

Secondary Angle-Closure Glaucoma

Mechanism/Etiology

With pupillary block: lens induced (phacomorphic [lens enlargement in elderly; urgent surgery needed to remove lens], dislocated lens, microspherophakia), seclusio pupillae, nanophthalmos, aphakic and pseudophakic pupillary block, silicone oil (prevent by performing an inferior PI because oil is lighter than water)

Without pupillary block:

Posterior "pushing" mechanism (mechanical/anterior displacement of lens–iris diaphragm; often from anterior rotation of ciliary body): inflammation (scleritis, uveitis, after scleral buckle or panretinal photocoagulation [PRP]), congestion (postscleral buckling, nanophthalmos), choroidal effusion (hypotony; uveal effusion, medication [topiramate, sulfonamides]), suprachoroidal hemorrhage, aqueous misdirection (malignant glaucoma), pressure from posterior segment (tumor, expanding gas, exudative RD), contraction of retrolental tissue (persistent hyperplastic primary vitreous [PHPV], retinopathy of prematurity [ROP])

Anterior "pulling" mechanism (adherence of iris to TM /membranes over TM): epithelial (epithelial downgrowth, fibrous ingrowth), endothelial (ICE syndrome, posterior polymorphous corneal dystrophy [PPCD]), PAS, adhesion from trauma, mesodermal dysgenesis syndromes, neovascular (NVG)

Mnemonic (etiology of NVG): **R(3)UBEITIC** (**R**etinopathy, **R**etinal vein occlusion [central retinal vein occlusion (CRVO)], **R**etinal detachment, **U**veitis, **B**ranch retinal vein occlusion [BRVO], **E**ales disease, ocular **I**schemic syndrome, **T**rauma, **I**ntraocular tumor, **C**arotid cavernous fistula)

Associated With RD Surgery

Anterior rotation of CB around the scleral spur secondary to swelling from excessive PRP or tight scleral buckle

Treatment: cycloplegics, PI, consider cutting encircling band

Nanophthalmos

>10 D hyperopia; small eye (<20 mm) with small cornea (mean diameter = 10.5 mm), shallow AC, narrow angle, and high lens/eye volume. Pupillary block or uveal effusion produces angle-closure glaucoma. Thick sclera (~2 × thicker than normal) may impede vortex venous drainage, as well as decrease uveoscleral outflow, and can also result in spontaneous uveal effusion with anterior rotation of CB leading to angle closure

Treatment: weak miotics, cycloplegics (if no angle crowding), laser PI, laser iridoplasty, trabeculectomy after prophylactic sclerotomy. Because there is a high complication rate with surgery (uveal effusion), first use medical therapy, then laser

Increased risk of complications with cataract surgery (RD, choroidal effusion, angle-closure glaucoma, flat AC, cystoid macular edema [CME], corneal decompensation, malignant glaucoma, IOL miscalculations). If shallow AC and thickened choroid preoperatively, perform prophylactic anterior sclerotomies with surgery

Malignant Glaucoma (Aqueous Misdirection Syndrome, Ciliolenticular or Ciliovitreal Block)

Mechanism: tips of ciliary processes rotate forward against lens (ciliolenticular block), causing anterior displacement of lens–iris diaphragm

Risk factors: uveitis, angle closure, nanophthalmos, hyperopia; occurs postoperatively (usually 5 days) following a variety of laser or incisional surgeries; usually in patients with PAS or chronic angle closure following intraocular surgery if the hyaloid face has not been broken (follows 2% of surgical cases for angle closure); can also occur in unoperated eye when mydriatics are stopped or miotics are added

Findings: entire AC shallow (vs. angle closure in which the AC is deeper centrally than peripherally), IOP higher than expected, presence of patent iridectomy, absence of suprachoroidal fluid or blood

DDx: pupillary block (no patent iridectomy; moderate depth of central AC), suprachoroidal hemorrhage (acute severe pain and choroidal elevation), choroidal effusion (usually low IOP and choroidal elevation), annular peripheral choroidal detachment

Treatment: 50% resolve within 5 days with medical therapy alone
   Medical: cycloplegic (relaxes ciliary muscle and pulls lens–iris diaphragm posteriorly; continued indefinitely to prevent recurrence), aqueous suppressants, peripheral iridotomy in both eyes (eliminate any component of pupillary block); miotics are contraindicated
   Surgical: argon laser photocoagulation of ciliary processes (requires shrinkage of at least 2–4 ciliary processes), Nd:YAG laser rupture of hyaloid face (for pseudophakic and aphakic patients; 4–6 mJ; best to perform peripherally [through PI]), combined iridectomy/zonulectomy/hyaloidectomy/vitrectomy often curative (for phakic patients)

Intraocular Tumors

Can push angle closed from posteriorly

Malignant melanoma of the anterior uveal tract can cause glaucoma by direct extension of tumor into TM, inducing neovascularization of the angle, obstructing TM with melanin-laden macrophages (melanomalytic), or seeding of tumor cells in outflow channels; other mechanisms include pigment dispersion, inflammation, and hemorrhage

PHPV

Contraction of retrolenticular membrane and swelling of cataract can cause angle closure

Treatment: remove lens and membrane via limbal approach (pars plana approach may be dangerous in that retina can extend up to the pars plicata)

Retinopathy of Prematurity (ROP)

Caused by contraction of retrolental tissue

Epithelial Downgrowth

Caused by epithelium growing over angle

Fibrous Ingrowth

Caused by fibrous proliferation through wound into AC

ICE Syndrome

Caused by descemetization of TM and angle closure from contraction of endothelial membrane; PAS are prominent but less responsible for glaucoma

Posterior Polymorphous Corneal Dystrophy (PPCD)

Caused by abnormal corneal endothelial cells that migrate into angle, causing glaucoma (15%)

Neovascular Glaucoma (NVG)

Caused by widespread retinal or ocular ischemia; clinically transparent fibrovascular membrane flattens anterior iris surface; myofibroblasts provide motive force for angle closure and ectropion uveae

Etiology: proliferative retinopathy (diabetes [33% of all forms of NVG], ischemic CRVO [33%], carotid occlusive disease [13%], ciliary artery occlusion, sickle cell, Norrie disease, ROP); intraocular inflammation (uveitis, postoperative); neoplasms (retinoblastoma [50% develop NVG], malignant melanoma, large cell lymphoma [reticulum cell sarcoma], metastatic); chronic retinal detachment

Treatment: aqueous suppressants and hyperosmotics; increase uveoscleral outflow (atropine; avoid miotics); panretinal photocoagulation; peripheral retinal cryotherapy (if poor visualization of retina; 50% develop phthisis with cyclocryotherapy); glaucoma drainage implant (70% success rate)

Normal-Tension Glaucoma (NTG)

Glaucoma with open angles and IOP <22 mm Hg

Proposed mechanisms:
   Nocturnal systemic hypotension: diurnal curve of blood pressure (BP) similar to IOP. 66% of patients will have a BP drop of greater than 10% during early-morning hours ("dippers"); patients with hypertension (HTN) have an even greater swing in BP (26% average drop); patients with HTN treated with β-blockers can have diastolic BP <50 mm Hg, which may compromise blood supply to ON

Autoimmune: increased incidence of proteinemia and autoantibodies in patients with NTG

Vasospasm

Previous hemodynamic crisis: excessive blood loss or shock

Findings: VF defects in NTG have steeper slopes, greater depths, and closer proximity to fixation than in POAG; splinter hemorrhages are more common

DDx: POAG with large diurnal variation, "burned-out" secondary open-angle glaucoma, chronic angle closure. Must rule out intracranial processes and other causes of optic neuropathy

Cupping can occur with neurologic disease: anterior ischemic optic neuropathy (AION; arteritic 50%; nonarteritic 10%), chiasmal compressive lesions (5%), optic neuritis (<5%), hereditary optic neuropathies, methanol toxicity. These entities are more likely to have early loss of central vision and color vision; pallor may be worse than cupping

Diagnosis: diurnal curve, neurologic workup (complete blood count [CBC], erythrocyte sedimentation rate [ESR], antinuclear antibody [ANA], Venereal Disease Research Laboratory [VDRL] and fluorescent treponemal antibody absorption [FTA-ABS], carotid evaluation, brain neuroimaging)

Prognosis: more difficult to treat than POAG

TREATMENT

Generally, medications are tried first, followed by laser treatment and then surgery; however, the choice and timing of various treatment modalities are dependent on the type of glaucoma, severity of ON damage, level of control, and many other factors. Therapy must also be directed to any preexisting or underlying process

Medication

Ocular hypotensive agents (see Chapter 2, Pharmacology)

Laser

Argon Laser Trabeculoplasty (ALT) (Fig. 9.16)

Power 400–1200 mW; spot size 50 μm; duration 0.1 s; titrate power to generate small bubble at junction of nonpigmented and pigmented TM; 50 applications/180°; average of 30% reduction in IOP; can be repeated

Iopidine immediately postoperatively to avoid pressure spike, and treat with steroids for 1 week. Assess efficacy of treatment at 6 weeks postoperatively

Anterior burns have poor effect; posterior burns more likely to develop PAS

Results: 25% fail to control IOP at 1 year; 10% per year failure rate thereafter. Repeating ALT may provide IOP control in 33%–50%, but sustained elevation in 10%

Best predictor of success is type of glaucoma: PXG (best) > PG > POAG > NTG > aphakic (worst)

The greater the amount of pigment in the angle, the better the result; poorer response in patients <50 years of age. ALT is ineffective (and may worsen IOP) in inflammatory glaucoma, angle recession, angle-closure glaucoma (membranes in angles), congenital glaucoma, and steroid-induced glaucoma. Contraindicated in patients with large amounts of PAS

Complications: IOP spike (increases with energy and number of laser burns), iritis, PAS

Selective Laser Trabeculoplasty (SLT)

Time and spot size (400 μm) are fixed, power 0.6–0.9 mJ; 50 confluent applications/180°, straddling TM

Produces less tissue destruction than ALT and is repeatable. Beware IOP spikes in patients with pigment dispersion syndrome and pigmentary glaucoma

Laser Iridotomy

Perform in eyes with narrow angles (prophylactically), iris bombe, synechial angle closure, pigmentary glaucoma (as a result of configuration of iris), plateau iris, and malignant glaucoma

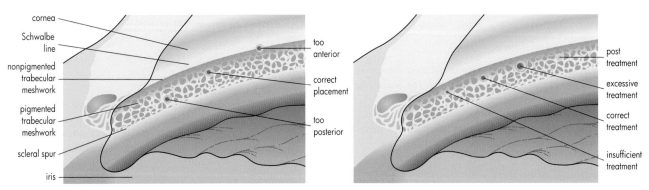

Figure 9.16 Argon laser trabeculoplasty. (From Schwartz AL. Argon laser trabeculoplasty in glaucoma: what's happening (survey results of American Glaucoma Society Members). *J Glaucoma.* 1993;2:329–336.)

Nd:YAG: power 1–12 mJ; bleed more, but close less than with argon

Argon: reaction is pigment related and requires more energy and total applications than with YAG; less bleeding because of thermal effect; extensive tissue destruction at margins of treatment; iritis more pronounced

Iridoplasty

For narrow angles; aim at peripheral iris; stretch iris away from angle; power 200–400 mW; spot size 500 μm; duration 0.5–1.0 s

Surgery

Trabeculectomy

Consider use of antimetabolite in patients at risk for bleb failure

Risk factors for bleb failure: previous surgical failure, darker skin pigmentation, history of keloid formation, neovascular changes, younger age, intraocular inflammation, scarred conjunctiva, high hyperopia, inability to use corticosteroids, shallow AC

Antimetabolites:
  Mitomycin C (MMC): antineoplastic antibiotic (isolated from *Streptomyces caespitosus*)
    MECHANISM: intercalates with DNA and prevents replication; suppresses fibrosis and vascular ingrowth after exposure to the filtration site. Toxic to fibroblasts in all stages of cell cycle; 100 × more potent than fluorouracil (5-FU)
    TOXICITY: intraocular causes corneal decompensation (damages endothelium), AC inflammation, and necrosis of CB and iris; can develop scleral necrosis; retinal toxicity with intravitreal injection
  5-FU: specifically affects the S-phase of the cell cycle; requires postoperative injections (30–35 mg in 5 mg doses over 1–3 weeks); corneal epithelial toxicity may occur

Complications: block ostium during surgery in hyperopia, nanophthalmos, or chronic angle closure, the ciliary processes can roll anteriorly

Treatment: suture wound and reinflate eye, allowing ciliary processes to revert to normal position; if still present, use cautery to remove the processes
  High IOP immediately postoperatively: attempt digital massage or laser suture lysis
  Shallow or flat AC: (Table 9.2)
  Blebitis: photophobia, discharge, marked conjunctival injection around an opalescent filtering bleb; often Seidel-positive, moderate AC cells and flare, but no involvement of the vitreous. Organism usually *Staphylococcus*
    TREATMENT: intensive topical antibiotics, repair wound leak, observe daily for endophthalmitis

Bleb-associated endophthalmitis: pain, decreased vision, AC cells and flare, hypopyon, and vitreous cells; often Seidel-positive. Organism usually *Streptococcus* species or *Haemophilus influenzae*
  TREATMENT: emergent, as for endophthalmitis
Suprachoroidal hemorrhage: usually occurs several days after trabeculectomy surgery with acute pain, often while straining; also, nausea, vomiting, and decreased vision
  MECHANISM: progressive serous choroidal detachment, stretching the long posterior ciliary artery until it ruptures
  RISK FACTORS: aphakia, hypertension, cardiovascular disease, and increased age
Hypotony: generally seen in young myopic patients, especially with antimetabolites
  DDX: wound leak, overfiltration, iridocyclitis, cyclodialysis, ciliochoroidal effusion, RD
  TREATMENT: wound revision
  COMPLICATIONS: corneal edema, cataract, choroidal effusion, optic disc edema, chorioretinal folds, maculopathy
Exuberant bleb: bleb can enlarge, spread onto cornea, and interfere with vision as a result of astigmatism, dellen, or encroachment into visual axis

TABLE 9.2 Treatment of shallow or flat anterior chamber following trabeculectomy

Bleb height	Intraocular pressure	Definitive diagnosis	Treatment
Elevated	Low	Excessive filtration	Bleb revision
Flat	Low	Choroidal detachment	Cycloplegic, steroid, drainage
		Bleb leak	Antibiotic, aqueous suppressants, stop steroid, anterior chamber reformation, pressure patch, Simmons scleral compression shell, large-diameter soft contact lens, trichloroacetic acid, glue, laser, or autologous blood injection Consider surgical intervention (drainage of choroidals and repair of wound) for impending failure of bleb, flat anterior chamber with corneal decompensation, kissing choroidals, progressive cataract
Flat	Elevated	Suprachoroidal hemorrhage	Drainage
		Pupillary block	Cycloplegic, steroid, peripheral iridotomy (PI)
		Malignant glaucoma	Cycloplegic, aqueous suppressants, PI, Nd:YAG anterior vitreolysis or vitrectomy
Elevated	Elevated	Encapsulated bleb	Needling, aqueous suppressants, bleb revision

Nd:YAG, Neodymium:yttrium aluminium garnet.

TREATMENT: recess or amputate bleb; usually a cleavage plane is present

Drainage Implants (Setons/Tubes)

Seton is from Latin *seta* or "bristle" (original surgery used horse hair)

Types:
  Nonvalve: Molteno (single or double plate), Schocket, Baerveldt; must temporarily occlude tube lumen with suture or biodegradable collagen plug
  Valve: Ahmed (one-way valve maintains IOP at 8 mm Hg or higher), Krupin, and Baerveldt (pressure-sensitive valve)
  Anterior chamber glaucoma drainage implant: for patients with scleral buckles who do not have adequate scleral surface for placement of a seton; a silicone implant shunts fluid from AC or posterior chamber to the fibrous capsule surrounding the episcleral encircling element

Nonpenetrating Filtration Surgery

Minimally invasive glaucoma surgery (MIGS): less invasive alternatives

Ab externo: Ex-Press minishunt, XEN gel, canaloplasty, viscocanalostomy

Ab interno: microstents (iStent, CyPass, XEN gel, Hydrus, DeepLight Gold micro-shunt, Preserflo), goniotomies (trabectome, Kahook dual blade), canaloplasty (Omni System)

Goniosynechialysis

Direct lysis of PAS with cyclodialysis spatula or other microinstrument; consider for angle-closure glaucoma of less than 12 months' duration

Cyclophotocoagulation

Laser treatment of ciliary body with argon (transpupillary or endoprobe), Nd:YAG (contact or noncontact), or diode (contact); useful in many types of refractory glaucomas, including aphakic, neovascular, and inflammatory, and in eyes with failed filtering blebs

Mechanism: reduced aqueous production by destruction of ciliary epithelium

Procedure is painful; therefore, requires peribulbar or retrobulbar block

Cyclocryotherapy

First treatment: 2.5 mm cryo tip, with anterior edge 1 mm from inferior limbus and 1.5 mm from superior limbus. Provide 6 freezes on the clock hours of the inferior 180°. Maintain each freeze for 60 seconds at −80°C. The ice ball will encroach upon cornea for ~0.5 mm. Wait 1 month for the IOP to reach new baseline

Second treatment: if first treatment does not lower IOP sufficiently, treat superior temporal quadrant with

2–4 freezes. Always leave at least 1 quadrant (usually superonasal) free to prevent hypotony. Give subconjunctival steroid postoperatively

Procedure is painful; therefore, requires peribulbar or retrobulbar block

Surgical Iridectomy

Perform through 3-mm clear corneal wound for angle-closure glaucoma

Indications: if severe corneal edema precludes adequate iris visualization, AC is extremely shallow, or patient is unable to cooperate for laser iridotomy

MAJOR GLAUCOMA CLINICAL STUDIES

Advanced Glaucoma Intervention Study (AGIS)

Objective: To evaluate argon laser trabeculoplasty (ALT) versus trabeculectomy as the initial surgery in patients with advanced open-angle glaucoma not controlled by medical treatment

Main outcome variable was visual function (field and acuity)

Results

7-year data

In African Americans, the best results were obtained when ALT was performed 1st, followed by trabeculectomy (ATT sequence)

In Caucasians, the best results occurred when trabeculectomy was performed 1st, followed by ALT, and finally by a 2nd trabeculectomy (TAT sequence)

Visual field defects were more severe in African American patients

Eyes with IOP <18 mm Hg at all visits had almost no progression of VF loss

Trabeculectomy increased relative risk of cataract by 78% (47% if no complications occurred vs. 104% if complications occurred, especially severe inflammation and flat AC)

Conclusions

In patients with advanced POAG, ALT should be considered as the first surgical treatment in African American patients; trabeculectomy should be considered first in Caucasians

Risk factors for ALT failure are younger age and higher IOP

Risk factors for trabeculectomy failure are younger age, higher IOP, diabetes, and postoperative complications (particularly elevated IOP and marked inflammation)

Risk factors for bleb encapsulation include male sex and previous ALT (but this was not statistically significant)

Low IOP reduces VF deterioration

IOP fluctuation is independent risk factor for progression in eyes with lower baseline IOP

For VF progression, repeat 6-month VF test confirmed defect in 72%, and 2nd confirmatory VF test verified defect in 84%

Trabeculectomy is associated with an increased risk of cataract formation

Ocular Hypertension Treatment Study (OHTS)

Objective: To evaluate the effect of topical medication in delaying or preventing POAG in patients with ocular hypertension (IOP between 24–32 mm Hg in one eye and between 21–32 mm Hg in the fellow eye; normal VFs and ONs)

The goal in the treatment group was to reduce the IOP by at least 20% from baseline and obtain a target pressure of ≤24 mm Hg

The primary outcome variable was VF loss or ON damage

Results

Mean IOP reduction in the medicine group was 22.5% versus 4.0% in the observation group

At 5 years, the cumulative risk of developing POAG was 4.4% in the medicine group versus 9.5% in the observation group

Conclusions:

Topical ocular hypotensive medication is effective in delaying or preventing POAG in eyes with ocular hypertension

Predictive factors (and relative risk) for developing POAG include higher baseline IOP (10% increase per 1 mm Hg increase), older age (22% increase per decade), larger vertical and horizontal C/D ratios (32% and 27% increase per 0.1 increase, respectively), higher pattern standard deviation on VF test (22% increase per 0.2 dB increase), and thinner central corneal thickness (CCT ≤555 μm; 81% increase per 40 μm decrease)

Collaborative Initial Glaucoma Treatment Study (CIGTS)

Objective: To evaluate medicine (stepped regimen) versus trabeculectomy (with or without 5-FU) for the treatment of newly diagnosed open-angle glaucoma (primary, pigmentary, or pseudoexfoliative)

The primary outcome variable was progression of VF loss

Secondary outcomes were quality of life, visual acuity, and intraocular pressure

Results

5-year data

VF loss was not significantly different with either treatment

Surgery had an initially increased risk of significant visual loss, but by 4 years, the average visual acuity was equal in the 2 groups; patients with worse baseline VF were less likely to progress with surgery; patients with diabetes were more likely to progress with surgery

IOP averaged 17–18 mm Hg (~38% reduction) in the medicine group versus 14–15 mm Hg (~46% reduction) in the surgery group; IOP fluctuation was risk factor for progression in medicine group but not surgery group

Quality of life was similar in both groups

The rate of visually significant cataract was greater in the surgery group

Conclusions

Initial treatment of open-angle glaucoma with medicine or surgery results in similar VF outcome

Although visual acuity loss was initially greater in the surgery group, the differences converged with time

Early Manifest Glaucoma Trial (EMGT)

Objective: to evaluate the effectiveness of reducing IOP (vs. no treatment) on the progression of newly diagnosed open-angle glaucoma

The treatment group received ALT plus topical betaxolol

The primary outcome measures were progression of VF loss and optic disc changes

A secondary aim was to assess risk factors for progression

Results

6-year data

53% of patients progressed

Treatment reduced the IOP on average 5.1 mm Hg (25%)

Progression was less common in the treatment group (45% vs. 62%) and occurred later

Each 1 mm Hg of IOP lowering from baseline to the first follow-up visit (3 months) reduced the risk of progression by 10%

Increased nuclear lens opacity occurred with treatment

Conclusions

Treatment of early glaucoma halves the risk of progression

Risk factors for progression included higher baseline IOP, pseudoexfoliation syndrome, bilateral disease, older age, worse mean deviation on VF test, and frequent disc hemorrhages

Glaucoma Laser Trial (GLT)

Objective: To evaluate the efficacy and safety of starting treatment for POAG with ALT versus topical medication (Timoptic 0.5% bid)

Results

Eyes treated initially with ALT had lower IOP and better VF and ON status than fellow eyes treated initially with topical medication

Conclusions

Initial treatment of POAG with ALT is at least as efficacious as initial treatment with Timoptic

Collaborative Normal Tension Glaucoma Study (CNTGS)

Objective: To evaluate whether IOP is a causative factor in NTG

The goal in the treatment group was to reduce the IOP by 30% with medication, laser, and/or surgery

Results

Lowering IOP by 30% or more reduced the rate of VF loss in NTG. However, the rate of progression without treatment is variable and usually slow—half of untreated patients showed no progression in 5 years

Factors that increase the rate of progression include female gender, migraine headaches, and presence of disc hemorrhage

Conclusions

IOP is a factor in the pathogenesis of NTG, and lowering the IOP by 30% is beneficial

REVIEW QUESTIONS *(Answers start on page 424)*

1. What is the most appropriate initial treatment of pupillary block in a patient with microspherophakia?
   a. acetazolamide
   b. laser iridotomy
   c. pilocarpine
   d. cyclopentolate

2. Which of the following statements is true?
   a. uveoscleral outflow is inversely proportional to intraocular pressure
   b. uveoscleral outflow is measured clinically by fluorophotometry
   c. uveoscleral outflow is increased by atropine
   d. uveoscleral outflow is responsible for about 10% of total outflow

3. Risk factors for angle-closure glaucoma include all of the following, *except*
   a. pseudoexfoliation
   b. myopia
   c. Eskimo ancestry
   d. nanophthalmos

4. Which of the following would cause the greatest elevation in IOP?
   a. blinking
   b. decreased blood cortisol levels
   c. change from supine to sitting position
   d. darkening the room

5. The most likely cause of a large filtering bleb and a shallow chamber is
   a. aqueous misdirection
   b. bleb leak
   c. pupillary block
   d. overfiltration

6. A change in Goldmann VF stimulus from I4e to II4e is equivalent to
   a. 1 log
   b. 2 log
   c. 3 log
   d. 4 log

7. An Amsler grid held at 33 cm measures approximately how many degrees of central vision?
   a. 5
   b. 10
   c. 20
   d. 30

8. The most decreased sensitivity in an arcuate scotoma occurs in which quadrant?
   a. inferotemporal
   b. superonasal
   c. superotemporal
   d. inferonasal

9. The best gonioscopy lens for distinguishing appositional from synechial angle closure is
   a. Goldmann three-mirror
   b. Zeiss
   c. Koeppe
   d. Goldmann one-mirror

10. Which is *not* a risk factor for POAG?
    a. myopia
    b. central retinal vein occlusion
    c. diabetes
    d. central retinal artery occlusion

11. ALT would be most effective in a patient with which type of glaucoma?
    a. congenital
    b. inflammatory
    c. pigmentary
    d. aphakic

12. In which direction should a patient look to aid the examiner's view of the angle during Zeiss gonioscopy?
    a. up
    b. toward the mirror
    c. away from the mirror
    d. down

13. The best parameter for determining the unreliability of a Humphrey VF is
    a. fixation losses
    b. false positives
    c. false negatives
    d. fluctuation

14. Which of the following does *not* cause angle-closure glaucoma?
    a. ICE syndrome
    b. PHPV
    c. RD
    d. choroidal effusion

15. Which of the following is *least* likely to cause increased IOP 2 days postoperatively?
    a. retained viscoelastic
    b. red blood cells
    c. macrophages
    d. steroid drops

16. Treatment of malignant glaucoma may include all of the following, *except*
    a. laser iridotomy
    b. pilocarpine
    c. atropine
    d. vitrectomy

17. The most common organism associated with bleb-related endophthalmitis is
    a. *Streptococcus* species
    b. *S. epidermidis*
    c. *H. influenzae*
    d. gram-negative organisms

18. Which VF defect is *least* characteristic of glaucoma?
    a. paracentral scotoma
    b. nasal defect
    c. central scotoma
    d. enlarged blind spot

19. The type of tonometer most greatly affected by scleral rigidity is
    a. Goldmann
    b. tonopen
    c. Schiøtz
    d. pneumotonometer

20. As compared with plasma, aqueous has a higher concentration of
    a. calcium
    b. protein
    c. ascorbate
    d. sodium

21. The rate of aqueous production per minute is approximately
    a. 0.26 μL
    b. 2.6 μL
    c. 26 μL
    d. 260 μL

22. Which location has the greatest resistance to aqueous outflow?
    a. corneoscleral meshwork
    b. uveal meshwork
    c. juxtacanalicular connective tissue
    d. Schlemm canal

23. The facility of aqueous outflow is best measured by
    a. tonography
    b. manometry
    c. tonometry
    d. fluorophotometry

24. A patient recently had an acute angle-closure attack in the right eye. What is the most appropriate treatment for her left eye?
    a. synechiolysis
    b. laser peripheral iridotomy
    c. laser iridoplasty
    d. pilocarpine

25. The most likely gonioscopic finding in a patient with glaucoma and radial midperipheral spokelike iris transillumination defects is
    a. concave peripheral iris
    b. anterior iris insertion
    c. peripheral anterior synechiae
    d. plateau iris configuration

26. A 60-year-old myope with early cataracts and enlarged C/D ratios of 0.6 OU is found to have an abnormal Humphrey VF test OS. He has no other risk factors for glaucoma. What is the most appropriate next step for this patient?
    a. repeat VF testing
    b. obtain diurnal curve (serial tonometry)
    c. start monocular trial of latanoprost
    d. perform laser trabeculoplasty

27. Bilateral scattered PAS in an elderly hyperope with no past ocular history is most likely a result of
    a. ICE syndrome
    b. uveitis
    c. chronic angle-closure glaucoma
    d. Axenfeld anomaly

28. According to the CIGTS 5-year results, initial treatment of POAG with which two methods had similar VF outcomes?
    a. medicine or laser trabeculoplasty
    b. medicine or trabeculectomy
    c. laser trabeculoplasty or trabeculectomy
    d. trabeculectomy or drainage implant

29. Which of the following medications should *not* be used to treat a patient with herpes simplex virus keratouveitis and elevated IOP?
    a. pilocarpine
    b. timolol
    c. brimonidine
    d. dorzolamide

30. A patient undergoes multiple subconjunctival injections of 5-FU after glaucoma filtration surgery. The most common reason for discontinuing these injections is if the patient develops toxicity of which tissue?
    a. lens
    b. sclera
    c. cornea
    d. conjunctiva

31. A patient with retinoblastoma develops glaucoma. The most likely mechanism is
    a. secondary angle closure
    b. uveitic
    c. neovascular
    d. tumor cell

32. Glaucoma resulting from elevated episcleral venous pressure occurs in all of the following, *except*
    a. carotid-cavernous fistula
    b. hyphema
    c. Sturge-Weber syndrome
    d. thyroid eye disease

33. The earliest color deficit in glaucoma is the loss of the
    a. yellow–green axis
    b. red–green axis
    c. red–blue axis
    d. blue–yellow axis

34. Blood in the Schlemm canal is *not* associated with
    a. Fuchs heterochromic iridocyclitis
    b. thyroid eye disease
    c. hypotony
    d. Sturge-Weber syndrome.

35. According to the OHTS conclusions, a predictive factor for the development of POAG is a central corneal thickness of less than or equal to how many microns?
    a. 565
    b. 555
    c. 545
    d. 535

36. Which index on Humphrey VF testing is most helpful for determining the progression of VF loss?
    a. false positive
    b. mean deviation
    c. pattern standard deviation
    d. short-term fluctuation

37. Which optic disc finding is most likely to indicate the progression of glaucoma?
    a. peripapillary atrophy
    b. focal notch
    c. pallor
    d. splinter hemorrhage

38. The most likely risk factor for phacomorphic glaucoma in a patient with brunescent cataracts and narrow angles is
    a. trauma
    b. pseudoexfoliation syndrome
    c. pigment dispersion syndrome
    d. hyperopia

39. A patient with an anterior chamber IOL presents with ciliary block. Exam shows a patent iridectomy. Which of the following is the most appropriate treatment option?
    a. topical cycloplegic
    b. topical β-blocker and carbonic anhydrase inhibitor
    c. laser iridoplasty
    d. anterior vitrectomy

40. A mechanic presents 1 week after an eye injury with decreased vision, redness, and eye pain. Exam reveals a self-sealing corneal laceration, elevated IOP, and white fluffy material in the anterior chamber. The most likely diagnosis is
    a. phacolytic glaucoma
    b. lens-particle glaucoma
    c. phacomorphic glaucoma
    d. ghost cell glaucoma

41. What VF defect would you expect to find in a patient with POAG and C/D ratio of 0.7 OD with an inferior notch?
    a. enlarged blind spot
    b. inferior nasal step
    c. superior arcuate
    d. temporal wedge

42. A 68-year-old man presents with IOP of 18 mm Hg, C/D ratio of 0.8, and nasal steps on VF testing OU. The next test to perform is
    a. magnetic resonance imaging
    b. carotid Doppler
    c. electrocardiogram
    d. tonometry

43. The GLT evaluated treatment with
    a. ALT and latanoprost
    b. ALT and timolol
    c. SLT and dorzolamide
    d. SLT and latanoprost

44. POAG and NTG are best differentiated with
    a. VF testing
    b. gonioscopy
    c. ON imaging
    d. serial tonometry

45. Angle closure without pupillary block is caused by
    a. aqueous misdirection
    b. dislocated lens
    c. seclusion pupillae
    d. silicone oil

Please visit the eBook for an interactive version of the review questions. See front cover for activation details.

SUGGESTED READINGS

Allingham, R. R., & Moroi, S. E. (2010). *Shields textbook of glaucoma* (6th ed.). Philadelphia: Lippincott Williams and Wilkins.

Anderson, D. R., & Patella, V. M. (1999). *Automated static perimetry* (2nd ed.). St Louis: Mosby.

Basic and Clinical Sciences Course. (2021). *Section 10: Glaucoma*. San Francisco: AAO.

Choplin, N. T., & Traverso, C. E. (2014). *Atlas of glaucoma* (3rd ed.). Boca Raton: CRC Press.

Higginbotham, E. J., & Lee, D. A. (2003). *Clinical guide to glaucoma management*. Amsterdam: Butterworth-Heinemann.

Ritch, R., Shields, M. B., & Krupin, T. (1996). *The glaucomas* (2nd ed.). St Louis: Mosby.

Weber, J., & Caprioli, J. (2000). *Atlas of computerized perimetry*. Philadelphia: WB Saunders.

Zimmerman, T. J., & Kooner, K. S. (2001). *Clinical pathways in glaucoma*. New York: Thieme Medical.

10

Anterior Segment

IRIS, CILIARY BODY (CB), AND ANTERIOR CHAMBER (AC) ANGLE
LENS

IRIS, CILIARY BODY (CB), AND ANTERIOR CHAMBER (AC) ANGLE

Anatomy

Limbus

Transition zone between cornea and sclera; 1–2 mm wide

Conjunctiva and Tenon capsule are fused over this area; contains corneal epithelial stem cells, goblet cells, lymphoid cells, Langerhans cells, mast cells

Definitions:

Anatomist's: termination of Descemet and Bowman membranes

Pathologist's: anterior limbus corresponds to termination of Bowman and Descemet membranes, and posterior limbus corresponds to line between iris root and Schlemm canal

Surgeon's: anterior blue zone (1 mm) and posterior white zone (1 mm); a perpendicular incision through the conjunctival insertion enters the AC through Descemet membrane; a perpendicular incision through the posterior aspect of the limbus will enter the AC through the trabecular meshwork (Fig. 10.1)

Iris

Anterior part of uvea; ciliary portion (peripheral 2/3) and pupillary portion (central 1/3) separated by collarette (thickest area where dilator and sphincter muscles overlap); pigment ruff at pupillary edge

Layers:

Stroma: anterior pigmented fibrovascular collagen matrix

Iris pigment epithelium (IPE): two cell layers aligned apex to apex, anterior nonpigmented and posterior pigmented; posterior epithelium continuous with nonpigmented epithelium of CB, apical surface attached to anterior iris epithelium, basal surface faces

posterior chamber and extends around pupil margin onto anterior iris stroma as pigment ruff

Muscles: neuroectoderm smooth muscle between stroma and IPE

DILATOR: originates from anterior pigment epithelium, extends radially into iris stroma

SPHINCTER: circular band in deep stroma near pupil

Vascular supply: radial vessels from major arterial circle (in CB) travel into iris stroma, anastomose with venous arcades at collarette to form minor vascular circle of iris

Innervation: sympathetic and parasympathetic to muscles

Dilator: sympathetic stimulation (α_1-adrenergic; from hypothalamus to ciliospinal center of Budge, superior cervical ganglion, and long ciliary nerves) causes contraction (dilation); parasympathetic stimulation (cholinergic) is inhibitory

Sphincter: parasympathetic (from Edinger-Westphal nucleus to cranial nerve [CN] 3, ciliary ganglion, and short ciliary nerves) stimulation (muscarinic) causes contraction (miosis); sympathetic stimulation is inhibitory (relaxes sphincter in dark)

Ciliary Body and Angle Structures

(See Chapter 9, Glaucoma)

Imaging

Ultrasound Biomicroscopy (UBM)

High-resolution acoustic imaging of anterior segment structures; axial and radial scans

Frequency = 50 MHz, axial resolution = 37 μm

Anterior Segment Optical Coherence Tomography (OCT)

High-resolution images of visible anterior segment structures; can also provide epithelial thickness map

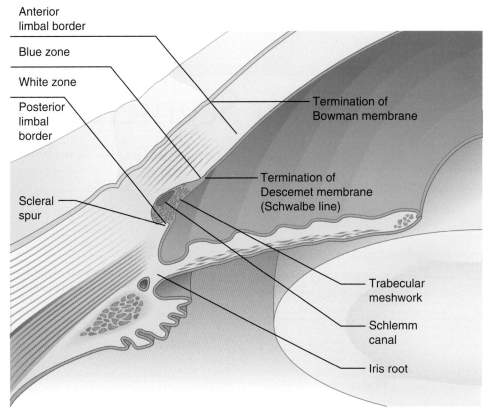

Anterior
limbal border

Blue zone

White zone

Posterior
limbal
border

Scleral
spur

Termination of
Bowman membrane

Termination of
Descemet membrane
(Schwalbe line)

Trabecular
meshwork

Schlemm
canal

Iris root

Figure 10.1 Anatomy of the surgical limbus.

Disorders

Trauma

Hyphema

Blood in AC

Etiology: trauma, surgery (incisional or laser, uveitis-glaucoma-hyphema [UGH] syndrome), spontaneous (neovascularization, Fuchs heterochromic iridocyclitis, intraocular tumors, juvenile xanthogranuloma), clotting abnormalities (leukemia, hemophilia, anemia, coumadin, aspirin, ethanol)

Findings: layer of blood and/or clot with suspended red blood cells (RBCs) in AC; graded by volume of blood (*microhyphema* if only circulating cells, grade I if <1/3 AC, grade II if 1/3-1/2 AC, grade III if >1/2 AC, grade IV if total AC) damage to other structures may be seen

Diagnosis: sickle prep, consider hemoglobin electrophoresis, rule out ruptured globe, gonioscopy (wait 4-6 weeks in traumatic cases)

Treatment: cycloplegic, topical steroid, control intraocular pressure (IOP; avoid miotics); consider Amicar (aminocaproic acid), protective shield; elevate head, bed rest, no aspirin-containing products, control systemic blood pressure (BP), antiemetics (if needed); may require surgery (AC washout) or intraocular lens (IOL) removal/exchange (UGH syndrome)

Indications for surgical intervention: large hyphema that persists for >10 days, total hyphema that persists for >5 days, corneal blood staining, uncontrolled IOP, rebleed, 8-ball hyphema; best to perform washout 4-7 days after injury (clot has time to solidify, reducing rate of rebleed)

Complications:
8-ball hyphema: hyphema that has clotted and taken on a black or purple color because of impaired aqueous circulation and deoxygenated blood, which prevents resorption; total hyphema is differentiated from 8-ball hyphema by retention of bright-red color, which indicates aqueous circulation
Corneal blood staining: passage of erythrocyte breakdown products into stroma, creates yellow–brown discoloration; occurs in ~5%, especially with recurrent hemorrhage, compromised endothelial cell function, large hyphemas that remain for extended periods, elevated IOP
Recurrent hemorrhage: usually larger than initial hyphema; incidence 5%–35%, with greatest risk at 2–5 days
Secondary glaucoma:
  EARLY: caused by trabecular meshwork (TM) obstruction, pupillary block by clot, hemolytic, steroid induced
  LATE: caused by angle recession, ghost cell, peripheral anterior synechiae (PAS) formation, posterior synechiae with iris bombe
Other: central retinal artery occlusion, optic atrophy

Sickle cell and hyphema: higher elevation in IOP (sickled RBCs cannot pass through TM), and higher risk of central retinal artery occlusion and optic nerve infarction as a result of vascular sludging

Factors that increase sickling: acidosis, hypoxia, hemoconcentration

Ocular hypotensive medications in sickle cell: β-blockers are safe; avoid carbonic anhydrase inhibitors (CAIs; increases concentration of ascorbic acid in aqueous, decreasing pH and leading to sickling), epinephrine and α-agonists (cause vasoconstriction with subsequent deoxygenation and sickling); hyperosmotics (lead to hemoconcentration with vascular sludging and sickling)

Iris and Angle Trauma (Fig. 10.2)

Iris sphincter tear: small tear at pupillary margin; asymptomatic

Traumatic mydriasis: dilated, poorly reactive pupil; may cause glare or photophobia; consider cosmetic contact lens or surgical repair

Iridodialysis: tear in iris root; consider cosmetic contact lens or surgical repair if large or symptomatic

Angle recession: tear in anterior face of CB between the longitudinal and circular ciliary muscles; most common source of hemorrhage in blunt trauma, occurs in >60% of hyphemas; 10% of patients with >180° of angle recession will develop chronic glaucoma

Cyclodialysis: separation of CB from scleral spur; allows free passage of aqueous into suprachoroidal space; can result in hypotony; treat with atropine, laser, and/or surgical repair

Open Globe/Intraocular Foreign Body

Full-thickness defect in cornea or sclera

Usually a result of trauma (penetrating or blunt); may also occur from melt (chemical injury, autoimmune disorder, infection)

Penetration: entrance wound only

Perforation: entrance and exit wounds (double-penetrating injury)

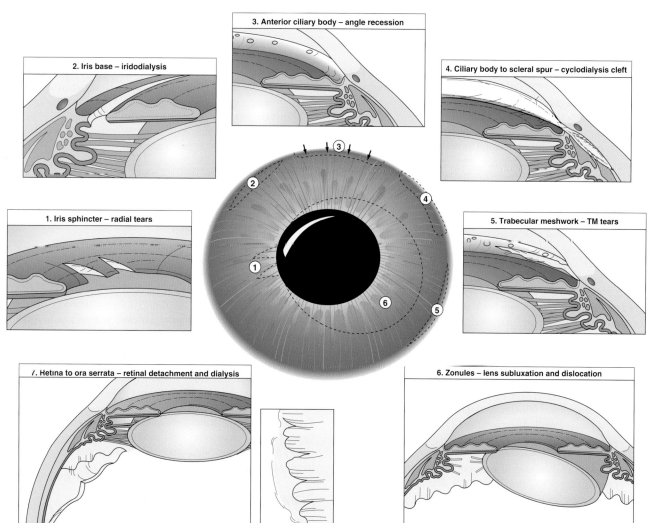

Figure 10.2 Seven areas of traumatic ocular tears *(shown in yellow)* with the resultant findings. (From Campbell DG. Traumatic glaucoma. In: Shingleton BJ, Hersh PS, Kenyon KR, eds. *Eye Trauma*. St Louis: Mosby; 1991.)

Risk of infectious endophthalmitis (2%–7%) increases if retained foreign body, delayed surgery (>24 hours), rural setting (soil contamination), and lens disruption

Staphylococcus is most common organism to cause posttraumatic endophthalmitis; *Bacillus cereus* is also common and causes severe damage (see Chapter 8, Uveitis)

Findings: wound with positive Seidel test, hemorrhage (conjunctiva, hyphema, vitreous, retina), decreased IOP, shallow or flat AC, peaked pupil (toward wound), cataract, retinal tear/detachment, prolapsed intraocular contents (uvea, vitreous), foreign body (small, high-velocity foreign body may cause self-sealing wound or intermittently positive Seidel; iris transillumination defect, capsule/lens disruption)

Types of foreign bodies:
  Inert: glass, plastic, sand, stone, ceramic, gold, platinum, silver, aluminum
  Reactive:
    COPPER: severity of inflammation is directly proportionate to amount of copper in foreign body (≥85% copper causes severe endophthalmitis; <85% causes chalcosis; <70% is relatively inert)
    CHALCOSIS: mild intraocular inflammation, deposition of copper in anterior lens capsule (sunflower cataract) and Descemet membrane (Kayser-Fleisher ring), retinal degeneration, iris may become green and sluggishly reactive to light
    ELECTRORETINOGRAM (ERG): decreased amplitude (suppressed by copper ions)
    IRON (siderosis): iris heterochromia (hyperchromatic on involved side), mid-dilated minimally reactive pupil, lens discoloration (brown–orange dots from iron deposition in lens epithelium, generalized yellowing from involvement of cortex), vitritis, pigmentary retinal pigment epithelium (RPE) degeneration with sclerosis of vessels, retinal thinning, and atrophy
    ERG: initial a-wave increased, may eventually become flat
    WOOD: significant inflammation; plant matter has higher risk of endophthalmitis

Treatment: rule out foreign body with computed tomography (CT) or magnetic resonance imaging (MRI) (contraindicated for metallic foreign body); surgical exploration and repair, remove reactive material as soon as possible
  Prophylactic antibiotics: intravenous (IV) (vancomycin 1 g q12h or cefazolin 1 g q8h; ceftazidime 1 g q12h) and intravitreal (vancomycin [1 mg/0.1 mL], amikacin [0.4 mg/0.1 mL], or ceftazidime [2.25 mg/0.1 mL]) reduces risk of endophthalmitis

Prognosis: variable; poor if endophthalmitis or proliferative vitreoretinopathy (PVR) develops (7–21 days later)

Congenital Abnormalities

(See Chapter 5, Pediatrics/Strabismus)

Mesodermal Dysgenesis Syndromes

(See Chapter 5, Pediatrics/Strabismus)

Other Disorders

Corectopia

Displacement of pupil

Isolated or associated with Axenfeld-Rieger syndrome, iridocorneal endothelial (ICE) syndrome, uveitis, trauma, or ectopia lentis et pupillae

Iris Heterochromia

Iris of different colors

May be congenital or acquired, unilateral (heterochromia iridis) or bilateral (heterochromia iridium)

DDx:
  Congenital:
    INVOLVED IRIS HYPOCHROMIC: Horner syndrome, Waardenburg syndrome, Hirschsprung disease, Parry-Romberg hemifacial atrophy
    INVOLVED IRIS HYPERCHROMIC: ocular or oculodermal melanocytosis, iris pigment epithelium hamartoma
  Acquired:
    INVOLVED IRIS HYPOCHROMIC: Horner syndrome, Fuchs heterochromic iridocyclitis, iris atrophy, metastatic carcinoma, juvenile xanthogranuloma
    INVOLVED IRIS HYPERCHROMIC: iris nevus or melanoma, ICE syndrome, rubeosis, siderosis, hemosiderosis, medication (prostaglandin analogues)

Treatment: rule out tumor or intraocular foreign body

Rubeosis Iridis

Neovascularization of the iris

Etiology: ischemia (usually proliferative diabetic retinopathy [PDR], central retinal vein occlusion [CRVO], carotid occlusive disease; also central retinal artery occlusion [CRAO], sickle cell retinopathy, anterior segment ischemia), tumor, uveitis, chronic retinal detachment (RD).

Findings: abnormal iris vessels; perform gonioscopy to assess presence of angle neovascularization; may have elevated IOP (neovascular glaucoma [NVG])

Treatment: intravitreal anti–vascular endothelial growth factor (VEGF); may require panretinal photocoagulation (PRP) for ischemia; NVG often needs glaucoma drainage implant for IOP control

Pigment Dispersion Syndrome

Pigment liberation from posterior iris surface (as a result of contact with zonules)

More common in young Caucasian males

Associated with myopia and lattice degeneration (20%)

Findings: pigment deposits on lens capsule, anterior iris, angle structures, and corneal endothelium (Krukenberg spindle); midperipheral, radial, iris transillumination defects; pigmentary glaucoma may develop

Iridocorneal Endothelial (ICE) Syndrome

Nonhereditary, progressive abnormality of corneal endothelium

Abnormal corneal endothelium grows across angle and iris, producing membrane that obstructs trabecular meshwork, distorts iris, and may contract around iris stroma to form nodules

Unilateral, mostly women, occurs during middle age

Findings: fine, beaten-metal appearance of endothelium; secondary angle-closure glaucoma may develop as a result of angle endothelialization and PAS

Syndromes: common features of iris distortion, corneal edema, secondary angle-closure glaucoma
  Iris nevus (Cogan-Reese) syndrome: flattening and effacement of iris stroma, pigmented iris nodules (pseudonevi) composed of normal iris cells that are bunched up from the overlying membrane, corectopia, ectropion uveae
  Chandler syndrome: corneal edema often with normal IOP, mild or no iris changes (minimal corectopia, iris atrophy, peripheral anterior synechiae)
  Essential iris atrophy: proliferating endothelium produces broad PAS, corectopia, ectropion uveae, and iris holes (stretch holes [area away from maximal pull of endothelial membrane is stretched so thin that holes develop] and melting holes [holes in areas without iris thinning as a result of iris ischemia])

Pathology: growth of endothelium and Descemet membrane over trabecular meshwork and onto iris

DDx: posterior polymorphous dystrophy, mesodermal dysgenesis syndromes

Iridoschisis

Separation of iris stroma as a result of senile changes

Bilateral; onset in 6th–7th decade of life

Glaucoma in 50%

Iris Nodules

Brushfield Spots

(See Chapter 5, Pediatrics/Strabismus)

Juvenile Xanthogranuloma (JXG)

(See Chapter 5, Pediatrics/Strabismus)

Epithelial Invasion, Serous Cyst, Implantation Membrane, Solid or Pearl Cyst

Serous or solid cysts after surgery or injury

Koeppe Nodules

Along pupillary border in granulomatous uveitis

Pathology: inflammatory cells and debris

Busacca Nodules

On anterior surface of the iris in granulomatous uveitis

Pathology: inflammatory cells and debris

Berlin Nodules

In AC angle in granulomatous uveitis

Pathology: inflammatory cells and debris

Iris Nevus Syndrome (Cogan-Reese)

(See above)

Iris Tumors

Perform transillumination to differentiate cyst from solid tumor

Freckle

No distortion of iris architecture

Nevus

Localized or diffuse variably pigmented lesion of stroma; obscures crypts

Pathology: usually low-grade spindle cells

Treatment: photo document; UBM and/or anterior segment OCT to evaluate extent and whether cystic or solid, radiation therapy (XRT) or surgical excision early for strong suspicion of melanoma

Prognosis: small risk of transformation into melanoma (~5% of suspicious iris lesions grow during first 5 years after detection). Only 4% suspicious iris nevi progress to melanoma in 10 years and 11% by 20 years

Risk factors for transformation (mnemonic **ABCDEF**): **A**ge (young, <40 years), **B**lood (hyphema), **C**lock hour inferiorly (4:00–9:00), **D**iffuse appearance, **E**ctropion uveae, **F**eathery margins

Melanocytosis

Congenital ocular: usually unilateral with diffuse iris nevus causing iris heterochromia

Oculodermal (nevus of Ota): ocular plus periorbital skin involvement

Melanocytoma

Form of nevus; darkly pigmented, very noncohesive (like black, wet sand)

May have necrotic center

5% risk of melanoma

Malignant Melanoma

4% of ocular melanomas (6% are CB, 90% are choroidal)

Elevated, vascular, darkly pigmented or amelanotic lesion; usually located inferiorly

Can be diffuse (appearing as iris heterochromia) and associated with glaucoma, localized, annular, or tapioca (dark tapioca appearance)

Common in Caucasians with light irides

Classification: American Joint Cancer Committee
- *T1* = limited to iris (1a = ≤3 clock hours, 1b = >3 clock hours, 1c = with secondary glaucoma)
- *T2* = confluent with or extending into CB, choroid, or both (2a = CB without secondary glaucoma, 2b = CB and choroid without secondary glaucoma, 2c = CB, choroid, or both with secondary glaucoma)
- *T3* = T2 with scleral extension
- *T4* = with extrascleral extension (4a = ≤5 mm in diameter, 4b = >5 mm in diameter)

Findings suggestive of melanoma: growth (only 6.5% of iris melanomas enlarge over 5-year period), spontaneous hyphema, large size, vascularity, ectropion uveae, iris heterochromia, elevated IOP, angle involvement, glaucoma, sectoral cataract

Pathology: low-grade spindle B cells; epithelioid cells are rare

B-scan ultrasound or UBM: rule out CB involvement and characterize lesion (≥3 mm basal diameter and ≥1 mm thickness replacing iris stroma with 3 or more of the following features: vascularity, ectropion uveae, secondary cataract, secondary glaucoma, and growth)

Treatment: resection (sector iridectomy), may require enucleation if extensive, radiotherapy (plaque or proton beam)

Prognosis: 3% mortality; risk of metastasis is 5% at 5 years, 7% at 10 years, and 11% at 20 years; risk increases with elevated intraocular pressure and extraocular extension

Tumors of Iris Pigment Epithelium

Adenoma (benign) or adenocarcinoma (malignant)

Rare compared with melanomas

Deeply pigmented, circumscribed or multinodular mass; can cause secondary glaucoma by involvement of angle

Treatment: chemotherapy, radiation, or excision

Lisch Nodules

Benign, tan, iris hamartomas; associated with neurofibromatosis type 1

Metastasis

Most commonly, breast, lung, lymphoma

Findings: fluffy, friable iris mass; may have pseudohypopyon, anterior uveitis, hyphema, rubeosis, and glaucoma

Leiomyoma

Well localized or pedunculated, often diffuse and flat

Pathology: very similar to amelanotic spindle cell melanoma

Leukemia

Rare nodular or diffuse milky lesions with intense hyperemia

Findings: iris thickening with loss of normal architecture; iris heterochromia and pseudohypopyon

Cystic Lesions

Iris pigment epithelium (IPE): can be autosomal dominant (AD); flocculi around pupillary margin; associated in certain families with aortic dissection; midperipheral cysts, peripheral cysts (usually clear; can push iris forward)

Stroma: congenital or acquired (after trauma or surgery)

Ciliary Body Tumors

Melanoma

6% of ocular melanomas

Pigmented mass

May be very large before detection, producing lenticular astigmatism, cataract, or shallow AC; may have classic sentinel vessel or nodule of extrascleral extension

Pathology: spindle, epithelioid, or mixed cells

Treatment: local resection, XRT, enucleation

Prognosis: poorer than other uveal melanoma because usually diagnosed at later stage; risk of metastasis is 25% at 5 years, 34% at 10 years, 55% at 20 years

Ciliary Body Leiomyoma

Similar to fibroid; myogenic origin

Schwannoma

Looks like amelanotic melanoma

Ciliary Body Adenoma or Adenocarcinoma

Arises from neuroepithelial cells

Occurs during adulthood

May metastasize

Fuchs Adenoma (Fuchs Reactive Hyperplasia, Benign Ciliary Epithelioma)

Proliferation of basement membrane material (type IV collagen and laminin) and nonpigmented CB epithelial cells located at ciliary crest

Occurs in 25% of older patients

Rarely causes localized occlusion of AC angle

Medulloepithelioma

(See Chapter 5, Pediatrics/Strabismus)

LENS

Anatomy/Physiology (Fig. 10.3)

Lens capsule: basement membrane secreted by epithelium, composed of type IV collagen and glycosaminoglycans; thickest peripherally near the equator, thinnest posteriorly (anterior thickness = 15.5 μm; posterior thickness = 2.8 μm) (Fig. 10.4). Thickening of lens capsule can occur with AC inflammation or pathologic proliferation of lens epithelium

Epithelium: single cell layer anteriorly, ending just posterior to the lens equator. Derived from cells of original lens vesicle. In the germinative zone, just anterior to equator, lens epithelial cells divide, elongate, and differentiate into lens fibers. During this transformation, epithelial cells lose

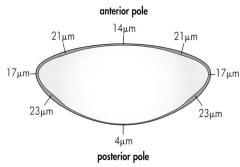

Figure 10.4 Thickness of the lens capsule. (From Saxby LA. Anatomy. In: Yanoff M, Duker JS, eds. *Ophthalmology.* London: Mosby; 1999.)

their nuclei and most organelles. Lens fibers do not contain nuclei except in rubella, Lowe syndrome, and trisomy 13. The embryonal nucleus develops by proliferation and migration of epithelial cells from the equator. Acute IOP elevation may cause patches of epithelium degeneration and necrosis beneath the capsule, which appear as white flecks (glaukomflecken). Chronic iritis may cause liquefaction of the nucleus, peripheral cortical changes, and degeneration and necrosis, as well as proliferation of anterior lens epithelium

Sutures: upright Y suture anteriorly and inverted Y suture posteriorly represent interdigitation of the ends of lens fibers; sutures appear during the 2nd month of gestation because of unequal growth of new lens fibers

Zonules: fibrillin fibers attach from pars plicata to anterior and posterior lens capsule in midperiphery (inserting more centrally on anterior capsule). During the 5th month of gestation, nonpigmented ciliary epithelium of CB secretes collagen fibers that become zonules. Equatorial zonules are lost with aging

Tunica vasculosa lentis: vascular network that surrounds lens during embryogenesis; derived from hyaloid and long ciliary arteries. Remnants of tunica vasculosa lentis include Mittendorf dot, epicapsular star, persistent pupillary membrane, and capsular whorls

Properties of the crystalline lens:
Composed of proteins: highest protein content in body (33% of its weight)
  WATER SOLUBLE:
    ALPHA CRYSTALLINS: largest of all water-soluble proteins, composed of 4 subunits, type of heat shock protein; ~35% of lens protein by weight; involved in transforming epithelial cells into lens fibers, and stabilizing and preventing aggregation of proteins
    BETA CRYSTALLINS: most abundant lens protein by weight; polymers composed of 3 subunits; ~55% of lens protein by weight; first appears in cortex
    GAMMA CRYSTALLINS: smallest lens protein, monomeric; concentrated in nucleus

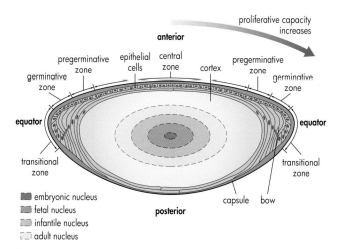

Figure 10.3 Gross anatomy of the adult human lens. (From Saxby LA: Anatomy. In: Yanoff M, Duker JS, eds. *Ophthalmology.* London: Mosby; 1999.)

WATER INSOLUBLE:

MAIN INTRINSIC PROTEIN: type of aquaporin, regulates water transport, role in cell adhesion; correlates with nuclear brunescence, mutations in *MIP* gene result in cataract

CYTOSKELETAL ELEMENTS: structural support filaments including actin, vimentin, tubulin, filensin, phakinin

Potassium-rich tissue: results from Na⁺/K⁺ pumps found on lens epithelial cells, which pump Na⁺ out and K⁺ in; concentrations of Na⁺ and K⁺ in aqueous are inverse to those in lens (10 × as much Na⁺ in aqueous as in lens)

Grows throughout life: weight at maturity is 3 × that at birth, anterior-posterior width increases from 3 mm at birth to 5 mm at maturity and 6 mm by 80 years old, equatorial length increases from 6.4 mm at birth to 9.0 mm at maturity; also increase in curvature with greater refractive power

Refractive index: high (1.390) owing to protein concentration; increase in lens curvature and thickness with age is offset by change in gradient of refractive index as a result of increased concentration of main intrinsic protein; associated with increased brunescence, resulting in greater absorption of blue and violet wavelengths, as well as ultraviolet (UV) light (aiding in retinal protection)

Metabolism: anaerobic; 80% of glucose metabolized by glycolysis, 10% metabolized by pentose phosphate pathway, 5% reduced to sorbitol, and 5% converted to glucuronic acid; highest metabolic rate is in cortex; energy is required for ion transport and glutathione production

Lens fiber structure: fibers contain few intracellular organelles and no nuclei; appear hexagonal in cross section

Average lens power: at birth = 37 diopters (D), at age 2 years = 23 D, at adulthood = 20 D

Protective mechanisms against free radical damage and oxidation: glutathione peroxidase, superoxide dismutase, catalase, and vitamins C and E; oxidation increases disulfide crosslinking of crystallins and protein aggregation (causes light scattering and cataract)

UV protection: lens blocks UV light ≤360 nm to protect retina (cornea and aqueous block light ≤300 nm), yellow chromophores accumulate with age protecting from shorter wavelengths

Accommodation: parasympathetic fibers of CN 3

Generally accepted theory is that of von Helmholtz: ciliary muscle contraction causes zonules to relax, allowing the lens to become more spherical and increasing its focusing power; presbyopia is therefore a result of loss of lens elasticity with age

Disorders

Congenital Anomalies

(See Chapter 5, Pediatrics/Strabismus)

Cataracts

Congenital Cataracts

(See Chapter 5, Pediatrics/Strabismus)

Acquired Cataracts

Classified by location or etiology

Mnemonic: **DAMAGED** (**D**iabetes, **A**ging, **M**yopia or **M**yotonic dystrophy, **A**nterior uveitis, **G**laucoma, **E**lectricity [radiation, trauma], **D**rugs)

Cortical: lens fiber fragments, degenerated protein, liquefaction

Spokes and vacuoles: radial lines and dots (Fig. 10.5)

Mature: completely white

Hypermature: leakage of degenerated cortical material, wrinkled capsule; may have calcium deposits

Morgagnian: total liquefaction of lens cortex; nucleus floats freely within capsule; lens material can leak through intact capsule (Fig 10.6)

Pathology: hydropic swelling of lens fibers; morgagnian globules (eosinophilic, globular material between lens fibers)

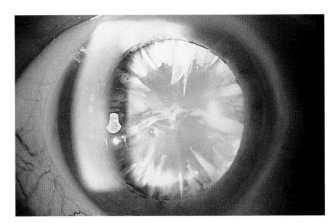

Figure 10.5 Cortical cataract. (From Collin J. The morphology and visual effects of lens opacities. In: Yanoff M, Duker JS, eds. *Ophthalmology.* London: Mosby; 1999.)

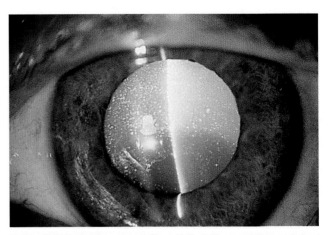

Figure 10.6 Morgagnian cataract. (From Collin J: The morphology and visual effects of lens opacities. In: Yanoff M, Duker JS, eds. *Ophthalmology.* London: Mosby; 1999.)

Nuclear sclerosis: increased nuclear density, then opacification occurs with aging; lenticular myopia results from increased index of refraction; "second sight" (presbyopes can often read again without spectacles)

Cataract brunescens (poor blue discrimination), cataract nigrans, calcium oxalate crystals in nucleus

Pathology: inwardly sequestered lens fibers degenerate (analogous to desquamating skin); homogenous loss of cellular laminations

Posterior subcapsular (PSC): posterior migration of lens epithelium, and bladder (Wedl) cell formation (eosinophilic globular cells with nuclei; swell to 5–6 × normal size)

Etiology: age, trauma, steroids, inflammation, ionizing radiation, retinitis pigmentosa, atopic dermatitis, Werner syndrome, Rothmund syndrome, diabetes

Symptoms: glare and poor vision from bright lights; affects near vision more than distance vision

Pathology: posterior migration of lens epithelial cells, which swell along posterior capsule (swollen cells are called Wedl cells)

Anterior subcapsular (ASC): fibrous plaque beneath folded anterior capsule, secreted by irritated metaplastic anterior epithelial cells (as a result of trauma or uveitis), can also occur in atopic dermatitis

Pathology: cells surrounded by basement membrane

Glaukomflecken: necrosis of lens epithelial cells as a result of ischemia from elevated IOP (angle closure); appears as central subcapsular small white dots and flecks

Traumatic and toxic cataracts:

Contusion: petalliform or rosette pattern resulting from separation of lens fibers around lens sutures

Vossius ring: with blunt injury, pigment from pupillary ruff is imprinted onto anterior lens capsule

Soemmerring ring: doughnut of residual equatorial cortex; after cataract surgery or trauma; can be associated with an adherent leukoma

Siderosis lentis: iron deposits in lens epithelium; anterior subcapsular orange deposits; photoreceptor and RPE degeneration resulting in pigmentary retinopathy with peripheral visual field loss; iris heterochromia (involved iris darker)

Chalcosis lentis: copper deposits in lens capsule; green discoloration of anterior lens capsule and cortex in petaloid configuration occurs in Wilson disease, forming a sunflower cataract; also Kayser-Fleischer ring (copper deposition in peripheral Descemet membrane); can also occur in multiple myeloma and lung carcinoma

Other intraocular foreign bodies: gold, silver, platinum, aluminum are inert; lead and zinc may cause mild nongranulomatous reaction

COPPER: if concentration ≥85%, an acute inflammatory reaction occurs; if concentration between 70%–85%, chalcosis develops; lesser concentrations are relatively inert

Mercurial lentis: mercury deposits in lens capsule (occupational)

Electrical: lens vacuoles in anterior midperiphery; linear opacities (stellate pattern) in anterior subcapsular cortex; burns >200 volts cause conjunctival hyperemia, iritis, hyphema, iris atrophy, sphincter changes

Argon laser: blue light absorbed by yellow sclerotic nucleus

Nonionizing radiation: infrared causes true exfoliation (glassblower's cataract) with splitting and scrolling of anterior lens capsule; ultraviolet (UV-B) causes cortical cataracts

Ionizing radiation: a threshold level of radiation is required to induce cataract development (posterior subcapsular cataract [PSC])

Medications: mnemonic **ABCD** (**A**miodarone, **B**usulphan, **C**hlorpromazine, **D**examethasone)

AMIODARONE AND PHENOTHIAZINES (including **C**hlorpromazine): pigmented deposits in anterior lens capsule; axial, spoke-like configuration; dose and duration dependent

BUSULFAN: PSC

CORTICOSTEROIDS (including **D**examethasone): PSC from long-term use of any form of steroids, most commonly topical; develop in 33% of patients on long-term daily dose of 10 mg; also associated with inhaled steroids

MIOTICS: echothiophate iodide and demecarium bromide cause anterior subcapsular vacuoles in adults (not children)

TAMOXIFEN: PSC

Cataracts associated with systemic disease:

Atopic dermatitis: PSC and anterior subcapsular cataract (ASC) shield-like plaque

Also associated with chronic keratoconjunctivitis, keratoconus, vernal keratoconjunctivitis

Diabetes: osmotic cataract resulting from high glucose levels and aldose reductase, which results in high sorbitol levels

Snowflake cataract (punctate white subcapsular opacities) can occur rapidly with high blood sugar

Myotonic dystrophy (AD): mapped to chromosome 19

FINDINGS: characteristic presenile "Christmas tree" cataract consisting of polychromatic cortical crystals; ptosis, lid lag, light-near dissociation, mild pigmentary retinopathy; ERG shows low voltage

OTHER FINDINGS: myotonia (bilateral facial weakness, difficulty relaxing grip, muscle wasting), testicular atrophy, frontal baldness, cardiac abnormalities, mental retardation; excessive contractility of muscles

Neurofibromatosis type 2: presenile PSC opacities

Werner syndrome: syndrome of premature aging, scleroderma-like matting of skin, and bilateral PSC cataracts in 3rd–4th decade of life

Wilson disease (hepatolenticular degeneration): deficiency of ceruloplasmin (alpha-2 globulin)

FINDINGS: green sunflower cataract resulting from deposition of copper in anterior lens capsule and cortex in petaloid configuration; Kayser-Fleischer ring (copper in peripheral Descemet membrane)

OTHER FINDINGS: cirrhosis, renal impairment, degeneration of basal ganglia

TREATMENT: penicillamine to lower serum copper

Lens Capsule Abnormalities

True Exfoliation

Delamination/schisis of anterior lens capsule, forming scrolls; often as a result of infrared radiation (glassblowers), can be an aging change; not associated with glaucoma

Pseudoexfoliation Syndrome (PXS)

Material produced by lens epithelial cells and extruded through lens capsule

Appears to be an ocular sign of systemic elastosis; also found in conjunctiva, skin, lung, and liver

Usually elderly, Caucasian females; increased incidence in Scandinavians and with increasing age

Findings: white fibrillar material on anterior lens capsule, iris, CB, zonules, anterior vitreous with characteristic pattern of deposition on lens surface (central disc, clear zone, then peripheral annulus, often with bridging strands to central disc); may see flakes on pupillary margin; Sampaolesi line (pigment band anterior to Schwalbe line) on gonioscopy; up to 50% develop glaucoma (PXG); poor dilation as a result of iris muscle degeneration or lack of iris stromal elasticity; peripapillary transillumination defects; weak zonules (phacodonesis, increased incidence of angle closure, lens subluxation, and complications during and after cataract surgery [vitreous loss, IOL and capsular dislocation])

Posterior Capsular Opacification (PCO; Secondary Cataract)

Proliferation of residual lens epithelial cells (Elschnig pearls) and fibrosis

Incidence: up to 50% of patients within 2 years of extracapsular cataract surgery; influenced by IOL optic material (acrylic < silicone < polymethylmethacrylate [PMMA]) and edge design (square edge < round edge); with newer IOLs, the incidence has decreased to ~10%. Incidence approaches 100% in children and patients with uveitis

Treatment: Nd:YAG laser posterior capsulotomy when visually significant

In young children, primary posterior capsulotomy and anterior vitrectomy are performed at the time of cataract surgery

Ectopia Lentis

Displacement of lens

Subluxation: partial displacement, remains in pupillary axis

Dislocation (luxation): complete displacement from pupil

Etiology: trauma (most common acquired cause), Marfan syndrome, homocystinuria, aniridia, congenital glaucoma, megalocornea, Ehlers-Danlos syndrome, hyperlysinemia, sulfite oxidase deficiency, hereditary ectopia lentis (AD >> autosomal recessive [AR]; bilateral; may not present until 3rd–5th decade), ectopia lentis et pupillae (AR; lens and pupil are displaced in opposite directions; bilateral, asymmetric), tertiary syphilis, congenital Zika syndrome, Weill-Marchesani syndrome, medulloepithelioma, Stickler syndrome, pseudoexfoliation (rare)

Mnemonic: **WATCH HIM SEE** (**W**eill-Marchesani, **A**niridia, **T**rauma, **C**ongenital glaucoma, **H**yperlysinemia, **H**omocystinuria, **I**ris coloboma, **M**arfan syndrome, **S**ulfite oxidase deficiency, **E**hlers-Danlos syndrome, **E**ctopia lentis et pupillae)

Findings: decreased vision, astigmatism, monocular diplopia, iridodonesis, phacodonesis, malpositioned lens

Marfan Syndrome (AD)

Mapped to chromosome 15q; defect in fibrillin (elastic microfibrillar glycoprotein, major constituent of zonules); 15% have no family history

Findings: ectopia lentis (65%; usually superotemporal); glaucoma, keratoconus, cornea plana, axial myopia, retinal degeneration (salt-and-pepper fundus), high risk of RD

Other findings: tall stature, spidery digits, arm span is larger than height, cardiac disease, dissecting aneurysm of the aorta

Homocystinuria (AR)

Deficiency of cystathionine β-synthase, which converts homocysteine to cystathionine; methionine and homocysteine accumulate; zonules are deficient in cysteine and weakened because of reduced sulfhydryl cross-linkage; degeneration of entire zonule occurs

Findings: bilateral ectopia lentis (90%; usually inferonasal; 30% in infancy, 80% by age 15), enlarged globe, myopia, peripheral RPE degeneration, increased risk of retinal detachment after cataract surgery, early loss of accommodation as a result of disintegration of zonules

Other findings: blonde, tall (marfanoid habitus with arachnodactyly), osteoporosis, fractures, seizures, mental retardation (50%), cardiomegaly, platelet abnormality with hypercoagulability (risk of thromboembolic problems, especially with general anesthesia); infants appear normal at birth; 75% mortality by age 30 years

Hyperhomocysteinemia: occurs in patients heterozygous for homocystinemia; high serum homocysteine increases risk of arterial and venous thrombosis (CRAO and central retinal vein occlusion [CRVO]) and cardiovascular disease, especially in patients with type 2 diabetes. In nondiabetic patients younger than 55 years of age who have had a stroke or myocardial infarction (MI), 25% have elevated homocysteine levels (5% in normal population)

Diagnosis: increased urinary excretion of homocysteine (nitroprusside urine test), amino acid assays; check renal function (homocysteine levels rise with elevated creatinine levels); subnormal or low levels of folate are associated with elevated levels of homocysteine

Treatment: vitamin B$_6$ (folate), methionine-restricted diet, supplementary cysteine (this diet can reduce lens dislocation); certain medications (methotrexate, phenytoin, carbamazepine) can elevate homocysteine levels by interfering with folate metabolism

Weill-Marchesani Syndrome (AR)

Findings: ectopia lentis (usually inferiorly or anteriorly), microspherophakia, high lenticular myopia, cataract, microcornea, glaucoma (pupillary block)

Other findings: short stature; short, stubby fingers with broad hands; hearing defects; inflexible joints; mental retardation

Ehlers-Danlos Syndrome (AD, AR, or X-Linked)

Defect in type III collagen; at least 9 types

Findings: ectopia lentis, easy lid eversion (Metenier sign), epicanthal folds, myopia, microcornea, blue sclera, keratoconus, angioid streaks, retinal detachment

Other findings: hyperextensible joints and skin, poor wound healing, easy bruising

Sulfite Oxidase Deficiency (AR)

Enzymatic defect causing molybdenum deficiency and increased urinary sulfite

Findings: ectopia lentis (50%), enophthalmos, Brushfield spots

Other findings: seizures, mental retardation, frontal bossing

Hyperlysinemia (AR)

Deficiency of lysine dehydrogenase

Findings: ectopia lentis, microspherophakia

Other findings: growth, motor, and mental retardation

Surgery

Nd:YAG Laser

Posterior Capsulotomy

Open visually significant posterior capsule opacity
> *Power:* 1.0–2.0 mJ; make an opening equal to the size of the pupil in ambient light
> *Treatment:* pretreat with Iopidine (apraclonidine); consider topical steroid qid × 1 week or longer for patients at risk for iritis or CME

Complications: increased IOP (glaucoma patients: 17% have rise after 2 hours, 14% with high IOP at 1 week; nonglaucoma patients: 6% have rise after 2 hours, 3% with high IOP at 1 week), RD (increased risk with axial length >25 mm), cystoid macular edema (CME), rupture of the anterior hyaloid face, IOL dislocation (increased risk with silicone plate IOL), iritis, pitting of IOL, corneal or retinal burn

Vitreolysis

Disrupt anterior vitreous face in aphakic and pseudophakic eyes with malignant glaucoma
> *Power:* 3–11 mJ, focused on anterior hyaloid; deepening of AC signifies success
> *Treatment:* topical steroid qid × 1 week and cycloplegic; vitrectomy if regimen described here fails and in phakic eyes

Relieve CME as a result of vitreous wick
> *Power:* 5–10 mJ bursts, often best to aim near wound or pigmented area of incarcerated vitreous; success occurs with a change in the pupil shape back to round
> *Treatment:* pretreat with pilocarpine to induce miosis and stretch the strand, then topical steroid × 1 week

Argon Laser

Iridoplasty

Align pupil with multifocal or extended depth of focus (EDOF) IOL in patients who have symptoms (i.e., reduced quality of vision, asymmetric glare/halo) from IOL-pupil misalignment
> *Parameters:* 500 mW power, 500 ms duration, 50 μm spot size
> *Treatment:* without a contact lens place 4 spots in midperipheral iris to enlarge pupil in that quadrant

Cataract Surgery

Indications: altered vision (based on patient's functional impairment; when patient is having visual difficulty performing tasks and does not achieve adequate improvement from corrective lenses), also medical indications (phacolytic glaucoma, phacomorphic glaucoma, phacoantigenic uveitis, narrow-angle glaucoma, dense cataract that obscures view of fundus in patients who require regular retinal evaluation [i.e., diabetes, glaucoma])

IOL Calculations

Formulas: rough estimation, use IOL power (D) = A constant of IOL – 2.5 (axial length) – 0.9 (average keratometry) (See Chapter 1, Optics)
> Anterior chamber depth (ACD) approximately 3.5 mm
> *First generation:* ACD is constant (represents estimated lens position [ELP])
> *Second generation:* ACD is based on axial length (AL)
> *Third generation* (Holladay 1, Hoffer Q, SRK/T): 2 variables: ACD is based on AL and keratometry (K)

Fourth generation (Holladay 2): 7 variables: AL, K,
    corneal diameter (HWTW), ACD, lens thickness (LT),
    refraction, and patient age
    (Haigis): 3 variables: AL, K, ACD
    (Olsen): ray tracing based on AL, K, ACD, LT
Fifth generation (Barrett Universal II): based on Gaussian
    optics, 5 variables: AL, K, HWTW, ACD, LT
    (Hoffer H-5): based on Holladay 2 and racial variations
Newer formulas (Hill-RBF): artificial intelligence
    (Ladas Super Formula): 3 variables, amalgam of
        existing formulas
Most accurate formulas according to axial length:
    Long eyes (AL >26.5 mm): Barrett, Hill RBF
    Medium-long eyes (AL 24.5–26.5 mm): Barrett, Hill RBF
    Medium eyes (AL 22.0–24.5 mm): Barrett, Hill RBF,
        Holladay 1 or 2, SRK/T, Haigis
    Short eyes (AL <22.0 mm): Hoffer Q, Holladay 2

A scan: error of 0.1 mm = 0.3 D error in lens power;
however, the shorter the axial length, the greater the effect of
a measurement error
    Myopia: 1.75 D error per mm of AL error
    Emmetropia: 2.35 D error per mm of AL error
    Hyperopia: 3.75 D error per mm of AL error
Ultrasound waves travel faster through lens (1640 m/s) than
either aqueous or vitreous (1532 m/s)

To correct any AL, use the formula:
$$AL_{corrected} = AL_{measured} \times (V_{correct}/V_{measured})$$

Average measurements:
    Axial length: 23.5 mm (22.0–24.5 mm)
    Keratometry: 43.0–44.0 D (anterior corneal curvature)
    Posterior corneal curvature: contributes approximately 0.4
        D against-the-rule astigmatism; measured directly with
        Scheimpflug imaging and ray tracing technologies
    Anterior chamber depth (ACD): 3.25 mm
    Lens thickness: 4.6 mm
    Ultrasound speeds:
        PHAKIC EYE = 1550 M/S
        APHAKIC EYE = 1532 M/S
        PSEUDOPHAKIC EYE (depends on IOL material and
            thickness) = 1556 m/s for PMMA lens, 1487 m/s for
            silicone lens, and 1549 m/s for acrylic lens
        More accurate method for calculating pseudophakic
            AL is to measure at 1532 m/s and to use correction
            factors:
                PMMA: $AL_{corrected} = AL_{1532} + 44\%$ IOL thickness + 0.04
                SILICONE: $AL_{corrected} = AL_{1532} - 56\%$ IOL
                    thickness + 0.04
                ACRYLIC: $AL_{corrected} = AL_{1532} + 75\%$ IOL
                    thickness + 0.04
        SILICONE OIL = 980 to 1040 m/s (this is only for the
            portion of the eye containing silicone); thus, to find
            the correct AL, the previous formula can be used, or
            the eye can be measured using an average velocity:
            phakic eye with silicone oil = 1140 m/s. Alternatively,
            use optical biometry (IOLMaster or Lenstar)
        If silicone oil is to be left in the eye, the index
            of refraction of the oil will cause a hyperopic
            refraction; therefore, adjust the IOL power by add-
            ing 3.0–3.5 D

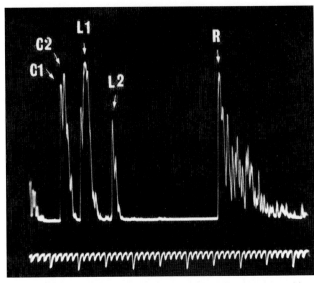

Figure 10.7 A-scan pattern of a phakic eye with the initial spike removed from the screen display. Identified are the two corneal peaks (*CI* and *C2*), the anterior lens spike (*L1*), the posterior lens spike (*L2*), and the retinal spike (*R*). (From Shammas HJ. Intraocular lens power calculations. In: Azar DT, ed. *Intraocular Lenses in Cataract and Refractive Surgery*. Philadelphia: WB Saunders; 2001.)

Immersion technique is more accurate than contact
    because of corneal compression (0.1–0.2 mm) for
    the later method. Optical biometry is most accurate

Contact A scan: 5 spikes corresponding to beam reflection
from interfaces: cornea, anterior lens surface, posterior lens
surface, retina, sclera (Fig. 10.7)
    Causes of falsely long axial length:
        Posterior staphyloma in high myopia (fovea may be
            located more anteriorly than the staphyloma)
        Measurement of the sclera rather than the retina
        Wrong ultrasonic velocity (too fast)
        Fluid meniscus between probe and cornea
        Wrong gate position (for ultrasound devices in which
            gates are manually set for the position of the differ-
            ent ocular structures)
    Causes of falsely short axial length:
        Excessive indentation of cornea with contact probe
        Nonperpendicular measurement
        Choroidal thickening or effusion
        Vitreous opacity
        Wrong ultrasonic velocity (too slow)
        Wrong gate position

**Keratometry in patient following refractive
surgery:** need to determine accurate central corneal
curvature; keratometer measures at 3 mm from center of
cornea
    Methods:
        CLINICAL HISTORY: K = preop K + (refraction
            preop – refraction postop)
            Convert for vertex distance: refraction (corneal
                surface) = refraction (spectacle plane)/(1–0.012
                refraction [spectacle plane])
        CONTACT LENS: use plano rigid gas-permeable contact
            lens with known base curve

K = base curve of CL + power + refraction (with CL) – refraction (without CL)

Convert for vertex distance

CORNEAL TOPOGRAPHY: use central 1 mm effective power reading from the Holladay diagnostic summary map (not sim K readings)

FORMULAS: numerous methods; online calculators available

Presence of cataract may induce myopia, causing error in first method, and may cause poor vision with inability to perform adequate CL overrefraction; therefore, a variety of methods should be used, then take flattest K to use in IOL calculation and consider using a final IOL 1–2 D stronger to avoid a hyperopic result

Piggyback IOL (Second IOL in Sulcus)

Different material from the IOL in the bag preferred to reduce the risk of interlenticular membrane formation between the two lens implants, and should have round edge to reduce risk of iris chafing with possible pigment dispersion, elevated IOP, or UGH syndrome

Hyperopia: Primary for patient requiring IOL power greater than maximum available IOL power

Secondary for refractive surprise; correct piggyback IOL power = 1.5 × spherical equivalent (i.e., if patient is +2.00 D, place a +3.00 D piggyback IOL)

Myopia: Secondary for refractive surprise; correct piggyback IOL power = 1.2 × spherical equivalent (i.e., if patient is –3.00, place a –3.50 D piggyback IOL)

Viscoelastic Agent (Ophthalmic Viscosurgical Device [OVD])

Variety of clear, gel-like materials composed of sodium hyaluronate and chondroitin sulfate

Used intraocularly to maintain and preserve space, displace and stabilize tissue, and coat and protect corneal endothelium

Vary in molecular weight, viscosity, clarity, ease of removal, and potential for IOP spike if retained in eye (peak usually 4–6 hours postoperatively)

Classification:

Cohesive agent (ability to adhere to itself): long chain, high molecular weight, high surface tension (low coating capability), high degree of pseudoplasticity (ability to transform from high viscosity at rest [zero shear rate] to lower viscosity at high shear rate)

ADVANTAGES: capsulorhexis, insert IOL, ease of viscoelastic removal

Examples: Healon, Healon GV, Amvisc, Amvisc Plus, Provisc

Dispersive agent: short chain, low molecular weight, low surface tension (high coating ability), low to moderate pseudoplasticity

ADVANTAGES: corneal coating, less IOP rise if retained, maintain space, move tissue

Examples: Viscoat, Vitrax, Ocucoat

Viscoadaptive agent: ultrahigh molecular weight, superviscous and cohesive at low shear rates, more dispersive at increasing shear rates; thus combines the advantages of cohesive and dispersive agents

Example: Healon 5

Phacodynamics

Irrigation: rate of fluid delivery; determined by bottle height above eye (34–110 cm); not adjusted by machine; depends on aspiration rate and wound leakage; maintains ACD

Flow (aspiration rate [AFR]): rate of fluid removal (0–60 mL/min); determines how quickly vacuum is created; attracts material to tip

Vacuum (aspiration level): negative pressure created at tip by pump (0–500 mmHg); holds material onto occluded tip

Pump systems:

Flow-based: independent, direct control of AFR and vacuum; vacuum rise requires tip occlusion; physically contacts and regulates aspiration line fluid

PERISTALTIC: rollers compress tubing; AFR not smooth because of peristaltic wave; less accurate, especially at higher vacuum levels

SCROLL: scroll element orbits against housing; more accurate; can act clinically like Venturi pump

Vacuum-based: direct control of vacuum only; AFR indirectly controlled by vacuum level; vacuum not affected by changes in tip occlusion; indirectly contacts aspiration line fluid by the induced vacuum in rigid drainage cassette between line and pump

VENTURI: compressed air flows through tube; rapid, precise aspiration and vacuum response; requires external air supply

DIAPHRAGM: flexible membrane moves like a piston; outmoded, large, noisy system

ROTARY VANE: wheel with vanes rotates; does not require external air supply

Hybrid: programmable like peristaltic or Venturi

Vacuum rise time: time for vacuum to reach preset limit; affected by aspiration rate; requires tip occlusion with peristaltic pump

Postocclusion surge (vacuum rush): collapse of AC resulting from an increase in aspiration rate to level of pump speed; during occlusion, vacuum builds to preset level, no flow occurs, and tubing collapses; when occlusion breaks, pump pulls fluid at preset rate and rebound of tubing pulls additional fluid through tip. Risk reduced by lowering maximum vacuum setting; prevented by venting, rigid tubing, microprocessor in pump

Followability: ability to bring material to tip; function of flow and vacuum

Holdability: ability to keep material at tip; function of vacuum and power

Phaco power (0%–100%): depends on frequency and stroke length; surgeon (linear) or panel control; pushes material away from tip; generates heat.

Power factors: amplitude (fixed vs. linear) and duration (continuous vs. intermittent)

Power modulation: pulse, burst, bimodal, dual linear

Ultrasound effect:

Fragmentation: mechanical (jackhammer effect)

Cavitation: sound waves expand and compress liquid, creating shock wave and microbubbles, which implode, forming cavity and dissolving nucleus in front of needle tip

Ultrasound instrument:

Handpiece: produces vibration of needle

MAGNETORESTRICTIVE: converts magnetic energy into motion

PIEZOELECTRIC CRYSTAL: converts electricity into motion

Needle: oscillation produces phaco power

FREQUENCY: rate of oscillation (25–62 kHz)

STROKE LENGTH: distance of travel (0.002–0.004 inch [0.05–0.1 mm])

BEVEL: occlusion versus cutting (0–45°)

TIP SIZE/BORE: 0.9, 1.1, flared

SHAPE: straight, angled

INNOVATIONS: microflow, microseal, aspiration bypass (ABS), torsional, elliptical

Foot pedal: usual settings; can be programmed differently

KICK LEFT: reflux

POSITION 0: resting

POSITION 1: irrigation

POSITION 2: aspiration

POSITION 3: ultrasound

Audible clues:

METALLIC CLICK: irrigation (plunger opens)

HUMMING: aspiration

BUZZING: ultrasound (harmonic overtones)

BELLS: occlusion (no flow)

Customized tones

Alternative systems: Sonic, Fluid, Laser

Complications of Cataract Surgery

Preoperative (retrobulbar/peribulbar injection):

Globe perforation

Retrobulbar hemorrhage

Strabismus (inferior rectus fibrosis or myotoxicity)

Central anesthesia

Intraoperative:

Wound burn

Iris prolapse

Iris damage

Intraoperative floppy iris syndrome (IFIS)

Descemet membrane detachment

Capsule damage (radial tear, posterior rupture, zonulolysis)

Retained material (nucleus, cortex)

Vitreous loss

Choroidal effusion

Suprachoroidal hemorrhage

Phototoxicity

Postoperative:

Wound leak

Inadvertent filtering bleb

Epithelial downgrowth

Corneal edema

Corneal melt

Toxic anterior segment syndrome (TASS)

Secondary glaucoma

UGH syndrome

Sputtering hyphema (vascularization of posterior wound lip; malpositioned IOL)

Pupillary capture of IOL

IOL decentration

Capsular block syndrome

Anterior capsular contraction syndrome

Posterior capsular opacification (PCO)

CME

RD

Endophthalmitis

Mydriasis

Ptosis

Retrobulbar Hemorrhage

May occur following retrobulbar injection or trauma; risk of CRAO as orbital pressure rises

Findings: marked proptosis, rapid orbital swelling and congestion, limited extraocular motility, hemorrhagic chemosis, lid ecchymosis and edema

Treatment: consider emergent surgical decompression with lateral canthotomy and cantholysis, hyperosmotic agents to lower IOP

Strabismus

Caused by inferior rectus damage

Paralysis or fibrosis result from anesthetic injection

Central Anesthesia Following Retrobulbar Block

Agent spreads along meningeal cuff of optic nerve to enter cerebrospinal fluid (CSF)

Increased risk with 4% lidocaine

Findings: mental confusion, dysphagia, dyspnea, apnea, amaurosis of fellow eye

Wound Burn

Thermal injury from phaco needle resulting from lack of irrigation

Etiology: excessively tight incision, low or empty infusion bottle, low-flow settings, occluded phaco tip (with dispersive viscoelastic agent or impaled nucleus), phaco needle without thermal protective design

Findings: wound whitening, distortion, and astigmatism; warning sign is lens milk/dust (milky substance) near phaco tip

Treatment: immediately stop phaco, check for incision tightness and phaco tip obstruction; scleral relaxing incision, horizontal suture, bandage contact lens; if severe, may require astigmatic surgery after stabilization or patch graft

Iris Prolapse During Phaco

Wound too large or too posterior, bottle too high, increased IOP, suprachoroidal hemorrhage

Intraoperative Floppy Iris Syndrome (IFIS)

Altered iris dilator tone resulting from systemic α_1 blocker medications (most commonly tamsulosin [Flomax]) with varying degrees of poor iris dilation and atonic floppy iris tissue (billows and prolapses), which may increase the risk of intraoperative complications during cataract surgery

Treatment: one or a combination of approaches depending on the severity of IFIS including preoperative topical atropine, intraoperative use of preservative free epinephrine or phenylephrine and ketorolac (Omidria), Healon 5, pupil expansion devices (i.e., Malyugin ring, Graether expander, Morcher dilator), iris hooks; manual pupil stretching does not help. Stopping the medication does not prevent IFIS and may lead to urinary retention

Descemet Membrane Detachment

Caused by inadvertent stripping of Descemet from instrument insertion during surgery or viscoelastic injection; causes corneal edema or decompensation

Treatment: air or gas bubble, may require repair with suture

Suprachoroidal Hemorrhage

May occur during intraocular surgery or days later

Risk factors: elderly patient, hypertension, atherosclerosis, diabetes, sudden drop in IOP during surgery, high myopia, vitreous loss or previous vitrectomy, previous expulsive hemorrhage in fellow eye, glaucoma, aphakia, postoperative Valsalva maneuver

Findings: forward movement of intraocular contents during surgery and loss of red reflex (ominous sign), extremely firm eye, subretinal hemorrhage, choroidal detachment, and extrusion of intraocular contents in most severe form (expulsive suprachoroidal hemorrhage); delayed hemorrhage presents with severe eye pain, nausea, vomiting, and rapid loss of vision

Treatment: close wound rapidly; may require surgical drainage

Prevention: decompress eye preoperatively, small wound, control BP during surgery, prevent bucking in patients under general anesthesia

Phototoxicity

Occurs in up to 39% for surgical time >100 minutes

Prevention: dim light, oblique light, pupil shield

Corneal Edema

Etiology: trauma to endothelium, elevated IOP, endothelial chemical toxicity, Descemet detachment, decompensation in patient with Fuchs corneal endothelial dystrophy

Corneal Ulceration and Melting

Occurs most commonly after cataract surgery in patients with keratoconjunctivitis sicca and rheumatoid arthritis; melting several weeks after uncomplicated cataract surgery as a result of collagenase release from surrounding inflammatory cells

Toxic Anterior Segment Syndrome (TASS)

Anterior segment inflammation following intraocular surgery; most commonly acute, within 24 hours of uncomplicated cataract extraction, and severe with corneal edema, AC reaction, and variable pain; may have increased IOP chemosis, keratic precipitates (KP), hypopyon, vitreous opacities, macular edema; can be mild and delayed (several months), and may occur after keratoplasty and posterior segment procedures

Etiology: form of sterile postoperative endophthalmitis resulting from toxicity from noninfectious exogenous contaminant (i.e., biofilm, endotoxins, enzymatic detergents, surgical instrument, intraocular solutions, compounded intraocular solutions, ophthalmic viscoelastic agents, IOL)

Treatment: rule out infectious endophthalmitis; treat promptly with frequent topical steroids to prevent damage to corneal endothelium, TM, and macula; consider topical nonsteroidal anti-inflammatory (NSAID); may require systemic steroids and topical ocular hypotensive medications; may require endothelial keratoplasty for corneal decompensation (wait at least 3 months), glaucoma surgery, or intravitreal steroid or anti-VEGF injections for CME

Uveitis-Glaucoma-Hyphema (UGH) Syndrome

Caused by repeated trauma to angle structures and iris by IOL; scarring and degeneration occur

Treatment: atropine, topical steroids, ocular hypotensive medications; consider argon laser of bleeding site; usually requires IOL explantation

Hyphema

Result of fine neovascularization of scleral incision (Swan syndrome) or mechanical trauma from IOL haptics

Occurs with more posteriorly located incisions

IOP can become dangerously elevated

Pupillary Capture

Portion of IOL optic anterior to iris

Risk factors: large or incomplete capsulorhexis, sulcus haptic placement, nonangulated IOL, upside-down IOL placement, vitreous pressure

Treatment: observe if long-standing and stable without symptoms; dilate and place patient supine if occurs early postoperatively; may require lens repositioning

IOL Decentration

Causes diplopia or polyopia because of prismatic effect

Sunset syndrome: inferior displacement of IOL within capsular bag; occurs with unrecognized zonular dialysis, capsular tears, or asymmetric IOL haptic implantation (1 in bag and other in sulcus)

Sunrise syndrome: superior displacement of IOL; occurs with asymmetric IOL haptic placement or capsular contraction

Treatment: consider pilocarpine; IOL repositioning or exchange may be required

Capsular Block Syndrome

Caused by retained viscoelastic behind IOL

Causes myopic shift

Treatment: Nd:YAG laser anterior capsulotomy

Anterior Capsular Contraction Syndrome (Capsular Phimosis)

Caused by small capsulorhexis with retention of lens epithelial cells

Treatment: Nd:YAG laser radial anterior capsulotomies

CME (Irvine-Gass Syndrome)

More common with intracapsular (ICCE) than extracapsular cataract extraction (ECCE)

50% angiographically for ICCE versus 15% for ECCE

Clinically significant (visual loss) in <1% of patients with ECCE

Risk factors: capsular rupture, dislocated IOL, iris-supported IOL, iris tuck, vitreous adhesion to pupil or wound; also patients with diabetes, epiretinal membrane, and retinal vein occlusion

Fluorescein angiography (FA): petaloid hyperfluorescence, late leakage; late staining of optic nerve

helps to differentiate postoperative CME from other forms of CME

OCT: increased foveal thickness; intraretinal cystoid spaces

Treatment: topical steroid and NSAID, consider posterior sub-Tenon steroid injection with Kenalog

Endophthalmitis

(See Chapter 8, Uveitis)

Rhegmatogenous Retinal Detachment

Incidence: 1%–2%

Risk factors: high myopia, lattice degeneration, no previous posterior vitreous detachment (PVD), history of RD in fellow eye, vitreous loss

Mydriasis

Caused by sphincter damage (mechanical from iris stretching or ischemic from elevated IOP [Urrets-Zavalia syndrome])

Ptosis

Caused by trauma from lid speculum

REVIEW QUESTIONS (Answers start on page 426)

1. The most helpful test for evaluating macular function in a patient with advanced cataract is
   a. blue field entoptic phenomenon
   b. 2-light separation
   c. red-light discrimination
   d. directional light projection
2. Ectopia lentis is *least* likely to be associated with
   a. cleft palate
   b. pectus excavatum
   c. short stature
   d. mental retardation
3. Anterior segment signs of CB melanoma include all of the following, *except*
   a. corneal edema
   b. increased IOP
   c. astigmatism
   d. cataract
4. Which of the following is *least* characteristic of ICE syndrome?
   a. corneal edema
   b. increased IOP
   c. ectropion uveae
   d. PAS
5. A stellate anterior subcapsular cataract is most likely to be found in a patient with
   a. Fabry disease
   b. atopic dermatitis
   c. myotonic dystrophy
   d. electrical injury

6. Which of the following does *not* occur in siderosis bulbi?
   a. glaucoma
   b. retinal atrophy
   c. sunflower cataract
   d. fixed pupil

7. A patient has a history of increased IOP with exercise; which finding is associated with this condition?
   a. Krukenberg spindle
   b. PAS
   c. phacodonesis
   d. pars plana snowbank

8. Separation between the longitudinal and circumferential fibers of the ciliary muscle is called
   a. iridoschisis
   b. angle recession
   c. iridodialysis
   d. cyclodialysis

9. Characteristics of pigment dispersion syndrome include all of the following, *except*
   a. increased IOP with exercise
   b. Krukenberg spindle
   c. phacodonesis
   d. radial iris transillumination defects

10. A patient with sickle cell with a hyphema develops increased IOP; which of the following treatment choices is best?
    a. pilocarpine
    b. acetazolamide
    c. hyperosmotic
    d. timolol

11. Of the following causes of iris heterochromia, the involved iris is hyperchromic in
    a. ICE syndrome
    b. Horner syndrome
    c. Waardenburg syndrome
    d. Fuchs heterochromic iridocyclitis

12. Which of the following iris lesions is a true tumor?
    a. Kunkmann-Wolffian body
    b. Koeppe nodule
    c. Lisch nodule
    d. JXG

13. At which location is the lens capsule the thinnest?
    a. anterior capsule
    b. posterior capsule
    c. equatorial capsule
    d. anterior paracentral capsule

14. Which of the following is *not* associated with sunset syndrome?
    a. asymmetric IOL haptic placement
    b. polyopia
    c. pseudoexfoliation
    d. hyphema

15. Lens epithelial cells differentiate into lens fibers
    a. anterior to the equator
    b. at the equator
    c. posterior to the equator
    d. in the fetal nucleus

16. Light of which wavelength is absorbed the greatest by a dense nuclear sclerotic cataract?
    a. red
    b. green
    c. yellow
    d. blue

17. A patient with background diabetic retinopathy and clinically significant macular edema desires cataract surgery. The most appropriate management is
    a. cataract surgery
    b. focal laser treatment, then cataract surgery
    c. cataract surgery, then panretinal photocoagulation
    d. cataract surgery with intraoperative laser treatment

18. After finishing phacoemulsification on a dense cataract, the surgeon notes whitening of the clear corneal incision. The most likely cause is
    a. tight incision
    b. high aspiration flow rate
    c. high phaco power
    d. 45° bevel phaco needle

19. Nuclear brunescence increases with higher concentrations of which lens protein?
    a. alpha crystallin
    b. beta crystallin
    c. gamma crystallin
    d. main intrinsic protein

20. Lens fibers contain nuclei in all of the following conditions, *except*
    a. trisomy 13
    b. syphilis
    c. rubella
    d. Lowe syndrome

21. The most likely cause of an intraoperative complication during cataract surgery in a patient with pseudoexfoliation syndrome is
    a. small pupil
    b. thin posterior capsule
    c. weak zonules
    d. shallow AC

22. The majority of glucose metabolism in the lens is by
    a. glycolysis
    b. pentose phosphate pathway
    c. reduction to sorbitol
    d. conversion to glucuronic acid

23. The most appropriate systemic treatment for a patient with a sunflower cataract is
    a. insulin
    b. penicillamine
    c. steroids
    d. methotrexate

24. Which of the following is the *least* likely cause of decreased vision 2 years after cataract surgery?
    a. subluxed IOL
    b. RD
    c. posterior capsular opacity
    d. CME

25. Which type of cataract is most closely associated with UV-B exposure?
    a. anterior subcapsular
    b. cortical
    c. nuclear sclerotic
    d. posterior subcapsular

26. Which of the following strategies is *least* likely to be effective for treating IFIS?
    a. atropine
    b. Healon 5
    c. manual pupil stretching
    d. Malyugin ring

27. Ocular melanoma is *least* likely to occur in which portion of the uvea?
    a. conjunctiva
    b. iris
    c. ciliary body
    d. choroid

28. A patient reports acute pain while hammering metal and presents with 20/20 vision, subconjunctival hemorrhage, and small hyphema OD. The most appropriate test to obtain is
    a. FA
    b. OCT
    c. MRI
    d. CT

29. A patient with a traumatic cataract requires cataract surgery. Which of the following is most helpful?
    a. laser interferometer
    b. Amsler grid
    c. brightness acuity test
    d. visual field

30. Pseudoexfoliation syndrome and pigment dispersion syndrome share which of the following findings?
    a. deep AC angles
    b. pigmented trabecular meshwork
    c. poor pupillary dilation
    d. phacodonesis

31. The most likely cause of monocular diplopia after blunt trauma is
    a. orbital fracture
    b. hyphema
    c. lens subluxation
    d. macular hole

32. Which of the following tests is most helpful in a patient with a Morgagnian cataract?
    a. ANCA
    b. HbA1c
    c. HLA-B27
    d. RPR

33. A truck driver desires the best range of vision after cataract surgery. Which IOL strategy is most appropriate?
    a. apodized diffractive lens
    b. zonal refractive lens
    c. mini-monovision with accommodating lens
    d. monovision with monofocal lens

34. One week after cataract surgery, a patient has increased AC cells and flare, IOP of 36 mm Hg, and a nuclear fragment in the inferior angle. Which is the most appropriate treatment option?
    a. increase the topical antibiotic
    b. increase the topical steroid
    c. perform a paracentesis
    d. remove the retained fragment

35. Which of the following tools is most helpful when performing surgery on a patient with a mature cataract?
    a. Trypan blue
    b. intracameral epinephrine
    c. cohesive OVD
    d. Malyugin ring

36. Glaukomflecken is caused by
    a. trauma
    b. steroids
    c. inflammation
    d. ischemia

37. Which of the following symptoms is *least* associated with posterior subcapsular cataracts?
    a. increased glare
    b. poor blue discrimination
    c. near vision affected more than distance vision
    d. reduced vision from bright lights

38. A piggyback IOL is most likely to be necessary in which of the following conditions?
    a. status post vitrectomy
    b. pseudoexfoliation syndrome
    c. high hyperopia
    d. diabetes

39. A 77-year-old woman with cataracts and macular degeneration is interested in cataract surgery. The most helpful test for evaluating this patient is
    a. Amsler grid
    b. brightness acuity test
    c. contrast sensitivity
    d. potential acuity meter

40. In which situation does optical biometry have the largest advantage over ultrasound biometry in determining an accurate measurement?
    a. keratoconus
    b. posterior subcapsular cataract
    c. high myopia
    d. after LASIK

41. During phacoemulsification a milky substance (lens milk) appears. What is the most appropriate next step?
    a. check for tight incision
    b. raise irrigation bottle
    c. increase aspiration and vacuum settings
    d. add more OVD

42. Which of the following is the most likely complication of Nd:YAG laser posterior capsulotomy?
    a. hypotony
    b. corneal burn
    c. retinal detachment
    d. epiretinal membrane

43. A patient with vitreous to the wound is most at risk for which postoperative complication?
    a. endophthalmitis
    b. retinal detachment
    c. increased IOP
    d. cystoid macular edema

44. On postop day 1 after cataract surgery, exam shows wound gape and a flat AC. The most appropriate treatment is
    a. cycloplegia
    b. bandage contact lens
    c. suture wound
    d. inject OVD

45. A silicone IOL should *not* be used in a patient with
    a. Fuchs corneal dystrophy
    b. proliferative diabetic retinopathy
    c. pseudoexfoliation syndrome
    d. macular degeneration

46. A patient with a posterior subcapsular cataract desires surgery. What is the most appropriate reason for performing cataract surgery?
    a. patient complains of glare and difficulty reading
    b. visual acuity at near is worse than at distance
    c. distance visual acuity is reduced in a bright room
    d. visual acuity improves after dilation

47. An anterior subcapsular cataract is most likely to develop in a patient with which skin condition?
    a. pemphigus
    b. Stevens-Johnson syndrome
    c. epidermolysis bullosa
    d. atopic dermatitis

48. Reduced color discrimination is most likely caused by which type of cataract?
    a. anterior subcapsular
    b. cortical
    c. nuclear sclerotic
    d. posterior polar

49. Which of the following is most likely to occur following cataract surgery in a patient with previous myopic LASIK?
    a. flap dislocation
    b. hyperopia
    c. diffuse lamellar keratitis
    d. corneal edema

50. A patient with no visual complaints is noted to have pupillary capture of an IOL. What is the most appropriate management?
    a. observation
    b. cycloplegia
    c. reposition IOL
    d. IOL exchange

51. One day after uncomplicated cataract surgery with phacoemulsification, the exam shows counting fingers vision, 3+ corneal edema with Descemet folds, and severe AC reaction with fibrinous material. The most likely diagnosis is
    a. vitreous in AC
    b. angle closure
    c. toxic anterior segment syndrome
    d. endophthalmitis

52. A patient with high hyperopia is at increased risk for which of the following complications of cataract surgery?
    a. posterior capsule tear
    b. CME
    c. RD
    d. choroidal effusion

53. The largest risk for capsule rupture during hydrodissection occurs with
    a. small pupil
    b. pseudoexfoliation syndrome
    c. posterior polar cataract
    d. mature cataract

54. After hydrodissection, you notice capsular block. The next step is to
    a. raise the irrigation bottle
    b. add OVD
    c. burp the wound
    d. decompress the nucleus and lift the anterior capsule

55. Which of the following measures is most likely to reduce the risk of postocclusion surge during phacoemulsification?
    a. increase the aspiration flow rate setting
    b. reduce the maximum vacuum setting
    c. lower the irrigation bottle height
    d. increase the tubing compliance

56. Which of the following IOL designs is most likely to be associated with a complication of laser posterior capsulotomy?
    a. PMMA one piece
    b. acrylic one piece
    c. silicone plate haptic
    d. silicone three piece

57. A patient with previous radial keratotomy surgery undergoes uncomplicated phacoemulsification. Two weeks after the cataract surgery, the patient states that her vision is blurry and unchanged. Her refraction is +2.00 +0.50 × 30, which improves her vision to 20/20. At this point, the most appropriate management options is
    a. observation
    b. conductive keratoplasty
    c. PRK with mitomycin C
    d. piggyback IOL

58. What is the most appropriate treatment for a patient with a hyphema and persistent elevated IOP for 1 week despite maximal medical therapy?
    a. oral steroids and aminocaproic acid
    b. hemoglobin electrophoresis
    c. paracentesis
    d. AC washout

59. A 32-year-old man presents 1 week after blunt trauma with 20/20 visual acuity and a dilated, unresponsive pupil OD. The most appropriate next step is
    a. careful slit lamp exam of iris
    b. hydroxyamphetamine test
    c. VDRL
    d. MRI

60. Which of the following IOL designs is most appropriate for placement in the sulcus?
    a. 1-piece acrylic
    b. truncated optic
    c. 5 mm optic
    d. 13.5 mm PMMA
61. One day after cataract surgery, a patient has an IOP of 6 mmHg. The AC is formed, and the 2.4 mm cataract incision is Seidel positive, demonstrating a slow, intermittent leak. Which of the following treatment options is most appropriate?
    a. observation
    b. timolol
    c. pilocarpine
    d. pressure patch
62. When performing a capsulorhexis in a patient with a mature cataract, which of the following is most helpful to prevent splitting of the anterior capsule?
    a. inject capsular dye to stain the capsule
    b. use a dispersive OVD to tamponade the lens
    c. create a can-opener capsulotomy
    d. aspirate liquid cortex from a small capsular opening and then enlarge
63. During phacoemulsification, the pupil is noted to suddenly dilate, and the AC deepens. What is the most likely cause?
    a. infusion misdirection syndrome
    b. posterior capsular rupture
    c. choroidal effusion
    d. suprachoroidal hemorrhage
64. Which type of IOL is best for sulcus placement?
    a. one-piece acrylic
    b. accommodating
    c. three-piece acrylic
    d. plate haptic
65. The type of cataract with the *least* effect on visual function is
    a. membranous
    b. cortical
    c. sutural
    d. posterior polar
66. All of the following are risk factors for the progression of an iris nevus, *except*
    a. older age
    b. ectropion uvea
    c. diffuse appearance
    d. hyphema
67. The retina is *least* protected from UV light by the
    a. cornea
    b. aqueous
    c. lens
    d. vitreous

Please visit the eBook for an interactive version of the review questions. See front cover for activation details.

SUGGESTED READINGS

Abelson, M. B. (2001). *Allergic diseases of the eye*. Philadelphia: WB Saunders.
Azar, D. T. (2019). *Refractive surgery* (3rd ed.). Philadelphia: Elsevier.
Basic and Clinical Sciences Course. (2021). *Section 11: Lens and cataract*. San Francisco: AAO.
Basic and Clinical Sciences Course. (2021). *Section 13: Refractive surgery*. San Francisco: AAO.
Boruchoff, S. A. (2001). *Anterior segment disorder: A diagnostic color atlas*. Boston: Butterworth-Heinemann.
Henderson, B. A. (2014). *Essentials of cataract surgery* (2nd ed.). Thorofare: SLACK.
Mackie, I. A. (2003). *External eye disease*. Boston: Butterworth-Heinemann.
Watson, P. G., Hazleman, B. L., McCluskey, P., & Pavesio, C. E. (2012). *Sclera and systemic disorders* (3rd ed.). London: JP Medical.

Posterior Segment

ANATOMY
PHYSIOLOGY
ELECTROPHYSIOLOGY
RETINAL IMAGING
DISORDERS
LASER TREATMENT

ANATOMY

Vitreous

Volume ~4 mL (~80% volume of globe), composed of ~98% water and 0.15% macromolecules (collagen, hyaluronan, and proteins); viscous, gel-like quality from mucopolysaccharide and hyaluronic acid that is folded into coiled chains and holds water like a sponge

Components: collagen fibers (type II [mainly], type IX, and type V/XI), chondroitin sulfate (main form is versican), opticin, VIT1, fibrillin, hyaluronidase, matrix metalloproteinase-2 (MMP-2), serum proteins and solutes (depend on integrity of blood–ocular barrier: iris vessel vascular endothelium, ciliary body [CB] nonpigmented epithelium, Schlemm canal inner wall endothelium, retinal vessel vascular endothelium, and retinal pigment epithelium [REP]); Na^+ and Cl^- concentrations similar to plasma, K^+ and ascorbate concentrations higher than plasma; few cells, hyalocytes, regulate immunologic response (also involved in epiretinal membrane formation); syneresis (liquefaction) occurs with aging (begins at approximately age 40 years), associated with loss of ascorbate (vitamin C eliminates oxygen reducing oxidative damage to lens, preventing cataract). After vitrectomy, lack of ascorbate allows increased oxygen diffusion and cataract formation. Mutations in *VCAN* gene (encodes versican) associated with optical empty vitreous (i.e., Wagner syndrome) (Figs. 11.1 and 11.2)

Vitreous base: portion of vitreous that attaches to peripheral retina and pars plana; 6-mm width (2 mm anterior and 4 mm posterior to the ora serrata); straddles ora serrata; avulsion is pathognomonic for trauma

Vitreoretinal junctions: arise from footplates of Müller cells at internal limiting membrane; provide firm vitreoretinal attachment, especially at vitreous base, macula, optic nerve, and retinal vessels; also at edge of lattice degeneration, chorioretinal scars, degenerative remodeling, enclosed ora bays; weak attachments at fovea and disc, and over areas of lattice. Adhesion of cortical vitreous collagen fibers and internal limiting membrane (ILM) is mediated by laminin, fibronectin, and chondroitin sulfate

Retina (Fig. 11.3)

Neurosensory retina (9 layers): inner refers to proximal or vitreous side of retina; composed of neurons (photoreceptor, bipolar, horizontal, amacrine, and ganglion cells) and glial cells (Müller cells, astrocytes, and microglia); converts light into electrical signal by phototransduction in rod and cone outer segments; information transmitted from retina to optic nerve via 3-neuron pathway (photoreceptor to bipolar to ganglion cell), horizontal and amacrine cells regulate flow; glial cells support the neurons. Retinal thickness ~0.23 mm at optic nerve, ~0.11 mm at ora serrata

1. *Internal limiting membrane (ILM):* foot processes of Müller cells (periodic acid-Schiff [PAS]-positive basement membrane); true basement membrane; clinically visible as small yellow–white spots (Gunn dots) at ora serrata; continuous with inner bordering membrane of CB
2. *Nerve fiber layer (NFL):* unmyelinated ganglion cell axons; also contains glial cells (astrocytes); myelination by oligodendrocytes occurs at lamina cribrosa; axons synapse with nuclei of cells in lateral geniculate body (LGB)
3. *Ganglion cell layer:* second neuron; usually a single cell layer with cells packed tightly near the optic disc and more scattered in the periphery; nuclei are multilayered in macula. Synapse with bipolar cells (on-bipolar to on-ganglion, and off-bipolar to off-ganglion); 3 types of ganglion cells: tonic from L or M cones, tonic from S cones, and phasic
4. *Inner plexiform layer:* synaptic processes between bipolar and ganglion cells, and amacrine and bipolar

335

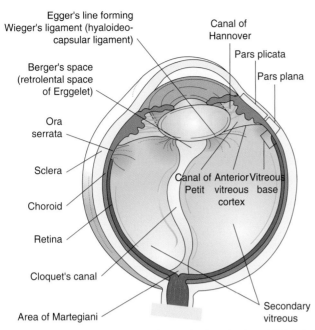

Egger's line forming Wieger's ligament (hyaloideo-capsular ligament)

Berger's space (retrolental space of Erggelet)

Canal of Hannover

Pars plicata

Pars plana

Ora serrata

Sclera

Choroid

Retina

Cloquet's canal

Area of Martegiani

Canal of Petit

Anterior vitreous

Vitreous base

Secondary vitreous

Figure 11.1 Vitreous anatomy according to classic anatomic and histologic studies. (From Schepens CL, Neetens A. *The Vitreous and Vitreoretinal Interface.* New York: Springer-Verlag; 1987.)

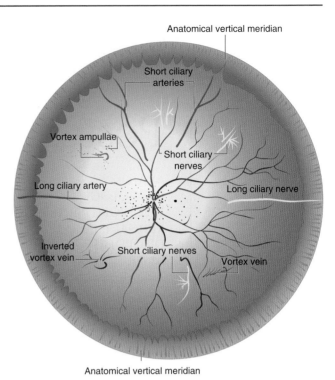

Anatomical vertical meridian

Short ciliary arteries

Vortex ampullae

Short ciliary nerves

Long ciliary artery

Long ciliary nerve

Inverted vortex vein

Short ciliary nerves

Vortex vein

Anatomical vertical meridian

Figure 11.3 Normal fundus as seen through indirect ophthalmoscope. (From Richard, JA, ed. *Practical Ophthalmology: A Manual for Beginning Residents,* 3rd ed. San Francisco: AAO; 1980, p. 122, Fig. 60.)

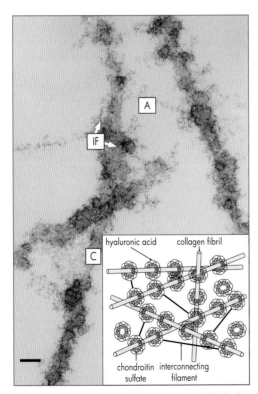

hyaluronic acid

collagen fibril

chondroitin sulfate

interconnecting filament

Figure 11.2 Ultrastructure of hyaluronan–collagen interaction in the vitreous. *C,* Collagen; *IF,* interconnecting filament. (Courtesy of Dr. Akiko Asakura. From Askura A. Histochemistry of hyaluronic acid of the bovine vitreous body as studied by electron microscopy. *Acta Soc Ophthalmol.* 1985;89:179–191.)

cells; outermost layer completely nourished by retinal arteries

5. ***Inner nuclear layer***: first neuron; inner 2/3 of retina receives its nourishment from retinal vasculature (outer 1/3 from choroid); contains superficial and deep capillaries; cell bodies of bipolar, horizontal (confined to outer surface), amacrine (confined to inner surface), and Müller (span from ILM [foot processes] to external limiting membrane [ELM; microvilli, which point toward RPE]) cells. Bipolar cells different for rods (1 type) and cones (9–12 types); cone bipolar cells are on-bipolar (excited by light, inhibited by dark) and off-bipolar (inhibited by light, excited by dark). Horizontal cells provide negative feedback to cones. Amacrine cells are inhibitory interneurons that delay the signals between bipolar and ganglion cells. Müller cells are supportive (regulate ionic in extracellular space, form ELM, may be involved in cone vitamin A metabolism)

6. ***Outer plexiform layer***: synaptic processes between photoreceptors and dendritic processes of bipolar cells; cone axons = Henle fibers

    MIDDLE LIMITING MEMBRANE (MLM): synapses; forms approximate border of vascular inner portion and avascular outer portion of the retina; barrier to exudates

    Central retinal artery supplies retina internally (MLM to ILM)

    Choriocapillaris supplies retina externally (MLM to RPE)

    Interior to MLM: dendrites of bipolar cells along with horizontally coursing processes of horizontal cells

External to MLM: basal aspect of photoreceptors

In macula, outer plexiform layer is called *Henle fiber layer*; radial orientation of fibers (responsible for macular star configuration and cystic spaces in cystoid macular edema)

7. *Outer nuclear layer*: photoreceptor cell bodies and nuclei; most cone nuclei lie in single layer immediately internal to ELM

8. *External limiting membrane (ELM)*: fenestrated intercellular bridges, situated external to photoreceptor nuclei; interconnects photoreceptor cells to Müller cells; not a true basement membrane but an illusion caused by tight junctions between Müller cells and photoreceptors

9. *Photoreceptor layer*: rods and cones; number equal in macula; 11-*cis* retinal converted to all-*trans* retinol in photoreceptor outer segments (not in RPE where it is converted back) (Fig. 11.4)

120 MILLION RODS: rods account for 95% of photoreceptors; rhodopsin; density maximal in a ring 20°–40° around fovea, no rods in center of fovea; when dark adapted, rods are 1000 x more sensitive than cones; rod disks are not attached to cell membrane, discrete structures; provide dark adapted vision

6 MILLION CONES (50% IN MACULA): 3 types of visual pigment (S [short-wavelength sensitive, blue, make up only 2%], M [middle-wavelength sensitive, green, 33%], and L [long-wavelength sensitive, red, 65%]); density maximal in fovea; cone disks are attached to cell membrane and undergo membranous replacement; provide high acuity and color vision

Peripheral retina: extends from macula to ora serrata, nonpigmented epithelium is contiguous with pars plana; defined as any area of the retina with a single layer of ganglion cells (Fig. 11.5). Equator is 14 mm, and vortex veins are 14-25 mm from limbus

Ora serrata: border between CB nonpigmented epithelium and peripheral retina, site of vitreous base attachment (2 mm wide), appears smooth temporally and serrated nasally, 8 mm posterior to limbus (approximated by spiral of Tillaux, the imaginary spiral line that passes through rectus muscle insertions)

Macula: central area of retina where ganglion cell layer is >1 cell thick (5.5 mm in diameter)

Centered 4 mm temporal and 0.8 mm inferior to optic nerve

Differentiation of the macula does not occur until age 4-6 months old

Predominantly red and green cones in macula

High levels of carotenoids (100–1000 × more than anywhere else): lutein (antioxidant) and zeaxanthin (light screening), create yellow color (macula lutea)

Blood supply from temporal short and long posterior ciliary vessels

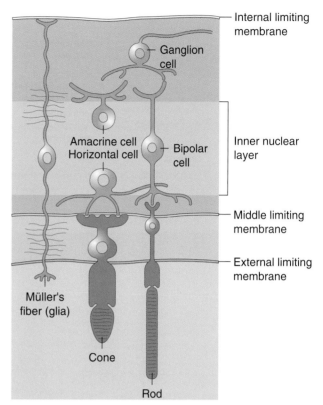

Figure 11.4 Neuronal connections in the retina and participating cells. (From Schubert HD. Structure and function of the neural retina. In: Yanoff M, Duker JS, eds. *Ophthalmology*. London: Mosby; 1999.)

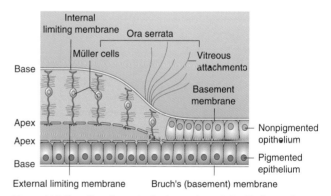

Figure 11.5 Transition of neural retina to nonpigmented epithelium at the ora serrata. (From Schubert HD. Structure and function of the neural retina. In: Yanoff M, Duker JS, eds. *Ophthalmology*. London: Mosby; 1999.)

Fovea (Figs. 11.6 and 11.7): central depression of inner retinal surface (1.5 mm in diameter; 0.55 mm thick at margin) within macula

Foveal avascular zone (FAZ) is 250-600 μm in diameter

Contains taller RPE cells and xanthophyll pigment (blocks choroidal fluorescence during fluorescein angiography)

Initially, ganglion cell nuclei are present in fovea but are gradually displaced peripherally, leaving fovea devoid of accessory neural elements

Floor of the fovea is made up of specialized Müller cells in inverted cone shape (Müller cell cone), likely a reservoir for concentrated xanthophyll and structural support for foveola

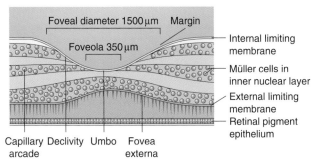

Figure 11.6 Foveal margin, foveal declivity, foveola, and umbo. (From Schubert HD. Structure and function of the neural retina. In: Yanoff M, Duker JS, eds. *Ophthalmology*. London: Mosby; 1999.)

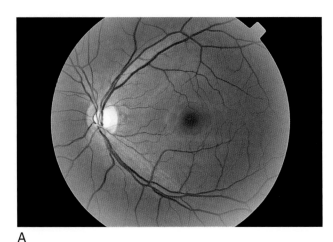

Figure 11.7 Normal fundus with macula encompassed by major vascular arcades. (From Schubert HD. Structure and function of the neural retina. In: Yanoff M, Duker JS, eds. *Ophthalmology*. London: Mosby; 1999.)

Foveola: central area of fovea (350 μm in diameter, 100 μm thick)

Absence of ganglion cells and other nucleated cells, only cones and elongated Müller cells, no rods; avascular, nourished by choroid

Mechanisms to prevent foveal detachment:

Microvilli of RPE, which surround tips of photoreceptors

Viscous mucopolysaccharides, which bathe photoreceptors and RPE

Intraocular pressure

Area around fovea: parafovea (0.5-mm belt), perifovea (1.5-mm belt)

Intercellular junctions:

Blood–retinal barrier:

INNER BARRIER: tight junctions (zonula occludens) between retinal vascular endothelial cells

OUTER BARRIER: tight junctions between RPE cells

Other intercellular junctions:

ZONULA ADHERENS (EXTERNAL LIMITING MEMBRANE): no barrier to passage of fluids

MACULA ADHERENS (DESMOSOMES): no barrier to passage of fluids

Collateral vessels: occur at site of obstruction, across horizontal raphe, and at disc

Hemorrhages:

Flame or splinter: superficial; blood tracks along NFL

Blot or dot: deep; blood confined by axons oriented perpendicular to Bruch membrane

Boat-shaped (scaphoid):

SUB-ILM: hemorrhagic detachment of ILM

SUB-HYALOID: blood between ILM and posterior hyaloid

Dark hemorrhage: sub-RPE; can be confused with choroidal melanoma

RPE: monolayer of hexagonal cells (4–6 million) with apical microvilli and basement membrane at base adherent to each other by system of tight junctions or terminal bars that make up blood–retinal barrier

RPE and outer segments of photoreceptors have apex-to-apex arrangement, resulting in a potential subretinal space

Merges anteriorly with pigmented epithelium of CB; more highly pigmented in central macula

Functions:

Helps with development of photoreceptors during embryogenesis

Involved in vitamin A cycle (uptake, transport, storage, metabolism, and isomerization), main function to generate 11-*cis*-retinal

Provides nourishment for outer half of retinal cells

Receives waste products: phagocytoses photoreceptor outer segments; photoreceptors renew outer segments every 10 days

Forms outer blood–retinal barrier (tight junctions between RPE cells)

Secretes basement membrane material (deposits on inner basal lamina of Bruch membrane)

Produces melanin granules in 6th week of gestation (first cells of body to melanize); melanization may induce further differentiation of retinal layers (may explain why macula fails to develop properly in albinism); melanin helps absorb excess light and is free-radical stabilizer; macular RPE cells contain larger and a greater number of melanosomes than those in periphery

Adenosine triphosphate (ATP)-dependent Na^+/K^+ pump on apical surface maintains environment of subretinal space

Contributes to adhesion of sensory retina (active transport of subretinal fluid and passive hydrostatic forces)

Heat exchange

Light absorption

RPE cells may undergo hypertrophy, hyperplasia, migration, atrophy, and metaplasia

Hypertrophy: flat, jet-black subretinal lesion

Hyperplasia: intraretinal pigment deposition

Migrate into retina to form bone spicules around blood vessels in retinitis pigmentosa

Migrate through retinal holes to form preretinal membranes in proliferative vitreoretinopathy

Metaplasia: nonspecific reaction, observed most often in phthisis; fibrous (component of disciform scars in age-related macular degeneration [AMD]) or osseous (intraocular ossification)

Bruch membrane: extracellular matrix between RPE and choriocapillaris; permeable to small molecules

Layers:

1. Basement membrane (inner basal lamina of RPE)
2. Inner collagenous zone (thick)
3. Elastic tissue
4. Outer collagenous zone (thin)
5. Basement membrane (outer basal lamina of choriocapillaris)

RPE and Bruch membrane are continuous with the pigmented ciliary epithelium

Neuroglial cells:

Astrocytes: branching neural cells in retina and central nervous system (CNS); proliferation leads to gliosis; cell of origin for optic nerve glioma; provide structural support to optic nerve and retina; contribute to nourishment of neuronal elements; foot processes ensheath blood vessels within nerve, contributing to blood–brain barrier

Müller cells: modified astrocytes; footplates form ILM, nuclei in inner nuclear layer; provide skeletal support; contribute to gliosis; extend from ILM to ELM

Microglia: phagocytic cells of the CNS

Arachnoidal cells: cell of origin for meningioma

Oligodendrocytes: produce myelin in the CNS; cell of origin for oligodendroglioma

Schwann cells: produce myelin in peripheral nervous system

Choroid

Posterior part of uveal tract that extends from ora serrata (outer layers end before inner) to optic nerve. Attached to sclera by strands of connective tissue at optic nerve, scleral spur, vortex veins, and long and short posterior ciliary vessels; derived from mesoderm and neuroectoderm; 0.25 mm thick posteriorly at optic nerve and 0.1-0.15 mm thick anteriorly at ora serrata

Layers:

1. *Bruch membrane* (innermost layer): PAS stain positive, 2 µm thick centrally and increases in thickness with age
2. *Choriocapillaris:* 40-60 µm diameter capillary layer with 600-800 Å wide fenestrations (leak fluorescein dye); fenestrations have thin covering diaphragm more numerous on internal side; lobular pattern in posterior pole, more parallel in periphery, at right angles anteriorly, forming ladder-like pattern (Fig. 11.8)
3. *Stroma:* mainly blood vessels; unfenestrated inner medium vessel layer (Sattler layer) and outer large vessel layer (Haller layer), lymphatics, nerves
4. *Suprachoroidal space* (outermost layer): 30 µm thick, darkly pigmented

Blood supply from 1-2 long and 15-20 short posterior ciliary arteries (from internal carotid to ophthalmic artery)

Endothelium is permeable to large molecules

Choriocapillaris arranged in segmental pattern; high blood flow, major source of nutrition for RPE and outer retinal layers

Drains via vortex veins to superior and inferior ophthalmic veins

Contain both parasympathetic and sympathetic nerves (autoregulatory function to keep blood flow constant) via short (mainly) and long posterior ciliary nerves

PHYSIOLOGY

Visual pigments: 4 types, each composed of 11-*cis*-retinal (vitamin A aldehyde) + a protein (opsin); 3 cone pigments and 1 rod pigment (Table 11.1)

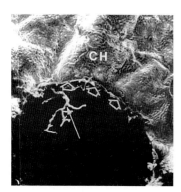 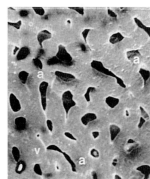 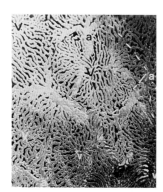 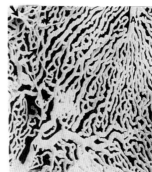

Figure 11.8 Human choriocapillaris, retinal view. (From Fryczkowski AW. Anatomical and functional choroidal lobuli. *Int Ophthalmol.* 1994;18:131–141.)

TABLE 11.1	Visual pigments	
Photoreceptor	**Pigment**	**Peak sensitivity**
Rod	Rhodopsin	505 nm
L (long-wavelength sensitive; red) cones	Erythrolabe (red sensitive)	560 nm
M (middle-wavelength sensitive; green) cones	Chlorolabe (green sensitive)	530 nm
S (short-wavelength sensitive; blue) cones	Cyanolabe (blue sensitive)	420 nm

Cone types:

S CONES (SHORT-WAVELENGTH SENSITIVE): detect color by comparing signal to M cones, responsible for blue-yellow color vision

M CONES (MIDDLE-WAVELENGTH SENSITIVE): detect high resolution (black and white) contrast

L CONES (LONG-WAVELENGTH SENSITIVE): enhance color vision, responsible for red–green color vision

L and M cone opsin genes on X chromosome (1 copy for L and 1–6 copies for M)

Unequal crossover between these genes produce hybrid opsins (with different spectral absorptions), causing most color vision abnormalities. Defects in one of these two genes produces red–green color deficiencies, defects in both genes cause monochromatism, and defects in all 3 color opsin genes cause achromatopsia or rod monochromatism (see Chapter 5, Pediatrics/Strabismus)

Phototransduction: photoreceptor outer segment membrane is lipid bilayer with light-activated opsins that control enzymatic cascade regulating cGMP-gated cation channels that control Na^+ and Ca^{++} flow. Rods contain rhodopsin; chromophore 11-*cis*-retinal (also called 11-*cis*-retinaldehyde) is oriented parallel to the lipid bilayer (perpendicular to the path of photons. Light converts the chromophore to all-*trans*-retinal, activating the visual pigment (opsin) as metarhodopsin II. This triggers transducin, which amplifies and regulates cGMP hydrolysis, controlling the ion channel and initiating an electrical impulse that travels to visual cortex; rhodopsin is then resynthesized; vitamin A is stored in liver and transported to RPE by serum retinol-binding protein and pre-albumin. Similar process occurs in cones

Rods shed outer segments during the day

Cones shed outer segments during the night

Inherited retinal dystrophies caused by mutations in genes regulating phototransduction pathway: rhodopsin gene *(RHO)* in retinitis pigmentosa, arrestin gene *(SAG)* and rhodopsin kinase gene *(GRK1)* in Oguchi disease, rod ABC transporter protein ABCA4 gene *(ABCR)* in Stargardt disease, Rab escort protein 1 gene *(CHM)* in choroideremia, ornithine aminotransferase gene *(OAT)* in gyrate atrophy, peroxin gene *(PEX1)* in Refsum disease

Luminosity curves:

Light adapted: cone peak sensitivity is to light of 555 nm; yellow, yellow–green, and orange appear brighter than blue, green, and red

Dark adapted: rod peak sensitivity is to light of 505 nm (blue)

Purkinje shift: shift in peak sensitivity that occurs from light- to dark-adapted states (Fig. 11.9)

ELECTROPHYSIOLOGY

Electroretinogram (ERG)

Electrical potential generated by retina in response to flash of light; measures mass retinal response; useful for processes affecting large areas of retina

Photoreceptors, bipolar and Müller cells contribute to flash ERG; ganglion cells do not

Light is delivered uniformly to entire retina in Ganzfeld bowl, and electrical discharges are measured with corneal contact lens electrodes and a ground electrode placed over ears

Components (Fig. 11.10):

a-wave: photoreceptor cell bodies (negative waveform)

b-wave: Müller and bipolar cells (positive waveform)

Amplitude: bottom of a-wave to top of b-wave; measured in microvolts

Measures response of entire retina; proportionate to area of functioning retina

Decreased in anoxic conditions (diabetes, central retinal artery occlusion [CRAO], ischemic central retinal vein occlusion [CRVO])

Implicit time: time from light flash to peak of b-wave; measured in milliseconds

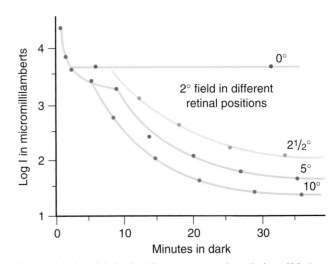

Figure 11.9 Normal dark-adaptation curves measuring retinal sensitivity to a small spot of light whose intensity is varied until the threshold value is found; a 2° test spot was placed at different distances from the foveal center. Note the cone–rod break at 9 minutes, middle graph. (From Hecht S, Haig C, Wald G. The dark adaptation of retinal fields of different size and location. *J Gen Physiol.* 1935;19:321–337.)

Increased in various hereditary conditions

Oscillatory potential: 4-10 high-frequency, low-amplitude wavelets superimposed on ascending b-wave of scotopic and photopic bright flash ERG

　Generated in middle retinal layers (inner plexiform layer): may be inhibitory potentials from amacrine cells

　Reduced in conditions of retinal hypoxia or microvascular disease

c-wave: RPE; late (2–4 seconds) positive deflection; occurs in dark-adapted state

Early receptor potential (ERP) (Fig. 11.11): outer segments of photoreceptors; completed within 1.5 ms

Represents bleaching of visual pigment; requires intense stimulus in dark-adapted state

Ganglion cells are not measured; therefore, flash ERG is not useful in glaucoma

Photopic (light adapted): strong flash in light adapted for 10-min state (bleach out rods); measures cone function

Flicker ERG: flashing light at 30 flashes/second (30 Hz) isolates cone response; photopic response to superstimulation

Small wave follows each flash

Cone response because rods cannot recycle rhodopsin this quickly

Poor response at 30 cycles/second indicates abnormal cone function; rods can respond up to 20 Hz

Cones also respond to repetitive light

Scotopic (dark adapted): weak flash in dark adapted for 30-min state (Fig. 11.12); measures rod function

Dim white or blue flash below cone threshold

At low intensity: small a- and b-waves

At increasing intensity: implicit time shortens, b-wave amplitude increases

Bright-flash ERG (in scotopic state; measures combined maximal rod and cone response): deep a-wave and large b-wave; oscillatory potentials are present (Fig. 11.13)

Indications:

Diagnose generalized retinal degeneration

Assess family members for heritable retinal degeneration

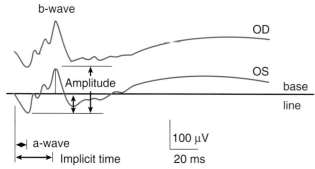

Figure 11.10 The photopic (cone-mediated) electroretinogram (ERG) is a light-adapted, bright-flash-evoked response from the cones of the retina; the rods do not respond in the light-adapted state.
(From Slamovits TL. *Basic and Clinical Science Course: Section 12: Orbit, Eyelids, and Lacrimal System.* San Francisco: American Academy of Ophthalmology.)

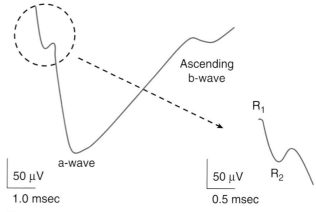

Figure 11.11 Normal human early receptor potential (ERP). This rapid response is complete within 1.5 ms and is believed to be generated by the outer segments. An intense, bright stimulus in the dark-adapted state is needed for an ERP to be obtained. (Redrawn from Berson EL, Goldstein EG. Early receptor potential in dominantly inherited retinitis pigmentosa. *Arch Ophthalmol.* 1970;83:412–420. From Slamovits TL. *Basic and Clinical Science Course: Section 12: Orbit, Eyelids, and Lacrimal System.* San Francisco: American Academy of Ophthalmology, 1993.)

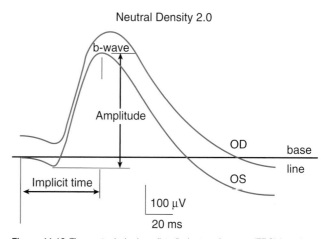

Figure 11.12 The scotopic (rod-mediated) electroretinogram (ERG) is a dark-adapted, dim-flash-evoked (below cone threshold) response that records the signal from the rods. The test should be performed after at least 30 minutes of dark adaptation. (From Slamovits TL. *Basic and Clinical Science Course: Section 12: Orbit, Eyelids, and Lacrimal System.* San Francisco, American Academy of Ophthalmology, 1993.)

Assess decreased vision and nystagmus present at birth

Assess retinal function in presence of opaque ocular media or vascular occlusion

Evaluate functional visual loss

Disease states (Fig. 11.14, Table 11.2):

CRAO: normal a-wave (perfused by choroid), absent b-wave

Ischemic CRVO: reduced b-wave amplitude, reduced ratio of b- to a-wave, prolonged b-wave implicit time

Retinitis pigmentosa (RP): early, reduced amplitude (usually b-wave) and prolonged implicit time; later, extinguished with no rod or cone response to bright flash

Female carriers of X-linked RP: prolonged photopic b-wave implicit time, reduced scotopic b-wave amplitude

Neutral Density 0.0

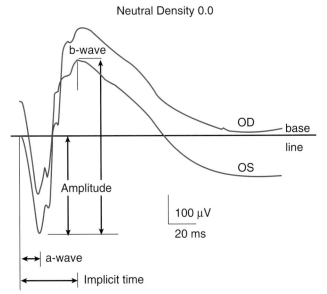

Figure 11.13 The bright-flash, dark-adapted electroretinogram (ERG) stimulates both the cone and rod systems and gives large a- and b-waves, with oscillatory potentials in the ascending b-wave. Some testing centers call this a "scotopic ERG," but the rods are not isolated by this method. (From Slamovits TL. *Basic and Clinical Science Course: Section 12: Orbit, Eyelids, and Lacrimal System.* San Francisco: American Academy of Ophthalmology, 1993.)

TABLE 11.2	Electroretinogram (ERG) patterns for various ocular diseases	
Extinguished ERG abnormal photopic, normal ERG	**Normal a-wave, reduced b-wave**	**Abnormal photopic, normal scotopic ERG**
RP	CSNB; Oguchi disease	Achromatopsia
Ophthalmic artery occlusion	X-linked juvenile retinoschisis	Cone dystrophy
DUSN	CVO	
Metallosis	CRAO	
RD	Myotonic dystrophy	
Drug toxicity (phenothiazine; chloroquine)	Quinine toxicity	
Cancer-associated retinopathy		

CRAO, *Central retinal artery occlusion;* CSNB, *congenital stationary night blindness;* CVO, *central vein occlusion;* DUSN, *diffuse unilateral subacute neuroretinitis;* RP, *retinitis pigmentosa.*

Sector RP: normal b-wave implicit time

Cone dystrophy: abnormal photopic and flicker, normal scotopic

X-linked foveal retinoschisis: normal a-wave until late, reduced b-wave (especially scotopic)

Retinal detachment (RD): reduction in amplitude corresponds to extent of neurosensory loss (50% decrease in amplitude = 50% of neurosensory retina is functionally detached)

Diffuse progressive retinal disease: increased b-wave implicit time

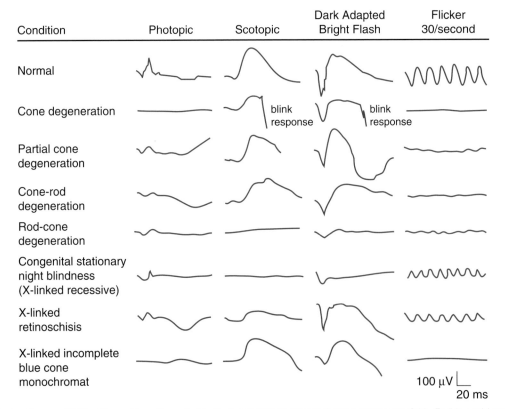

Figure 11.14 Electroretinogram (ERG) patterns. (From Slamovits TL. *Basic and Clinical Science Course: Section 12: Orbit, Eyelids, and Lacrimal System.* San Francisco: American Academy of Ophthalmology, 1993.)

Nonprogressive retinal disease: decreased b-wave amplitude

Multiple evanescent white dot syndrome (MEWDS): reduced a-wave

Chalcosis: reduced amplitude (suppressed by intraocular copper ions)

Retinal microvascular disease (diabetes, hypertension, CVO): loss of oscillatory potentials

Achromatopsia: absent cone function; normal rod function

Leber congenital amaurosis: flat ERG

Congenital stationary night blindness (CSNB): normal a-wave, poor b-wave

Congenital rubella: normal ERG

Glaucoma: normal ERG

Optic neuropathy/atrophy: normal ERG

Pattern ERG (PERG): waveform similar to flash ERG, but different test to measure ganglion cell activity; stimulus is an alternating checkerboard pattern that gives a constant illumination to the retina (Fig. 11.15)

Normal response is composed of 3 waves:

N_{35}: cornea-negative wave at 35 ms

P_{50}: cornea-positive wave peak at 50 ms

N_{95}: negative trough at 95 ms

Multifocal ERG (mfERG): topographic representation of electrophysiologic function; retina stimulated with array of hexagonal elements that are illuminated in pseudorandom pattern; mathematical extraction of recorded signal is displayed as three-peak waveform (N1, P1, and N2); N1 includes same cells as full-field cone ERG a-wave; P1 includes same cells as cone b-wave and oscillatory potentials

Useful in disorders of posterior pole, such as cone dystrophy

Electro-Oculogram (EOG)

Indirect measure of standing potential of eye (voltage difference between inner and outer retina) (Fig. 11.16)

Depolarization of basal portion of RPE produces light peak; normal result requires that both RPE and sensory retina be normal

Arden ratio: ratio of light-to-dark peak (2:1 is normal; <1.65 is abnormal); decreased ratio is a result of photoreceptor or RPE disorder

Procedure: light adaptation × 5 minutes, recording during dark adaptation × 20 min, and another recording under standard light adaptation × 10 min; electrode placed on cornea and another on body in Ganzfeld bowl, and electrodes placed on canthi of eye; measurement is based on eye movement dependent voltage generation from patient looking back and forth between two fixation lights; both eyes are recorded simultaneously

Dark adaptation causes progressive decrease in response, reaching a trough (dark trough) at 8-12 minutes

Light adaptation causes progressive rise in amplitude over 6-9 minutes (light peak)

Measure lowest voltage with dark adaptation and highest voltage with light adaptation

Amplitude is higher with light adaptation than dark adaptation

ERG is abnormal in all cases in which EOG is abnormal except:

Best disease and carriers: normal ERG but abnormal EOG

Pattern dystrophies

Chloroquine toxicity

Abnormal ERG, normal EOG: conditions with abnormal bipolar region but normal rods

CSNB

X-linked retinoschisis

RETINAL IMAGING

Optical Coherence Tomography (OCT)

Creates cross-sectional image of tissue from reflections of broad bandwidth light based on low-coherence interferometry

Provides retinal thickness measurements, optic nerve measurements, and cross-sectional retinal imaging to ~3-10 μm, depending on light source; anterior segment spectral domain OCT is useful to image anterior segment, in particular the cornea and angle. Using specialized techniques evaluation of flow can produce images of vasculature (OCT angiography [OCTA])

Superluminescent diodes or short-pulse lasers create beams of infrared light through a Michelson interferometer at both the eye and a reference mirror; the reflected light from the retina is compared with the light from the reference mirror and analyzed so that the tissue reflectivity (similar to ultrasound) and density can be determined;

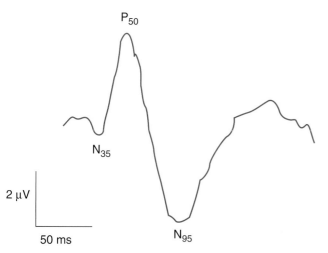

Figure 11.15 Pattern electroretinogram (ERG) with components labeled. This waveform measures retinal ganglion cell function and is not related to the flash ERG test. (After Treat GL. The pattern electroretinogram in glaucoma and ocular hypertension. In: Heckenlively JR, Arden GB, eds. *Principles and Practice of Clinical Electrophysiology of Vision.* St Louis: Mosby-Yearbook, 1991.)

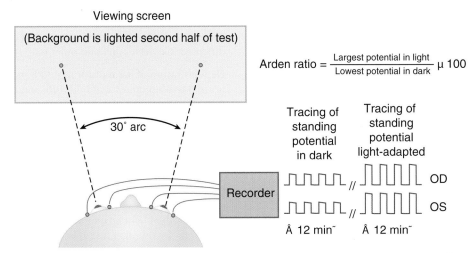

Figure 11.16 Diagram illustrating technique used in recording the electro-oculogram test; the patient is positioned so that the eyes will traverse a 30° arc between 2 blinking red lights. The skin electrodes are positioned at the lateral and inner canthi. The standing potential is measured as the patient moves his eyes between the lights, first in the dark and then in the light. The maximum amplitude from the light condition is compared with minimum value from the dark to give a light peak-to-dark trough ratio. (From Heckenlively JR. *Retinitis Pigmentosa*. Philadelphia: JB Lippincott, 1988.)

more reflective areas create greater interference; with time-domain OCT (TDOCT), the reference mirror moves; with spectral-domain or spatially encoded frequency domain OCT (SDOCT), the mirror does not move, and the broadband interference is evaluated by a Fourier transform to obtain reflectance information (this makes SDOCT much faster than TDOCT). Swept-source OCT (time-encoded frequency domain) uses even longer wavelength laser source and photodetectors to further increase scan speed

Useful for optic nerve (glaucoma) and macular pathology (edema, hole, pucker, choroidal neovascularization [CNV]); can compare thickness in cases of macular edema from one visit to next; can diagnose and differentiate vitreomacular pathology (e.g., stage 1 macular hole/vitreomacular traction vs. full-thickness hole vs. pseudohole or lamellar holes) (Figs. 11.17 and 11.18)

Heidelberg Retinal Tomograph (HRT)

Laser tomography

Confocal scanning laser produces 3-dimensional (3D) sections of optic nerve and retina through undilated pupil

Diode laser (670 nm) that is periodically deflected by oscillating mirrors; laser scans retina, and instrument measures reflectance and constructs series of 2-dimensional (2D) images at different depths, which are combined to create a multilayer 3D topographic image

Measures surface height to within 20 μm

Retinal Thickness Analyzer (RTA)

Creates thickness contour map

HeNe laser scans central 2 × 2 mm area; receives 2 reflections, 1 from ILM and 1 from RPE, then maps distance between these layers

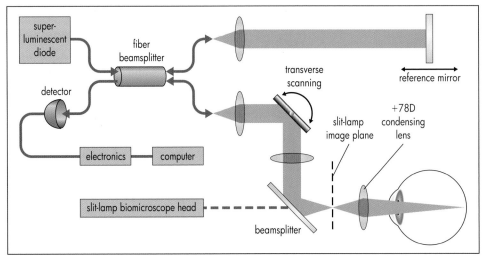

Figure 11.17 Optical coherence tomography principle. (Adapted from Shuman JS, Hee MR, Puliafito CA, et al. Quantification of nerve fiber layer thickness in normal and glaucomatous eyes using optical coherence tomography. *Arch Ophthalmol.* 1995;113:586–596. From Yanoff M, Duker JS, eds. *Ophthalmology*. London; Mosby, 1999.)

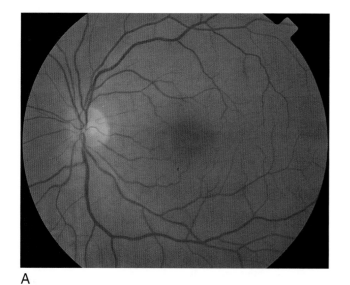

A

B

Figure 11.18 Full-thickness macular hole. (A) Fundus photograph. (B) Time-domain optical coherence tomography (OCT). (From Yanoff M, Duker JS, eds. *Ophthalmology*. London: Mosby; 1999.)

Scanning Laser Ophthalmoscope (SLO)

Modulated red-light laser (633 nm)

Performs funduscopy and automated perimetry simultaneously

Ultrasound

Acoustic imaging of globe and orbit

Uses echoes to image tissue: piezoelectric crystal converts electric energy into sound waves that are emitted by probe, changed by tissue surface/interfaces, and reflected; signal generated depends on amplitude, frequency, and travel time of reflected echoes

Penetration depth and image resolution depend on ultrasound frequency, inversely related (higher frequency provides higher resolution but less penetration)

A-scan: frequency = 8-12 MHz; 1-dimensional display (amplitude of echoes plotted as vertical height against distance) (Figs. 11.19–11.21)

B-scan: frequency = 10 MHz, axial resolution = 100 μm; 2D display (amplitude of echoes represented by brightness on a grayscale image), 3 types of scans: axial, transverse, longitudinal; 3D information by combining data from 2 orthogonal scans (Fig. 11.22)

Reflectivity: height of spike on A-scan and signal brightness on B-scan

Internal reflectivity refers to amplitude of echoes within a lesion or tissue

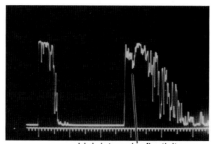

high internal reflectivity

Figure 11.19 A-scan ultrasound demonstrating high internal reflectivity. (From Friedman NJ, Kaiser PK, Pineda R II. *The Massachusetts Eye and Ear Infirmary Illustrated Manual of Ophthalmology*, 3rd ed. Philadelphia: Elsevier; 2009.)

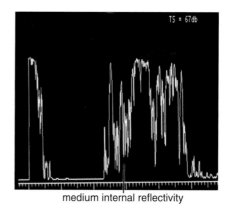

medium internal reflectivity

Figure 11.20 A-scan ultrasound demonstrating medium internal reflectivity. (From Friedman NJ, Kaiser PK, Pineda R II. *The Massachusetts Eye and Ear Infirmary Illustrated Manual of Ophthalmology*, 3rd ed. Philadelphia: Elsevier; 2009.)

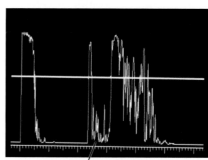

low internal reflectivity

Figure 11.21 A-scan ultrasound demonstrating low internal reflectivity. (From Friedman NJ, Kaiser PK, Pineda R II. *The Massachusetts Eye and Ear Infirmary Illustrated Manual of Ophthalmology*, 3rd ed. Philadelphia: Elsevier; 2009.)

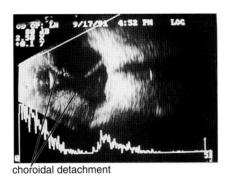

choroidal detachment

Figure 11.22 B-scan ultrasound demonstrating choroidal detachment. (From Kaiser PK, Friedman NJ, Pineda R II. *The Massachusetts Eye and Ear Infirmary Illustrated Manual of Ophthalmology*, 3rd ed. Philadelphia: Elsevier; 2009.)

Internal structure: degree of variation in histologic architecture within a mass lesion
  Regular internal structure indicates homogenous architecture (minimal or no variation in the heights of spikes in A-scan and uniform appearance of echoes on B-scan)

Sound attenuation: occurs when acoustic wave is scattered, reflected, or absorbed by tissue
  Decrease in strength of echoes within or posterior to lesion; may produce a void posterior to lesion called "shadowing" (caused by dense substances [bone, calcium, foreign body])

After movement: dynamic features of lesion echoes
  Observe B-scan echoes for motion after cessation of eye movements (i.e., rapid movement of vitreous hemorrhage [VH] distinguished from slower, undulating movement of rhegmatogenous retinal detachment [RRD])

Vascularity: spontaneous motion of echoes within lesion corresponds to blood flow; may be visualized with color Doppler

Specific lesions: (Tables 11.3 and 11.4) (Figs. 11.22–11.27)
  Asteroid hyalosis:
    A-SCAN: medium to high internal reflectivity
    B-SCAN: bright echoes in vitreous as a result of calcium soaps; area of clear vitreous usually present between opacities and posterior hyaloid face
  Intraocular foreign body:
    B-SCAN: high reflectivity when ultrasound probe is perpendicular to reflective surface of foreign body; bright echo persists when gain turned down; shadowing often present
  Intraocular calcification:
    A-SCAN: high-amplitude peak as a result of strong acoustic interface
    B-SCAN: white echoes; partial or complete shadowing

TABLE 11.3 Ultrasound characteristics of select retinal lesions

Pathology	Location	Shape	Internal reflectivity	Internal structure	Vascularity
Melanoma	Choroid and/or ciliary body	Dome or collar button	Low to medium	Regular	Yes
Choroidal hemangioma	Choroid; posterior pole	Dome	High	Regular	Yes
Metastasis	Choroid; posterior pole	Diffuse, irregular	Medium to high	Irregular	No
Choroidal nevus	Choroid	Dome or flat	High	Regular	No
Choroidal hemorrhage	Choroid	Dome	Variable	Variable	No
Disciform lesion	Macula	Dome, irregular	High	Variable	No

TABLE 11.4 Ultrasound characteristics of different types of retinal detachments

Pathology	Topographic (B-scan)	Quantitative (A-scan)	After movement
Retinal detachment	Smooth or folded surface Open or closed funnel Inserts at ON and ora serrata May see intraretinal cysts	Steep spike (100% high)	Moderate to none
Posterior vitreous detachment	Smooth surface Open funnel With or without ON or fundus insertion Inserts at ora serrata or ciliary body	Variable spike height (<100%)	Marked to moderate
Choroidal detachment	Smooth, dome, or flat surface No ON insertion Inserts at ciliary body and vortex veins	Steeply rising, thick, double-peaked spike (100% high)	Mild to none

ON, *Optic nerve.*

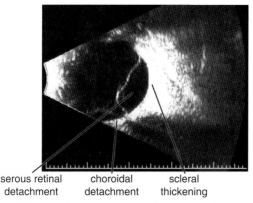

serous retinal   choroidal   scleral
detachment   detachment   thickening

Figure 11.23 B-scan ultrasound demonstrating serous retinal detachment with shifting fluid, shallow peripheral choroidal detachment, and diffuse scleral thickening. (From Kaiser PK, Friedman NJ, Pineda R II. *The Massachusetts Eye and Ear Infirmary Illustrated Manual of Ophthalmology,* 3rd ed. Philadelphia: Elsevier; 2009.)

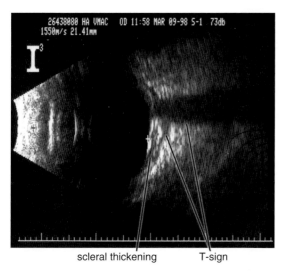

scleral thickening   T-sign

Figure 11.24 B-scan ultrasound demonstrating scleral thickening and the characteristic peripapillary T sign. (From Kaiser PK, Friedman NJ, Pineda R II. *The Massachusetts Eye and Ear Infirmary Illustrated Manual of Ophthalmology,* 2nd ed. Philadelphia: Saunders; 2004.)

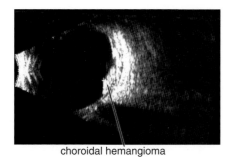

choroidal hemangioma

Figure 11.25 B-scan ultrasound demonstrating elevated mass with underlying thickened choroid. (From Kaiser PK, Friedman NJ, Pineda R II. *The Massachusetts Eye and Ear Infirmary Illustrated Manual of Ophthalmology,* 2nd ed. Philadelphia: Saunders; 2004.)

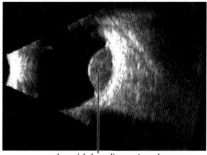

choroidal malignant melanoma

Figure 11.26 B-scan ultrasound demonstrating dome-shaped choroidal mass. (From Kaiser PK, Friedman NJ, Pineda R II. *The Massachusetts Eye and Ear Infirmary Illustrated Manual of Ophthalmology,* 2nd ed. Philadelphia: Saunders; 2004.)

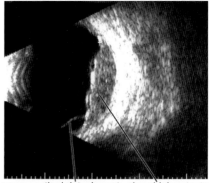

serous retinal detachment   choroidal metastasis

Figure 11.27 B-scan ultrasound of a patient with choroidal metastasis demonstrating elevated choroidal mass with irregular surface and overlying serous retinal detachment. (From Kaiser PK, Friedman NJ, Pineda R II. *The Massachusetts Eye and Ear Infirmary Illustrated Manual of Ophthalmology,* 2nd ed. Philadelphia: Saunders; 2004.)

DDX: tumors (retinoblastoma, choroidal osteoma, optic nerve meningioma, choroidal hemangioma, choroidal melanoma), *Toxocara* granuloma, chronic RD, optic nerve head drusen, vascular occlusive disease of optic nerve, phthisis bulbi, intumescent cataractous lens

Fluorescein Angiogram (FA)

Phases: choroidal filling, arterial, venous, recirculation

Sodium fluorescein in a hydrocarbon-based yellow–red dye with a molecular weight of 376 daltons (Da). Dye enters choroidal circulation via short posterior ciliary arteries 10-15 seconds after injection; choroidal flow is very rapid; choriocapillaris filling is usually completed in the atrioventricular (AV) or early venous phase; cilioretinal artery is filled at time of choroidal filling; central retinal artery takes more circuitous route, resulting in dye arriving 1-2 seconds after choroidal filling; AV phase occurs 1-2 seconds after arterial phase; veins fill in 10-12 seconds (Figs. 11.28–11.32)

Fluorescein absorbs light at 465-490 nm (blue), emits at 520-530 nm (yellow–green); to produce an image, two filters are required: an exciter filter that emits blue

347

light, which stimulates fluorescein to emit yellow–green light (barrier filter transmits only green light), so image produced by what returns through filter

80% bound to albumin and other serum proteins

90% excreted from kidney (also liver) within 24-36 hours

Transient yellowing of skin and conjunctiva that lasts 8-12 hours; most common adverse events: nausea (3%–15%), vomiting (5%), pruritus (5%); anaphylactic reaction in 1 in 100,000; death occurs in 1 in 220,000; pregnancy in first trimester is a relative contraindication

Characteristics:

Hyperfluorescence: leakage (fenestrated choriocapillaris, iris vessels), staining (structures such as collagen), pooling (pockets of fluid), window defects (RPE defects)

Hypofluorescence: blockage (opacity that reduces fluorescence (e.g., RPE, blood, xanthophyll) or filling defect (ischemia)

Macular dark spot is a result of blockage by xanthophyll in outer plexiform layer and tall RPE cells with increased melanin and lipofuscin

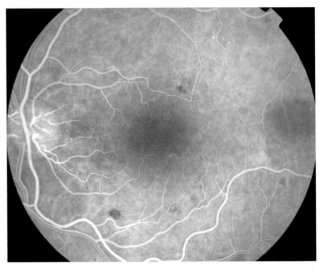

Figure 11.30 Fluorescein angiogram demonstrating early venous phase with laminar filling.

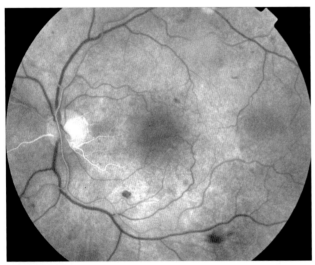

Figure 11.28 Fluorescein angiogram demonstrating choroidal and early arterial filling.

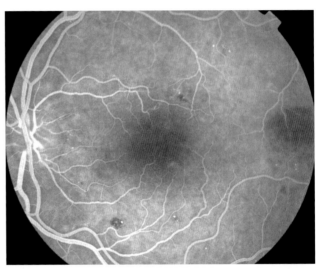

Figure 11.31 Fluorescein angiogram demonstrating peak atrioventricular (AV) transit.

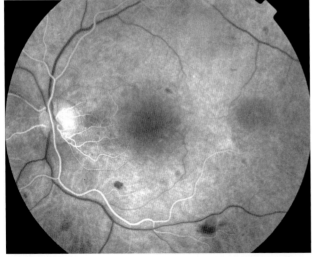

Figure 11.29 Fluorescein angiogram demonstrating arterial phase.

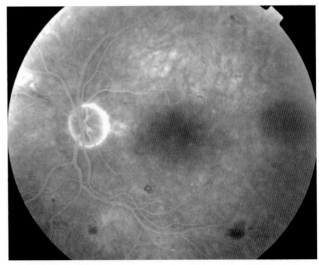

Figure 11.32 Fluorescein angiogram demonstrating late phase.

Fluorescein passes through Bruch membrane, cannot pass through RPE or retinal capillaries

Autofluorescence: fluorescence prior to fluorescein dye injection; seen in optic nerve drusen, astrocytic hamartomas, and large deposits of lipofuscin

Choroidal filling: choroidal lesions (malignant melanoma, cavernous hemangioma) and cilioretinal artery

Arterial phase filling: retinal lesions (capillary hemangioma, neovascularization of the optic disc [NVD])

Indocyanine Green (ICG)

Sterile, water-soluble, tricarbocyanine dye with a molecular weight of 775 Da. Absorbs light in near-infrared range (790–805 nm), emits at range of 770-880 nm (peak at 835 nm), which penetrates RPE, blood, and other ocular pigments to greater extent than visible light and fluorescein (60%–75% of blue light absorbed by RPE and choroid)

98% bound to serum proteins (80% to globulins such as alpha-lipoproteins); therefore, less dye escapes through choriocapillaris fenestrations, allowing enhanced imaging of the choroidal circulation; CNV often appears as hot spot (bright area; occurs within 3–5 min, lasts 20 min) (Fig. 11.33)

Excreted via liver into bile

Safer than fluorescein angiography; nausea and vomiting less common; should not be done in patients allergic to iodine, uremic, or with liver disease

DISORDERS

Vitreous Abnormalities

Asteroid Hyalosis

Refractile particles (calcium soaps) suspended in vitreous

More common in older patients and those with diabetes; 25% bilateral

Rarely affects vision, but may prevent visualization of posterior pole; use FA to look for abnormalities in these patients

Pathology: gray spheres with "Maltese cross" birefringence on polarization

Synchysis Scintillans (Cholesterol Bulbi)

Cholesterol crystals derived from old VH; with posterior vitreous detachment (PVD) crystals settle inferiorly

Rare, unilateral

Occurs after blunt or penetrating trauma in blind eyes

Crystals sink to bottom of globe because no fixed vitreous framework

Primary Amyloidosis

Vitreous involvement in familial amyloidotic polyneuropathies (FAP I and II get systemic manifestations)

Amyloid enters via retinal vessels

Patients have cardiac disease and amyloid neuropathy

Posterior Vitreous Detachment (PVD)

Separation of posterior hyaloid face from retina

Mechanism: vitreous syneresis (liquefaction) and contraction with age

Symptoms: floaters; may see flashes (resulting from traction on retina)

Findings: acute symptomatic PVD may have retinal tear (10%–15% of acute symptomatic PVDs), VH (hemorrhagic PVD; 7.5% of PVDs) if vessel is torn during vitreous separation (70% risk of retinal tear); RD, especially when pigmented vitreous cell is present (Schaffer sign)

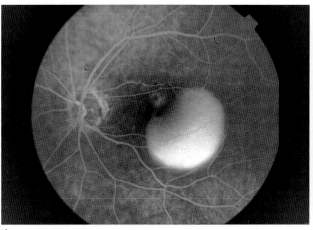
A

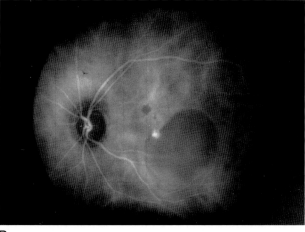
B

Figure 11.33 (A) Serous retinal pigment epithelial detachment seen on fluorescein angiogram. (B) Associated hot spot seen on indocyanine green. (From Reichel E. Indocyanine green angiography. In: Yanoff M, Duker JS, eds. *Ophthalmology*. London: Mosby; 1999.)

Vitreous Hemorrhage (VH)

Etiology: diabetes (most common), other proliferative retinopathies, trauma, PVD, Terson syndrome (blood from subarachnoid hemorrhage travels along optic nerve and into eye), ruptured retinal arterial macroaneurysm, retinal angioma; in children, consider child abuse, pars planitis, X-linked retinoschisis

Ochre membrane: results from chronic hemorrhage accumulating on posterior surface of detached vitreous

Persistent Hyperplastic Primary Vitreous (PHPV)

(See Chapter 5, Pediatrics/Strabismus)

Retinal Abnormalities

Congenital

(See Chapter 5, Pediatrics/Strabismus)

Trauma

Commotio Retinae (Berlin Edema)

Transient retinal whitening at level of deep sensory retina resulting from disruption (probably photoreceptor outer segments) with photoreceptor loss and thinning of outer nuclear and plexiform layers; not true edema

Pigmentary changes can occur (RPE hyperplasia); traumatic macular hole may develop; usually resolves without sequelae (Fig. 11.34)

Contusion of RPE

Blunt trauma can cause RPE edema with overlying serous RD

Choroidal Rupture

Tear in choroid, Bruch membrane, and RPE as a result of blunt or penetrating trauma

Mechanism: mechanical deformation results in rupture of choroid; sclera is resistant because of its high tensile strength, retina is resistant because of its elasticity; Bruch membrane is less elastic and breaks with choroid and RPE

Direct: occurs anteriorly at site of impact; oriented parallel to ora serrata

Indirect: occurs posteriorly away from site of impact; usually crescent-shaped, concentric with and temporal to optic disc; often associated with VH

Findings: choroidal neovascular membrane (CNV) can develop during healing process (months to years after trauma; can regress spontaneously), scar forms by 3-4 weeks, hyperplasia of RPE at margin of lesion (Fig. 11.35)

Retina Sclopetaria

Trauma to retina and choroid caused by transmitted shock waves and necrosis from high-velocity projectile

Findings: rupture of choroid and retina with hemorrhage and commotio; VH can occur; lesion heals with white fibrous scar and RPE changes (Fig. 11.36)

Low risk of RD in young patients with formed vitreous; posterior vitreous face usually intact; choroid and retina tightly adherent

Traumatic Retinal Break

Most patients are young with formed vitreous that tamponades the break

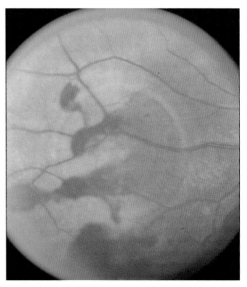

Figure 11.34 Berlin edema (commotio retinae) in a patient after blunt ocular trauma. (From Rubsamen PE. Posterior segment ocular trauma. In: Yanoff M, Duker JS, eds. *Ophthalmology*. London: Mosby; 1999.)

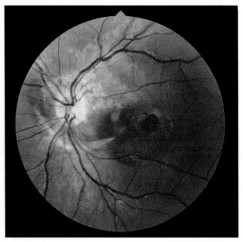

Figure 11.35 Choroidal rupture after blunt trauma. (From Rubsamen PE. Posterior segment ocular trauma. In: Yanoff M, Duker JS, eds. *Ophthalmology*. London: Mosby; 1999.)

As vitreous liquefies over time, fluid passes through breaks, causing retina to detach

Trauma is associated with 10%-20% of all phakic RDs

4 types: horseshoe tear, operculated tear, retinal dialysis, macular hole (rare)

Dialysis: most common type of retinal tear associated with traumatic RD; usually inferotemporal (31%) or superonasal (22%); 50% have demarcation line; 10% of dialysis-related RDs are present on initial examination, 30% occur within 1 month, 50% within 8 months, 80% within 2 years

Avulsion of vitreous base: separation of vitreous base from ora serrata; pathognomonic for trauma

Oral tear: at ora serrata; results from split of vitreous; fish-mouth appearance

Preoral tear: anterior border of vitreous base; most often superotemporal

Treatment: laser therapy or cryotherapy for horseshoe tear, operculated tear, and retinal dialysis without RD; vitrectomy with gas for macular hole; scleral buckle for RD as a result of retinal tear; proliferative vitreoretinopathy (PVR) is uncommon

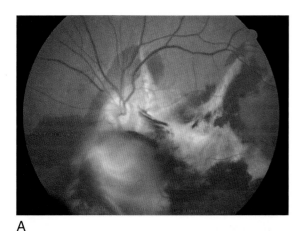

A

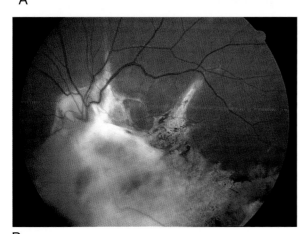

B

Figure 11.36 Gunshot wound to the periocular region demonstrating appearance of retina sclopetaria. (A) Acute. (B) Chronic. (From Rubsamen PE. Posterior segment ocular trauma. In: Yanoff M, Duker JS, eds. *Ophthalmology*. London: Mosby; 1999.)

Purtscher Retinopathy

Caused by head trauma or compressive injury to trunk

Unilateral or bilateral

Findings: retinal whitening, hemorrhages, cotton-wool spots, papillitis; may have positive relative afferent pupillary defect (RAPD) (Fig. 11.37)

DDx: pancreatitis, fat emboli, lupus, leukemia, amniotic fluid emboli, dermatomyositis

FA: leakage from retinal vasculature, late venous staining

May take up to 3 months to resolve

Terson Syndrome

Vitreous hemorrhage following subarachnoid or subdural hemorrhage as a result of intracranial hypertension blocking venous return from eye; patients have acute neck stiffness

20% of patients with spontaneous or traumatic subarachnoid hemorrhage will present with VH; bleeding can also occur between ILM and NFL (Fig. 11.38)

Valsalva Retinopathy

Rise in intrathoracic or intra-abdominal pressure against a closed glottis (Valsalva maneuver) causes superficial veins to rupture with hemorrhage under ILM

Preretinal hemorrhage in macula causes sudden decreased vision

Fat Emboli Syndrome

Follows fracture of medullated bones; occurs in 5% of patients with long-bone fractures

Affects multiple organ systems

Findings (in 50%): cotton-wool spots, small blot hemorrhages; rarely intravenous fat or CRAO 20% mortality

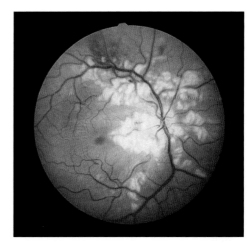

Figure 11.37 Purtscher retinopathy. (From Regillo CD. Distant trauma with posterior segment effects. In: Yanoff M, Duker JS, eds. *Ophthalmology*. London: Mosby; 1999.)

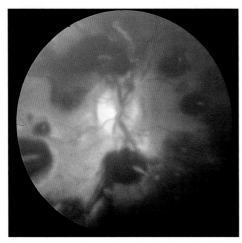

Figure 11.38 Terson syndrome. (From Regillo CD. Distant trauma with posterior segment effects. In: Yanoff M, Duker JS, eds. *Ophthalmology*. London: Mosby; 1999.)

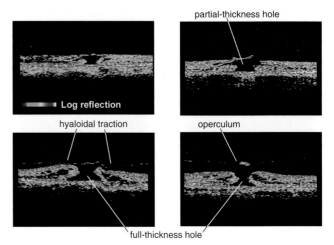

Figure 11.39 Optical coherence tomography scans demonstrating cross-sectional image of all stages of macular hole formation and the full-thickness retinal defect. (From Kaiser PK, Friedman NJ, Pineda R II. *The Massachusetts Eye and Ear Infirmary Illustrated Manual of Ophthalmology*, 2nd ed. Philadelphia: Saunders; 2004.)

Whiplash Retinopathy

Associated with severe flexion/extension of head and neck without direct eye injury

Findings: mild reduction in vision (to 20/30); gray swelling of fovea, foveal pit (50–100 µm)

FA: may have tiny focal area of early hyperfluorescence

Macular Diseases

Epiretinal Membrane (Cellophane Maculopathy, Macular Pucker)

Proliferations at vitreoretinal junction, may contract and cause retinal striae, folds, and macular edema

12% prevalence in individuals 43-86 years old; 20% bilateral; 2% associated with retinal folds (decreased vision)

Associated with diabetes, retinal vascular occlusions, anomalous, PVD, high myopia, retinal hole/tear, previous ocular or laser surgery, and increasing age

OCT: epiretinal membrane visible on surface of retina, distortion of retinal surface evident in 3D map; may produce intraretinal cysts and fluid, as well as localized traction RD

Treatment: consider surgery for decreased vision (<20/50), marked retinal distortion, or metamorphopsia

Full-Thickness Macular Hole

Caused by tangential traction on foveal region by posterior cortical vitreous

Most commonly idiopathic (senile); may develop after trauma, surgery, cystoid macular edema (CME), or inflammation

Female > male; bilateral in 25%-30%; prevalence = 0.33%; average age of onset is 67 years; risk of developing in fellow

eye <1% (no risk if PVD present); if traction is present risk rises to 40% (also known as stage 0 macular hole)

Gass classification (Fig. 11.39):
  Stage 1: premacular or impending hole with foveal detachment and macular cyst (yellow spot [1a] or ring [1b])
  Stage 2: full-thickness eccentric hole; usually <400 µm in width
  Stage 3: full-thickness hole with operculum, cuff of subretinal fluid, yellow deposits at base, positive
  Stage 4: Watzke-Allen sign
  Stage 5: full-thickness hole with PVD

Can also be classified by OCT findings, with subclassification based on size of smallest retinal aperture, presence/absence of traction, and presence/absence of other conditions (e.g., trauma, high myopia):
  1. *Small:* <250 µm
  2. *Medium:* 250-400 µm
  3. *Large:* >400 µm

Watzke-Allen sign: shine narrow-slit beam over macular hole, positive if patient perceives "break" in slit beam

DDx: epiretinal membrane with pseudohole, lamellar hole, vitreomacular traction/detachment

FA: window defect corresponding to the full-thickness macular hole (hyperfluorescence during choroidal filling)

OCT: differentiates between various stages and other disease, hole always evident on scan; often have rim of subretinal fluid (SRF) and cysts within edges of hole, occasionally operculum can be seen over the hole

Treatment: stage 1 also known as *vitreomacular traction (VMT)*, so no full-thickness hole is present; may close spontaneously, so observation; if it worsens, can consider intravitreal injection of recombinant microplasmin (ocriplasmin [Jetrea]) or 0.3 mL of 100% C_3F_8 gas (Diabetic

Retinopathy Clinical Research Network [DRCR] Protocol AG); consider vitrectomy with peeling of posterior hyaloid and gas tamponade for stage 2 through stage 4; ocriplasmin (Jetrea) can also close smaller macular hole in presence of VMT in up to 40% of cases. In DRCR Protocol AH, 29% of small full-thickness macular holes closed with injection of 0.3 mL of 100% C_3F_8 gas, but 12% of cases developed a retinal tear or detachment so this is not recommended

> *Complications of surgery:* increased size of hole, RPE mottling, light toxicity, cataract, retinal tear, RD, endophthalmitis

Prognosis: good if recent onset and hole width <400 μm, poor if >1 year duration and larger holes

Traumatic Macular Hole

Rare (5%); caused by disruption and necrosis of retinal photoreceptors with subsequent loss of retinal tissue; results from preexisting commotio retinae in macula

Solar Retinopathy

Photochemical retinal damage can occur after ~90 seconds or longer of sungazing, thought to be caused by blue (441 nm) and near-ultraviolet (UV) light (325–250 nm)

With foveal fixation, retinal image of sun is 160 μm and is usually within the foveola and FAZ

Associated with solar eclipse, psychiatric disorders, religious rituals, or ingestion of hallucinogens

Symptoms: vision can range from normal to 20/100; usually returns to 20/20-20/40 within 6 months

Findings: yellow–white spot in fovea; later, red foveolar depression or lamellar hole (Fig. 11.40)

FA: intense staining of damaged RPE, particularly in acute phase of injury, but no leakage; as RPE heals, window defects develop (Fig. 11.41)

Central Serous Retinopathy/Chorioretinopathy (CSR, CSC; Idiopathic Central Serous Choroidopathy [ICSC])

Serous RD ± retinal pigment epithelium detachment (PED) (Fig. 11.42)

Males (80%), typically in 4th-5th decade

Associated with hypertension, steroid use, psychiatric medication use, and type A personality

Findings: blurred vision, micropsia, paracentral scotoma; poor color vision; induced hyperopia, absent foveal reflex; after resolution, may have yellow subretinal deposits, RPE changes

DDx: AMD, Vogt-Koyanagi-Harada (VKH) syndrome, uveal effusion syndrome, toxemia of pregnancy, optic nerve pit, pigment epithelial detachment from other causes (CNV)

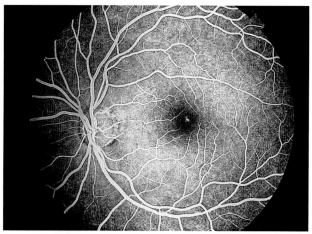

Figure 11.41 Fluorescein angiography of solar retinopathy in the left eye. (Courtesy of William E. Benson. From Baumal CR. Light toxicity and laser burns. In: Yanoff M, Duker JS, eds. *Ophthalmology*. London: Mosby; 1999.)

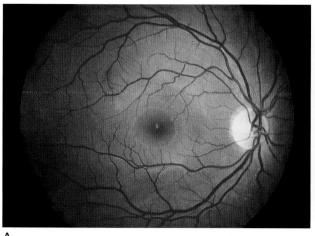 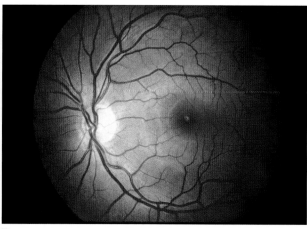

A   B

Figure 11.40 Solar retinopathy of both eyes. (Courtesy of William E. Benson. From Baumal CR. Light toxicity and laser burns. In: Yanoff M, Duker JS, eds. *Ophthalmology*. London: Mosby; 1999.)

FA: small focal hyperfluorescent dot (leakage of dye from choroid through RPE); later, dye accumulates beneath neurosensory detachment; "smokestack" appearance in 10%; expanding dot of hyperfluorescence in 80%, diffuse leakage in the rest (Fig. 11.43)

OCT: sensory retinal elevation, may have PED (usually within or near subretinal fluid accumulation); thickened choroid

ICG: can be useful in helping to distinguish atypical diffuse CSR in older patients from occult CNV in exudative AMD and idiopathic polypoidal choroidal vasculopathy (PCV)

Fundus autofluorescence (FAF): teardrop-shaped area of hyperautofluoresence corresponding to dependent migration of fluid

Treatment: observation in most cases, consider laser to focal hot spots outside fovea or verteporfin (Visudyne) ocular photodynamic therapy (PDT) for subfoveal spots or diffuse leakage (off-label); recently mineralocorticoid antagonists have been shown to be beneficial, especially in chronic cases including spironolactone or eplerenone (off-label)

Treatment indications:
1. Persistent serous detachment (>3 months)
2. Previous episode of CSR, with permanent vision reduction

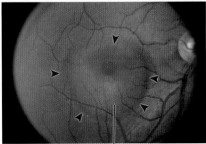

pigment epithelial detachment

Figure 11.42 Idiopathic central serous retinopathy with large serous retinal detachment. (From Kaiser PK, Friedman NJ, Pineda R II. *The Massachusetts Eye and Ear Infirmary Illustrated Manual of Ophthalmology*, 2nd ed. Philadelphia: Saunders; 2004.)

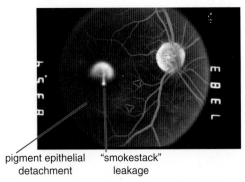

pigment epithelial   "smokestack"
detachment   leakage

Figure 11.43 Fluorescein angiogram demonstrating classic smokestack appearance in central serous chorioretinopathy. (From Kaiser PK, Friedman NJ, Pineda R II. *The Massachusetts Eye and Ear Infirmary Illustrated Manual of Ophthalmology*, 2nd ed. Philadelphia: Saunders; 2004.)

3. Episode in fellow eye with vision loss
4. Demand for rapid recovery of binocular function for occupational reasons

Laser and PDT accelerate resolution of fluid, but do not result in better final vision or reduce rate of recurrence; laser may rarely cause CNV

Prognosis: 90% spontaneous resorption in 1-6 months; 50% recur; 66% achieve 20/20; 14% with bilateral vision loss over 10 years

Retinal Pigment Epithelial Detachment (PED)

Appears as discrete, blister-like elevation; sometimes outlined by orange–pink rim of subretinal fluid

DDx:
In patient <50 years old: probably a result of central serous retinopathy
In patient >50 years old: PED associated with drusen may indicate occult CNV, especially if PED has a notch

FA: discrete early hyperfluorescence of entire serous PED with late pooling into PED

Complications: 33% develop CNV (FA shows slower, more homogenous filling with sharp border) termed *pachychoroidal neovascularization*

Age-Related Macular Degeneration (ARMD, AMD)

Leading cause of central visual loss in patients >60 years old in the United States and Western world

Risk factors: age, heredity, sex (female), race (white), smoking, nutrition, photic exposure, hypertension, light iris color, hyperopia

Symptoms: decreased vision, central scotoma, metamorphopsia

Forms:
Nonexudative or dry (80%–90%): drusen, pigment changes, RPE atrophy (Figs. 11.44–11.47)
Exudative, neovascular, or wet (10%–20%): characterized by CNV (Figs. 11.48–11.50)

Drusen: focal deposits of extracellular debris located between basal lamina of RPE and inner collagenous layer of Bruch membrane; clinical marker for sick RPE; PAS-positive, mildly eosinophilic hyaline excrescences of abnormal basement membrane material; found to contain lipid, mainly esterified cholesterol, unesterified cholesterol, and phosphatidylcholine; carbohydrates, zinc, and nearly 150 proteins, including vitronectin, apolipoproteins E and B, and numerous components of complement system

Types of drusen:
Hard (nodular/cuticular/hyaline): small yellow–white spots 50 μm in diameter
Soft: larger (63–1000 μm), less dense, more fluffy, with tapered edges; may resemble PED; associated with thickened inner Bruch membrane and wet AMD

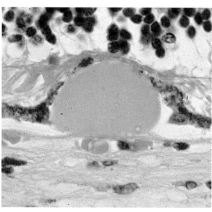

Figure 11.44 Nodular "hard" drusen. (From Edwards MG, Bressler NM, Raja SC. Age-related macular degeneration. In: Yanoff M, Duker JS, eds. *Ophthalmology*. London: Mosby; 1999.)

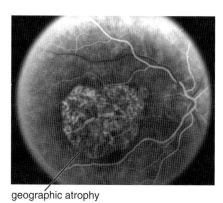

geographic atrophy

Figure 11.47 Fluorescein angiogram of same patient as in Fig. 11.46, demonstrating well-defined window defect corresponding to the area of geographic atrophy. (From Kaiser PK, Friedman NJ, Pineda R II. *The Massachusetts Eye and Ear Infirmary Illustrated Manual of Ophthalmology,* 2nd ed. Philadelphia: Saunders; 2004.)

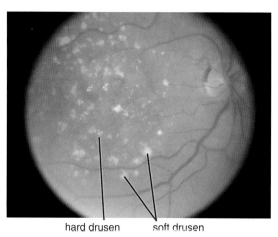

hard drusen   soft drusen

Figure 11.45 Dry, age-related macular degeneration demonstrating drusen and pigmentary changes (category 3). (From Kaiser PK, Friedman NJ, Pineda R II. *The Massachusetts Eye and Ear Infirmary Illustrated Manual of Ophthalmology,* 2nd ed. Philadelphia: Saunders; 2004.)

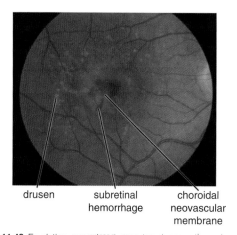

drusen   subretinal hemorrhage   choroidal neovascular membrane

Figure 11.48 Exudative age-related macular degeneration, demonstrating subretinal hemorrhage from classic choroidal neovascular membrane. (From Kaiser PK, Friedman NJ, Pineda R II. *The Massachusetts Eye and Ear Infirmary Illustrated Manual of Ophthalmology,* 2nd ed. Philadelphia: Saunders; 2004.)

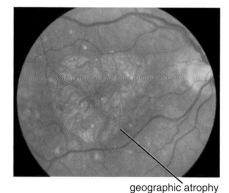

geographic atrophy

Figure 11.46 Advanced, atrophic, nonexudative, age-related macular degeneration demonstrating subfoveal geographic atrophy (category 4). (From Kaiser PK, Friedman NJ, Pineda R II. *The Massachusetts Eye and Ear Infirmary Illustrated Manual of Ophthalmology,* 2nd ed. Philadelphia: Saunders; 2004.)

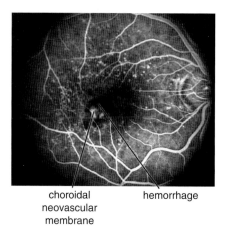

choroidal neovascular membrane   hemorrhage

Figure 11.49 Fluorescein angiogram of same patient as in Fig. 11.48, demonstrating leakage from the choroidal neovascularization (CNV) and blockage from the surrounding subretinal blood. (From Kaiser PK, Friedman NJ, Pineda R II. *The Massachusetts Eye and Ear Infirmary Illustrated Manual of Ophthalmology,* 2nd ed. Philadelphia: Saunders; 2004.)

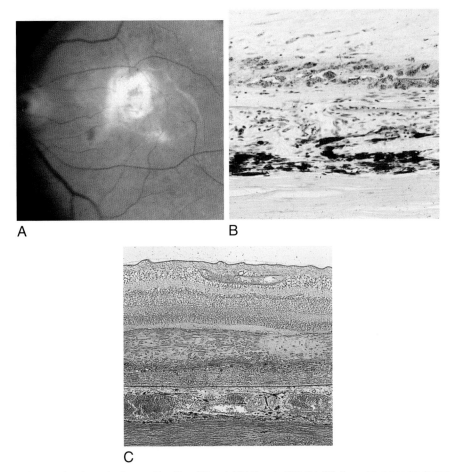

Figure 11.50 (A–C) Neovascular, age-related macular degeneration. (From Edwards MG, Bressler NM, Raja SC: Age-related macular degeneration. In: Yanoff M, Duker JS, eds. *Ophthalmology*. London: Mosby, 1999.)

Basal laminar (cuticular): diffuse, confluent, densely packed small yellow–white (blocks early, stains late on FA, "starry sky" appearance) produces sawtooth pattern of small blunted triangles that sit on Bruch membrane on OCT

Calcific: sharply demarcated, glistening; associated with RPE/geographic atrophy (GA)

Reticular pseudodrusen or subretinal drusenoid debris: located in subretinal space not sub-RPE

Drusen classification: based on size and extent

Small: <64 μm in diameter

Intermediate: 64-124 μm in diameter

Large: ≥125 μm in diameter (approximately equal to vein width at disk margin)

Small drusen considered extensive if the cumulative area within 2 disc diameters (DD) of the center of the macula equal to at least that of the AREDS standard circle C-1 (with diameter $^1/_{12}$ that of the average disc); this corresponds to ~15 small drusen from stereo photographs or 5-10 small drusen

Intermediate drusen considered extensive if soft, indistinct drusen are present and the total area occupied by the drusen is equivalent to the area that would be occupied by 20 drusen each having a diameter of 100 μm. If no soft indistinct drusen are present, intermediate drusen are considered to be extensive when they occupy an area equivalent to at least 1/5 of a disc area (~65 100-μm diameter drusen)

DDx of yellow foveal spot: solar maculopathy, adult vitelliform dystrophy, Best disease, stage 1a macular hole, CSR, old subfoveal hemorrhage, CME, pattern dystrophy

FA: hyperfluorescence of drusen resulting from window defects (from degeneration of overlying RPE) and uptake of dye within drusen (staining)

OCT: drusen appear as elevations of RPE; useful to differentiate dry from wet AMD where the CNV, as well as intraretinal, subretinal, or sub-RPE fluid, is evident

Signs of CNV: subretinal blood, fluid, and/or lipid; RPE detachment (PED); gray–green subretinal discoloration

Types of CNV: historically defined by appearance of leakage on FA

Classic:

EARLY PHASE: bright, fairly uniform hyperfluorescence that progressively intensifies throughout the transit phase

LATE PHASE: progressive leakage of dye that extends beyond the margins of the CNV seen in early stages

Occult (2 types):

FIBROVASCULAR PED:

EARLY PHASE: irregular mottled hyperfluorescence at level of RPE

LATE PHASE: stippled hyperfluorescent leakage that is not as bright or extensive as classic lesions

LATE LEAKAGE OF UNDETERMINED ORIGIN:

EARLY PHASE: no apparent leakage

LATE PHASE: stippled hyperfluorescence at level of RPE

Can also be defined by lesion location:

TYPE 1: CNV under RPE; PCV is a variant of type 1

TYPE 2: CNV above RPE

TYPE 3: retinal angiomatous proliferation (RAP) = often bilateral with small intraretinal hemorrhages and associated PED; develop retinal-choroidal anastomosis

Location of CNV:

Extrafoveal: posterior border of CNV is 200-2500 μm from center of FAZ

Juxtafoveal: 1-199 μm from center of FAZ, or CNV 200-2500 μm from center of FAZ with blood or blocked fluorescence within 200 μm of FAZ center

Subfoveal: under center of FAZ

ICG: helpful for visualizing CNV that is not well seen on FA; CNV appears as focal hot spots or plaque of late hyperfluorescence; can demonstrate CNV under thin hemorrhage that would be blocked on FA; high-speed ICG useful to delineate feeder vessels of CNV. Also useful to visualize polyps and branching vascular network of PCV

Treatment: follow Amsler grid, low-vision aids, vitamin supplements; consider intravitreal injections (anti–vascular endothelial growth factor [VEGF] agents), focal laser, or PDT for CNV

Age-Related Eye Disease Study (AREDS):

Supplements with high-dose antioxidants and zinc are helpful in reducing vision loss and the progression of disease in patients with category 3 and 4 AMD; AREDS2 study evaluated lutein, zeaxanthin, and omega-3 fatty acids in addition to the original AREDS formulation; formulations had almost equal efficacy, so AREDS2 recommended for smokers to avoid beta-carotene

Vitamins C and E can increase risk of myocardial infarction (MI) in postmenopausal women

Zinc is associated with benign prostate hypertrophy in men and stress incontinence in women

Macular Photocoagulation Study (MPS):

Treatment of well-demarcated extrafoveal or juxtafoveal CNV with uniform laser. After 5 years, 64% of untreated eyes had >6 lines of vision loss; 46% of treated eyes had >6 lines of vision loss; >50% recurrence rate. However, many patients do not qualify because of subfoveal CNV and occult lesions

Treatment of Age-Related Macular Degeneration with Photodynamic Therapy (TAP) Trial:

Photodynamic therapy with verteporfin (Visudyne) can prevent vision loss in eyes with subfoveal, predominantly classic and occult AMD, with no classic CNV

Verteporfin in Photodynamic Therapy (VIP) Trial:

Photodynamic therapy with verteporfin (Visudyne) can prevent vision loss in eyes with occult and no classic CNV, especially if <4 MPS disc areas in size or baseline vision <20/50

Pegaptanib (Macugen) VISION Trial:

Aptamer approved by the US Food and Drug Administration (FDA) that is a selective VEGF antagonist binding to the 165 isoform of VEGF-A while sparing other isoforms; no longer commonly used; intravitreal injection every 6 weeks.

Ranibizumab (Lucentis) MARINA and ANCHOR Trials:

FDA approved, humanized, antigen-binding fragment (Fab) designed to bind and inhibit all VEGF isoforms; intravitreal injection monthly or as needed (Complications of Age-Related Macular Degeneration Treatment Trials [CATT] finding was equal efficacy when delivered monthly or as needed)

Bevacizumab (Avastin):

Off-label, full-length antibody that binds and inhibits all VEGF isoforms (FDA approved for colorectal cancer); the CATT study reported that monthly Avastin was noninferior to monthly Lucentis, but as-needed Avastin was not equal. There were significantly greater serious systemic adverse events in the Avastin groups than Lucentis; intravitreal injection monthly. Other comparison studies, including IVAN, MANTA, GEFAL, and LUCAS, have reported similar finding that Lucentis and Avastin efficacy are very similar

Aflibercept (Eylea) VIEW 1 and 2 Trials:

Fusion receptor decoy containing domain 2 from VEGF receptor 1 and domain 3 from VEGFR-2 fused to human Fc fragment that blocks all isoforms of VEGF-A, VEGF-B, and placental growth factor (PLGF); labeled indication is injected every 2 months after a loading dose of 3 monthly injections

Brolucizumab (Beovu) HAWK and HARRIER Studies:

Single-chain antibody fragment that blocks all isoforms of VEGF-A. Labeled indication is 3 monthly injections for loading dose, then based on disease activity, either 8- or 12-week dosing. Intraocular inflammation was seen in ~5% of cases, including cases of retinal occlusive vasculitis

Faricimab, TENAYA and LUCERNE Studies:

Bispecific antibody that blocks all isoforms of VEGF-A and angiopoietin 2 (Ang2)

Anti-VEGF safety: all anti-VEGF agents can get into the systemic circulation, putting patients at risk of arteriothrombotic events (ATEs), such as hypertension, MI, and stroke

Combination treatment: Combination therapy with PDT and anti-VEGF agents has been shown to be safe, with similar visual results and decreased injections (DENALI and MT BLANC Studies). In particular, the best therapy for PCV is combination therapy PDT and anti-VEGF agents (EVEREST Study). Combination therapy with other drugs, such as anti-PDGF, is being evaluated in phase III

Radiation: internal (strontium-90; CABERNET Study— failed) or external (low-dose x-ray radiation) combined with anti-VEGF agents (experimental)

Surgery: in certain cases, consider submacular surgery to remove CNV or displace hemorrhage in cases with large submacular hemorrhage, or macular translocation (experimental)

Prognosis:

Rate of Progression to Advanced AMD (AREDS) over 5 years: 1.3% have many small or few medium drusen (if both eyes have many intermediate drusen, but no large drusen, then patient score = 1 in scale below) 18% many medium or any large drusen 43% unilateral advanced AMD

AREDS Clinical Severity Scale (AREDS) for AMD: Based on giving 1 point for the presence of ≥1 large drusen and/or pigment changes (hyper-, hypo-, or noncentral GA) per eye, or 2 points for advanced AMD in 1 eye, then total 2 eyes to come up with a point score that shows patient's risk of developing advanced AMD in 5 years:
0 points = 0.5%
1 point = 3%
2 points = 12%
3 points = 25%
4 points = 50%

Risk of CNV in fellow eye at 5 years: if drusen is present
Hard (nodular) = 10%
Soft = 30%
Pigmented = 30%
Soft and pigmented = 60%

Risk of fellow eye developing CNV: 4%-12% per year; increased risk with multiple soft drusen, RPE clumping, densely packed drusen, PED

MAJOR AGE-RELATED MACULAR DEGENERATION CLINICAL STUDIES

Macular Photocoagulation Study (MPS)

Objective: to evaluate efficacy of laser photocoagulation in preventing visual loss from CNV

Methods: patients were randomly assigned to laser photocoagulation vs. observation in the following groups:

Extrafoveal Study: well-demarcated CNV resulting from AMD or ocular histoplasmosis syndrome (OHS), or idiopathic, that was 200-2500 μm from center of FAZ with vision >20/100. Patients who received previous photocoagulation were excluded. Patients were randomly assigned to

argon blue–green treatment to the entire CNV and 100-125 μm beyond the borders of the lesion vs. observation

Juxtafoveal (Krypton) Study: well-demarcated CNV as a result of AMD or OHS, or idiopathic, that was 1-199 μm from center of FAZ, or with a CNV >200 μm with blood or pigment extending within 200 μm and with vision >20/400. Patients were randomly assigned to Krypton red treatment of entire CNV and 100 μm beyond the borders of the lesion except on the foveal side of the lesion vs. observation

Subfoveal, New CNV AMD Study: well-demarcated CNV resulting from AMD under the center of FAZ with vision between 20/40-20/320. The entire lesion had to measure less than 3.5 MPS disc areas in size and could be classic or occult CNV. Patients were randomly assigned to argon green or krypton red treatment of entire CNV and 100 μm beyond the borders of the lesion vs. observation

Subfoveal Recurrent CNV Study: well-demarcated CNV resulting from AMD under the center of FAZ contiguous with previous laser treatment scar and with vision between 20/40-20/320. The entire lesion had to measure <6 MPS disc areas in size and could be classic or occult CNV. Patients randomly assigned to argon green or krypton red treatment of entire CNV and 100 μm beyond the borders of the lesion vs. observation

DEFINITIONS:
EXTRAFOVEAL: 200-2500 μm from center of FAZ
JUXTAFOVEAL: 1-199 μm from center of FAZ
SUBFOVEAL: extends beneath center of fovea

MAIN OUTCOME MEASURES: visual acuity (VA), contrast sensitivity, reading speed, persistent and/or recurrent CNV, treatment complications

Results:

Extrafoveal study:

After 18 months:
AMD: 25% of treated vs. 60% of untreated eyes had lost ≥6 lines of vision (a quadrupling of the visual angle [i.e., 20/50-20/200])
PRESUMED OCULAR HISTOPLASMOSIS SYNDROME (POHS): 9.4% of treated vs. 34.2% of untreated eyes had lost ≥6 lines of vision
IDIOPATHIC: sample size (67) was too small to reach clinical significance, but trend was similar to results for AMD and POHS
Recurrence of CNV after argon laser was 52% with AMD, 28% with POHS, 28% with idiopathic CNV

After 3 years:
Relative risk of severe vision loss (≥6 lines) for no treatment vs. treatment was 1.4 for AMD, 5.5 for POHS, and 2.3 for idiopathic CNV

After 5 years:

AMD: treated eyes lost 5.2 lines of vision vs. 7.1 lines in untreated eyes; recurrence in 54% of treated eyes; 26% developed CNV in fellow eye

POHS: treated eyes lost 0.9 lines of vision vs. 4.4 lines in untreated eyes; recurrence in 26% of treated eyes

IDIOPATHIC: treated eyes lost 2.7 lines of vision vs. 4.4 lines in untreated eyes; recurrence in 34% of treated eyes

Juxtafoveal study:

After 3 years:

POHS: 4.6% of treated vs. 24.6% of untreated eyes had lost ≥6 lines of vision

IDIOPATHIC: 10% of treated vs. 37% of untreated eyes had lost ≥6 lines of vision

After 5 years:

Relative risk of severe vision loss (≥6 lines) for no treatment vs. treatment was 1.2 for AMD (hypertensive patients had little or no benefit), 4.26 for POHS, and intermediate between AMD and POHS for idiopathic CNV

Subfoveal new CNV AMD study:

After 3 months:

AMD: 20% of treated vs. 11% of untreated eyes had lost ≥6 lines of vision

After 2 years:

AMD: 20% of treated vs. 37% of untreated eyes had lost ≥6 lines of vision; recurrence in 51% of treated eyes

After 4 years:

AMD: 22% of treated vs. 47% of untreated eyes had lost ≥6 lines of vision

Subfoveal recurrent CNV AMD study:

After 3 years: 12% of treated vs. 36% of untreated eyes had lost ≥6 lines of vision

Conclusions: treat extrafoveal CNV in patients with AMD, POHS, and idiopathic lesions

Patients with juxtafoveal CNV (AMD, POHS, and idiopathic) benefit from krypton laser photocoagulation, except for hypertensive AMD patients

Patients with AMD with subfoveal CNV (new or recurrent) benefit equally from argon green or krypton red laser treatment

For unilateral CNV, large drusen and focal hyperpigmentation are risk factors for development of CNV in fellow eye

Treatment of AMD patients with juxtafoveal CNV is beneficial when the lesion is classic, even though CNV recurs; treatment of classic CNV alone in lesions with both classic and occult CNV was not beneficial

Treatment of Age-Related Macular Degeneration with Photodynamic Therapy (TAP) Trial

Objective: to evaluate verteporfin (Visudyne) ocular photodynamic therapy (OPT) in the management of subfoveal CNV with some classic characteristics

Methods: patients with evidence of AMD, age > 50 years, evidence of new or recurrent subfoveal "classic" (can have occult features) CNV by fluorescein angiography with greatest linear dimension of CNV < 5400 μm (9 MPS disc areas), Early Treatment Diabetic Retinopathy Study (ETDRS) VA of 20/40-20/200, and the ability to return every 3 months for 2 years. Patients were excluded who had other ocular diseases that could compromise VA, history of previous experimental treatment for CNV, porphyrin allergy, liver problems, or intraocular surgery within the previous 2 months. Two-thirds of patients in both studies were randomly assigned (2:1 randomization scheme) to receive verteporfin (Visudyne 6 mg/m^2) and one-third to control vehicle (D$_5$W IV infusion) infused over a 10-minute period. All patients were then irradiated with a 689-nm diode laser (light dose: 50 J/cm^2; power density: 600 mW/cm^2; duration: 83 seconds) 15 minutes after the start of infusion

Results: 609 patients enrolled (311 in Study A and 298 in Study B). Vision was stabilized or improved in 61.4% of patients treated with Visudyne OPT compared with 45.9% treated with placebo at 12 months. The difference was sustained at 24 and 60 months (TAP Extension Study). In subgroup analysis, VA benefit was most pronounced for lesions in which area of classic CNV occupied more than 50% of entire area of lesion (predominantly classic). Specifically, 33% of Visudyne-treated eyes compared with 61% of placebo-treated eyes sustained moderate visual loss. No difference in VA was noted when area of classic CNV was greater than 0% but less than 50% of entire lesion (minimally classic). Sixteen percent of patients experienced an improvement in vision (1 or more lines) in Visudyne-treated group compared with 7.2% in control group. Overall, Visudyne group was 34% more likely to retain vision. Most patients required periodic retreatments with an average of 3.4 (of a possible 4) being required in first year, 2.1 in second year (5.5 total over 24 months), and 1.5 in third year (7 total over 36 months)

Conclusions: Visudyne ocular photodynamic therapy is recommended for subfoveal, predominantly classic, CNV

Verteporfin in Photodynamic Therapy (VIP) Trial; Verteporfin in Photodynamic Therapy–Pathologic Myopia (VIP-PM) Trial

Objective: to evaluate Visudyne OPT in the management of subfoveal CNV not included in original TAP investigation

Methods: patients with evidence of AMD, age >50 years, evidence of subfoveal "occult" only CNV by FA with recent disease progression, defined as evidence of hemorrhage, loss of ≥1 line of vision, or increased size of the lesion by 10% during the preceding 3 months, and ETDRS VA ≥20/100; or subfoveal "classic" CNV with ETDRS VA of ≥20/40, greatest linear dimension of CNV < 5400 µm (9 MPS disc areas), and the ability to return every 3 months for 2 years. Patients were excluded who had other ocular diseases that could compromise VA, history of previous experimental treatment for CNV, porphyrin allergy, liver problems, or intraocular surgery within previous 2 months. Two-thirds of the patients in both studies were randomly assigned (2:1 randomization scheme) to receive verteporfin (Visudyne 6 mg/m^2) and one-third to control vehicle (D$_5$W IV infusion) infused over a 10-minute period. All patients were then irradiated with the use of a 689-nm diode laser (light dose: 50 J/cm^2; power density: 600 mW/cm^2; duration: 83 seconds) 15 minutes after the start of the infusion

Results: 459 patients enrolled. 1-year results showed no statistically significant difference between Visudyne-treated patients and placebo (difference 4.2%). However, by 24 months, a statistically significant difference was seen that was attributable to a decline in vision in control group (difference 13.7%). Moreover, this difference was most pronounced in patients with "occult"-only CNV lesions measuring <4 MPS disc areas in size at baseline, or who had baseline VA of ≤20/50

Few ocular or other systemic adverse events were seen with Visudyne therapy. In 4.4% of patients, an immediate severe visual decrease within 7 days of treatment was observed

Conclusions: Visudyne OPT is recommended in the management of subfoveal occult but not classic CNV when there is evidence of recent disease progression, especially if baseline lesion size is <4 MPS disc areas or the baseline vision is <20/50

Age-Related Eye Disease Study (AREDS)

Objective: to evaluate the effect of high-dose supplements on the progression of AMD and on the development and progression of cataracts

Methods: patients aged 55-80 years with ≥20/32 vision OU, or ≥20/32 in one eye and AMD in fellow eye, received antioxidants (vitamin C [500 mg], vitamin E [400 IU], beta-carotene [vitamin A, 15 mg]), zinc (80 mg plus 2 mg copper), both, or placebo

Categorized into 4 groups:
Category 1: <5 small (<63-µm) drusen
Category 2 (mild AMD): multiple small drusen or single or nonextensive intermediate (63-124 µm) drusen, or pigment abnormalities

Category 3 (intermediate AMD): extensive intermediate-sized drusen, or ≥1 large (>125 µm) drusen, or noncentral GA
Category 4 (advanced AMD): vision loss (<20/32) as a result of AMD in 1 eye (as a result of either central/subfoveal geographic atrophy or exudative macular degeneration
Primary outcomes:
Progression to advanced AMD: treatment for CNV or photographic evidence (geographic atrophy of center of macula, nondrusenoid RPE detachment, serous or hemorrhagic RD, subretinal hemorrhage or fibrosis)
Moderate vision loss: ≥15-letter loss (doubling of visual angle)
Development and progression of lens opacities

Results: 4757 patients enrolled
Antioxidants plus zinc: reduced the risk of progression to advanced AMD and vision loss over 6 years in 25% of high-risk patients
High-risk patients: intermediate AMD (many intermediate drusen [63–124 µm] or 1 large drusen [≥125 µm] in 1 or both eyes) or advanced AMD (in 1 eye only)
Zinc alone: reduced risk of vision loss by 21%
Antioxidants alone: reduced risk of vision loss by 17%

Conclusions: high-dose supplements are beneficial in reducing risk of vision loss in patients with high-risk AMD (categories 3 and 4). Caution should be exercised in smokers or recent smokers in use of high-dose beta-carotene because of possible increased risk of lung cancer

Treatment is of no benefit in patients with no AMD or early AMD (several small or intermediate drusen)

Treatment does not affect development or progression of cataract

Age-Related Eye Disease Study (AREDS2)

Objective: to evaluate the effect of high-dose supplements, macular carotenoids, and omega-3-fatty acid on the progression of AMD

Methods: 4203 patients randomized to receive various combinations of vitamin C (500 mg), vitamin E (400 IU), beta-carotene (vitamin A, 15 mg), zinc (80 mg plus 2 mg copper), lutein (10 mg), zeaxanthin (2 mg), omega-3 long-chain polyunsaturated fatty acids (LCPUFAs) in the form of docosahexaenoic acid (DHA) (350 mg) and eicosapentaenoic acid (EPA) (650 mg)

Results: original AREDS formula reduced risk of progression to advanced AMD. Adding lutein and zeaxanthin provided about 20% reduction in progression beyond original AREDS, in those who had the lowest dietary intake of lutein and zeaxanthin. Addition of omega-3 did not reduce risk of progression

Conclusions: National Eye Institute recommends AREDS formula be adjusted by removal of betacarotene and addition of lutein and zeaxanthin

VEGF Inhibition Study in Ocular Neovascularization (VISION) Trial

Objective: to evaluate intravitreal pegaptanib for subfoveal CNV as a result of neovascular AMD

Methods: 2 concurrent randomized, double-masked clinical trials; 1208 patients received either pegaptanib intravitreal injection (0.3 mg, 1.0 mg, or 3.0 mg) or a sham injection into study eye every 6 weeks for total of 48 weeks. Patients were eligible for trial if they were ≥50 years old and had subfoveal classic, minimally classic, and/or occult CNV as a result of wet AMD with best-corrected VA of 20/40-20/320 in study eye

Results: on average, patients treated with pegaptanib 0.3 mg and sham-treated patients continued to experience vision loss. However, rate of VA decline in pegaptanib-treated group was slower than rate in patients who received sham treatment; 70% of patients treated with pegaptanib sodium injection (0.3 mg; $n = 294$) lost <15 letters of VA compared with 55% in control group ($n = 296$; $P < 0.001$); 10% of patients treated with pegaptanib sodium injection (0.3 mg; $n = 294$) had severe VA loss (≥30 letters) compared with 22% in the control group ($n = 296$; $P < 0.001$). Beneficial effect was observed for all subtypes of neovascularization (NV) and was sustained for up to 2 years of follow-up

Conclusions: pegaptanib was better than sham and PDT for neovascular AMD

Minimally Classic/Occult Trial of the Anti-VEGF Antibody Ranibizumab in the Treatment of Neovascular AMD (MARINA) Trial

Objective: pivotal phase III, multicenter, double-blind 24-month study that compared monthly intravitreal injections of ranibizumab 0.3 or 0.5 mg or sham injections ($n = 716$) in patients with subfoveal occult only or minimally classic CNV as a result of wet AMD

Results: enrolled 716 patients with minimally classic and occult subfoveal CNV associated with AMD. Primary outcome was prevention of moderate visual loss (≤15 letters loss of vision), which was seen in 94.5% with ranibizumab 0.3 mg, 94.6% with ranibizumab 0.5 mg, and 62.2% of patients receiving sham injections

($P < 0.001$). Vision improved by ≥15 letters for a significantly greater number of ranibizumab-treated patients (24.8% for 0.3 mg and 33.8% for 0.5 mg) vs. sham-treated patients (5.0%). Mean increases in VA from baseline were +6.5 letters for ranibizumab 0.3-mg group and +7.2 letters for ranibizumab 0.5-mg group, whereas sham-injected patients had a mean decrease of −10.4 letters. This benefit in VA in ranibizumab-treated patients was maintained through 24 months. At 24 months, 90% of ranibizumab-treated patients in MARINA study lost <15 letters of VA; 33% gained ≥15 letters of VA. Ranibizumab-treated patients exhibited a statistically significant improvement compared with sham-treated patients in all subgroups for all outcome measures

Conclusions: ranibizumab was better than sham for occult with no classic and minimally classic CNV resulting from neovascular AMD

Anti-Vascular Endothelial Growth Factor (VEGF) Antibody for The Treatment of Predominantly Classic Choroidal Neovascularization (CNV) in Age-Related Macular Degeneration (ANCHOR) Trial

Objective: second pivotal phase III, multicenter, randomized, double-masked 24-month clinical trial to compare ranibizumab with the active control verteporfin PDT in subfoveal predominantly classic CNV resulting from wet AMD

Results: enrolled 423 patients with predominantly classic subfoveal CNV associated with AMD. Primary outcome was prevention of moderate visual loss (≤15 letters loss of vision), which was seen in 94.3% with ranibizumab 0.3 mg, 96.4% with ranibizumab 0.5 mg and 64.3% of patients receiving PDT. Vision improved by ≥15 letters in significantly more ranibizumab treated patients (35.7% for 0.3 mg and 40.3% for 0.5 mg) than PDT-treated patients (5.6%). At 12 months, mean change in VA increased by +8.5 letters in ranibizumab 0.3-mg group and by +11.3 letters in 0.5-mg group but decreased by −9.5 letters in sham group

Conclusions: ranibizumab was superior to verteporfin for treatment of predominantly classic CNV resulting from neovascular AMD

Aflibercept for Age-Related Macular Degeneration Study (VIEW 1/2)

Objective: phase II studies to evaluate 3 different dosing regimens of aflibercept, 0.5 mg every 4 weeks, 2 mg every 4 weeks, and 2 mg every 8 weeks (following 3 initial monthly injections), compared with ranibizumab 0.5 mg every 4 weeks; 2-year study

Results: integrated analysis of VIEW 1 and VIEW 2 studies, VA gain from baseline in aflibercept 2 mg every-8-week group at week 96 was 7.6 letters compared with 8.4 letters at week 52, with an average of 11.2 injections over 2 years and 4.2 injections during the second year. VA gain from baseline in monthly ranibizumab group at week 96 was 7.9 letters compared with 8.7 letters at week 52, with an average of 16.5 injections over 2 years and 4.7 injections during the second year. Safety results between drugs were similar

Conclusions: VIEW studies found that aflibercept injected every 2 months was equivalent to ranibizumab injected monthly after 3 monthly loading doses; 94% (VIEW 1) and 95% (VIEW 2) of patients treated with aflibercept or ranibizumab maintained vision (<15 letters loss) at 2 years

Comparison of AMD Treatment Trials (CATT)

Objective: to compare Avastin vs. Lucentis with monthly and as-needed treatment schedules for 2 years. After year 1, patients initially assigned to monthly treatment were randomly reassigned to monthly or as-needed treatment without changing their drug assignment

Results: 1107 patients included. After 2 years, differences in VA outcomes between drugs when given monthly or as needed were not statistically significant; mean gain in VA was similar for both drugs (bevacizumab-ranibizumab difference, 1.4 letters). Mean gain was greater for monthly treatment than for as-needed treatment (difference, –2.4 letters). However, many of the secondary anatomic outcomes suggested that bevacizumab is biologically inferior to ranibizumab. Proportion of patients who were completely dry as measured by OCT was 13.9% with PRN bevacizumab vs. 30.2% with monthly bevacizumab, and 22.3% with PRN ranibizumab vs. 45.5% with monthly ranibizumab. Eyes receiving PRN bevacizumab required mean of 14.1 injections vs. 12.6 with PRN ranibizumab. Macular atrophy was found to be greater in groups that received monthly treatment (19% with bevacizumab and 30% with ranibizumab) than PRN treatment groups (14% with bevacizumab and 16% with ranibizumab). The significance of this is unknown. Arterial thrombotic event rates were similar between the 2 drugs, but proportion of patients with ≥1 serious systemic adverse events was significantly greater with bevacizumab than with ranibizumab: 39.9% vs. 31.7%

The Alternative Treatments to Inhibit VEGF in Age-Related Choroidal Neovascularization (IVAN) Study

Objective: to evaluate ranibizumab vs. bevacizumab to treat neovascular AMD. Patients randomized into 4 groups: ranibizumab or bevacizumab, given either every month (continuous) or as needed (discontinuous), with monthly evaluations. Performed in the UK by National Health Service. Unlike CATT, patients received 3 monthly injections at outset of trial

Results: 610 patients included; 1-year results reported that comparison between bevacizumab and ranibizumab was "inconclusive." Discontinuous treatment was equivalent to continuous treatment. Fewer participants receiving bevacizumab had an arteriothrombotic event or heart failure. There was no difference between drugs in proportion experiencing a serious systemic adverse event. Serum VEGF levels were lower with bevacizumab and higher with discontinuous treatment; bevacizumab was less costly for both treatment regimens; 2-year results showed no difference in vision between the drugs. For best-corrected visual acuity (BCVA), bevacizumab was neither noninferior nor inferior to ranibizumab. Discontinuous treatment was neither noninferior nor inferior to continuous treatment. Monthly treatment resulted in slightly better levels of vision, detected through testing of near VA and contrast sensitivity. Discontinuous group received on average 13 injections over the 2-year period compared with 23 for monthly treatment group. Frequency of arterial thrombotic events or hospital admission for heart failure did not differ between drugs, but mortality was lower with continuous than discontinuous treatment

Conclusions: CATT, IVAN, MANTA LUCAS, and GEFAL found that either monthly or PRN treatment with bevacizumab or ranibizumab was equally effective in treating neovascular AMD at up to 2 years. However, there are concerns that bevacizumab may have worse side-effect profile because of its greater systemic bioavailability. In addition, PRN dosing was not as efficacious as fixed dosing, especially with bevacizumab

HAWK and HARRIER Studies

Objective: to evaluate brolucizumab vs. aflibercept in treatment of naïve wet AMD patients with subfoveal CNV in a 48-week, noninferiority (4-letter margin) study. Aflibercept was dosed per label with 3 monthly loading doses, then every-8-weeks dosing. Brolucizumab was dosed with 3 monthly loading doses, then evaluated for evidence of disease activity at weeks 16, 20, 32, and 44. If no disease activity seen, patients were dosed at 12-week intervals. If disease activity was seen, the patients were dosed at 8-week intervals. Disease activity was based on VA decline or increase in retinal thickness or increased leakage on OCT

Results: 1083 patients (360 in 3 mg, 361 in 6 mg, and 361 in the aflibercept arms) were enrolled in HAWK and 743 patients (372 in 6 mg and 371 in aflibercept arms) in HARRIER. The noninferiority margin was met with a treatment difference of –0.2 letters in HAWK ($P < 0.0001$) and –0.7 letters vs. aflibercept in HARRIER

($P < 0.0001$). The mean change in vision was +6.7/6.5 letters in the 6-mg brolucizumab arms and +6.7/7.7 letters in the aflibercept arms in HAWK and HARRIER, respectively; 57%/52% of brolucizumab patients were maintained at 12-week dosing intervals in HAWK and HARRIER, respectively. Significantly fewer patients in the brolucizumab arms had disease activity at the head-to-head assessment points. In the second years of the study, the mean change in vision from baseline was +5.9/+6.1 in the 6-mg brolucizumab arms and +5.3/+6.6 letters in the aflibercept arms in HAWK and HARRIER, respectively. Brolucizumab had superior reduction in central retinal thickness, intraretinal fluid, and/or subretinal fluid. The safety of the two drugs was similar, except for an imbalance in the rate of intraocular inflammation. A post hoc safety review revealed 4.6% of patients had intraocular inflammation (IOI), with 3.3% having retinal vasculitis and 2.1% having retinal occlusive vasculitis

Conclusions: although the VA noninferiority efficacy outcomes were met, the safety issue with 4.6% of patients receiving brolucizumab having intraocular inflammation and 2.1% having retinal occlusive vasculitis was problematic. In addition, a study with monthly dosing (MERLIN) in wet AMD revealed even higher levels of IOI and retinal occlusive vasculitis, leading to termination of all studies with more frequent dosing than q8 weeks

TENAYA and LUCERNE Studies

Objective: to evaluate faricimab vs. aflibercept in treatment-naïve patients with wet AMD with subfoveal CNV in a 48-week, noninferiority study. Aflibercept was dosed per label with 3 monthly loading doses then every-8-weeks dosing. Faricimab was dosed with 4 monthly loading doses, then evaluated for evidence of disease activity at weeks 20 and 24. If no disease activity seen, patients were dosed at 16-week intervals. If disease activity seen, patients were dosed at 8- or 12-week intervals. Disease activity was based on VA decline or increase in retinal thickness or increased leakage on OCT

Results: 671 patients enrolled (334 in faricimab arm, 337 in aflibercept arm) in TENAYA and 658 in LUCERNE (331 in faricimab arm, 327 in aflibercept arm). The noninferiority margin was met with a treatment difference of +0.7 letters in TENAYA and 0 letters in LUCERNE. In TENAYA, 45.7% were dosed at every 16 weeks, 34.0% at every 12 weeks, and 20.3% at every 8 weeks. In LUCERNE, 454.9% were dosed at every 16 weeks, 32.9% at every 12 weeks, and 22.2% at every 8 weeks. After 48 weeks, the mean change in vision was +5.8/+6.6 letters in the faricimab arm and +5.1/6.6 letters in the aflibercept arm in TENAYA and LUCERNE, respectively. The safety analysis was similar between groups. IOI was 1.5%/2.4% in the faricimab arms and 0.6%/1.8% in the aflibercept arms in TENAYA and

LUCERNE, respectively. No cases of retinal occlusive vasculitis were seen. The AVONELLE-X is the long-term extension study to follow patients up to 4 years

Conclusions: the primary endpoint of noninferiority of VA results was met, with faricimab demonstrating ≥ every-12-weeks dosing in ~80% of patients at 48 weeks. Similar reductions in central retinal thickness were seen in both arms. The drugs were well tolerated, with no vasculitis or retinal occlusive vasculitis seen

Other Disorders Associated With Choroidal Neovascular Membrane (CNV)

Mnemonic: **HAMMAR** (**H**istoplasmosis, **A**MD, **M**ultifocal choroiditis, **M**yopia, **A**ngioid streaks, **R**upture of choroid)

Treatment for all CNV: consider laser only for extrafoveal lesions (MPS showed that laser treatment for juxtafoveal and extrafoveal CNV was beneficial); juxtafoveal and subfoveal lesions are treated with anti-VEGF agents or photodynamic therapy (see above)

Presumed Ocular Histoplasmosis Syndrome (POHS) (See Chapter 8, Uveitis)

Etiology: caused by infection with *Histoplasma capsulatum*, endemic to Mississippi and Ohio River valleys

Macular involvement associated with HLA-B7, HLA-DRw2

Findings: triad of peripapillary atrophy, multiple punched-out chorioretinal scars ("histo spots"), and maculopathy. CNV can occur different from that in AMD in that vessels penetrate Bruch membrane and extend over RPE; a second layer of RPE forms (basal side up) and attempts to encircle the CNV (Fig. 11.51)

Complications: risk of CNV is 1% if no signs of POHS in fellow eye, 5% if no histo spots in macula, and 15% (within 5 years) if histo spots in macula

Treatment: anti-VEGF injections similar to CNV secondary to wet AMD, except fewer injections required

Angioid Streaks

Peripapillary linear cracks in thickened, degenerated, and calcified Bruch membrane (Fig. 11.52)

Subretinal hemorrhage can occur with minor trauma; patients should consider safety glasses

Etiology: 50% associated with systemic condition, 50% idiopathic

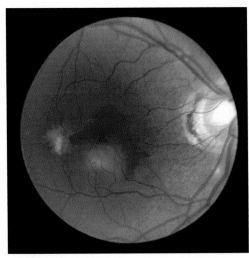

Figure 11.51 Presumed ocular histoplasmosis syndrome (POHS) demonstrating peripapillary scarring and macular, juxtafoveal choroidal neovascular membrane with surrounding subretinal hemorrhage. (From Noorthy RS, Fountain JS. Fungal uveitis. In: Yanoff M, Duker JS, eds. *Ophthalmology.* London: Mosby; 1999.)

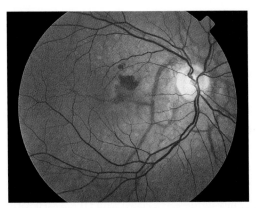

Figure 11.52 Peripapillary angioid streaks. (From Vander JF: Angioid streaks. In: Yanoff M, Duker JS, eds. *Ophthalmology.* London: Mosby; 1999.)

Mnemonic **PEPSI:**

Pseudoxanthoma elasticum (PXE) (autosomal recessive [AR] >> autosomal dominant [AD]): female > male; peau d'orange appearance to retina; redundant skin with waxy, yellow, papule-like lesions ("plucked chicken" skin); increased elastic tissue; vascular malformations; abnormal mucosal vasculature may cause gastrointestinal (GI) bleeds; may have optic nerve head drusen; angioid streaks present in 85%

Ehlers-Danlos syndrome (fibrodysplasia hyperelastica) (AD): hyperextensible skin as a result of deficient collagen matrix; other eye findings include subluxed lens, high myopia, keratoconus, blue sclera, RD

Paget disease: increased bone production and destruction; increased serum alkaline phosphatase; prone to basal skull and long bone fractures; other bone disorders (acromegaly, calcinosis)

Sickle cell: risk for autoinfarction of spleen and thrombotic episodes; other hematologic diseases (thalassemia, hereditary spherocytosis, acanthocytosis [Bassen-Kornzweig syndrome]); angioid streaks present in 1%

Idiopathic: 50%

Others: senile elastosis, calcinosis, abetalipoproteinemia, thalassemia, hereditary spherocytosis; also associated

with optic disc drusen, acromegaly, homocystinuria, lead poisoning, Marfan syndrome, and retinitis pigmentosa

DDx: lacquer cracks in myopia

Pathologic Myopia

High myopia = axial length ≥ 26.5 mm; > −6 D of myopia

Pathologic myopia refers to posterior segment structural changes from increased axial length

~3% of population; female > male; progressive, irreversible

Increased risk of glaucoma, cataract, RRD

Findings: RPE attenuation causes tessellated fundus appearance and peri-papillary atrophy,

Posterior staphyloma: ~50%; eye wall bulges outward, caused by scleral weakness; 6 types: wide macular (most common, ~75%), narrow macular, peripapillary, nasal, inferior (associated with tilted disc syndrome), other configurations; often leads to atrophic, traction, or neovascular maculopathy

Myopic choroidal neovascularization (CNV): 5%-11%, often near fovea (65%); commonly in young patients, bilateral ~15%; risk factors: lacquer cracks (breaks in Bruch membrane; incidence of 4%-9% in high myopia; sudden decrease in vision, metamorphopsia, often in teenagers; focal subretinal hemorrhage, dense, round, deep, and often centered on fovea; blood may obscure crack; 29% develop CNV), choroidal thinning, impaired choroidal circulation, and patchy retinal atrophy

  TREATMENT: anti-VEGF injections, better outcome than AMD-related CNV, regresses faster, fewer injections required (67% have only 1 injection), recurrence usually within 1 year

  PROGNOSIS: poor; without treatment VA ≤20/200 within 5 years; even with treatment 90% have significant reduced vision over 5-10 years from progression of chorioretinal atrophy

Myopic maculopathy: progressive chorioretinal atrophy; associated with age, AL, posterior staphyloma, and myopic CNV

  META-ANALYSIS OF PATHOLOGIC MYOPIA (META-PM) CLASSIFICATION:

    CATEGORY 0: no myopic retinal degenerative lesion

    CATEGORY 1: tessellated fundus

    CATEGORY 2: diffuse chorioretinal atrophy

    CATEGORY 3: patchy chorioretinal atrophy

    CATEGORY 4: macular atrophy

    "PLUS" SIGNS: lacquer cracks, myopic CNV, Fuchs spot (RPE hyperplasia in area of regressed CNV)

    PATHOLOGIC MYOPIA: ≥ category 2 or "plus" lesion or posterior staphyloma

  ATN CLASSIFICATION: based on 3 factors (atrophy, traction, neovascularization)

    ATROPHIC COMPONENT (SAME AS META-PM CATEGORIES)

      A0: no myopic retinal lesions

      A1: tessellated fundus only

      A2: diffuse chorioretinal atrophy

A3: patchy chorioretinal atrophy

A4: complete macular atrophy

TRACTIONAL COMPONENT:

T0: no macular schisis

T1: inner or outer foveoschisis

T2: inner + outer foveoschisis

T3: foveal detachment

T4: full-thickness macular hole (MH)

T5: MH + RD

NEOVASCULAR COMPONENT:

N0: no myopic CNV

N1: macular lacquer cracks

N2a: active CNV

N2s: scar/Fuchs spot

Myopic subretinal hemorrhage: ~3%; usually from lacquer crack; hemorrhage resolves without treatment

Dome-shaped macula: macula bulges inward; associated with subretinal fluid, RPE detachment, CNV, and polypoidal choroidal vasculopathy at apex of dome

Myopic traction maculopathy (MTM): findings include retinal thickening, retinoschisis, lamellar macular hole, and foveal detachment

TREATMENT: vitrectomy with ILM peeling

Macular hole retinal detachment: more common in females and Asians

TREATMENT: vitrectomy

PROGNOSIS: poor, VA <20/200

Other Causes of Macular CNV

Idiopathic, optic nerve head drusen, choroidal rupture, choroidal nevus, sympathetic ophthalmia, VKH disease, serpiginous choroiditis, other posterior uveitides (choroidal inflammation may enhance production of angiogenic factors; when coupled with RPE–Bruch membrane disruption, CNV can develop)

Vascular Diseases

Damage to vessel walls causes leakage of serum and blood into plexiform layers, causing edema, exudates, and hemorrhages

Edema: histologically appears as clear cystoid spaces

Lipid: appears as yellow lesion; histologically, hard exudates are eosinophilic and PAS-positive

DDx: diabetes, hypertensive retinopathy, CNV, vein occlusion, macular telangiectasia, Coats disease, radiation retinopathy, CSR, trauma, macroaneurysm, papilledema, angiomatosis retinae

Microaneurysm: fusiform outpouching of capillary wall

Cotton-wool spot: microinfarction of NFL (usually secondary to occlusion of retinal arteriole) with cessation of axoplasmic flow, mitochondria accumulate (resemble a nucleus, so lesion appears like a cell ["cytoid body"])

Hemorrhage: shape of intraretinal blood depends on layer in which it occurs (dot/blot in plexiform layer where cells are oriented vertically; flame-shaped/feathery border in NFL where cells are oriented horizontally)

Roth spot: white-centered hemorrhage

DDx: ischemia (anemia, anoxia, carbon monoxide poisoning), elevated venous pressure (birth trauma, shaken baby syndrome, intracranial hemorrhage), capillary fragility (hypertension, diabetes), infection (bacterial endocarditis, HIV), leukemia, collagen vascular disease

Neovascularization: growth of new vessels on vitreous side of ILM; new vessels grow along posterior hyaloid

Vascular tortuosity: may be congenital (arterial and venous) or acquired (venous)

DDx: hypertension, high venous pressure (occlusion), papilledema, high viscosity, AV fistula; associated with fetal alcohol syndrome, Peter anomaly, optic nerve hypoplasia

Retinal Vasculitis

Involvement of retinal arterioles (arteritis), veins (phlebitis), or both (periphlebitis)

Findings: sheathing of vessels, hemorrhage

DDx: temporal arteritis, polyarteritis nodosa, lupus, Behçet disease, inflammatory bowel syndrome, multiple sclerosis, pars planitis, granulomatosis with polyangiitis, Eales disease, sarcoidosis, syphilis, toxoplasmosis, viral retinitis (herpes simplex virus [HSV], varicella-zoster virus [VZV]), IV drug abuse, Lyme disease, tuberculosis

Cystoid Macular Edema (CME)

Intraretinal edema in honeycomb-like spaces; flower-petal pattern as a result of Henle layer

Etiology: mnemonic **DEPRIVEN**

Diabetes

Epinephrine

Pars planitis

Retinitis pigmentosa

Irvine-Gass syndrome

Venous occlusion

E$_2$ prostaglandin

Nicotinic acid maculopathy (does not leak)

Others: uveitis, hypertensive retinopathy, retinal vasculitis, epiretinal membrane, radiation retinopathy, post laser or cryo treatment, hypotony, occult rhegmatogenous RD, intraocular tumors, macular telangiectasia, CNV (rare), juvenile retinoschisis (does not leak), Goldmann-Favre syndrome (does not leak), latanoprost (Xalatan), vitreous wick

Pathophysiology: abnormal perifoveal retinal capillary permeability; initial fluid accumulation may be within Müller cells (rather than in spaces of outer plexiform and inner nuclear layers)

Findings: CME, optic nerve swelling, vitreous cell (Fig. 11.53)

FA: multiple small focal fluorescein leaks early; late pooling of dye in cystoid spaces; classically, flower-petal ("petalloid") pattern; staining of optic nerve (Fig. 11.54)

OCT: cystic intraretinal spaces (Fig. 11.55)

DDx of cystic macular changes (looks like CME clinically, but no fluorescein filling of cysts):
1. Juvenile retinoschisis
2. Goldmann-Favre syndrome
3. Some types of retinitis pigmentosa
4. Nicotinic acid maculopathy

Treatment: depends on etiology; focal laser treatment, topical steroids and NSAID, oral Diamox, sub-Tenon or intravitreal steroid injection

Congenital Retinal Telangiectasia/Coats Disease (Leber Miliary Aneurysms)

(See Chapter 5, Pediatrics/Strabismus)

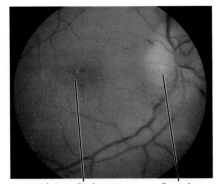

intraretinal cysts   disc edema

Figure 11.53 Cystoid macular edema with decreased foveal reflex, cystic changes in fovea, and intraretinal hemorrhages. (From Kaiser PK, Friedman NJ, Pineda R II. *The Massachusetts Eye and Ear Infirmary Illustrated Manual of Ophthalmology*, 2nd ed. Philadelphia: Saunders; 2004.)

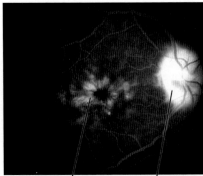

petalloid leakage   disc leakage

Figure 11.54 Fluorescein angiogram of same patient as in Fig. 11.53, demonstrating characteristic petalloid appearance with optic nerve leakage. (From Kaiser PK, Friedman NJ, Pineda R II. *The Massachusetts Eye and Ear Infirmary Illustrated Manual of Ophthalmology*, 2nd ed. Philadelphia: Saunders; 2004.)

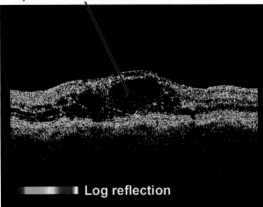

cystoid macular edema

Log reflection

Figure 11.55 Optical coherence tomography of cystoid macular edema, demonstrating intraretinal cystoid spaces and dome-shaped configuration of fovea. (From Kaiser PK, Friedman NJ, Pineda R II. *The Massachusetts Eye and Ear Infirmary Illustrated Manual of Ophthalmology*, 2nd ed. Philadelphia: Saunders; 2004.)

Macular Telangiectasia (MacTel)

Microaneurysmal and saccular dilation of parafoveal vessels

Formerly called parafoveal/juxtafoveal telangiectasia

Classification:
  Type 1: unilateral, male > female (10:1); onset during middle age; in spectrum of Coats disease
    TYPE 1A: congenital; confined to temporal half of fovea; macular edema and exudation (lipid)
    TYPE 1B: idiopathic; capillary telangiectasia confined to 1 clock hour at edge of FAZ; minimal leakage on FA; occasional hard exudates; vision usually >20/25; can be treated with laser
  Type 2A (most common): bilateral, acquired; male = female; 5th-6th decade of life; symmetric, involving area <1 DD; minimal macular edema; occasionally, superficial glistening white dots (Singerman spots); right-angle retinal venules dive deep into choroid; eventually develop RPE hyperplasia; occasionally, yellow lesion measuring 1/3 DD centered on FAZ (pseudovitelliform macular degeneration); may develop macular edema that is a result of ischemia (not amenable to laser treatment); 1/3 have abnormal glucose tolerance test
    FA: parafoveal capillary leakage; risk of CNV
  Type 3: bilateral, idiopathic; male = female; capillary occlusion predominates
    TYPE 3A: occlusive idiopathic
    TYPE 3B: occlusive idiopathic; associated with central nervous system vasculopathy
Structural abnormalities in types 2 and 3 are similar to diabetic microangiopathy (but no risk of neovascularization elsewhere in retina [NVE])

DDx: diabetes, vein occlusion, radiation retinopathy, Coats disease, Eales disease, Best disease, sickle cell, Irvine-Gass syndrome, ocular ischemia

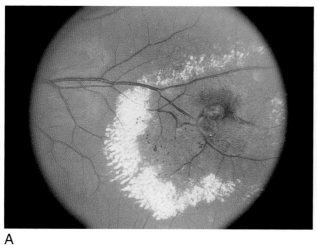

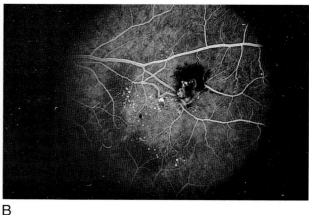

A   B

Figure 11.56 Macroaneurysm with surrounding dilated and telangiectatic capillary bed. (A) Fundus photograph. (B) Fluorescein angiogram. (Courtesy Susan Fowell, MD. From Mittra RA, Mieler WF, Pollack JS. Retinal arterial macroaneurysms. In: Yanoff M, Duker JS, eds. *Ophthalmology*. London: Mosby; 1999.)

Complications: macular edema, exudates, CNV, intraretinal NV, retinal–retinal anastomosis

Retinal Arterial Macroaneurysm (RAM)

May bleed, then autoinfarcts

Usually, elderly females; most common along temporal arcades; 10% bilateral

Mechanism: arteriosclerosis (fibrosis, thinning, decreased elasticity of vessel wall), hypertension (increased pressure on thin wall)

Findings: blood in every retinal layer, lipid exudate, artery occlusion downstream (especially following laser treatment), CME (Fig. 11.56)

DDx of blood in every retinal layer (subretinal, intraretinal, and preretinal): macroaneurysm, trauma, sickle cell retinopathy, choroidal melanoma, vein occlusion (rare), CNV (rare)

Pathology: overall thickening of vessel wall with hypertrophy of muscularis

Treatment: observation; consider focal laser (risk of hemorrhage)

Hypertensive Retinopathy

Focal or generalized vasoconstriction, breakdown of blood–retinal barrier with subsequent hemorrhage and exudate

Associated with microaneurysms or macroaneurysms

Classification systems:

Keith-Wagener-Barker Classification:
  GRADE 1: minimal constriction and tortuosity of arterioles
  GRADE 2: moderate constriction of arterioles; focal narrowing and arteriovenous nicking
  GRADE 3: grade 2 plus cotton-wool spots, hemorrhages, and exudates

  GRADE 4: grade 3 plus optic disc edema
Modified Scheie Classification:
  GRADE 0: no visible changes
  GRADE 1: diffuse arteriolar narrowing
  GRADE 2: pronounced arteriolar narrowing and focal constriction
  GRADE 3: grade 2 plus retinal hemorrhages
  GRADE 4: grade 3 plus optic disc edema

Findings:

Retinopathy: AV nicking, "copper or silver wire" arterial changes, hemorrhages, exudates, cotton-wool spots
Choroidopathy: fibrinoid necrosis of choroidal arterioles; may have Elschnig spots (zone of nonperfusion of choriocapillaris; pale white or red patches of RPE), Siegrist streak (reactive RPE hyperplasia along sclerosed choroidal vessel), and exudative RD; caused by acute hypertensive episode (pre-eclampsia, eclampsia, or pheochromocytoma); FA shows early hypoperfusion and late staining
Optic neuropathy: florid disc edema with macular exudate, linear flame hemorrhages

Pathology: thickening of arteriolar walls leads to nicking of venules; endothelial hyperplasia

Complications: retinal vein occlusion, retinal macroaneurysm, nonarteritic anterior ischemic optic neuropathy (AION), ocular motor nerve palsies, worsening of diabetic retinopathy

Diabetic Retinopathy (DR)

Leading cause of new blindness in United States, adults aged 20-74 years

Classification:

Background (BDR) or nonproliferative (NPDR): hemorrhages, exudates, cotton-wool spots, microaneurysms (MA), intraretinal microvascular abnormalities (IRMA), venous beading (Fig. 11.57)
Severe NPDR ("4-2-1 rule") (15% progress to PDR in 1 year): defined as any one of the following:

367

4 quadrants of hemorrhages/MA

2 quadrants of venous beading

1 quadrant of IRMA (Fig. 11.58)

Very severe NPDR (50% progress to PDR in 1 year): defined as ≥2 of the above

Proliferative (PDR): NV of disc or elsewhere (Fig. 11.59)

High-risk proliferative (HR-PDR): defined as any one of the following:

1. NVD ≥ 1/4 to 1/3 disc area
2. Any NVD with VH
3. Surface neovascularization (NVE) ≥ 1/2 disc area with VH

Epidemiology:

Type 1 diabetes mellitus (DM):

AT DIAGNOSIS: no NPDR

AT 5 YEARS: 25% NPDR, PDR rare

AT 20 YEARS: 98% NPDR, 60% PDR, 30% clinically significant macular edema (CSME)

Type 2 insulin-dependent diabetes mellitus (IDDM):

AT DIAGNOSIS: 30% NPDR

AT 5 YEARS: 40% NPDR, 2% PDR

AT 20 YEARS: 90% NPDR, 25% PDR, 40% CSME

Type 2 non–insulin-dependent diabetes mellitus (NIDDM):

AT DIAGNOSIS: 20% NPDR

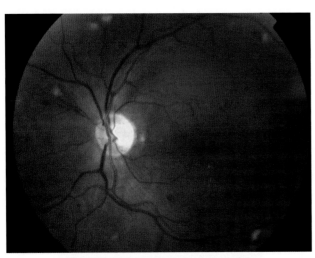

Figure 11.57 Nonproliferative diabetic retinopathy.

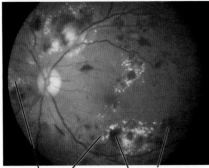

lipid exudate   intraretinal hemorrhages

Figure 11.58 Severe nonproliferative diabetic retinopathy with extensive hemorrhages, microaneurysms, and exudates. (From Kaiser PK, Friedman NJ, Pineda R II. *The Massachusetts Eye and Ear Infirmary Illustrated Manual of Ophthalmology,* 2nd ed. Philadelphia: Saunders; 2004.)

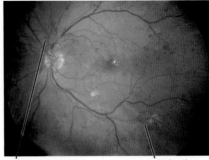

neovascularization   neovascularization
of the disc   elsewhere

Figure 11.59 Proliferative diabetic retinopathy demonstrating florid neovascularization of the disc and elsewhere. (From Kaiser PK, Friedman NJ, Pineda R II. *The Massachusetts Eye and Ear Infirmary Illustrated Manual of Ophthalmology,* 2nd ed. Philadelphia: Saunders; 2004.)

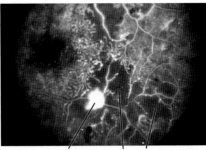

neovascularization   capillary nonperfusion

Figure 11.60 Fluorescein angiogram of a patient with proliferative diabetic retinopathy, showing extensive capillary nonperfusion, neovascularization elsewhere, and vascular leakage. (From Kaiser PK, Friedman NJ, Pineda R II. *The Massachusetts Eye and Ear Infirmary Illustrated Manual of Ophthalmology,* 2nd ed. Philadelphia: Saunders; 2004.)

AT 5 YEARS: 30% NPDR, 2% PDR

AT 20 YEARS: 50% NPDR, 10% PDR, 20% CSME

Findings: cotton-wool spots, lipid exudates (may appear as circinate exudate [ring of hard exudate surrounding leaky focus] or macular star [pattern reflects radial orientation of Henle fibers]), hemorrhages (blot [outer plexiform layer], flame [tracks along NFL]), microaneurysms, IRMA; shunts [arteriole to venule]), venous beading and loops, neovascularization (disc [NVD], elsewhere in retina [NVE], iris [NVI]) (Fig. 11.60)

Clinically significant macular edema (CSME) definition: one of the following:

1. Thickening within 500 µm of the macular center
2. Hard exudate within 500 µm of the macular center with associated thickening of adjacent retina
3. Zone of retinal thickening 1 disc *area* in size, any part of which is within 1 disc *diameter* of the macular center

Asymmetric diabetic retinopathy is usually a result of carotid disease (on either side)

Main cause of vision loss in NPDR: macular edema or ischemia

Main causes of vision loss in PDR: tractional RD (TRD), neovascular glaucoma (NVG), VH

Other sequelae:

Diabetic cataract: aldose reductase pathway converts glucose into sorbitol and fructose; causes osmotic effect; aldose reductase also converts galactose into galactitol (which causes cataracts in galactosemia)

Diabetic iridopathy: iris NV; lacy vacuolization of iris pigment epithelium in 40%; glycogen-filled cysts in iris pigment epithelium (PAS+)

Papillitis: acute disc swelling; vision usually ≥20/50; 50% bilateral; may have VF defect; most recover to ≥20/30

Isolated cranial nerve palsies: CN 3, 4, 6 (including pupil-sparing CN 3 palsy)

Pupillary abnormalities: light-near dissociation

Fluctuation in refractive error: results from osmotic effect on crystalline lens from unstable blood sugar levels

Pathology: selective loss of pericytes, no endothelial cells or pericytes in nonperfused areas; thickening of retinal capillary basement membranes; microaneurysm formation; retinal capillary closure; breakdown of blood–retinal barrier; lacy vacuolization of iris pigment epithelium; intraepithelial vacuoles contain glycogen; gitter cells (lipid-laden macrophages) (Figs. 11.61 and 11.62)

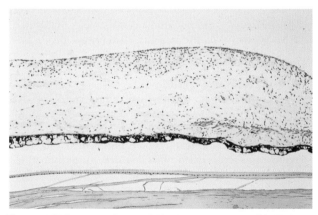

Figure 11.61 Lacy vacuolization of iris pigment epithelium. (Modified from Yanoff M, et al. Diabetic lacy vacuolization of iris pigment epithelium. *Am J Ophthalmol.* 1970,09.201–210. From Yanoff M, Fine BS. *Ocular pathology,* 5th ed. St Louis: Mosby; 2002.)

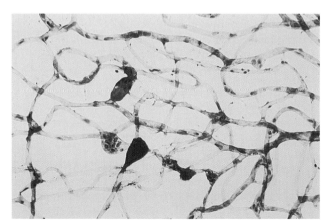

Figure 11.62 Microaneurysms, pericyte dropout, and acellular capillaries are seen. (From Benson WE. Diabetic retinopathy. In: Yanoff M, Duker JS, eds. *Ophthalmology.* London: Mosby; 1999.)

DDx: ocular ischemic syndrome, radiation retinopathy, hypertensive retinopathy, retinal vein occlusion, proliferative retinopathies (sarcoidosis, sickle cell), macular telangiectasia

FA: to identify macular ischemia, localize microaneurysms to guide focal laser treatment, identify areas of NVE, identify areas of capillary nonperfusion

OCT: macular edema appears as increased retinal thickness, cysts, and subretinal fluid; can identify vitreous traction

B-scan ultrasound: to identify TRD if VH present

Treatment: based on results from important studies

Diabetes Control and Complications Trial (DCCT):
Tight control of blood sugar slows progression of retinopathy, diabetic macular edema (DME), and visual loss in patients with type 1 DM; patients with Hb A1c <8% had a significantly reduced risk of retinopathy

Rapid normalization and tight control of blood sugar after a period of prolonged hyperglycemia can lead to worsening of retinopathy

United Kingdom Prospective Diabetes Study (UKPDS):
Tight control of blood sugar and blood pressure slows progression of retinopathy and development of macular edema in patients with type 2 DM

Early Treatment Diabetic Retinopathy Study (ETDRS):
Focal laser decreases vision loss from macular edema by 50%

No benefit from aspirin

Focal laser: for CSME (VA is not part of treatment criteria); argon green preferred; yellow (577 nm) is also used because it is well absorbed by hemoglobin within microaneurysms; reexamine every 3-4 months

Diabetic Retinopathy Study (DRS):
PRP reduces incidence of severe vision loss in high-risk PDR by 60%

CRITERIA: HR-PDR
1. NVD ≥ 1/4 to 1/3 disc area
2. Any NVD with VH
3. NVE ≥ 1/2 disc area with VH

COMPLICATIONS: decreased night vision (destruction of extramacular rods), angle-closure glaucoma (choroidal effusion), RD (regression of NV fronds can cause contracture, leading to retinal tear and rhegmatogenous or traction RD), central scotoma (worsening of CSME), progression of cataract

Up to 33% of patients will not respond to PRP

Anti-VEGF agents: for center-involving macular edema (no CSME definition in the anti-VEGF trials) bevacizumab, ranibizumab or aflibercept injections with immediate or deferred laser were significantly better than laser therapy alone (DRCR, RISE, RIDE, VIVID, VISTA, RESOLVE, RESTORE, YOSEMITE, and RHINE studies; see below)

Steroids: triamcinolone acetonide intravitreal injections found to be effective in pseudophakic patients, but not in overall group (see DRCR Protocol B below). Iluvien is a sustained drug delivery system that uses a drug matrix in a tiny cylindrical tube that is injected intravitreally via a 25-g needle, releasing 0.2 µg/day of the corticosteroid fluocinolone acetonide over 2-3 years (found to be effective in the phase III FAME studies); dexamethasone polymer implant (Ozurdex) releases dexamethasone from poly-lactic-co-glycolic acid (PLGA) polymer that is completely biodegradable over several months

Diabetic Retinopathy Vitrectomy Study (DRVS):
Early vitrectomy for VH in patients with type 1 DM only, can defer in type 2 (however, indications for vitrectomy have changed from these DRVS study conclusions largely owing to better vitrectomy systems, improved instrumentation, and the use of endolaser)

INDICATIONS FOR VITRECTOMY:
Nonclearing VH
Combined tractional-rhegmatogenous RD
Traction RD of the fovea. If tractional detachment is extramacular, watch closely; if macula is threatened or detaches, perform vitrectomy
Anterior hyaloidal fibrovascular proliferation
Refractory macular edema: patients with taut posterior hyaloid face can have chronic macular edema that does not resolve with laser. Chronic traction of vitreous face on macula appears to produce persistent leakage; can resolve after traction is relieved with vitrectomy
Progressive fibrovascular proliferation despite complete PRP
Ghost cell glaucoma
Consider for refractory DME (also consider injecting steroids, or intravitreal anti-VEGF agents)

Prognosis: risk of progression without treatment from preproliferative to proliferative DR over 2 years is 50%

Severe NPDR has 50% risk of progression to proliferative disease in 12-18 months

Conditions that exacerbate DR: hypertension, puberty, pregnancy (at conception, if no BDR, 88% have no retinopathy; if mild BDR, 47% worsen, 5% develop PDR; if PDR, 46% have progression), renal disease, anemia

Follow Hb A1c (serum glycosylated hemoglobin [provides 3-month view of blood sugar levels])

MAJOR DIABETIC RETINOPATHY CLINICAL STUDIES

Diabetic Retinopathy Study (DRS)

Objective: to evaluate whether photocoagulation prevents severe visual loss in eyes with diabetic retinopathy

Methods: patients had PDR in at least 1 eye or severe NPDR in both eyes, or ≥20/100 vision in each eye, and were randomly assigned to treatment with scatter laser photocoagulation (randomly assigned to either xenon arc [200–400, 4.5° spots] or argon blue-green laser [800–1600, 500-µm spots]) in 1

eye and no treatment in fellow eye (protocol later amended to allow deferred laser photocoagulation). Surface neovascularization (NVE) treated directly with confluent burns, and NVD treated directly only in argon laser–treated eyes. Patients were excluded if they had previous panretinal photocoagulation or traction RD-threatening macula

Severe NPDR defined as having at least 3 of the following:
Cotton-wool spots
Venous beading
IRMA in ≥2 of 4 contiguous overlapping photographic fields
Moderate to severe retinal hemorrhages and/or microaneurysms in ≥1 standard photographic field

Results: 1727 patients enrolled
PRP reduced the risk of severe vision loss (VA < 5/200 on 2 consecutive visits 4 months apart) by 50%-60% in patients with high-risk characteristics (see later discussion)

Conclusions: perform PRP for patients with high-risk proliferative retinopathy (HR-PDR) regardless of vision

NVD (new vessels on or within 1 disc diameter of the disc) ≥ 1/4 to 1/3 of disc area (standard photo 10A)

Any NVD with vitreous or preretinal hemorrhage

NVE (new vessels elsewhere) ≥ 1/2 of disc area (standard photo 7) with vitreous or preretinal hemorrhage

PRP is also indicated for NVI

DRS did not report a clear benefit for immediate PRP in patients with severe nonproliferative diabetic retinopathy and proliferative diabetic retinopathy without high-risk characteristics. However, older-onset patients with diabetes should be considered for earlier PRP

Early Treatment Diabetic Retinopathy Study (ETDRS)

Objective: to evaluate
1. Whether photocoagulation is effective for DME
2. Effect of aspirin on the course of DR
3. When to initiate PRP treatment for DR

Methods: patients had mild, moderate, or severe NPDR or early PDR (does not meet high-risk criteria of PDR) in both eyes, and ≥20/200 vision in each eye, and were randomly assigned to receive 650 mg daily aspirin or not *and* 1 of the following:
1. Moderate to severe NPDR or early PDR with no macular edema = immediate PRP (further randomly assigned to full [1200–1600, 500-µm spots] scatter or mild [400–650, 500-µm spots] scatter PRP) vs. deferred PRP until high-risk characteristics developed
2. Mild or moderate NPDR and macular edema = immediate laser (further randomly

assigned to immediate focal laser photocoagulation and deferred full scatter or mild scatter when high-risk characteristics developed; or immediate mild or full scatter PRP and deferred focal laser photocoagulation) vs. deferred laser photocoagulation

3. Severe NPDR or early PDR and macular edema = immediate laser (further randomly assigned to immediate mild or full PRP and immediate or deferred focal laser photocoagulation) vs. deferred laser photocoagulation

Patients were excluded if they had high-risk proliferative DR

Mild NPDR, defined as:

At least 1 microaneurysm, but not enough to qualify as moderate NPDR

Moderate NPDR, defined as:

Extensive intraretinal hemorrhages and/or microaneurysms, cotton-wool spots, IRMA, venous beading, but not enough to qualify as severe NPDR

Severe NPDR, defined with "4-2-1 rule" as any one of the following:

Intraretinal hemorrhages and/or microaneurysms in all 4 quadrants

Venous beading in at least 2 quadrants

IRMA in at least 1 quadrant

CSME, defined as one of the following:

1. Retinal thickening at or within 500 μm of the center of the macula
2. Hard exudates at or within 500 μm of the center of the macula with associated thickening of the adjacent retina
3. Retinal thickening ≥1 disc *area* in size ≤1 disc *diameter* from the center of the macula

Results: 3711 patients enrolled

Immediate focal laser decreased moderate vision loss in patients with clinically significant macular edema by ~50%

Early PRP reduced the risk of development of high-risk PDR in patients with NPDR and early PDR, but difference in severe visual loss was minimal

Immediate focal laser and deferred scatter PRP reduced moderate visual loss by 50% in patients with mild or moderate NPDR and macular edema

Immediate focal laser and scatter PRP reduced severe visual loss by 50% in patients with severe NPDR or early PDR and macular edema

Aspirin had no effect on progression or complications of diabetic retinopathy

Conclusions: treat all patients with CSME, regardless of vision

Immediate PRP should be reserved for patients with high-risk PDR and possibly those with severe NPDR in both eyes

No benefit from aspirin (650 mg/day)

Diabetic Retinopathy Vitrectomy Study (DRVS)

Objective: to observe patients with severe DR in type 1 and type 2 diabetes over 2 years to determine visual outcomes

Methods: patients with severe NPDR or early PDR (do not meet high-risk criteria of PDR) were placed into 1 of 3 groups

Group N: natural history study with 744 eyes of 644 patients enrolled

Group NH: to evaluate early surgical intervention vs. delayed surgery (for at least 1 year) in eyes with severe DR and active NV or fibrovascular proliferation but without severe visual loss (vision >10/200); 370 eyes enrolled. Amount of new vessel severity was quantified

NVC-1 (least severe): new vessel severity no worse than moderate in only 1 photographic field

NVC-2 (moderately severe): moderate new vessels in 2 or more fields, but not severe in any field

NVC-3 (severe): severe NVD or NVE in at least 1 field

NVC-4 (very severe): severe NVD and NVE in at least 1 field

Group H: to evaluate early surgical intervention (within days) vs. delayed surgery (for at least 1 year, unless TRD of macula detected on ultrasound examination) in eyes with severe diabetic retinopathy and active NV or fibrovascular proliferation, with history of sudden visual loss from severe VH within 6 months (vision <5/200, not NLP); 616 eyes enrolled. (Note: endophotocoagulation was not used in DRVS)

Patients were excluded if they had previous vitrectomy, photocoagulation within 3 months, intraocular pressure (IOP) > 29 mmHg on medications, severe iris NV, or neovascular glaucoma

Results:

Group NR:

4-YEAR RESULTS: patients in early-vitrectomy group had better vision than those in deferral group

Up to 18 months, early-vitrectomy group had a higher risk of no light perception vision; this was not seen at later time points

Patients with type 1 DM had an increased chance of obtaining good vision with early vitrectomy

Previous PRP increased chances of good vision

With increasing severity of vessels, early intervention was better than deferred intervention

Group H:

2-YEAR RESULTS: patients in early-vitrectomy group had better vision than those in deferral group

Patients with type 1 DM had superior outcomes from early vitrectomy, no advantage seen in type 2 DM

Conclusions: early vitrectomy for eyes with severe visual loss as a result of nonclearing VH (at least 1 month) is helpful in patients with type 1 DM and monocular patients despite the type of diabetes. Early vitrectomy is also recommended for eyes with useful vision and advanced active PDR, especially when extensive NV is present

NLP was seen in 20% of eyes, regardless of intervention once severe VH had occurred

Eyes with traction RD not involving fovea can be observed until fovea becomes detached, provided that fibrovascular proliferation is not severe

Diabetes Control and Complications Trial (DCCT)

Objective: to evaluate effect of tight vs. conventional control of blood sugar on diabetic complications in patients with type 1 DM

Methods: patients with insulin dependence defined by C-peptide secretion were randomly assigned to either intensive therapy or conventional therapy

> *Intensive therapy:* ≥3 daily insulin injections or implantation of an insulin pump
> Self-monitoring of glucose levels at least 4 times a day
> Adjust insulin dose based on glucose level
> Preprandial glucose = 70-120 mg/dL (3.9 and 6.7 mmol/L)
> Postprandial glucose <180 mg/dL (10.0 mmol/L)
> Weekly 3 AM glucose > 65 mg/dL (3.6 mmol/L)
> Monthly Hb A1c < 6.05% (nondiabetic range)
> *Conventional therapy:* 1 or 2 daily insulin injections
> Daily self-monitoring of glucose levels
> Did not adjust insulin dose daily
> Education about diet and exercise
> Followed every 3 months
> No glycosuria or ketonuria
> Absence of hyperglycemic or hypoglycemic symptoms

Results: 1441 patients included, study stopped after average follow-up of 6.5 years by independent safety and monitoring committee
> Average difference in Hb A1c was >2% between groups; however, <5% of intensive group kept <6.05%
> Incidence of DR was the same up to 36 months
> At baseline, 726 patients had no retinopathy, and 715 had mild retinopathy. After 5 years, incidence of retinopathy was approximately 50% less with intensive therapy
> Patients with Hb A1c < 8% had significantly reduced risk of retinopathy
> *Intensive control:*
> Reduced the risk of development of DR by 76%
> Slowed the progression of DR by 54% and reduced the development of severe NPDR or PDR by 47%
> Reduced the risk of macular edema by 23%
> Reduced the risk of laser treatment by 56%
> Reduced albuminuria by 54%

> Reduced clinical neuropathy by 60%
> *Adverse effect:* 2-3 × increase in severe hypoglycemia

Conclusions: tight control is beneficial; however, rapid normalization and tight control of blood sugar after a period of prolonged hyperglycemia can lead to an initial worsening of retinopathy

Epidemiology of Diabetes Interventions and Complications (EDIC) Trial

Objective: to gain further follow-up of patients from DCCT

Methods: 1208 patients from DCCT, all of whom received intensive therapy and were followed for an additional 4 years

Results: intensive therapy reduced the risk of
> Progression of retinopathy by 75%
> Any macular edema by 58%
> Laser treatment by 52%

Conclusions: tight control is still beneficial

United Kingdom Prospective Diabetes Study (UKPDS)

Objective: to compare effects on risk of microvascular and macrovascular complications of intensive blood glucose control with oral hypoglycemics and/or insulin and conventional treatment with diet therapy

Methods: 4209 newly diagnosed patients with type 2 diabetes, median age 54 years (range, 25–65 years), were randomly assigned to intensive therapy with a sulfonylurea (chlorpropamide, glibenclamide [glyburide], or glipizide) or with insulin, or conventional therapy using diet control

Results: after median duration of therapy of 11 years, intensive treatment with sulfonylurea, insulin, and/or metformin was equally effective in reducing fasting plasma glucose concentrations.

Over 10 years, Hb A1c was 7.0% (range 6.2–8.2) in intensive group compared with 7.9% (range, 6.9–8.8) in conventional group—an 11% reduction. No difference in Hb A1c was seen among agents in intensive group.

Compared with conventional group, risk in intensive group was 12% lower for any diabetes-related endpoint; 10% lower for any diabetes-related death; and 6% lower for all-cause mortality.

The reduction in Hb A1c was associated with a 25% overall reduction in microvascular complications, including retinopathy (21% reduction) and nephropathy (34% reduction); 37% of patients had microaneurysms in 1 eye at diagnosis and random assignment

Conclusions: patients with type 2 DM benefit from intensive glycemic control, as do patients with type 1 DM

The United Kingdom Prospective Diabetes Study—Hypertension in Diabetes Study (UKPDS-HDS)

Objective: to compare effects of intensive blood pressure control on the risk of microvascular and macrovascular complications

Methods: 1148 patients with type 2 DM and mild to moderate hypertension to determine if "tight blood pressure control (150/85 mmHg)" using an angiotensin-converting enzyme (ACE) inhibitor or a β-blocker vs. "less tight control (<180/105 mmHg)" would prevent diabetic complications.

Patients were randomly assigned to captopril (ACE inhibitor) or atenolol (β-blocker) and followed for a median of 8.4 years

Results: tight control of blood pressure in patients with hypertension and type 2 DM reduced risk of death related to diabetes by 32%

In addition, there was a 34% reduction in risk of deterioration of retinopathy by ≥2 ETDRS steps from baseline, and a 47% reduction in risk of deterioration of VA by 3 ETDRS lines with tight blood pressure control

Lowering of blood pressure with captopril or atenolol was similarly effective in reducing incidence of diabetic complications, suggesting that blood pressure reduction in itself may be more important than the treatment used

Conclusions: tight blood pressure control reduced the risk of complications from DR

A Study of Ranibizumab Injection in Subjects With CSME With Center Involvement Secondary to Diabetes (RIDE)

Objective: to compare efficacy of ranibizumab vs. sham with laser rescue in patients with DME

Methods: multicenter, randomized, double-masked, sham-injection-controlled, 36-month (sham injection controlled for 24 months) phase III study designed to assess the efficacy and safety profile of ranibizumab in 382 patients with DME. Patients randomized to receive monthly injections of either 0.3 mg ranibizumab (n = 125), 0.5 mg ranibizumab (n = 127), or monthly sham injections (n = 130). Beginning at 3 months, macular laser rescue treatment was made available to all patients, if needed, based on prespecified criteria. After month 24, patients in the sham injection group were eligible to receive monthly injections of 0.5 mg ranibizumab, and all patients will continue to be followed and dosed monthly for a total of 36 months. The study then continues in an open-label extension phase.

Results: at 24 months, 33.6% of patients who received 0.3 mg ranibizumab and 45.7% of patients who received 0.5 mg ranibizumab were able to read ≥15 letters compared with baseline, compared with 12.3% of patients who received sham injections with laser rescue.

Conclusions: ranibizumab injections are effective in diabetic macular edema

A Study of Ranibizumab Injection in Subjects With CSME With Center Involvement Secondary to Diabetes (RISE)

Objective: to compare efficacy of ranibizumab vs. sham with laser rescue in patients with diabetic macular edema

Methods: multicenter, randomized, double-masked, sham-injection-controlled, 36-month phase III study designed to assess the safety and efficacy profile of ranibizumab in 377 patients with DME. Primary endpoint compared the proportion of ranibizumab and sham-treated patients who gained ≥15 letters in BCVA at month 24, relative to baseline. Patients were randomized to receive monthly injections of either 0.3 mg ranibizumab (n = 125), 0.5 mg ranibizumab (n = 125), or monthly sham injections (n = 127). At 3 months, rescue laser treatment was made available to all patients, if needed, based on prespecified criteria. After month 24, patients in the control group are eligible to receive monthly injections of 0.5 mg ranibizumab, and all patients will continue to be followed for 36 months

Results: patients receiving monthly ranibizumab achieved an improvement in vision (BCVA) of ≥15 letters at 24 months, compared with those in control group, who received placebo (sham) injection.

Conclusions: ranibizumab injections are effective in DME

Safety and Efficacy of Ranibizumab in Diabetic Macular Edema (RESTORE/RESOLVE) Studies

Objective: to compare efficacy of ranibizumab with or without laser vs. laser alone in patients with DME

Methods: randomized, double-masked, multicenter, laser-controlled phase III trial (n = 345) with patients randomized to either ranibizumab 0.5 mg with 3-monthly loading dose followed by PRN ranibizumab alone; focal laser and ranibizumab 0.5 mg with 3-monthly loading dose followed by PRN ranibizumab; or focal laser alone. Primary outcome was mean change in vision from baseline at month 12

Results: at month 12, ranibizumab alone group (n = 115) gained +6.1 letters, ranibizumab plus laser (n = 118) gained +5.9 letters, and the laser alone (n = 110) gained +0.8

letters. There was a mean of 2.1 laser treatments in the laser alone group. The groups gained ≥15 letters in 22.6%, 22.9%, and 8.2%, respectively. Central retinal thickness improved in all groups: the ranibizumab alone group decreased by –118.7 μm, ranibizumab plus laser decreased by –128.3 μm, and the laser group decreased by –61.3 μm. A companion study RESOLVE reported that ranibizumab-treated patients achieved an average +11.7 letters gain in VA at 12 months compared with sham-treated patients, some of whom received laser treatment.

Conclusions: ranibizumab therapy with or without laser resulted in significant visual gain over laser treatment alone.

Diabetic Retinopathy Clinical Research Network (DRCR) Studies: Major Protocols Only

Protocol B

Objectives: to compare intravitreal triamcinolone acetonide (TA) injections at doses of 1 mg or 4 mg and macular laser photocoagulation in treatment of DME

Methods: patients aged ≥18 years. Study eye with center-involved DME present on clinical exam and on OCT based on mean retinal thickness on two OCT measurements ≥250 microns in central subfield, and best-corrected E-ETDRS acuity ≥24 letters (≥20/320) and ≤73 letters (<20/40). Patients randomized to either 1- or 4-mg TA or focal laser photocoagulation. Primary outcome was ≥15-letter improvement in VA from baseline at 2 years

Results: 840 eyes (693 subjects) enrolled. Primary outcome was mean improvement in vision at 24 months: +1 letters in the laser group (*n* = 330); –2 letters in the 1-mg triamcinolone group (*N* = 256); –3 letters in the 4-mg triamcinolone group (*n* = 254). Increased IOP > 30 mmHg was seen in 4% of laser treated group, 9% of 1-mg TA group and 21% in 4-mg TA group. Cataract surgery was required in 13% of laser-treated group, 23% of 1-mg TA patients, and 51% in 4-mg TA group.

Conclusions: TA injections were not superior to focal/grid photocoagulation and resulted in more adverse events

Protocol I

Objectives: to evaluate safety and efficacy of (1) intravitreal ranibizumab in combination with focal laser photocoagulation, (2) intravitreal ranibizumab treatment alone, and (3) intravitreal triamcinolone acetonide in combination with focal laser photocoagulation in eyes with center-involved DME

Methods: patients aged ≥18 years. Study eye with center-involved DME present on clinical exam and on OCT based on mean retinal thickness on two OCT measurements ≥250 μm in central subfield, and BCVA ≤20/32. Patients were randomized to 1 of 4 groups: Group A: sham injection plus focal (macular) photocoagulation; Group

B: 0.5-mg injection of intravitreal ranibizumab plus focal photocoagulation; Group C: 0.5-mg injection of intravitreal ranibizumab plus deferred focal photocoagulation; Group D: 4-mg intravitreal triamcinolone plus focal photocoagulation. Primary outcome was ≥15-letter improvement in VA from baseline at 1 year

Results: 854 patients randomized. Primary outcome was mean improvement in vision at 12 months: +3 letters in the laser group (*n* = 293); +9 letters in the ranibizumab with prompt laser group (*n* = 187); +9 letters in the ranibizumab with deferred laser group (*n* = 188); and +4 letters in the triamcinolone plus laser group (*n* = 186). Only 28% of patients in ranibizumab plus deferred laser group received laser in first year and 42% by year 2. At 24 months, mean improvement in vision was +2 letters in laser group; +7 letters in ranibizumab with prompt laser group; +10 letters in ranibizumab with deferred laser group; and +0 letters in triamcinolone plus laser group. Mean change in retinal thickness was –102 μm in laser group; –131 μm in ranibizumab with prompt laser group; –137 μm in ranibizumab with deferred laser group; and –127 μm in triamcinolone plus laser group; 5-year extended follow-up report noted that number of visits declined in years 2 through 5 (interval could be extended up to 16 weeks starting in year 2). Of maximum of 65 visits, prompt laser group had mean of 38 visits and deferred laser group had 40, and median of 13 injections was given in prompt laser group and 17 in deferred laser group

Conclusions: intravitreal ranibizumab with prompt or deferred (≥24 weeks) focal/grid laser had superior VA and OCT outcomes compared with focal/grid laser treatment alone

Although intravitreal triamcinolone combined with focal/grid laser did not result in superior VA outcomes compared with laser alone, an analysis limited to pseudophakic eyes showed that triamcinolone group's outcome for VA appeared to be of similar magnitude to that of 2 ranibizumab groups

Protocol S

Objective: to evaluate noninferiority of intravitreous ranibizumab compared with PRP for VA outcomes in patients with proliferative diabetic retinopathy

Methods: eyes were randomly assigned to receive PRP treatment, completed in 1-3 visits (*n* = 203 eyes), or ranibizumab, 0.5 mg, by intravitreous injection at baseline and as frequently as every 4 weeks based on a structured re-treatment protocol (*n* = 191 eyes). Eyes in both treatment groups could receive ranibizumab for DME

Results: 394 patients (191 in ranibizumab and 203 in PRP group) enrolled. The mean VA letter improvement at 2 years was +2.8 in the ranibizumab group vs. +0.2 in the PRP group. Mean peripheral visual field sensitivity loss was worse (–23 dB vs. –422 dB), vitrectomy was more frequent (15% vs. 4%), and DME development was more frequent (28% vs. 9%) in PRP group vs. ranibizumab group, respectively. Eyes without active or regressed NV at 2 years were not significantly different (35% in the ranibizumab group vs. 30% in the PRP group). One eye in ranibizumab group developed endophthalmitis. No significant differences between groups in rates of major cardiovascular events. After 5 years, there was no difference in mean change in vision

Conclusions: among eyes with PDR, treatment with ranibizumab resulted in VA that was noninferior to (not worse than) PRP treatment at 2 years

There was less VF loss, vitrectomies, center-involved DME in the ranibizumab groups

Protocol T

Objective: to compare aflibercept, bevacizumab, and ranibizumab for the treatment of center-involving DME

Results: 660 patients randomly assigned and followed for 2 years. At 1 year, mean VA score (range, 0 - 100, with higher scores indicating better VA; a score of 85 is approximately 20/20) improved by 13.3 with aflibercept, by 9.7 with bevacizumab, and by 11.2 with ranibizumab. When initial VA letter score was 78 to 69 (equivalent to approximately 20/32-20/40) (51% of participants), mean improvement was 8.0 with aflibercept, 7.5 with bevacizumab, and 8.3 with ranibizumab. When initial letter score was less than 69 (approximately ≤20/50), mean improvement was 18.9 with aflibercept, 11.8 with bevacizumab, and 14.2 with ranibizumab. There were no significant differences among study groups in rates of serious adverse events, hospitalization, death, or major cardiovascular events. Median numbers of injections were 5, 6, and 6 in year 2 and 15, 16, and 15 over 2 years in aflibercept, bevacizumab, and ranibizumab groups, respectively. Focal/grid laser was administered in 41%, 64%, and 52%, respectively. At 2 years, mean VA improved by 12.8, 10.0, and 12.3 letters, respectively. With worse baseline VA (20/50-20/320), mean improvement was 18.3, 13.3, and 16.1 letters, respectively. With better baseline VA (20/32-20/40), mean improvement was 7.8, 6.8, and 8.6 letters, respectively. Anti-Platelet Trialists' Collaboration (APTC) events occurred in 5% with aflibercept, 8% with bevacizumab, and 12% with ranibizumab

Conclusions: aflibercept, bevacizumab, or ranibizumab improved vision in eyes with center-involved diabetic macular edema, but the relative effect depended on baseline VA

When initial VA loss was mild, there were no apparent differences, on average, among study groups

At worse levels of initial VA, aflibercept and ranibizumab was more effective at improving vision than bevacizumab

Protocol V

Objective: to compare aflibercept vs. laser vs. observation in patients with center-involved DME and good vision (≥20/25). The primary outcome was percentage of patients with >5 letter VA loss

Results: 702 patients (226 in prompt aflibercept, 240 in laser with deferred aflibercept, and 236 in observation arms) enrolled. The primary outcome of >5 letter VA loss was seen in 27%, 25%, and 21% of patients in the aflibercept, laser with deferred aflibercept, and observation groups, respectively, at 2 years. The mean change in central retinal thickness was similar between groups. Patients with fellow eye receiving treatment for DME, baseline CST ≥300 μm, and Diabetic Retinopathy Severity Scale (DRSS) ≥47 (moderate to severe NPDR) were more likely to lose vision

Conclusions: eyes with center-involved DME and good vision (≥20/25) can be observed unless vision worsens

Protocol W

Objective: to evaluate the prevention of PDR and DME in patients with aflibercept vs. sham

Results: center-involved DME with vision loss or developing PDR was seen in 16.3% of aflibercept patients and 43.5% of sham patients. There was a 3 x reduction in the development of DME and a 2 x reduction in the development of PDR. On average, 8 aflibercept injections were given. There was no difference in VA outcomes. The study will continue for 4 years

Conclusions: proactive intervention prevented complications but had no effect on visual outcomes

Intravitreal Aflibercept for Diabetic Macular Edema (VIVID/VISTA) Trials

Objective: to evaluate aflibercept vs. laser therapy for center-involving DME

Results: 872 eyes randomized to receive aflibercept 2 mg every 4 weeks (2q4) (n - 155), aflibercept 2 mg every 8 weeks (2q8) (n = 152), or laser photocoagulation (n = 154). Mean vision gains from baseline to week 52 in aflibercept 2q4 and 2q8 groups versus laser group were 12.5 and 10.7 vs. 0.2 letters in VISTA, and 10.5 and 10.7 vs. 1.2 letters in VIVID. Mean reductions in central retinal thickness were 185.9 and 183.1 vs. 73.3 μm in VISTA, and 195.0 and 192.4 vs. 66.2 μm in VIVID. After 2 years, mean vision improved 11.5 letters in aflibercept 2q4 group and 11.1 letters in 2q8 group. Patients in laser photocoagulation group had mean BCVA improvement of 0.9 letters. After 3 years, patients receiving aflibercept every month had mean gain in BCVA from baseline of 10.3 letters, patients receiving aflibercept every 2 months had mean gain in BCVA from baseline of 11.7 letters. Patients in the laser photocoagulation treatment group had mean change in BCVA from baseline of 1.6 letters. Safety was similar among groups

Conclusions: at week 52, aflibercept demonstrated significant superiority in functional and anatomic endpoints over laser, with similar efficacy in 2q4 and 2q8 groups. Results held for 3 years of follow-up

PANORAMA Study

Objective: to evaluate the effect of aflibercept dosed at every-8-weeks or every-16-weeks intervals on DRSS in patients with moderately severe to severe NPDR (DRSS levels 47 or 53) in whom PRP could be deferred for at least 6 months. The primary outcome was the proportion of patients with ≥2-step improvement on DRSS at 24 weeks

Results: 402 patients (135 in q16 weeks, 134 in q8 weeks, and 133 in sham arms) were enrolled. Greater than 2-step improvement in DRSS was seen in 55.2%, 61.5%, and 6% of patients in the q8, q16, and sham groups, respectively ($P < 0.0001$). Patients developing PDR was 25.6%, 3.7%, and 5.2% in the sham, q16, and q8 week arms, respectively. Center-involved DME developed in 14.4%, 2.3%, and 4.7% in the sham, q16, and q8 week arms, respectively. Safety was excellent

Conclusions: in patients with moderately severe to severe NPDR aflibercept dosed either at every-8-weeks or every-16-weeks intervals significantly improved DRSS scores at 24 weeks

Vision-threatening complications occurred at higher rates in the sham group

RHINE and YOSEMITE Studies

Objective: to evaluate the noninferiority of faricimab vs. aflibercept in center-involved DME with center subfield thickness ≥325 μm. Patients were randomized to two different 6.0-mg faricimab groups: 6-monthly loading dose, then every 8 weeks, and 4-monthly loading dose, then a personalized treatment interval (PTI) based on a treat and extend paradigm, vs. aflibercept with 5-monthly loading dose, then every-8-weeks dosing

Results: 940 patients (315 in every-8-weeks arm, 313 in the PTI arm, and 312 in the aflibercept arm) enrolled in YOSEMITE, and 951 patients (317 in every-8-weeks arm, 319 in the PTI arm, and 315 in the aflibercept arms) enrolled in RHINE. The noninferiority primary endpoint was met with a –0.2/+0.7 difference from aflibercept in the every-8-weeks and PTI groups, respectively, in YOSEMITE, and +1.5/+0.5 in RHINE. The mean change in vision was similar between the groups in both studies. In the PTI groups, 52.8% were dosed at every 16 weeks in YOSEMITE and 51% in RHINE. Safety was similar between groups, with low rates of IOI and no cases of retinal vasculitis. The RHONE-X extension study will follow patients for 4 years

Conclusions: VA gains were similar between faricimab dosed every 8 weeks or up to every 16 weeks and aflibercept dosed every 8 weeks

There were better anatomic outcomes with faricimab

Safety was excellent

Sickle Cell (SC) Retinopathy

Proliferative retinopathy, usually equatorial or pre-equatorial

Most severe in hemoglobin sickle cell (HbSC) disease; SC > S Thal > SS > SA

Incidence in African American population: SS = 1%; sickle trait = 8%; SC < 0.5%;

20%-60% autoinfarct; unlike DR, NV can regress spontaneously and involute

Findings: salmon patch (intraretinal hemorrhage following peripheral retinal arteriolar occlusion), black sunburst (chorioretinal scar with RPE proliferation as a result of old hemorrhage), sea fan (peripheral NV), refractile spots (old, resorbed hemorrhages), silver wiring of peripheral vessels, angioid streaks, vascular occlusions (macular arteriolar occlusions [wedge sign], CRAO, retinal vein occlusion [RVO], choroid; CRAO can develop in patients with hyphema), venous tortuosity, comma-shaped conjunctival vessels, VH, rhegmatogenous and traction RD (resulting from contracture of NV fronds) (Figs. 11.63–11.65)
  Stage 1: peripheral arterial occlusions
  Stage 2: peripheral anastomoses
  Stage 3: neovascularization (sea fan) at posterior border of areas of nonperfusion
  Stage 4: vitreous hemorrhage
  Stage 5: vitreous traction with RD

Diagnosis: sickle cell prep, Hgb electrophoresis

FA: capillary nonperfusion, AV anastomoses, NV (Fig. 11.66)

Treatment: laser (PRP) or consider cryotherapy (controversial) for NV; surgery for RD and chronic VH; risk of anterior segment ischemia if encircling scleral buckle placed or large volume of intraocular gas; try to avoid epinephrine in infusion fluid during surgery

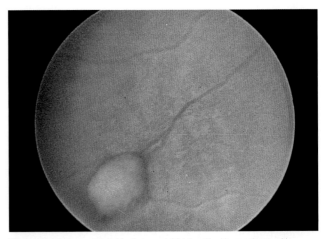

Figure 11.63 An equatorial "salmon patch" intraretinal hemorrhage with periarteriolar hemorrhage. (Courtesy of William Tasman, MD. From Ho AC. Hemoglobinopathies. In: Yanoff M, Duker JS, eds. *Ophthalmology.* London: Mosby; 1999.)

Eales Disease

Idiopathic retinal perivasculitis and peripheral nonperfusion with NV
Occurs in healthy young men; 90% bilateral
More common in Middle East and India
Increased risk of branch vein occlusion (BVO)

Findings: NV (80%, NVD or NVE), recurrent VH, rubeosis, neovascular glaucoma, cataract, vascular sheathing (80%) with leakage on FA, vascular tortuosity, collateral formation around occluded vessels, peripheral nonperfusion; may have AC reaction, KP, vitreous cells, macular edema

> *Stage 1:* sheathing of retinal venules, retinal edema, hemorrhages
> *Stage 2:* more severe involvement and vitreous haze
> *Stage 3:* peripheral NV
> *Stage 4:* proliferative retinopathy with VH and TRD

Other findings: vestibulocochlear involvement (sensorineural hearing loss and vestibular dysfunction), purified protein derivative (PPD)-positive, cerebral vasculitis (rare), epistaxis

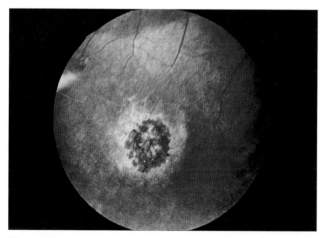

Figure 11.64 A black "sunburst" retinal lesion. (From Ho AC. Hemoglobinopathies. In: Yanoff M, Duker JS, eds. *Ophthalmology.* London: Mosby; 1999.)

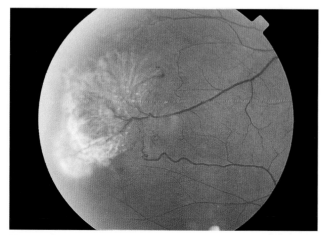

Figure 11.65 A sea fan in a patient with hemoglobin sickle cell disease. (From Ho AC. Hemoglobinopathies. In: Yanoff M, Duker JS, eds. *Ophthalmology.* London: Mosby; 1999.)

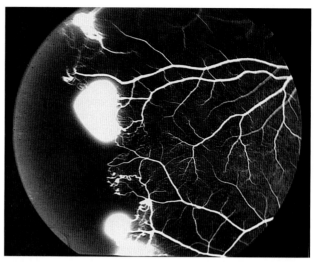

Figure 11.66 Fluorescein angiography of sea fans with peripheral nonperfusion. (From Ho AC. Hemoglobinopathies. In: Yanoff M, Duker JS, eds. *Ophthalmology.* London: Mosby; 1999.)

DDx of peripheral neovascularization:

hemoglobinopathies, diabetes, retinal vein occlusions, retinopathy of prematurity (ROP), familial exudative vitreoretinopathy (FEVR), retinal emboli (talc), hyperviscosity syndromes, carotid-cavernous sinus fistula, ocular ischemia, sarcoidosis, lupus, inflammatory bowel disease, retinal vasculitis, uveitis, VKH syndrome, pars planitis, Norrie disease, incontinentia pigmenti

Retinopathy of Prematurity (ROP; Retrolental Fibroplasia)

(See Chapter 5, Pediatrics/Strabismus)

Familial Exudative Vitreoretinopathy (FEVR)

(See Chapter 5, Pediatrics/Strabismus)

Branch Retinal Vein Occlusion (BRVO)

Site of occlusion is at AV crossing (usually thickened artery compresses vein in common adventitial sheath); generally superotemporal (63%)

Associated with increased age (>60 years), cardiovascular disease, hypertension, increased body mass index (BMI) at age 20, glaucoma, papilledema, optic disc drusen, and high serum alpha$_2$-globulin. Note: diabetes is not a risk factor. Decreased incidence with high levels of high-density lipoprotein (HDL) cholesterol and light to moderate alcohol consumption (especially after ophthalmology board exams)

Types:

> *Nonischemic:* <5 DD of capillary nonperfusion
> *Ischemic:* ≥5 DD of capillary nonperfusion

Findings: numerous deep and superficial hemorrhages (in a wedge-shaped distribution with the tip pointing toward the etiologic crossing), cotton-wool spots, CME, disc edema (Figs. 11.67 and 11.68)

Complications:

Nonischemic BVO: macular edema can develop

Ischemic BVO: macular edema, ischemic maculopathy, NV, VH, tractional or rhegmatogenous RD; 40% risk of developing NV (NVI rare)

Treatment: sector PRP for NV and VH, grid laser for macular edema when vision < 20/40 for at least 3 months and no macular ischemia on FA; recent studies with intravitreal anti-VEGF and steroids agents have shown better results than laser

Branch Vein Occlusion Study (BVOS):

Perform grid argon laser for macular edema and vision < 20/40 for >3 months (treated eyes more likely to have improved vision: +6.7 letters vs. +1 letter with observation)

Perform PRP for ≥5 DD of nonperfusion if NV develops (treated eyes less likely to develop NV and VH)

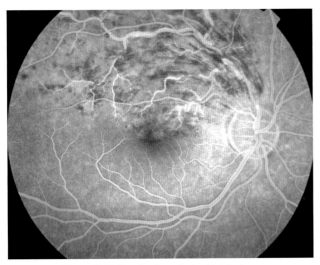

Figure 11.67 Branch vein occlusion. Early leakage.

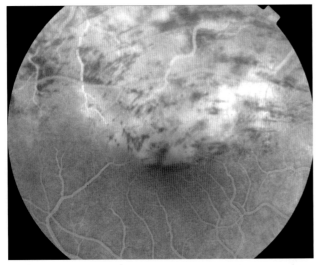

Figure 11.68 Branch vein occlusion. Late leakage.

Branch Retinal Vein Occlusion (BRAVO) Study:

Intravitreal injection of ranibizumab (Lucentis) for macular edema

Intravitreal Aflibercept for Macular Edema Following Branch Retinal Vein Occlusion (VIBRANT) Study:

Intravitreal injection of aflibercept for macular edema

Global Evaluation of Implantable Dexamethasone in Retinal Vein Occlusion with Macular Edema (GENEVA) Study:

Intravitreal injection of sustained-release dexamethasone intravitreal implant (Ozurdex) for macular edema

Prognosis: 30% have spontaneous recovery; >50% maintain vision >20/40 after 1 year; 10% have episode in fellow eye

Central Retinal Vein Occlusion (CRVO)

Thrombosis of central retinal vein at or posterior to the lamina cribrosa

Types:

Perfused/non-ischemic (70%): vision > 20/200, 16% progress to nonperfused; 50% resolve completely without treatment; defined as <10 DD of capillary nonperfusion (Fig. 11.69)

Non-perfused/ischemic (30%): ≥10 DD non-perfusion; patients are older and have worse vision; 60% develop iris NV; up to 33% develop neovascular glaucoma (NVG; "90-day" glaucoma because it occurs 3–5 months after occlusion); extensive hemorrhage with marked venous dilation and cotton-wool spots; very poor prognosis, with only 10% having >20/400 vision (Fig. 11.70)

10% combined with branch retinal artery occlusion (BRAO) (usually cilioretinal artery as a result of low perfusion pressure of choroidal system)

Risk factors: age (>50 years old in 90%), hypertension (61%), diabetes (unlike BVO), heart disease, glaucoma, increased erythrocyte sedimentation rate (ESR) in women, syphilis, sarcoidosis, vasculitis, increased intraorbital or intraocular pressure, hyphema, hyperviscosity syndromes (multiple myeloma, Waldenström macroglobulinemia, leukemia), high homocysteine levels, sickle cell, HIV

Findings: venous dilation and tortuosity, hemorrhages in all 4 quadrants, may have disc edema and macular edema

High-risk characteristics: marked vision loss, numerous cotton-wool spots, positive RAPD, dense central scotoma with peripheral field changes on VF, widespread capillary nonperfusion on FA, reduced ratio of b-wave to a-wave on ERG

Pathology: marked retinal edema, focal retinal necrosis, gliosis; subretinal, intraretinal, and preretinal hemorrhages

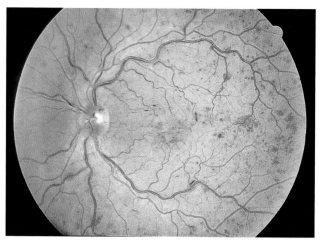

Figure 11.69 Nonischemic central retinal vein occlusion. (From Heier JS, Morley MG. Venous obstructive disease of the retina. In: Yanoff M, Duker JS, eds. *Ophthalmology*. London: Mosby; 1999.)

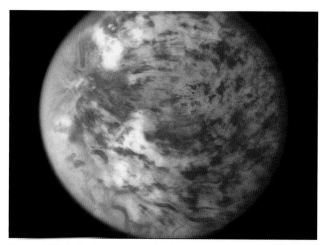

Figure 11.70 Ischemic central retinal vein occlusion. (From Heier JS, Morley MG. Venous obstructive disease of the retina. In: Yanoff M, Duker JS, eds. *Ophthalmology*. London: Mosby; 1999.)

Workup: younger patients require more extensive workup including systemic vascular disease (hypertension, diabetes mellitus, cardiovascular disease), blood dyscrasias (polycythemia vera, lymphoma, and leukemia), clotting disorders (activated protein C resistance, lupus anticoagulant, anticardiolipin antibodies, protein C and protein S, antithrombin III) paraproteinemia and dysproteinemias, multiple myeloma, cryoglobulinemia, vasculitis, syphilis, sarcoidosis, autoimmune disease, systemic lupus erythematosus, oral contraceptive use in women, other rare associations (closed-head trauma, optic disc drusen, AV malformations of retina)

Complications: iris NV (more common than NVD or NVE), NVG, TRD, VH, and macular edema

Treatment: follow every month for first 6 months, including gonioscopy; intravitreal steroids or anti-VEGF agents for macular edema

Central Vein Occlusion Study (CVOS):
    No benefit from early PRP (to prevent iris NV) in ischemic CVO; therefore, wait until first sign of NV
    No benefit from focal laser for macular edema

Central Retinal Vein Occlusion (CRUISE) Study:
    Intravitreal injection of ranibizumab (Lucentis) for macular edema

Intravitreal Aflibercept Injection for Macular Edema Resulting from Central Retinal Vein Occlusion (COPERNICUS/GALILEO) Studies:
    Intravitreal injection of aflibercept (Eylea) for macular edema

Global Evaluation of Implantable Dexamethasone in Retinal Vein Occlusion with Macular Edema (GENEVA) Study:
    Intravitreal injection of dexamethasone sustained-release intravitreal implant (Ozurdex) for macular edema; time to first gain of ≥15 letters was faster with the biodegradable implant compared with observation with 20%-30% 3-line gainers. Watch IOP because increased in 25% of eyes

Prognosis: >75% have disease progression

Hemiretinal Vein Occlusion (HRVO)

Risk factors: hypertension, diabetes, glaucoma

Ischemic HRVO: higher risk of NVD (30%) or NVE (40%) than with either an ischemic CVO or a BVO; NVI in 10%

MAJOR RETINAL VEIN OCCLUSION CLINICAL STUDIES

Branch Vein Occlusion Study (BVOS)

Objective: to evaluate photocoagulation in patients with BVO for:
1. Prevention of NV
2. Prevention of VH
3. Improvement of vision in eyes with macular edema, reducing vision to 20/40 or worse

Methods:

Group I (at risk for NV): patients with BVO occurring within 3-18 months with an area of retinal involvement ≥5 DD in size, with no NV present and vision >5/200, were randomly assigned to peripheral scatter laser photocoagulation vs. observation
Group II (at risk for VH): patients with BVO occurring within 3-18 months with disc or peripheral NV and

vision >5/200 were randomly assigned to peripheral scatter laser photocoagulation vs. observation

Group III (at risk for vision loss as a result of macular edema): patients with BVO occurring within 3-18 months with macular edema involving the fovea and vision <20/40 were randomly assigned to grid pattern laser photocoagulation with argon laser vs. observation

Group X (at high risk for NV): patients with BVO occurring within 3-18 months with ≥5 DD of capillary nonperfusion were followed. Note: This group was recruited after group I recruitment had ended

Results:

Group 1: 319 patients enrolled. After average follow-up of 3.7 years, development of NV was significantly less in laser-treated eyes. Treated eyes were less likely to develop NV (12% vs. 24% of untreated)

Group II: 82 eyes enrolled. After average follow-up of 2.8 years, development of VH was significantly less in laser-treated eyes. Treated eyes were less likely to develop VH (29% vs. 61% of untreated)

Group III: 139 patients enrolled. After an average follow-up of 3.1 years, treated eyes were more likely to have improved vision (gain of ≥2 lines in 65% vs. 37% of untreated), vision > 20/40, and final average vision better than untreated eyes

Group X: eyes with ≥5 DD of nonperfusion were considered nonperfused and showed greater risk of developing NV

Conclusions: grid pattern laser photocoagulation recommended for eyes with a BVO of 3-18 months duration if VA is ≤20/40 and if FA documents macular edema without foveal hemorrhage as cause of visual loss Perform PRP if retinal NV develops, especially if ≥5 DD of nonperfusion exists

The Standard Care Versus Corticosteroid for Retinal Vein Occlusion (SCORE) Study

Objective: to compare intravitreal triamcinolone to observation in retinal vein occlusion

Methods: Patients >18 years old with center-involved macular edema as a result of CVO or BVO of at least 3 months' duration but no longer than 18 months with central retinal thickness >250 µm on OCT and ETDRS VA score 20/40-20/200 randomized to either 1-mg or 4-mg doses of preservative-free intravitreal TA vs. standard of care (observation in CVO and focal laser in BVO). The primary outcome was ≥3-line gainers at month 12. All patients will be followed and retreated as needed every 4 months for 3 years

Results: 271 patients enrolled. For CVO, patients with ≥3-line gain in vision at month 12 (primary outcome) was 7% in observation group (*n* = 73), 27% in 1-mg TA group (*n* = 83), and 26% in 4-mg TA group (*n* = 82). Mean change in vision at 12 months was −12.1 letters in observation group, −1.2 letters in the 1-mg TA group and −1.2 letters in 4-mg TA group. For BVO, the patients with ≥3-line gain in vision at month 12 (primary outcome) was 29% in the laser group, 26% in the 1-mg TA group, and 27% in the 4-mg TA group. Overall, IOP-lowering medications were required in 8% in the laser group, 20% in the 1-mg TA group and 35% in the 4-mg TA group. Cataract progression was seen in 18% in standard-of-care group, 26% in 1-mg TA group, and 33% in 4-mg TA group

Conclusions: TA was superior to observation in CVO (5 x greater chance of gaining 3 lines) but not to laser in BVO. Complications were higher in the 4-mg TA group than the 1-mg TA group, so 1 mg is preferred.

Study of COmparative Treatments for REtinal Vein Occlusion 2 (SCORE2)

Objective: noninferiority (5-letter margin) 6-month trial to compare monthly bevacizumab vs. aflibercept for treatment of center-involving macular edema resulting from CRVO

Methods: 362 patients enrolled; study eyes randomized 1:1 to intravitreal bevacizumab (1.25 mg) every 4 weeks vs. intravitreal aflibercept (2.0 mg) every 4 weeks for treatment of CRVO. Ozurdex (dexamethasone) will be offered as rescue therapy in one study arm

Results: 362 patients enrolled. The mean change in vision was +18.6 letters in the bevacizumab group and +18.9 letters in the aflibercept group. The mean difference was −0.14 letters meeting the noninferiority outcome (*P* = 0.001). Adverse events were similar between groups

Conclusions: outcomes in patients with macular edema resulting from CRVO were similar between bevacizumab and aflibercept

BRAnch Retinal Vein Occlusion (BRAVO) Study

Objective: to assess the safety and efficacy profile of ranibizumab in macular edema secondary to branch retinal vein occlusion

Methods: multicenter, randomized, double-masked, sham-injection-controlled phase III study of 397 patients designed to assess safety and efficacy profile of ranibizumab in macular edema secondary to branch RVO. Patients were included if they were ≥18 years of age with foveal center-involved macular edema secondary to branch/hemi-RVO diagnosed within 12 months prior to screening. BCVA 20/40-20/400 and retinal thickness ≥250 μm. Patients were randomized to 0.3 mg ranibizumab, 0.5 mg, or sham injections. Laser rescue after 3 months. Primary endpoint was mean change in vision from baseline at 6 months. In next 6 months, monthly ranibizumab PRN was allowed for all patients with rescue laser at month 9

Results: At 6 months, mean change in vision (primary outcome) was +7.3 letters in the sham group ($n = 132$), +16.6 letters in 0.3-mg ranibizumab group ($n = 134$), and +18.3 letters in 0.5-mg ranibizumab group ($n = 131$). In addition, 55% (74/134) of patients who received 0.3 mg of ranibizumab and 61% (80/131) who received 0.5 mg of ranibizumab had their vision improved by ≥15 letters, compared with 29% (38/132) of patients receiving sham injections. Mean gain in BCVA was observed beginning at day 7 with a +7.6-letter and +7.4-letter gain in the 0.3-mg and 0.5-mg study arms of ranibizumab, respectively (compared with +1.9 letters in the sham injection arm)

Conclusions: ranibizumab injections are safe and effective in BRVO

Intravitreal Aflibercept for Macular Edema Following Branch Retinal Vein Occlusion (VIBRANT) Study

Objective: to compare efficacy and safety of intravitreal aflibercept injection (IAI) with macular grid laser photocoagulation for treatment of macular edema after BRVO

Methods: eyes that gained ≥15 ETDRS letters from baseline at 6 months was 52.7% in IAI group compared with 26.7% in laser group. Mean improvement from baseline BCVA at week 24 was 17.0 ETDRS letters in IAI group and 6.9 ETDRS letters in laser group. Mean reduction in CRT from baseline at week 24 was 280.5 μm in IAI group and 128.0 μm in laser group

Conclusions: monthly aflibercept provided significantly greater visual benefit and reduction in CRT at 24 weeks than grid laser photocoagulation in eyes with macular edema after BRVO

Central Vein Occlusion Study (CVOS)

Objective: to evaluate patients with CVO for:

1. Natural history of eyes with perfused (<10 disc areas of nonperfusion) CVO
2. Improvement of vision in eyes with perfused macular edema
3. Eyes with nonperfused CVO; does early PRP prevent NVI?
4. Eyes with nonperfused CVO; is early PRP more effective than delayed PRP in preventing NVG?

Methods:

Group P (perfused): patients with CVO occurring for <1 year with intraretinal hemorrhages in all 4 quadrants and with capillary nonperfusion <10 DD in size and with no iris or angle NV. These patients were observed; 547 patients enrolled

Group N (nonperfused): patients with CVO occurring for <1 year with intraretinal hemorrhages in all 4 quadrants and with capillary nonperfusion >10 DD in size and with no iris or angle NV were randomly assigned to immediate PRP or observation; 180 patients enrolled

Group I (indeterminate): patients with CVO occurring for <1 year with intraretinal hemorrhages in all 4 quadrants and with retinal hemorrhages that prevent measurement of the area of capillary nonperfusion and with no iris or angle NV. These patients were followed; 52 eyes enrolled

Group M (macular edema): patients with CVO occurring for ≥3 months with macular edema that involves the fovea and with VA of 20/50-5/200 were randomly assigned to grid pattern laser photocoagulation or observation; 155 eyes enrolled

Results:

Group P: 34% became nonperfused at 3 years
   RISK FACTORS FOR PROGRESSION TO NON-PERFUSED: CVO of <1-month duration, VA <20/200, presence of >5 disc areas of nonperfusion

Group N: prophylactic PRP did not prevent iris or angle NV (18 of 90 eyes [20%] with prophylactic PRP developed iris or angle NV, vs. 32 of 91 eyes [35%] that did not receive prophylactic PRP), eyes prophylactically treated with PRP did not respond well to supplemental PRP (18 of 32 [56%] observation eyes responded to PRP following development of iris or angle NV, vs. 4 of 18 eyes [22%] that received prophylactic PRP responded to supplemental PRP)
   RISK FACTORS FOR DEVELOPING NVI: amount of nonperfused retina, extent of retinal hemorrhages, male sex, CVO of <1-month duration

Group M: grid pattern photocoagulation did not preserve or improve VA (but reduced angiographic evidence of macular edema)

Conclusions: no benefit from early PRP in nonperfused CVO; therefore, wait until first sign of NVI before initiating PRP

PRP for nonperfused CVO when 2 clock hours of NVI or any angle NV present

Monthly follow-up with gonioscopy during first 6 months after CVO

No benefit from focal laser for treatment of macular edema after CVO

Central Retinal Vein Occlusion (CRUISE) Study

Objective: to assess safety and efficacy profile of ranibizumab in macular edema secondary to CRVO

Methods: multicenter, randomized, double-masked, sham-injection-controlled phase III study designed to assess safety and efficacy profile of ranibizumab in 392 patients with macular edema secondary to CRVO. Patients were included if they were ≥18 years of age with foveal center-involved ME secondary CRVO diagnosed within 12 months prior to screening. BCVA 20/40-20/400 and baseline retinal thickness ≥250 μm. Patients were randomized to 0.3 mg ranibizumab, 0.5 mg, or sham injections. Primary endpoint was mean change in vision from baseline at 6 months. In the next 6 months, monthly ranibizumab PRN was allowed for all patients

Results: at 6 months, mean change in vision (primary outcome) was +0.8 letters in sham group ($n = 130$), +12.7 letters in 0.3-mg ranibizumab group ($n = 132$), and +14.9 letters in 0.5-mg ranibizumab group ($n = 130$). In addition, 46% (61/132) of patients given 0.3 mg of ranibizumab and 48% (62/130) given 0.5 mg of ranibizumab had their vision improved by ≥15 letters compared with 17% (22/130) of patients receiving sham injections. Mean gain in BCVA was observed beginning at day 7 with a +8.8-letter and +9.3-letter gain in the 0.3-mg and 0.5-mg study arms of ranibizumab, respectively, compared with +1.1 letters in sham injection arm

Conclusions: ranibizumab injections are safe and effective in CRVO

Intravitreal Aflibercept Injection for Macular Edema Resulting from Central Retinal Vein Occlusion (COPERNICUS)

Objective: phase III studies to determine efficacy of aflibercept injected into the eye on vision function in subjects with macular edema resulting from CRVO

Methods: 189 patients randomized in COPERNICUS. Patients received IAI 2 mg (IAI 2q4) ($n = 114$) or sham injections ($n = 74$) every 4 weeks up to week 24. During weeks 24-52, patients from both arms were evaluated monthly and received IAI as needed, or PRN (IAI 2q4 + PRN and sham + IAI PRN). During weeks 52-100, patients were evaluated at least quarterly and received IAI PRN

Results: proportion of patients gaining ≥15 letters was 56.1% vs. 12.3% at week 24, 55.3% vs. 30.1% at week 52, and 49.1% vs. 23.3% at week 100 in the aflibercept 2q4 + PRN and sham + IAI PRN groups, respectively. Mean change from baseline BCVA was also significantly higher in IAI 2q4 + PRN group compared with sham + IAI PRN group at week 24 (+17.3 vs. −4.0 letters), week 52 (+16.2 vs. +3.8 letters), and week 100 (+13.0 vs. +1.5 letters). Mean reduction from baseline in central retinal thickness was 457.2 vs. 144.8 μm at week 24, 413.0 vs. 381.8 μm at week 52, and 390.0 vs. 343.3 μm at week 100 in IAI 2q4 + PRN and sham + IAI PRN groups, respectively. Mean number (standard deviation) of PRN injections in IAI 2q4 + PRN and sham + IAI PRN groups was 2.7 ± 1.7 vs. 3.9 ± 2.0 during weeks 24-52 and 3.3 ± 2.1 vs. 2.9 ± 2.0 during weeks 52-100, respectively

Conclusions: visual and anatomic improvements after fixed IAI dosing through week 24 and PRN dosing with monthly monitoring from weeks 24 to 52 were diminished after continued PRN dosing, with a reduced monitoring frequency from weeks 52 to 100

Intravitreal Aflibercept Injection for Macular Edema Resulting from Central Retinal Vein Occlusion (GALILEO)

Objective: phase III studies to determine efficacy of aflibercept injected into the eye on vision function in subjects with macular edema resulting from CRVO

Methods: patients received either 2 mg intravitreal aflibercept or sham injections every 4 weeks for 20 weeks. From week 24 to 48, aflibercept group received aflibercept PRN, and sham group continued receiving sham injections

Results: 177 patients in GALILEO. At week 52, mean percentage of patients gaining 15 letters or more was 60.2% in aflibercept group and 32.4% in sham group. Aflibercept patients, compared with sham patients, had significantly higher mean improvement in BCVA (+16.9 letters vs. +3.8 letters, respectively) and reduction in central retinal thickness (−423.5 μm vs. −219.3 μm, respectively) at week 52. Aflibercept patients received a mean of 2.5 injections (standard deviation, 1.7 injections) during PRN dosing

Conclusions: treatment with intravitreal aflibercept provided significant visual and anatomic benefits after 52 weeks as compared with sham. Improvements achieved after 6 monthly doses at week 24 largely were maintained until week 52 with PRN dosing

Branch Retinal Artery Occlusion (BRAO)

90% caused by emboli (cholesterol, calcium, fibrin, platelets)

Most commonly at retinal arterial bifurcations

10% risk of episode in fellow eye

Central Retinal Artery Occlusion (CRAO)

Most common cause of cherry-red spot (thin transparent foveal tissue surrounded by opacified ischemic retina)

Etiology:

Atherosclerosis: of CRA at lamina cribrosa

Emboli: cholesterol (73%), platelet fibrin (15%) from carotid plaque, calcific (from heart, especially valves), tumor (atrial myxoma), lipid emboli (pancreatitis), talc

Vasculitis: giant cell arteritis (GCA) in elderly patient (always check ESR)

Trauma: retrobulbar injection, orbital surgery, penetrating injury

Coagulopathy: oral contraceptives, pregnancy, sickle cell (especially after hyphema), platelet or factor abnormalities, homocystinuria, hyperhomocysteinemia, protein S deficiency, antiphospholipid antibody (check anticardiolipin antibody panel; also at risk for deep vein thrombosis [DVT], pulmonary embolism, cardiac vessel blockage, and spontaneous abortion; treat with Coumadin; steroids do not decrease risk of thromboembolism)

Ocular abnormalities: optic disc drusen, prepapillary loops, elevated IOP

Collagen vascular disease: lupus, polyarteritis nodosa, granulomatosis with polyangiitis

Migraine: in young patients

Orbital mucor

Fibromuscular hyperplasia

Behçet disease

Leukemia

Findings: severe visual loss (light perception [LP] to counting fingers [CF] vision in 90%), retinal whitening in posterior pole with cherry-red spot, box-carring (interruption of blood column), emboli, positive RAPD; whitening resolves after 4 to 6 weeks, and pale disc and attenuated vessels develop

Pathology: atrophy of inner retinal layers (those supplied by retinal circulation) (Fig. 11.71)

DDx: ophthalmic artery occlusion, inadvertent intraocular injection of gentamicin, arteritic AION (check ESR and C-reactive protein)

DDx of cherry red spot: sphingolipidosis (Tay-Sachs, Niemann-Pick, Gaucher, Farber disease), quinine toxicity, commotio retinae, macular hole with surrounding RD, macular hemorrhage, subacute sclerosing panencephalitis, ocular ischemia, methanol toxicity

Diagnosis:

Lab tests: complete blood count (CBC), ESR, complete cardiovascular workup; consider workup for clotting disorders: serum protein electrophoresis, protein C, activated protein C resistance (factor V Leiden deficiency), protein S, antithrombin III, anticardiolipin antibodies, lupus anticoagulant, plasma homocysteine, C-ANCA

FA: delayed filling, increased AV transit time, focal staining at obstruction, collateral or retrograde flow (Fig. 11.72)

ERG: depressed b-wave (inner retina), normal/supernormal a-wave, loss of oscillatory potentials

Treatment: irreversible damage occurs after 90 minutes; therefore, emergent lowering of IOP to allow arterial pressure to reestablish blood flow: paracentesis, ocular massage, carbogen (95% O_2, 5% CO_2) or breath into paper bag, oral and topical ocular hypotensive agents may be tried; PRP for neovascular complications

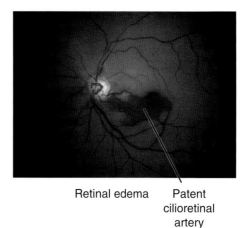

Retinal edema   Patent cilioretinal artery

Figure 11.71 Cilioretinal artery-sparing central retinal artery occlusion with patent cilioretinal artery, allowing perfusion (thus no edema) in a small section of the macula. (From Kaiser PK, Friedman NJ, Pineda R II. *The Massachusetts Eye and Ear Infirmary Illustrated Manual of Ophthalmology*, 2nd ed. Philadelphia: Saunders; 2004.)

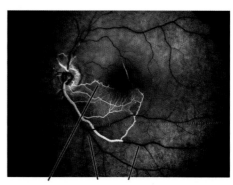

Patent   Absent flow
cilioretinal
artery

Figure 11.72 Fluorescein angiogram of the same patient as in Fig. 11.71, demonstrating no filling of retinal vessels except in cilioretinal artery and surrounding branches. (From Kaiser PK, Friedman NJ, Pineda R II. *The Massachusetts Eye and Ear Infirmary Illustrated Manual of Ophthalmology*, 2nd ed. Philadelphia: Saunders; 2004.)

Complications: rubeosis (15%)

Prognosis: 10% recover vision (usually from cilioretinal artery [in 25% of population]), 18% have vision ≥ 20/40, 66% have vision ≤ 20/400; <5% develop neovascular glaucoma; 1% with bilateral disease; 10% risk of episode in fellow eye

Ophthalmic Artery Occlusion

No light perception (NLP) vision and no cherry-red spot; RPE pigmentary changes develop

May occur with orbital mucormycosis

FA: absent choroidal and retinal filling

ERG: absent a-wave

Ocular Ischemic Syndrome

Reduced blood flow to globe produces anterior and/or posterior segment ischemia

Etiology: carotid occlusion (most common, usually >90% obstruction), carotid dissection, arteritis (rare) Associated with diabetes (56%), hypertension (50%), coronary artery disease (38%), CVA/TIA (31%)

Symptoms: amaurosis fugax, gradual or sudden visual loss, dull pain (improves on lying down); may experience transient visual loss, sometimes precipitated by exposure to bright light (resulting from impaired photoreceptor regeneration)

Findings:
Anterior segment: chronic conjunctival injection, rubeosis and NV of the iris (NVI) common (IOP often not elevated as a result of CB shutdown), PAS, AC cells and flare, corneal edema, cataract, altered IOP, hypopyon (rare)
Posterior segment: vitreous cells, NV, optic disc pallor (40%), optic nerve swelling (8%), superficial hemorrhages in midperiphery, CME, cherry red spot (18%), altered vessels (attenuated, box-carring, dilated, nontortuous veins) (Fig. 11.73)

DDx: aortic arch disease, Takayasu disease

Diagnosis: digital pressure on eye causes arterial pulsation
FA: delayed filling (retina and choroid), diffuse leakage (Fig. 11.74)
Ophthalmodynamometry: decreased retinal arterial pressure
Carotid ultrasound: severe stenosis (>80%)

Treatment: lower IOP to increase perfusion pressure, carotid surgery; PRP (controversial because anterior segment ischemia can possibly be caused by uveal ischemia without retinal ischemia); carotid endarterectomy (CEA) beneficial when carotid stenosis 70%-99% (not possible when 100%)—may lead to increased IOP from improved CB perfusion

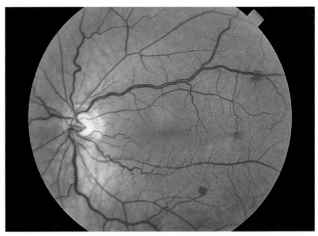

Figure 11.73 Retinal vascular changes in ocular ischemic syndrome. (From Fox GM, Sivalingham A, Brown CG. Ocular ischemic syndrome. In: Yanoff M, Duker JS, eds. *Ophthalmology.* London: Mosby; 1999.)

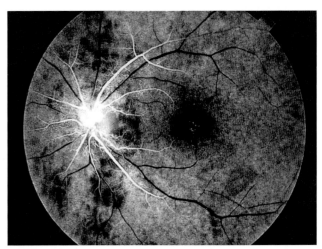

Figure 11.74 Fluorescein angiography, ocular ischemic syndrome. (From Fox GM, Sivalingham A, Brown CG. Ocular ischemic syndrome. In: Yanoff M, Duker JS, eds. *Ophthalmology.* London: Mosby; 1999.)

Radiation Retinopathy

Slowly progressive microangiopathy following exposure to radiation (6 months to 3 years after radiation treatment)

Threshold dose is 300 rads (3 Gy); occurs 4-32 months following plaque brachytherapy with mean dose of 15,000 rads (150 Gy); occurs 36 months after external beam radiation with mean dose of 5000 rads (50 Gy)

Findings: hemorrhage, exudate, microaneurysms, capillary nonperfusion, cotton-wool spots, NV, optic disc swelling, optic neuropathy; gradual occlusion of larger retinal vessels, eventually proliferative retinopathy; may have cataract, dry eye disease, lid abnormalities

Pathology: vascular decompensation with focal loss of capillary endothelial cells and pericytes; radiation-induced optic neuropathy: ischemic demyelination with obliterative endarteritis of nerve sheath vasculature

Treatment: focal laser for macular edema, PRP for NV; hyperbaric O$_2$ (controversial)

Certain types of chemotherapy and preexisting vascular compromise (e.g., diabetic or hypertensive retinopathy) can worsen radiation retinopathy

Hypercoagulable States

Etiology: antiphospholipid antibodies (lupus anticoagulant) and anticardiolipins, Waldenström macroglobulinemia, leukemia

Findings: cotton-wool spots, blot hemorrhages, box-carring, capillary nonperfusion, arteriolar attenuation

Disseminated Intravascular Coagulation

May cause fibrinoid necrosis of choriocapillaris, serous RDs, and multiple areas of RPE changes

Phakomatoses

(See Chapter 5, Pediatrics/Strabismus)

Inflammatory/Immune Disease

(See Chapter 8, Uveitis)

Infections

(See Chapter 8, Uveitis)

Neuroretinitis

Usually unilateral

50% have viral prodrome

Symptoms: decreased vision; colors appear washed out; rarely, retrobulbar pain, pain associated with eye movement, or headache

Findings: optic nerve swelling (optic atrophy can develop), peripapillary NFL hemorrhages, serous RD; iritis, vitritis, and/or scleritis (rare); vascular occlusions may develop

Etiology:

Noninfectious: cerebral AV malformation, elevated ICP, malignant hypertension, ischemic optic neuropathy, polyarteritis nodosa, Leber idiopathic stellate neuroretinitis

LEBER IDIOPATHIC STELLATE NEURORETINITIS (LISN):

Affects individuals aged 8-55 years (usually in 3rd decade); male = female; >70% unilateral

Viral prodrome in 5%

FINDINGS: decreased vision; positive RAPD (75%); cecocentral or central scotoma; vitreous cells; optic disc edema (resolves over 8–12 weeks); optic atrophy is rare; macular star develops in second week; exudative peripapillary RD can occur; RPE defects late; rarely develop chorioretinitis with elevated yellow–white spots in deep retina

FA: hot disc; no perifoveal capillary leakage or macular abnormalities

Prognosis: excellent

Infectious: (suggested by multiple areas of retinitis): syphilis, Lyme disease, viral (influenza A, mumps, coxsackie B, Epstein-Barr virus [EBV]), cat-scratch disease *(Bartonella henselae),* tuberculosis (TB), *Salmonella typhi,* parasites *(Toxocara, Toxoplasma,* DUSN)

DIFFUSE UNILATERAL SUBACUTE NEURORETINITIS (DUSN):

Caused by infection with subretinal nematode: *Ancylostoma caninum* (dog hookworm), *Baylisascaris procyonis* (raccoon worm)

Chronic course

Does not have characteristic neuroretinitis appearance

FINDINGS: multifocal pigmentary changes resulting from movement of the worm, minimal intraocular inflammation, decreased vision (typically out of proportion to findings); may have positive RAPD. Late findings include visual field defects, optic nerve pallor, chorioretinal atrophy, and narrowed retinal vessels

DIAGNOSIS: stool for ova and parasites, CBC with differential (eosinophilia sometimes present); lactate dehydrogenase (LDH) and serum glutamic-oxaloacetic transaminase (SGOT) sometimes elevated

FA: early hypofluorescence and late staining of lesions, perivascular leakage, and disc staining; multifocal window defects in late disease

ERG: subnormal, loss of b-wave

TREATMENT: laser photocoagulation of the worm; rarely subretinal surgery to remove worm (controversial)

Systemic antihelmintic medications (thiabendazole, diethylcarbamazine, pyrantel pamoate) are controversial and often not effective; steroids are usually added because worm death may increase inflammation

PROGNOSIS: poor without treatment; variable if worm can be killed with treatment

DDx of optic nerve swelling and macular star:

LISN, syphilis, hypertension, trauma, acute febrile illness (measles, influenza), TB, coccidiomycosis, cat-scratch disease, papillitis, papilledema, AION (macular star rare), DUSN (macular star rare)

Diagnosis:

Lab tests: ESR, VDRL, fluorescent treponemal antibody absorption (FTA-ABS), Lyme titer, *Bartonella* serology, *Toxoplasma* and *Toxocara* titers, PPD

FA: diffuse leakage from disc, peripapillary capillary staining; 10% have disc leakage in fellow eye; no leakage in macula

Treatment: treat underlying disease, observe idiopathic form; most recover ≥20/50 after 3 months; only 3%-5% have permanent severe visual loss

HIV Retinopathy

Microangiopathy in up to 50% of human immunodeficiency virus (RNA retrovirus) infected individuals as a result of complement deposition (not infectious)

Asymptomatic, nonprogressive

Findings: cotton-wool spots, Roth spots, hemorrhages, and microaneurysms in posterior pole; many HIV-positive patients have early presbyopia caused by inflammation of CB with loss of accommodative amplitude

Diagnosis: HIV antibody test, CD4 count, HIV viral load

Treatment: none; spontaneous resolution within 1-2 months

Toxic Retinopathies

Aminoglycosides (Gentamicin/Tobramycin/Amikacin)

Toxic dose: seen after injecting 0.1 mg of gentamicin (also described after diffusion through cataract wound from subconjunctival injection)

Findings: acute, severe, permanent visual loss after intraocular injection of toxic doses with marked retinal whitening (especially in macula) and retinal hemorrhages; optic atrophy and pigmentary changes occur later

FA: sharp zones of capillary nonperfusion corresponding to the areas of ischemic retina

No effective treatment with poor visual prognosis

Chloroquine (Aralen)/Hydroxychloroquine (Plaquenil)

Binds to melanin in RPE; ganglion cells are also directly affected

Toxic dose: >2.3 mg/kg real weight for chloroquine, >5.0 mg/kg real weight for hydroxychloroquine. Hydroxychloroquine appears safer because it does not readily cross blood–retinal barrier

Daily dosage is most important risk factor for retinal toxicity. Other major risk factors for hydroxychloroquine toxicity: duration of use (>5 years with no other risk factors), renal disease, concomitant tamoxifen use (5 × increase risk), and retinal/macular disease (interfere with interpretation of screening tests); lesser risk factors are liver disease and older age. Toxicity in 7.5% of long-term users; risk of toxicity at recommended doses (<5.0 mg/kg/day) is <1% up to 5 years, <2% up to 10 years, and ~20% after 20 years.

Findings: early, mild mottling of perifoveal RPE with decreased foveal reflex; progresses to bull's-eye maculopathy; peripheral pigmentary retinopathy, eyelash whitening, and cornea vortex keratopathy may develop

DDx of bull's-eye maculopathy: cone dystrophy, AMD, Stargardt disease, fundus flavimaculatus,

Spielmeyer-Vogt disease, albinism, fenestrated sheen macular dystrophy, central areolar choroidal dystrophy, benign concentric annular macular dystrophy, clofazimine toxicity, fucosidosis

VF: decreased; paracentral scotomas

ERG: enlarged a-wave, depressed b-wave

EOG: depressed

OCT: ring of outer retinal thinning (UFO sign)

FAF: bull's-eye pattern is often seen

Progression of retinopathy can occur after cessation of medication; vision loss rarely recovers

Pentosan Polysulfate (Elmiron)

Used to treat interstitial cystitis/bladder pain syndrome; produces pigmentary retinopathy with chronic exposure

Occurs in female patients, median age 60 years

Findings: paracentral hyperpigmented spots, yellow or orange deposits in macula

Dark adaptation: prolonged

FAF: well-circumscribed, central area of hyper- and hypo-autofluorescence

OCT: focal areas of hyperreflectance at the level of the RPE, thickening of RPE; CME can be seen

Thioridazine (Mellaril)

Concentrates in uveal tissue with RPE damage, decreased vision, nyctalopia, and sometimes altered color vision

Toxic dose: >1200 mg/day

Findings: peripheral pigmentary retinopathy, pigment deposition in eyelids, cornea, and lens (Fig. 11.75)

ERG: depressed a- and b-waves
Progression of retinopathy can occur after cessation of medication

Chlorpromazine (Thorazine)

Toxic dose: 1200-2400 mg/day for at least 12 months

Findings: pigment deposition in eyelids, cornea, lens, and retina

Chloramphenicol

Atrophy of maculopapular bundle

VF: cecocentral scotoma

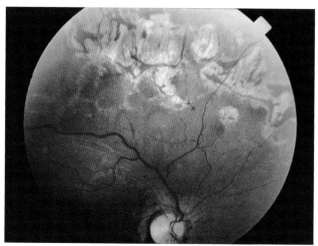

Figure 11.75 Thioridazine retinopathy associated with chronic use (nummular retinopathy). (From Weinberg DV, D'Amico DJ. Retinal toxicity of systemic drugs. In: Albert DM, Jakobiec FA, eds. *Principles and Practice of Ophthalmology.* Philadelphia: WB Saunders; 1994.)

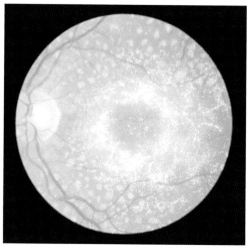

Figure 11.76 Severe tamoxifen retinopathy. (From McKeown CA, Swartz M, Blom J, et al. Tamoxifen retinopathy. *Br J Ophthalmol.* 1981;65:177–179.)

Quinine

Toxicity causes blurred vision, visual field loss, photophobia, nyctalopia sometimes transient blindness; may have neurologic symptoms, dilated pupils, nausea, hearing loss, drowsiness, and become comatose

Acute overdose: single dose ≥4 g; may cause irreversible blindness

Findings: retinal opacification with cherry-red spot, dilated retinal vessels; later develop fine RPE mottling, retinal vascular attenuation, disc pallor; end-stage appears like vascular occlusion

Tamoxifen

Toxic dose: >30 mg/day

Symptoms: asymptomatic

Findings: fleck-like crystalline retinopathy with refractile retinal deposits, typically in ring around macula; may develop pigmentary retinal changes and mild CME (Fig. 11.76)

FA: macular edema

Canthaxanthin

Toxic dose: >35 g (cumulative) of this oral tanning agent

Symptoms: asymptomatic, or mild metamorphopsia

Findings: refractile yellow deposits in a ring around the fovea; "gold-dust" retinopathy (Fig. 11.77)

Methoxyflurane

Crystalline retinopathy resulting from oxalate crystals

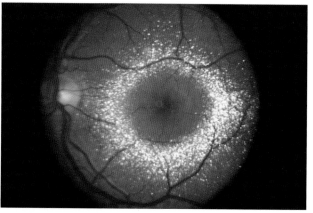

Figure 11.77 Canthaxanthin retinopathy. (From Weinberg DV, D'Amico DJ. Retinal toxicity of systemic drugs. In: Albert DM, Jakobiec FA, eds. *Principles and Practice of Ophthalmology.* Philadelphia: WB Saunders; 1994.)

Methoxyflurane is metabolized to oxalate, which binds with calcium to form insoluble calcium oxalate salt

Crystals are permanent

Talc

Particles deposit in blood vessels of IV drug users; appear as tiny crystals

Talc deposits in lungs; with prolonged abuse pulmonary AV shunts develop, and talc passes into systemic circulation

Talc emboli can cause arteriolar occlusions, resulting in ischemic maculopathy, retinal NV, and VH

Treatment: consider PRP for NV

Nicotinic Acid Maculopathy

Atypical nonleaking CME resulting from intracellular edema of Müller cells

Symptoms: blurred vision with metamorphopsia

FA: CME does not leak

Digoxin

Direct effect on cones; causes visual disturbance with minimal fundus changes

Symptoms: xanthopsia (yellow vision), blurred vision

Findings: poor color vision, paracentral scotomas, and reduced vision with increased background light

Ergotamine

Vasoconstriction of retinal vessels, CME, CVO, papillitis, optic disc pallor; orthostatic hypotension, postpartum hemorrhages

Oral Contraceptives

Associated with thromboembolic disease

May develop CME, retinal hemorrhages, vascular occlusions

Vancomycin

Intraocular/intracameral (1 mg/0.1 mL) rarely associated with hemorrhagic occlusive retinal vasculitis (HORV); probably immune hypersensitivity reaction (type III) rather than direct toxicity

Delayed onset (1–26 days) of severe vision loss, mild anterior chamber and vitreous reaction, large patches of intraretinal hemorrhages in sectors of retinal vascular occlusion; often develop NVG

Immediate and intensive treatment with steroids (topical, oral, and consider intravitreal), intravitreal anti-VEGF injections, and panretinal photocoagulation may limit visual loss

Interferon

Presumed to result from immune complex deposition in retinal vasculature, followed by white blood cell infiltration with eventual vascular closure

Findings: cotton-wool spots, hemorrhages, macular edema, capillary nonperfusion, vascular occlusions

May exacerbate autoimmune thyroiditis and polyarthropathy

Sildenafil (Viagra)/Tadalafil (Cialis)/Vardenafil (Levitra)

May cause transient blue hue to vision 1-2 hours after ingestion possibly by changing the transduction cascade in photoreceptors

ERG: mildly reduced photopic and scotopic b-wave amplitudes and less than 10% decrease in photopic a- and b-wave implicit times during acute episode, reverts back to normal over time

For Viagra, occurs in 3% of individuals taking a dose of 25-50 mg, 11% of patients taking 100-mg dose, and in 50% taking >100 mg; no permanent effects seen

Inherited Retinal Diseases

(See Chapter 5, Pediatrics/Strabismus)

Metabolic Diseases

(See Chapter 5, Pediatrics/Strabismus)

Vitreoretinal Disorders

(See Chapter 5, Pediatrics/Strabismus)

Degenerations

(Table 11.5)

Oral Bay

Oval island of pars plana epithelium immediately posterior to ora serrata (Fig. 11.78); retinal break may occur

TABLE 11.5	Classification of select retinal degenerations
Benign	**Predisposing to retinal detachment**
White without pressure	Lattice degeneration
Pigment clumping	Snail track degeneration
Diffuse chorioretinal atrophy	Zonuloretinal traction tufts
Peripheral microcystoid changes	Snowflake degeneration
Pavingstone degeneration	
Oral pigmentary degeneration	
Degenerative "senile" retinoschisis	

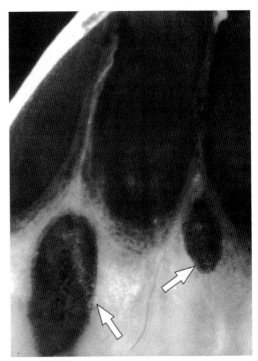

Figure 11.78 Enclosed oral bays. (From Tasman WS. Peripheral retinal lesions. In: Yanoff M, Duker JS, eds. *Ophthalmology.* London: Mosby; 1999.)

Meridional Fold

Elevated fold of retina in upper nasal quadrant

20% prevalence

Retinal break may occur (Fig. 11.79)

Meridional Complex

Meridional fold extending to posterior aspect of a ciliary process

Retinal break may occur

Normal variation of anatomy at ora serrata

Vitreoretinal Tuft

Small internal projection of retinal tissue

Noncystic retinal tuft: short, thin (base < 0.1 mm) projection of fibroglial tissue; can break off, leaving fragments in vitreous; usually inferonasal; not associated with retinal break; not present at birth

Cystic retinal tuft: chalky white, nodular projection (base 0.1–1.0 mm) of fibroglial tissue; usually nasal; may have pigment at base; increased vitreous adhesion predisposes to tractional tears from PVD; present at birth; occurs in 5% of population; <1% risk of RD; therefore, no prophylactic treatment; associated with 10% of RDs; second to lattice degeneration as visible peripheral retinal lesion associated with RD

Zonular traction tuft: thin strand of fibroglial tissue extending from peripheral retina anteriorly to a zonule; usually nasal; present at birth; break occurs in 2%-10%

Pars Plana Cyst

Clear cystoid space between pigmented and nonpigmented ciliary epithelium of pars plana; filled with mucopolysaccharides (hyaluronic acid) (Fig. 11.80)

Not a true cyst (not lined with epithelium)

Occurs in 17% of autopsied eyes

Analogous to detachment of sensory retina from underlying RPE; caused by traction by vitreous base and zonules; no increased risk of RD

Stains with Alcian blue

Also seen in conditions with formation of abnormal proteins (multiple myeloma)

Ora Serrata Pearl

Glistening opacity over oral tooth

Increased prevalence with age

Resembles drusen

White With/Without Pressure

Geographic areas of peripheral retinal whitening

More common in young individuals, African Americans, and myopes

White with pressure: visible only with scleral depression

White without pressure: visible without scleral depression

Peripheral Microcystoid Degeneration

Typical/"senile" (Blessing-Iwanoff cysts): outer plexiform layer; bubble-like appearance behind ora serrata; lined by Müller cells; may coalesce and progress to typical degenerative ("senile") retinoschisis

Reticular: NFL; linear or reticular pattern, corresponding to retinal vessels; finely stippled internal surface; continuous with and posterior to typical type (therefore, does not reach the ora); may progress to reticular degenerative retinoschisis

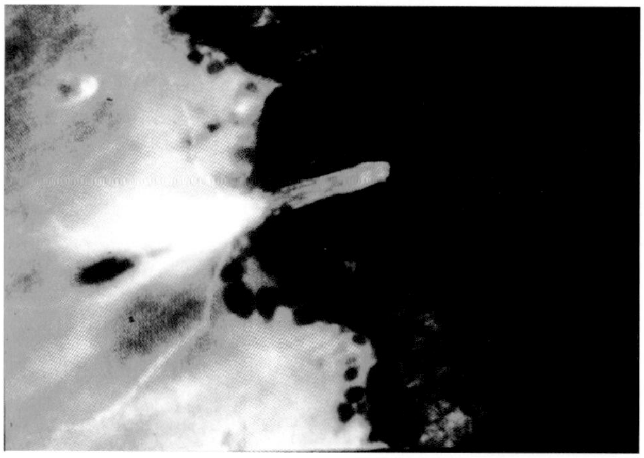

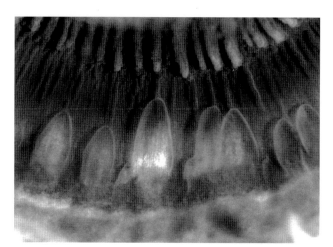

Figure 11.79 Meridional fold with a small break at the base of the fold. (From Tasman WS. Peripheral retinal lesions. In: Yanoff M, Duker JS, eds. *Ophthalmology.* London: Mosby; 1999.)

Figure 11.80 Pars plana cysts. (Courtesy of Dr. Ralph Eagle. From Tasman WS. Peripheral retinal lesions. In: Yanoff M, Duker JS, eds. *Ophthalmology.* London: Mosby; 1999.)

Degenerative (Involutional) "Senile" Retinoschisis

Occurs in 7%-31% of individuals >40 years old, 50%-80% bilateral, often symmetric; 70% inferotemporal, 25% superotemporal

Usually asymptomatic and nonprogressive; hyperopia in 70%

Findings: splits or cysts within neurosensory retinal layers; typical peripheral cystoid degeneration is precursor
  Inner wall: smooth, dome-shaped surface; may be markedly elevated in reticular type; sheathed retinal vessels; holes uncommon (small if present)
  Outer wall: pock-marked on scleral depression; holes (16%–23%) are larger and well delineated, more common in reticular type, have rolled margins (Fig. 11.81)
  Typical: splitting of OPL; bilateral; elderly patients; 1% of adult population; follows coalescence of cavities of microcystoid degeneration; beaten-metal appearance; white spots (Müller cell remnants [Gunn dots]) in stippled pattern along edge appear as glistening dots or snowflakes; inner-layer holes can occur; no risk of RD unless outer-layer hole is also present; intact outer retinal layer whitens/blanches with scleral depression
  Reticular: splitting of NFL; 41% bilateral; 18% of adult population; always posterior to peripheral cystoid; fine, delicately stippled surface

Differentiate from RD: no underlying RPE degeneration, no tobacco dust; absolute scotoma (relative scotoma in RD); laser treatment blanches underlying RPE (RD will not blanch); no shifting fluid; dome shaped

Pathology: cavity contains hyaluronic acid, Müller cell remnants on inner and outer surfaces of cavity, fibrous thickening of vessel walls with patent lumen

Complications: RD (from outer layer holes; slowly progressive, unless both outer and inner holes), progression (toward posterior pole; rare through fovea), hemorrhage (into vitreous or schisis cavity)

Treatment: laser barrier, treat tears and RD

Pavingstone/Cobblestone Degeneration

Usually inferior; 33% bilateral

Occlusion of choriocapillaris causes loss of outer retinal layers and RPE

Increased incidence with age and myopia (27% in those >20 years old)

No symptoms or complications

Findings: yellow-white spots 1/2 to 2 DD in size adjacent to ora; traverse retinal and choroidal vessels; may have irregular black pigmentation at margins

Pathology: degeneration of choroid and retina; loss of outer retinal layers; RPE absent; firm adhesion between retina and Bruch membrane/choroid (no predisposition to RD) (Fig. 11.82)

Lattice Degeneration

Occurs in 7% of population; more common in myopic eyes; no sex predilection

Often bilateral; usually superotemporal

Present in 20%-35% of eyes with RD; 0.5% risk that patient with lattice will develop an RD

Findings: peripheral circumferential cigar-shaped atrophic retinal patches; crisscrossing pattern of sclerosed vessels (fine white lines) within lesion in 12%; superficial white dots in 80% (ILM and inner retina); pigmentary disturbance in 82%; firm adhesions of vitreous at margins; clear pockets of vitreous fluid over central thin portion; retinal breaks (round or atrophic holes) in 18%, horseshoe tear in 1.4% at

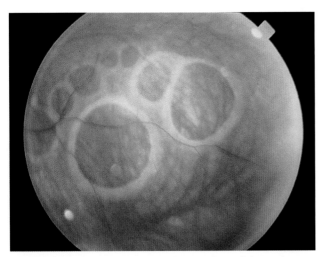

Figure 11.81 Degenerative retinoschisis demonstrating multiple outer layer breaks. (From Tasman WS. Peripheral retinal lesions. In: Yanoff M, Duker JS, eds. *Ophthalmology*. London: Mosby; 1999.)

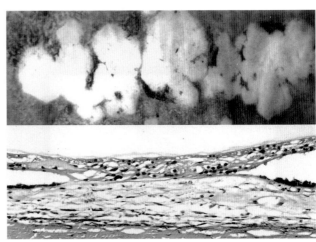

Figure 11.82 Pavingstone degeneration. (Courtesy of Dr. Ralph Eagle. From Tasman WS. Peripheral retinal lesions. In: Yanoff M, Duker JS, eds. *Ophthalmology*. London: Mosby; 1999.)

posterior or lateral edge as a result of severe vitreous traction (Fig. 11.83)

Pathology: discontinuity of ILM, overlying pocket of liquid vitreous, condensation and adherence of vitreous at margin of lesion, focal area of retinal thinning with loss of inner retinal layers, melanin-laden macrophages, fibrous thickening of retinal vessel walls

Treatment: no proof that prophylactic treatment prevents RD; consider treatment of fellow eye if history of RD from lattice

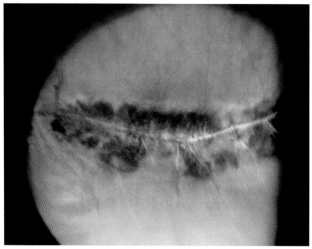

Figure 11.83 Lattice degeneration showing the typical white lines. (From Tasman WS. Peripheral retinal lesions. In: Yanoff M, Duker JS, eds. *Ophthalmology.* London: Mosby; 1999.)

Detachments

Rhegmatogenous Retinal Detachment (RD)

Etiology: retinal break allows liquid vitreous access to subretinal space (Figs.11.84 and 11.85)

1 in 10,000/year; retinal break can be found in 97%

Most tears (70%) are located superiorly between 10 and 2 o'clock positions

Types of breaks:
Horseshoe tear
Atrophic hole: myopia, increasing age

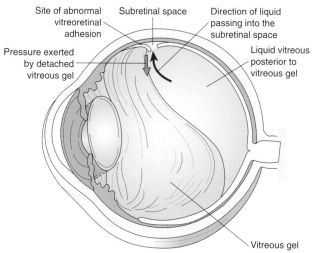

Figure 11.85 Classic pathogenesis of rhegmatogenous retinal detachment. (From Wilkinson CP. Rhegmatogenous retinal ophthalmology. In: Yanoff M, Duker JS, eds. *Ophthalmology.* London: Mosby; 1999.)

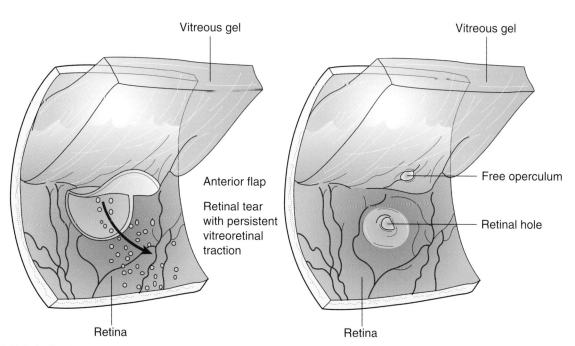

Figure 11.84 Retinal breaks demonstrating horseshoe tear and operculated hole. From Wilkinson CP. Rhegmatogenous retinal ophthalmology. In: Yanoff M, Duker JS, eds. *Ophthalmology.* London: Mosby; 1999.)

Dialysis: splitting of vitreous base (usually inferotemporally, second-most-common site is superonasal); traumatic or idiopathic

Giant tear: >3 clock hours or 90°; trauma (≥90%), myopia; 50% risk of RD in fellow eye

Operculated hole: fragment of retinal tissue found in overlying vitreous

Risk factors: age, history of RD in fellow eye (15%), high myopia/axial length (7%), family history, lattice degeneration, trauma, cataract surgery (1% after intracapsular cataract extraction [ICCE]; 0.1% after extracapsular cataract extraction [ECCE] with intact posterior capsule), diabetes, Nd:YAG laser posterior capsulotomy

After blunt trauma, dialysis is most common form of tear, followed by giant retinal tear, flap tear, and tear around lattice degeneration

Symptoms: flashes and floaters in 50%

Findings: retinal break; detached retina is opaque, corrugated, and undulates; tobacco dust (pigment in vitreous); decreased IOP; VH; nonshifting subretinal fluid

Long-standing RD: thin retina, small breaks or dialysis, demarcation lines, underlying RPE atrophy, subretinal precipitates, macrocysts; may have increased IOP (photoreceptor outer segments in AC [Schwartz-Matsuo syndrome]), PVR

DDx: exudative or traction RD

Complications: PVR

Treatment:

Pneumatic retinopexy: ideal if RD caused by single break in superior 8 clock hours or multiple breaks within 1-2 clock hours; phakic patients tend to do better than aphakic patients

Injection of inert gas or sterile air into vitreous cavity; strict positioning of patient's head allows gas bubble to contact retinal break and form barrier (RPE pumps subretinal fluid into choroid, allowing retina to reattach); break is sealed with cryo at time of gas injection or sealed with laser once subretinal fluid has resorbed

INTRAOCULAR GASES (in order of decreasing time gas remains in eye): perfluoropropane (C_3F_8), perfluoroethane (C_2F_6), sulfur hexafluoride (SF_6), air

Surgery: scleral buckle and/or vitrectomy, with laser therapy or cryotherapy

GOALS: identify all retinal breaks

Close all retinal breaks

Place scleral buckle to support all retinal breaks and bring retina and choroid into contact; retinal tears should be flat on buckle (Fig. 11.86)

Reduce vitreous traction on retinal breaks

Complications of cryotherapy: proliferative vitreoretinopathy (PVR), uveitis, CME, intraocular hemorrhage, chorioretinal necrosis

Complications of scleral buckle surgery: ischemia (anterior or posterior segments), infection, perforation,

strabismus, erosion or extrusion of explant, change in refractive error (induced myopia from increased axial length), macular pucker, cataract, glaucoma, new retinal tears (1.6%), PVR (4%), failure (5%–10%)

Complications of SRF drainage: hemorrhage, retinal tear, retinal incarceration, hypotony, vitreous loss, infection

Silicone oil: specific gravity less than water; surface tension less than that of all gases; buoyant when placed in eye; therefore, make iridectomy inferiorly; complications: cataract (100%), band keratopathy (24%), glaucoma (19%), corneal decompensation (8%)

Prognosis: scleral buckle has 91% success rate

Final vision depends on macular involvement: worse prognosis if macular detached; timing of macular detachment is also important: if <1 week, 75% recover vision > 20/70; if >1 week, 50% > 20/70

Proliferative Vitreoretinopathy (PVR)

Retinal break allows cells (RPE, glial, myofibroblasts) to proliferate on inner and outer surfaces of retina along scaffold of detached vitreous (Fig. 11.87)

Membranes contract, causing fixed folds and tractional RD

Risk of PVR: following ocular perforation = 43%, following rupture = 21%, following penetration = 15%; associated with intraocular foreign body in 11%

Most common reason for failure of retinal reattachment surgery; usually occurs 4-6 weeks after initial repair

Classification system: 3 grades (A–C) in order of increasing severity

B-scan ultrasound: detached retina with triangle sign (transvitreal membrane connecting the 2 sides)

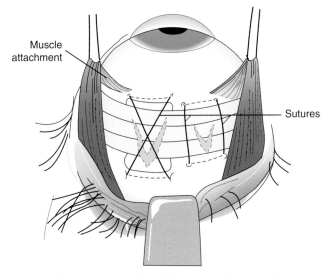

Muscle attachment

Sutures

Figure 11.86 Suture placement for both tire and meridional elements. (From Williams GA. Scleral buckling surgery. In: Yanoff M, Duker JS, eds. *Ophthalmology*. London: Mosby; 1999.)

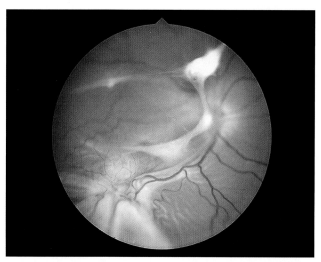

Figure 11.87 Star fold from proliferative vitreoretinopathy. (From Aylward GW. Proliferative vitreoretinopathy. In: Yanoff M, Duker JS, eds. *Ophthalmology.* London: Mosby; 1999.)

Treatment: vitreoretinal surgery is successful in approximately 70% of cases, leading to anatomic success

Exudative RD

Etiology: uveitis (VKH syndrome, sympathetic ophthalmia, pars planitis, viral retinitis), tumors, glomerulonephritis, hypertension, eclampsia/pre-eclampsia, hypothyroidism, Coats disease, nanophthalmos, scleritis, CSR (Fig. 11.88)

Findings: shifting fluid, smooth retinal surface, no retinal break, retina behind the lens (pathognomonic)

Traction RD

Etiology: penetrating trauma (PVR), proliferative retinopathies, PHPV, toxoplasmosis, vitreous degenerations

Findings: taut retinal surface, immobile, concave shape, no retinal break; does not extend to the ora serrata

Pathology: subretinal fluid, photoreceptor degeneration, cystoid degeneration, glial membrane formation

Folds of Neurosensory Retina

Caused by epiretinal membrane or rhegmatogenous RD

Not visible on FA; can be seen on OCT

Choroidal Abnormalities

Choroidal Folds

Results from shrinkage of inner choroid or Bruch membrane, causing undulations of overlying RPE and outer retina

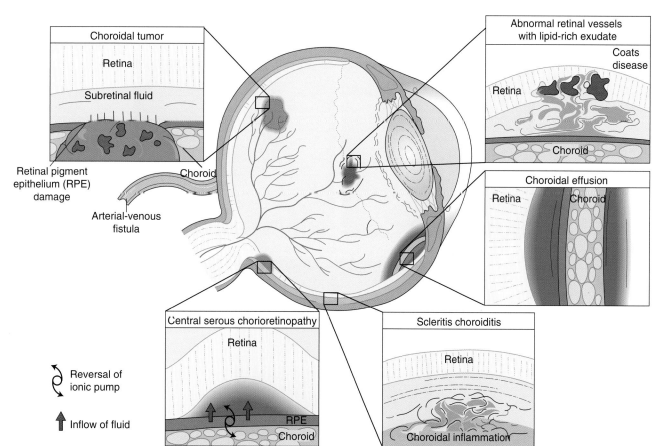

Figure 11.88 Pathologic processes that result in serous detachment of the neural retina. (From Anand R. Serous detachment of the neural retina. In: Yanoff M, Duker JS, eds. *Ophthalmology.* London: Mosby; 1999.)

Etiology: mnemonic **THIN RPE** (**T**umors, **H**ypotony, **I**nflammation/**I**diopathic, **N**eovascular membrane, **R**etrobulbar mass, **P**apilledema, **E**xtraocular hardware)

Findings: yellow elevated crests alternating with darker bands between crests

FA: light bands/crests contain thinner RPE, producing prominent choroidal fluorescence; dark bands/troughs contain compressed RPE, producing relative hypofluorescence

Choroidal Detachment

Caused by fluid (choroidal effusion) or blood (choroidal hemorrhage) in suprachoroidal space

Etiology: hypotony, uveitis, idiopathic, uremia, nanophthalmos (thickened sclera impedes vortex venous drainage), intraocular surgery (rapid change in IOP shears choroidal perforating arteries), intense PRP

Hemorrhage is caused by rupture of small vessels with sudden decrease of IOP (opening globe for surgery); may be expulsive with loss of intraocular contents through wound

Findings: dark dome-shaped appearance (Fig. 11.89)

B-scan ultrasound: echogenic convexity attached at scleral spur and vortex veins (not at optic nerve)

Treatment: treat underlying disorder; consider partial-thickness scleral windows near vortex vein exit sites in 3 or 4 quadrants; if it occurs during surgery, immediately close globe and give mannitol IV; may require drainage (sclerotomies)

Choroidal Ischemia

May occur with hypertensive retinopathy

Elschnig spot: zone of nonperfusion of choriocapillaris, which appears as atrophic area of RPE overlying infarcted choroidal lobule

Siegrist streak: reactive RPE hyperplasia along sclerosed choroidal vessel

Polypoidal Choroidal Vasculopathy (PCV)/ Posterior Uveal Bleeding Syndrome (PUBS)

Branching inner choroidal vessels external to the choriocapillaris with polyp-like terminal dilations; classified as type 1 CNV; PCV is idiopathic and peripapillary

More common in African Americans and Asians

Risk factors include hypertension; smoking; and genetic mutations in *ARMS2*, *HTRA1*, *Y402H*, *C2*, and *CFH* genes

May leak fluid or bleed, causing serous and hemorrhagic RPE detachments (often notched); best seen with ICG angiography

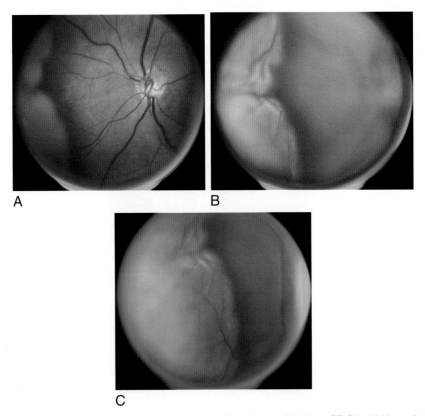

Figure 11.89 (A–C) Hemorrhagic choroidal detachment viewed ophthalmoscopically. (From Kapusta MA, Lopez PF: Choroidal hemorrhage. In: Yanoff M, Duker JS, eds. *Ophthalmology*. London: Mosby; 1999.)

Treatment is with anti-VEGF and/or verteporfin PDT; rates of complete polyp closure: aflibercept = PDT + ranibizumab > ranibizumab alone (EVEREST 1 and 2, PLANET studies)

Miscellaneous

Albinism, Aicardi syndrome, color blindness (see Chapter 5, Pediatrics/Strabismus)

Tumors

Benign Tumors

Choroidal Nevus

Neoplasm of choroidal melanocytes; most common primary intraocular tumor

Can also arise within iris, CB, or optic disc

Usually unilateral and unifocal; increased frequency with age; prevalence of 6.5% in US population >49 years old

Multifocal nevi: associated with neurofibromatosis

Findings: flat slate-gray to dark-brown choroidal lesion with ill-defined margins; surface drusen common; subretinal fluid and orange clumps of pigment rare (Fig. 11.90)

Risk factors for malignant transformation:
  Mnemonic: **To Find Small Ocular Melanoma Doing Imaging (TFSOM-DIM)**
    Thickness (>2 mm)
    Fluid (subretinal)
    Symptoms (visual symptoms, often flashes or floaters)
    Orange pigment (lipofuscin)
    Melanoma hollow on ultrasound
    DIaMeter (>5 mm on fundus photography)
  Mnemonic: **MOLES** (**M**ushroom shape, **O**range pigment, **L**arge size (>2 mm thickness, >5 mm diameter), **E**nlarging tumor, **S**ubretinal fluid)

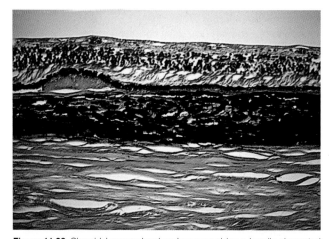

Figure 11.90 Choroidal nevus showing drusen overlying a heavily pigmented choroidal nevus composed almost completely of plump polyhedral nevus cells. (Modified From Naumann G, et al. *Arch Ophthalmol.* 1966;76:784. From Yanoff M, Fine BS. *Ocular Pathology,* 5th ed. St Louis: Mosby; 2002.)

Pathology: benign spindle cells with pigment

DDx: Congenital hypertrophy of the retinal pigment epithelium (CHRPE), melanoma, melanocytoma

FA: hyperfluorescence

Choroidal Cavernous Hemangioma

Congenital, unilateral vascular tumor

Types:
    Diffuse: associated with Sturge-Weber syndrome
    Circumscribed: not associated with systemic disease

Symptoms: blurred vision, micropsia, metamorphopsia; vision loss as a result of cystic macular retinal degeneration or adjacent exudative RD

Findings:
    Diffuse type: generalized red–orange choroidal thickening ("tomato catsup" fundus); may have elevated IOP
    Circumscribed type: red–orange dome-shaped choroidal mass within 2 DD of optic disc or fovea

Pathology: lakes of erythrocytes separated by thin, fibrous septa; large-caliber vascular channels lined by mature endothelium. Circumscribed type has sharply demarcated borders and compresses surrounding melanocytes and choroidal lamellae (seen clinically as ring of hyperpigmentation at periphery of lesion and on FA as ring of blockage of underlying choroidal fluorescence) (Fig. 11.91)

FA: early hyperfluorescent filling of lesion at same time as retinal vessels, late leakage/staining of entire lesion

ICG: early hyperfluorescent filling of intralesional vessels (Fig. 11.92)

Ultrasound: A-scan shows high initial spike with high internal reflectivity; B-scan shows sonoreflective tissue, often with choroidal thickening (Fig. 11.93)

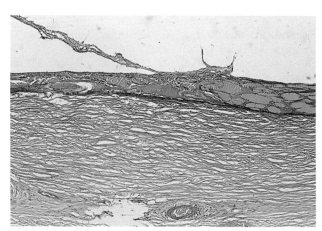

Figure 11.91 Hemangioma of choroid. (From Yanoff M, Fine BS. *Ocular Pathology,* 5th ed. St Louis: Mosby; 2002.)

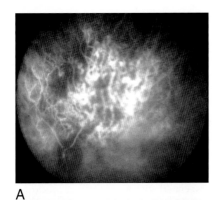

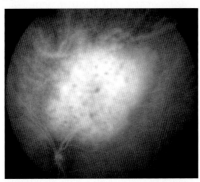

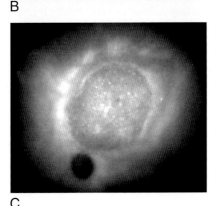

Figure 11.92 (A–C) Indocyanine green angiography of circumscribed choroidal hemangioma. (From Augsburger JJ, Anand R, Sanborn GE. Choroidal hemangiomas. Yanoff M, Duker JS, eds. *Ophthalmology*. London: Mosby; 1999.)

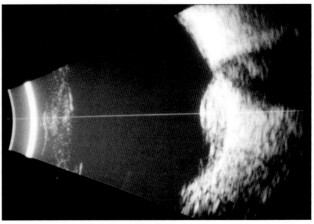

Figure 11.93 B-scan ultrasonography of circumscribed choroidal hemangioma. (From Augsburger JJ, Anand R, Sanborn GE. Choroidal hemangiomas. In: Yanoff M, Duker JS, eds. *Ophthalmology*. London: Mosby; 1999.)

Treatment: laser therapy, photodynamic therapy, or low-dose external beam XRT for exudative RD

Choroidal Osteoma

Tumor composed of bone

Sporadic, unifocal, bilateral in 20%

Arises in late childhood to early adulthood; more common in women (90%)

Symptoms: blurred vision, central scotoma

Findings: yellow–white to pale-orange circumpapillary lesion with well-defined pseudopod-like margins; CNV and RPE disruption can cause progressive visual impairment

Pathology: plaque of mature bone involving full-thickness choroid, usually sparing RPE

FA: patchy early hyperfluorescence and late staining of lesion

ICG: hypofluorescence of lesion with hyperfluorescent intralesional vessels, late leakage of lesion

B-scan ultrasound: highly reflective plate-like lesion with orbital shadowing beyond lesion (Fig. 11.94)

Computed tomography (CT) scan: plate-like thickening of eyewall

Treatment: for CNV if present

Retinal Capillary Hemangioma

Vascular tumor (hemangioblastoma); AD, sporadic, or associated with von Hippel-Lindau disease (bilateral retinal capillary hemangiomas [40%–60%], cystic cerebellar hemangioblastoma [60%, most common cause of death], renal cell carcinoma, pheochromocytoma, liver, pancreas, and epididymis cysts = chromosome 3p26-p25; mutation in the *VHL* tumor-suppressor gene)

Arises in older children and young adults

Symptoms: blurred vision, visual field loss

Findings: red globular mass with prominent dilated tortuous afferent and efferent retinal blood vessels, exudative RD may develop

FA: feeding arteriole fills rapidly; dye leaks into vitreous and subretinal space

Treatment: slowly progressive if untreated; can treat with laser, cryotherapy, or photodynamic therapy (PDT)

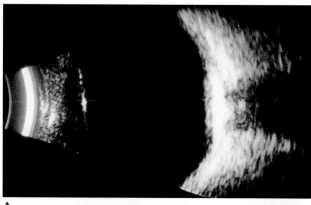

A

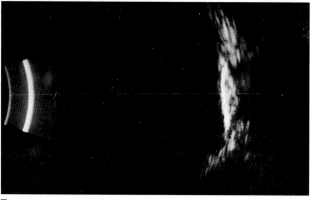

B

Figure 11.94 B-scan ultrasonography of choroidal osteoma. (A) At 77 dB, the osteoma appears as an intensely white plate in the posterior eyewall. (B) At 55 dB, the lesion persists, but most of the normal tissues are no longer evident. (From Yanoff M, Duker JS, eds. *Ophthalmology.* London: Mosby; 1999.)

Retinal Cavernous Hemangioma

Vascular tumor; probably congenital; occasionally associated with similar CNS or skin vascular lesions

Usually unilateral, unifocal; rarely progressive

Findings: cluster of dark red intraretinal vascular sacs ("bunch of grapes" appearance), typically associated with an anomalous retinal vein; associated overlying retinal gliosis; no intraretinal exudates or detachment; may have VH

FA: fluid levels within the vascular sacs

Treatment: vitrectomy for nonclearing VH

Retinal Astrocytoma (Astrocytic Hamartoma)

Glioma arising from retinal glial cells

Occurs in older children and young adults; can be unilateral or bilateral, unifocal or multifocal; usually stable

Rarely associated with tuberous sclerosis (multifocal, bilateral) and NF

Symptoms: blurred vision, visual field loss, or asymptomatic

Findings: 1 or more yellow–white masses that obscure retinal vessels; occasionally exudative RD; calcification in some larger lesions; may have glistening, mulberry appearance or softer, fluffy appearance

Combined Hamartoma of the Retina and RPE

Tumor composed of neurosensory retina and RPE; probably congenital; associated with neurofibromatosis type 2

Usually unilateral, unifocal; minimal progression

Symptoms: blurred vision

Findings: gray, juxtapapillary lesion with surface gliosis and prominent intralesional retinal vascular tortuosity; amblyopia (Fig. 11.95)

Pathology: cords of proliferated pigment epithelium with excess blood vessels and glial tissue

Treatment: none

Adenoma and Adenocarcinoma

Tumor composed of RPE cells, rarely arise from nonpigmented ciliary epithelium; seldom undergoes malignant transformation

Findings: elevated dark black lesion, may resemble deeply pigmented melanoma; may have iridocyclitis, secondary cataract, subluxated lens

Pathology: massive proliferation of RPE cells

Treatment: excision

Racemose Hemangioma

Congenital AV malformation

Associated with Wyburn-Mason syndrome when associated with AV malformation of midbrain

No exudate or leakage

Malignant Tumors

Retinoblastoma (RB)

(See Chapter 5, Pediatrics/Strabismus)

Choroidal Malignant Melanoma

Malignant neoplasm of uveal melanocytes; unilateral, unifocal; 85% of ocular melanomas arise in choroid, less common in CB (10%) or iris (5%)

Most common primary intraocular malignant tumor in Caucasian adults (1 in 2000)

Uncommon before age 40 years

Risk factors: ocular melanocytosis, sunlight exposure, uveal nevi, race (Caucasian; only 1%–2% in African

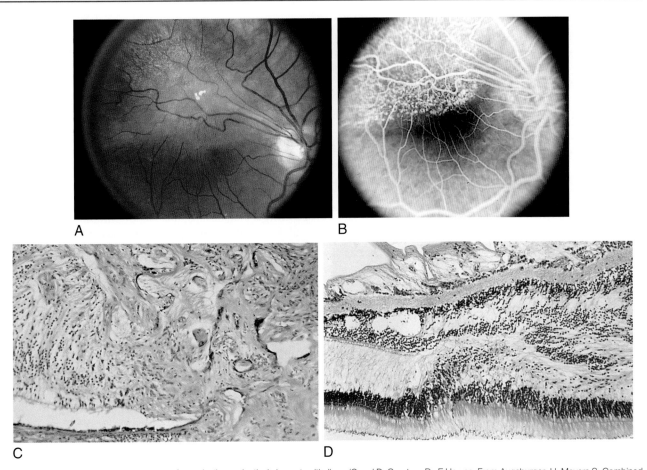

Figure 11.95 (A–D) Combined hamartoma of neural retina and retinal pigment epithelium. (C and D, Courtesy Dr. E Howes. From Augsburger JJ, Meyers S. Combined hamartoma of retina. In: Yanoff M, Duker JS, eds. *Ophthalmology*. London: Mosby; 1999.)

Americans or Asians), cigarette smoking, neurofibromatosis, dysplastic nevus syndrome, bilateral diffuse uveal melanocytic proliferation (BDUMP) syndrome

Symptoms: blurred vision, visual field loss, flashes and floaters

Findings: brown, domed-shaped or mushroom-shaped tumor; orange pigment clumps (accumulation of lipofuscin in RPE), adjacent exudative RD, sentinel vessel (dilated tortuous episcleral vessel); secondary glaucoma; may be amelanotic and appear as a pale mass

Pathology: Callender classification (Figs. 11.96–11.99)
  Spindle A cells: slender, cigar-shaped nucleus with finely dispersed chromatin; low nuclear-to-cytoplasmic ratio; absent or inconspicuous nucleolus; no mitotic figures; tumors composed exclusively of spindle A cells are considered benign nevi
  Spindle B cells: oval (larger) nucleus with coarser chromatin and prominent nucleolus; mitotic figures; tumors with spindle A and B cells are called spindle cell melanomas. Spindle A and B cells grow as a syncytium with indistinct cytoplasmic borders
  Epithelioid cells: polyhedral with abundant cytoplasm; poorly cohesive; distinct borders; most malignant;

large, round to oval nucleus with peripheral margination of chromatin; prominent eosinophilic or purple nucleolus (epithelioid cells "look back at you"); worst prognosis
  Mixed cell melanoma: composed of spindle and epithelioid cells
  Gross examination requires identification of vortex veins to rule out tumor extension

Transillumination: most melanomas cast shadow

Ultrasound: A-scan shows low internal reflectivity with characteristic reduction in amplitude from front to back, high-amplitude spikes consistent with break in Bruch membrane; B-scan shows solid tumor with mushroom shape or biconvex shape (Fig. 11.100)

FA: "double" circulation (choroidal and retinal vessels), mass is hypofluorescent early, pinpoint leakage late (Fig. 11.101)

OCT: subretinal fluid

FAF: orange pigment (lipofuscin)

Magnetic resonance imaging (MRI): bright on T1; dark on T2

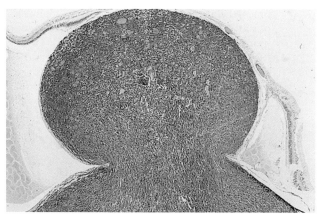

Figure 11.96 Uveal mushroom melanoma. (From Yanoff M, Fine BS. *Ocular Pathology*, 5th ed. St Louis: Mosby; 2002.)

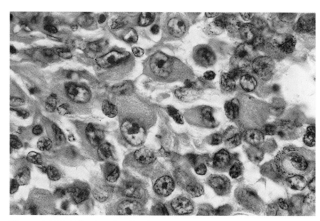

Figure 11.99 Callender classification. Histologic section of epithelioid cells. (From Yanoff M, Fine BS. *Ocular Pathology*, 5th ed. St Louis: Mosby; 2002.)

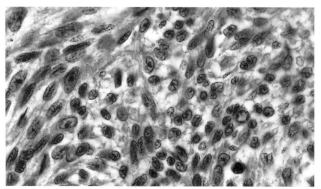

Figure 11.97 Callender classification. Spindle A cells, identified by a dark stripe parallel to the long axis of the nucleus, are seen in longitudinal section. They are identified in transverse cross section by the infolding of the nuclear membrane that causes the dark stripe. (From Yanoff M, Fine BS. *Ocular Pathology*, 5th ed. St Louis: Mosby; 2002.)

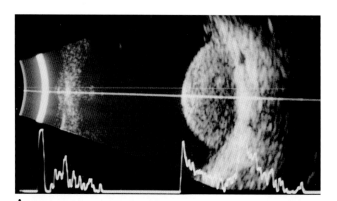

A

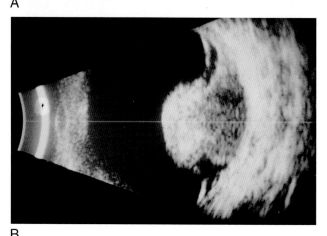

B

Figure 11.100 (A and B) Ultrasonography of posterior uveal melanoma. (From Augsburger JJ, Damato BE, Bornfield N. Uveal melanoma. In: Yanoff M, Duker JS, eds. *Ophthalmology*. London: Mosby; 1999.)

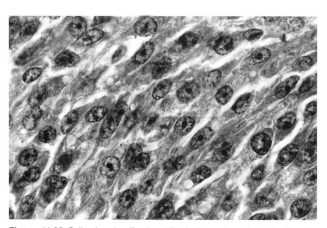

Figure 11.98 Callender classification. Histologic section of spindle B cells. (From Yanoff M, Fine BS. *Ocular Pathology*, 5th ed. St Louis: Mosby; 2002.)

Treatment:

Enucleation: large tumor, optic nerve invasion, painful eye with poor visual potential

Plaque brachytherapy: most eyes with medium-sized tumors with visual potential, or failure of laser

HIGH ENERGY: cobalt-60, iridium-192

LOW ENERGY: iodine-125 ([I-125] sphere of radiation), palladium-106 (25% less energy than I-125), ruthenium-106 (β-particles, travel only 5 mm; therefore, use for small tumors)

Charged particle radiation: proton beam (cylinder of radiation); large anterior segment dose, low macular dose (reverse of plaque)

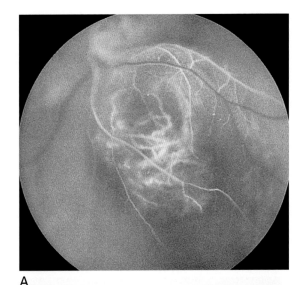

A

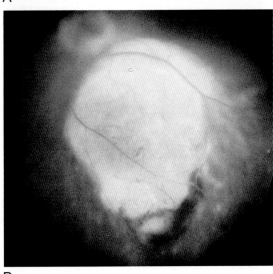

B

Figure 11.101 (A and B) Fluorescein angiograms of mushroom-shaped choroidal melanoma. (From Augsburger JJ, Damato BE, Bornfield N. Uveal melanoma. In: Yanoff M, Duker JS, eds. *Ophthalmology*. London: Mosby; 1999.)

Resection: most iris and iridociliary tumors; some CB and choroidal tumors

Transpupillary thermotherapy: small tumors

Zimmerman hypothesis: manipulation of tumor during enucleation causes metastasis and increases mortality; not true. Derived from plotting of life table data, which showed bell-shaped curve for death rate; specifically, mortality rate increased to 8% following enucleation (vs. 1% per year in patients with untreated tumors)

Complications of treatment: radiation retinopathy (if severe, treat with PRP to prevent NVG); cataracts (PSC in 42% within 3 years of proton beam therapy); dry eye

Collaborative Ocular Melanoma Study (COMS):
SMALL TUMOR TRIAL (apical height = 1.5–2.4 mm and basal diameter = 5–16 mm): 1/3 grew; 5-year tumor mortality = 1%
MEDIUM TUMOR TRIAL (apical height = 2.5–10 mm and basal diameter ≤16 mm): survival rates similar between enucleation and I-125 plaque

brachytherapy; I-125 brachytherapy has a high risk of substantial visual loss (up to 49%); 5-year tumor mortality ~10%
LARGE TUMOR TRIAL (apical height >10 mm and basal diameter >16 mm; without metastasis): pre-enucleation radiation does not change the survival rate in patients with large choroidal melanomas with or without metastases over enucleation alone; 5-year tumor mortality ~27%
Updated definition of large tumor is apical height >2 mm and basal diameter >16 mm, or apical height >10 mm regardless of basal diameter, or apical height >8 mm and <2 mm from optic disc

Prognosis:
Factors:
CELL TYPE: epithelioid has worst prognosis (5-year survival <30%); presence of epithelioid cells is important in survivability; 5-year survival rate for spindle A cell is 95%, 15-year survival rate for mixed tumor is 37%, 15-year survival for pure spindle cell melanoma with no epithelioid cells is 72%
SIZE: larger and diffuse tumors have a worse prognosis
LOCATION
VARIABILITY IN NUCLEOLAR SIZE
PRESENCE OF INTRATUMOR VASCULAR NET-WORKS
PRESENCE OF NECROSIS
METALLOTHIONEIN LEVELS: may indicate metastatic potential and poor survival
GENETICS: monosomy 3 associated with higher death rates; gene expression profiling can also predict melanoma-related mortality
~50% with large tumors have metastasis within 5 years
Mean survival after metastasis is 9 months

Metastasis: hematogenous spread via vortex veins; risks include elevation (>2 mm), proximity to optic nerve, visual symptoms, growth; 92% of metastases are to liver, also skin, lungs, other organs; local extension into optic nerve and brain
Metastatic workup: abdominal examination (hepatosplenomegaly), liver function tests (LFTs), chest x-ray (CXR); 2% have evidence of metastasis at diagnosis; if any abnormal, then liver/abdomen/chest CT and MRI

MAJOR CLINICAL STUDY

Collaborative Ocular Melanoma Study (COMS)

Objective: to evaluate treatment options for choroidal malignant melanomas

Methods:
Small tumor study (not large enough for COMS trial) (apical height = 1.5–2.4 mm and basal diameter

5–16 mm): not randomized; observation vs. treatment at discretion of investigator

Medium tumor trial (apical height = 2.5–10 mm and basal diameter ≤16 mm): randomized to enucleation vs. radiation (I-125 plaque brachytherapy)

Large tumor trial (apical height >10 mm and basal diameter >16 mm; no metastasis): randomized enucleation alone vs. 20-Gy external beam radiation for 5 days and then enucleation (preoperative external beam radiation therapy [PERT])

Primary outcome was survival; secondary outcomes included tumor growth, visual function, time to metastasis, and quality of life

Results:

Small tumor study: 21% grew by 2 years and 31% by 5 years; 6 deaths resulted from metastatic melanoma; 5-year all-cause mortality was 6%, and 8-year all-cause mortality was 14.9%; risk factors for growth included initial tumor thickness and diameter, presence of orange pigment, absence of drusen, and absence of adjacent RPE changes

Medium tumor trial: after 3 years, 43%-49% of I-125–treated eyes had poor vision outcomes (loss of ≥6 lines of VA or VA of ≤20/200), and this was strongly associated with larger tumor apical height and smaller distance from the foveal avascular zone; other risk factors for poor visual outcome included diabetes, tumor-related RD, and tumors that were not dome-shaped; estimated 5-year survival rates were 81% for the enucleation group and 82% for the I-125 group

Large tumor trial: 1003 patients enrolled. Estimated 5-year survival rates were 57% for enucleation alone and 62% for radiation followed by enucleation, and for patients with metastases at the time of death, the 5-year survival was 72% vs. 74%; prognostic risk factors were age and basal diameter

Conclusions:

Small tumor study: otherwise-healthy patients with small choroidal melanomas have a low risk of death within 5 years

Medium tumor trial: there is a high risk of substantial visual loss from I-125 brachytherapy (up to 49%); I-125 brachytherapy does not change the survival rate (for up to 12 years) in patients with medium choroidal melanomas

Large tumor trial: pre-enucleation radiation does not change the survival rate in patients with large choroidal melanomas with or without metastases

Primary Intraocular Lymphoma (Reticulum Cell Sarcoma)

Non-Hodgkin B-cell lymphoma, large cell type

Affects older (mean age 70 years) and immunocompromised patients; usually bilateral and multifocal

No systemic involvement outside of CNS

Increased risk of development of concurrent primary CNS lymphoma

Symptoms (precede CNS signs in 80%): blurred vision, floaters; dementia may occur

Findings: creamy white, diffuse sub-RPE and vitreous infiltrates; AC reaction, hypopyon, vitritis, secondary glaucoma; may have multifocal atrophic or punched-out lesions, and exudative RD; choroidal form manifests with choroidal nodules or detachments of RPE and is associated with systemic lymphoma (Fig. 11.102)

Diagnosis: MRI, lumbar puncture (LP) (positive in 25%), vitreous biopsy (low yield; atypical lymphocytes with prominent nucleoli, mitoses; cellular necrosis) (Fig. 11.103)

FA: leopard spots

Treatment: chemotherapy or XRT

Prognosis: poor, mortality often within 2 years (mean survival is 22 months)

Reactive Lymphoid Hyperplasia of the Choroid

Benign counterpart

Findings: diffuse or multiple yellow choroidal lesions; overlying RD may occur; often similar infiltrates in conjunctiva and orbit (check conjunctiva for salmon patch)

Associated with systemic lymphoma (vs. retinovitreous lymphoma, which is associated with CNS lesions)

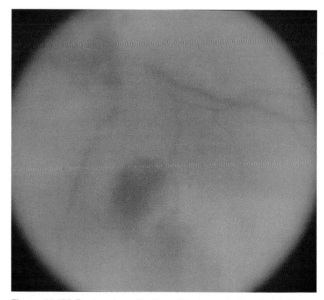

Figure 11.102 Fundus view of yellow–white hemorrhagic retinal infiltrates. (From Burnier MN, Blanco G. Intraocular lymphoma. In: Yanoff M, Duker JS, eds. *Ophthalmology*. London: Mosby; 1999.)

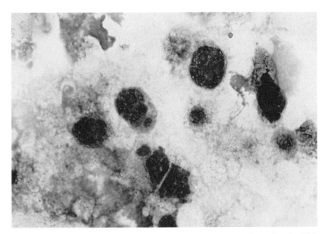

Figure 11.103 Large neoplastic cells in a vitreous specimen. (From Burnier MN, Blanco G. Intraocular lymphoma. In: Yanoff M, Duker JS, eds. *Ophthalmology.* London: Mosby; 1999.)

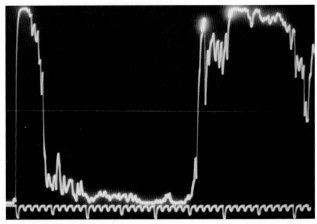

A

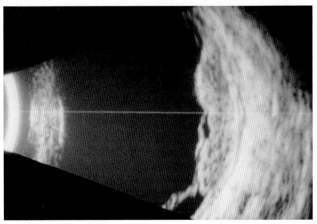

B

Figure 11.104 Ultrasonography of metastatic carcinoma to choroid. (A) A-scan. (B) B-scan. (From Augsburger JJ, Guthoff R. Metastatic cancer to the eye. In: Yanoff M, Duker JS, eds. *Ophthalmology.* London: Mosby; 1999.)

Pathology: mass of benign lymphocytes, plasma cells, and Dutcher bodies

Treatment: low-dose XRT

Intraocular Leukemia

(See Chapter 5, Pediatrics/Strabismus)

Metastases

Most common intraocular malignancy (including cases evident only at autopsy)

Most commonly breast carcinoma in women (most have previous mastectomy), lung carcinoma in men (often occult)

Bilateral and multifocal in 20%; 25% have no previous history of cancer

93% to choroid; 2% to CB; 5% to iris; can also metastasize to optic nerve; retina is rare

Symptoms: blurred vision, visual field defects, flashes and floaters

Findings: ≥1 golden-yellow, thin, dome-shaped choroidal tumors or creamy yellow amelanotic tumors with placoid or nummular configuration; may produce extensive exudative RD; usually metastasize to macula (richest blood supply)

DDx of amelanotic choroidal mass: amelanotic melanoma, old subretinal hemorrhage, choroidal osteoma, granuloma, posterior scleritis

FA: early hyperfluorescence with late staining of lesions

Ultrasound: A-scan shows medium to high internal reflectivity; B-scan is sonoreflective (Fig. 11.104)

Treatment: chemotherapy, external beam XRT, or combination

Carcinoma-Associated Retinopathy (CAR)

Rare, paraneoplastic syndrome (mainly small cell lung carcinoma, breast cancer, and gynecologic cancer; also reported in other types of lung cancer, colon cancer, mixed Müllerian tumor, squamous skin cancer, kidney cancer, pancreatic, lymphoma, basal cell tumor, and prostate cancer); loss of photoreceptors without inflammation

Findings: severe decreased vision, visual field defects, nyctalopia, APD if asymmetric (but usually bilateral) that clinically appears normal in early cases, but may later develop uveitis, chorioretinal atrophy, retinal pigment degeneration, narrowed retinal vessels, optic atrophy, and vitreous cells; antibodies to retinal proteins, including recoverin, carbonic anhydrase II, transducin B, α-enolase, Tubby-like Protein 1 (TULP1), PNR photoreceptor cell-specific nuclear receptor, heat shock cognate protein HSC 70, arrestin, and glyceraldehyde 3-phosphate dehydrogenase, have been described

ERG: extinguished

FAF: parafoveal ring of enhanced autofluorescence with normal autofluorescence within the ring and hypoautofluorescence outside the ring

Treatment: systematic immunosuppression (high-dose steroid with methylprednisolone and prednisone, cyclosporin, azathioprine, alemtuzumab), intravenous immunoglobulin, plasmapheresis, and combination of these treatments have been tried; find and treat primary cancer

Prognosis: poor

Bilateral Diffuse Uveal Melanocytic Proliferation Syndrome (BDUMPS)

Paraneoplastic syndrome (ovarian, uterine, lung cancer most common); unknown etiology

Diffuse uveal thickening from benign nevoid or spindle-shaped cells; also involves sclera

Findings: acute decreased vision, multiple orange or pigmented choroidal nodules, iris thickening and pigmentation, exudative RDs, cataracts (may appear similar to VKH syndrome)

ERG: markedly reduced

FA: orange spots hyperfluorescence

Treatment: none; treat underlying primary cancer

LASER TREATMENT

Thermal burn (photocoagulation) of inner retina will occur with argon blue–green or xenon arc

Retinal structures that absorb laser:
Melanin: primary site of light absorption and heat emission; absorbs argon blue–green, argon green, and krypton red
Hemoglobin: absorbs argon blue–green, argon green; does not absorb krypton (used to penetrate hemorrhage)
Xanthophyll: absorbs blue wavelengths

Wavelengths:
Blue–green (488 and 514 nm): blue light is absorbed by cornea and lens, heavily absorbed by nuclear sclerotic cataracts and absorbed by xanthophyll pigment
Green (514 nm): absorbed by blood, melanin; preferred for treatment of CNV in cases in which RPE has little pigment
Yellow (577 nm): may be better for treatment of microaneurysms; be careful of blood vessels
Red (647 nm): penetrates cataracts better; not absorbed by blood; causes less inner retinal damage; absorbed by melanin; poorly absorbed by xanthophyll (safer near fovea); passes through mild VH and nuclear sclerotic cataracts better than argon

Infrared (810 nm): has similar characteristics as red, but with deeper penetration
Xenon arc: polychromatic white light; not as precisely focused as monochromatic light; emits considerable amount of blue light, which can be harmful to retina and lens
Nd:YAG (532 nm): pattern-scanning laser (PASCAL); causes less damage

Panretinal Photocoagulation (PRP)

Indications: treatment of NV and peripheral nonperfusion, most commonly in retinal vascular diseases (PDR, CVO, BVO, sickle cell, radiation, and hypertensive retinopathy); DRCR Protocol S reported that intravitreal ranibizumab injections for PDR were associated with superior vision over the course of 2 years, reduced the incidence of center-involving DME (9% vs. 28%), less peripheral visual field loss, fewer vitrectomies (4% vs. 15%), and no major ocular or systemic safety differences except for one case of endophthalmitis versus prompt PRP

Parameters: 500-µm spot size, 0.1- 0.5-s duration, 1200-2000 spots; moderate white burn, 1 burn-width apart, 2 DD from fovea and 1 DD from optic nerve; 2 or more sessions. Best to avoid ciliary nerves at 3 and 9 o'clock

Adverse effects: decreased acuity (worsened by 1 line in 11%; worsened by 2 lines in 3%), constricted visual field, loss of color vision in 10%

Retreat at 4 weeks if NVD fails to regress or develops, new NVE develops, iris or angle NV develops, further regression of NV desired

Complications: choroidal effusion, exudative RD, permanent mydriasis and impairment of accommodation (ciliary nerve damage), VH, lens or corneal damage, foveal or optic nerve damage, CME, CNV, retinal vascular occlusion, angle closure

Focal Laser

Indication: treatment of macular edema (CSME, BVO, juxtafoveal telangiectasia [JXT])

Parameters: 50- to 100-µm spot size, 0.1-s duration; burns that slightly blanch the RPE, should be barely visible immediately after treatment, grid pattern 1 burn-width apart, in areas of diffuse edema; focal treatment of leaking vessels and microaneurysms; whiten/darken microaneurysms and/or cause mild depigmentation of RPE; do not treat over hemorrhage; identify leaking microaneurysms by FA; subthreshold micropulse laser with 810 nm divides laser pulse into short, repetitive pulses that persist for 0.1-0.5 s ("on" time is duration of each micropulse [typically 100–300 µs] and "off" time [1700–1900 µs] is interval between successive micropulses) has also been used successfully

Decreases risk of moderate visual loss over 3 years by 50% in CSME; DRCR Protocol I 5-year results suggest that focal laser treatment at initiation of intravitreal ranibizumab injections is no better than deferring laser treatment for ≥24 weeks in eyes with center-involving DME with vision impairment; thus, focal laser is second-line therapy for center-involving edema

Retreat at 3 months if CSME still present or treatable areas seen on repeat FA

REVIEW QUESTIONS *(Answers start on page 429)*

1. Which substance does *not* cause crystalline deposits in the retina?
   a. thioridazine
   b. canthaxanthin
   c. tamoxifen
   d. talc

2. The finding most predictive of VA in a patient with PDR is
   a. microaneurysms
   b. macular edema
   c. cotton-wool spots
   d. intraretinal microvascular abnormalities

3. The MPS showed the best prognosis for laser treatment of CNV in which disorder?
   a. AMD
   b. myopia
   c. idiopathic
   d. POHS

4. Which of the following is *not* a feature of Stickler syndrome?
   a. Pierre-Robin malformation
   b. AD inheritance
   c. retinoschisis
   d. marfanoid habitus

5. Sites at which the uvea is attached to the sclera include all of the following, *except*
   a. vortex veins
   b. optic nerve
   c. scleral spur
   d. ora serrata

6. A patient with multifocal choroiditis and retinal vasculitis is most likely to have
   a. VKH disease
   b. tuberculosis
   c. cat-scratch disease
   d. sarcoidosis

7. All three types of retinal hemorrhage (preretinal, intraretinal, and subretinal) may occur simultaneously in all of the following conditions, *except*
   a. macroaneurysm
   b. AMD
   c. diabetes
   d. capillary hemangioma

8. Characteristics of choroidal melanoma include all of the following, *except*
   a. choroidal excavation
   b. high internal reflectivity
   c. double circulation
   d. orbital shadowing

9. Which of the following statements regarding the ETDRS is *false*?
   a. the ETDRS concluded that PRP reduces the risk of severe visual loss in patients with high-risk PDR
   b. the ETDRS identified the risk factors for the development of PDR
   c. the ETDRS defined CSME
   d. the ETDRS showed that aspirin does not affect disease progression

10. The DRVS found that early vitrectomy for VH was helpful in which patients?
    a. patients with type 1 diabetes
    b. patients with type 2 diabetes
    c. patients with type 1 and 2 diabetes
    d. none of the above

11. Which of the following treatments is a CVOS recommendation?
    a. focal laser for macular edema of >3 to 6 months' duration with VA < 20/40
    b. PRP for >10 disc areas of nonperfusion
    c. PRP for iris or angle NV
    d. macular grid photocoagulation for CME

12. Which peripheral retinal lesion has the greatest risk of an RD?
    a. cystic retinal tuft
    b. asymptomatic retinal hole
    c. senile retinoschisis
    d. lattice degeneration

13. The intraocular structure most commonly affected by leukemia is the
    a. iris
    b. choroid
    c. retina
    d. optic nerve

14. Which is *not* a function of the RPE?
    a. conversion of vitamin A alcohol to aldehyde
    b. concentration of taurine
    c. inactivation of toxic products of oxygen metabolism
    d. phagocytosis of rod outer segments

15. Which of the following best describes the cellular reaction when light strikes a photoreceptor?
    a. increased cGMP, closed Na channel
    b. increased cGMP, open Na channel
    c. decreased cGMP, closed Na channel
    d. decreased cGMP, open Na channel

16. Prognostic factors for choroidal melanoma include all of the following, *except*
    a. size
    b. location
    c. cell type
    d. pigmentation

17. Which of the following does *not* involve the outer plexiform layer of the retina?
    a. degenerative retinoschisis
    b. cystoid macular edema
    c. Henle fiber layer
    d. diabetic microaneurysm

18. The best test for distinguishing between a subretinal hemorrhage and a choroidal melanoma is
    a. FA
    b. B-scan
    c. A-scan
    d. ERG
19. Which of the following is the *least* radiosensitive lesion?
    a. metastases
    b. lymphoma
    c. RB
    d. melanoma
20. Which of the following is the *least* common complication of PRP?
    a. iritis
    b. increased IOP
    c. RD
    d. narrow angle
21. A cluster of pigmented lesions is seen in the peripheral retina of a patient's left eye during routine ophthalmoscopy. Which of the following tests would be most helpful in detecting an associated hereditary disorder?
    a. electrocardiogram
    b. colonoscopy
    c. brain MRI
    d. chest CT scan
22. Which of the following is *not* associated with a typical angiographic appearance of CME?
    a. nicotinic acid
    b. epinephrine
    c. Irvine-Gass syndrome
    d. pars planitis
23. The *least* likely finding in a patient with a chronic detachment of the inferotemporal retina is
    a. retinal thinning
    b. macrocysts
    c. fixed folds
    d. RPE atrophy
24. In a patient with AMD, which type of drusen is most associated with the development of CNV?
    a. soft
    b. basal laminar
    c. hard
    d. calcific
25. The ERG oscillatory potential is caused by which cell type?
    a. Müller
    b. amacrine
    c. bipolar
    d. RPE
26. Chloroquine retinopathy
    a. is reversible with discontinuation of the medication
    b. can be associated with other CNS reactions
    c. is best diagnosed with red-free photographs
    d. is more likely with higher cumulative doses rather than higher daily doses
27. Proven systemic control for diabetic retinopathy includes
    a. lowering serum cholesterol
    b. aspirin use
    c. ACE inhibitors
    d. blood pressure control
28. Retinal artery macroaneursysms
    a. are usually located in the macula
    b. produce multilayered hemorrhages
    c. are best seen on ICG angiography
    d. should be treated with focal laser photocoagulation to prevent bleeding
29. The Branch Vein Occlusion Study reported that
    a. aspirin prevented recurrent episodes
    b. focal laser photocoagulation decreased visual loss
    c. panretinal photocoagulation should be applied in ischemic patients
    d. photocoagulation should be delayed in the presence of extensive macular ischemia
30. True statements about ocular photodynamic therapy include all of the following, *except*
    a. requires light precautions for 48 hours after treatment
    b. is indicated for occult with no classic CNV lesions
    c. often requires retreatment every 6 weeks
    d. stabilizes but rarely improves vision
31. Cystoid macular edema
    a. does not leak fluorescein when associated with nicotinic acid
    b. responds to nonsteroidal anti-inflammatory drops
    c. is associated with β-blockers
    d. has a petalloid appearance on FA
32. PDR is most likely to develop if which one of the following findings is present on fundus exam?
    a. exudates
    b. hemorrhages
    c. microaneurysms
    d. venous beading
33. Which of the following is the biggest risk factor for AMD?
    a. smoking
    b. elevated serum cholesterol level
    c. dark iris color
    d. myopia
34. The most important visual prognostic factor for a rhegmatogenous RD is
    a. the size of the break
    b. the extent of the detachment
    c. macular involvement
    d. the type of surgery
35. The earliest sign of a macular hole is
    a. RPE atrophy in the fovea
    b. vitreous detachment at the fovea
    c. yellow spot in the fovea
    d. partial-thickness eccentric hole in the fovea
36. Focal laser treatment is indicated for diabetic macular edema when there is
    a. hard exudates with retinal thickening 1000 μm from the center of the fovea
    b. NVE >1/3 disc area in size
    c. ischemia within 250 μm of the center of the fovea
    d. retinal edema within 500 μm of the center of the fovea
37. Reduced IOP would be most unexpected in a patient with
    a. choroidal effusion
    b. choroidal hemorrhage
    c. serous RD
    d. rhegmatogenous RD

38. Which of the following is the correct indication for treating macular edema from a BRVO?
    a. ≥5 DD of capillary nonperfusion
    b. thickening within 500 μm of the fovea
    c. exudates in the fovea
    d. vision <20/40 for >3 months

39. Which test is best for distinguishing a choroidal melanoma from a choroidal hemangioma?
    a. transillumination
    b. red-free photo
    c. ultrasound
    d. CT scan

40. The etiology of vitreous hemorrhage in Terson syndrome is
    a. intracranial hypertension
    b. hypercoagulability
    c. embolus
    d. neovascularization

41. Which is the most common site of metastasis for a choroidal melanoma?
    a. brain
    b. liver
    c. lungs
    d. skin

42. Which of the following is *least* characteristic of Eales disease?
    a. vascular sheathing
    b. vitreous hemorrhage
    c. neovascularization
    d. macular edema

43. Crystalline retinopathy is *not* associated with
    a. tamoxifen
    b. methoxyflurane
    c. thioridazine
    d. canthaxanthin

44. Combined hamartoma of the retina and RPE has been associated with all of the following, *except*
    a. neurofibromatosis
    b. tuberous sclerosis
    c. Gorlin syndrome
    d. Gardner syndrome

45. Which of the following statements regarding uveal metastases is *false*?
    a. the most common primary sites are the breast and lung
    b. the most common ocular location is the anterior choroid
    c. they often have an exudative RD
    d. FA usually demonstrates early hyperfluorescence

46. The most worrisome sign in a patient with an acute PVD is
    a. pigment in the vitreous
    b. multiple vitreous floaters
    c. lattice degeneration
    d. Weiss ring

47. The most likely diagnosis in a patient with choroidal neovascular membrane in the macula, peripapillary atrophy, and punched-out chorioretinal scars is
    a. toxocariasis
    b. toxoplasmosis
    c. POHS
    d. syphilis

48. Which is the most common complication of an epiretinal membrane?
    a. macular hole
    b. CME
    c. RD
    d. choroidal neovascular membrane

49. Which is the most helpful test to obtain in a patient with a branch retinal artery occlusion?
    a. electrocardiogram
    b. ERG
    c. OCT
    d. carotid ultrasound

50. Angioid streaks are associated with all of the following systemic conditions, *except*
    a. Ehlers-Danlos syndrome
    b. Paget disease
    c. syphilis
    d. pseudoxanthoma elasticum

51. An elderly hypertensive man with a sudden change in vision is found to have hemorrhages and cotton-wool spots in the superior temporal retina and a reduced foveal reflex. The most appropriate initial management is to obtain a(n)
    a. B-scan ultrasound
    b. FA
    c. ESR
    d. carotid Doppler

52. Which of the following is *not* a type of visual pigment?
    a. L
    b. M
    c. P
    d. S

Please visit the eBook for an interactive version of the review questions. See front cover for activation details.

SUGGESTED READINGS

Agarwal, A. (2012). *Gass' atlas of macular diseases* (5th ed.). Philadelphia: Saunders.

Basic and Clinical Sciences Course. (2021). *Section 12: Retina and vitreous*. San Francisco: American Academy of Ophthalmology.

Byrne, S. F., & Green, R. L. (1992). *Ultrasound of the eye and orbit* (2nd ed.). St Louis: Mosby.

Freund, K. B., Sarraf, D., & Mieler, W. F. (2016). *The retinal atlas* (2nd ed.). Philadelphia: Saunders.

Guyer, D. R., Yannuzzi, L. A., Chang, A., et al. (1999). *Retina-vitreous-macula*. Philadelphia: WB Saunders.

Schachat, A. P., Wilkinson, C. P., Hinton, D. R., Sadda, S. R., & Wiedemann, P. (2017). *Ryan's retina* (6th ed.). Philadelphia: Elsevier.

Schuman, J. S., Puliafito, C. A., Fujimoto, J. G., & Duker, J. S. (2012). *Optical coherence tomography of ocular diseases* (3rd ed). Thorofare, NJ: Slack.

Shields, J. A., & Shields, C. L. (2015). *Intraocular tumors: An atlas and textbook* (3rd ed.). Philadelphia: Lippincott Williams & Wilkins.

Wilkinson, C. P., & Rice, T. A. (1997). *Michels's retinal detachment* (2nd ed.). St Louis: Mosby.

Answers to Questions

CHAPTER 1 OPTICS

1. A Prince rule is helpful in determining all of the following, *except*
   d. accommodative convergence

2. A myope who pushes his spectacles closer to his face and tilts them is
   d. increasing effectivity, increasing cylinder

3. The Prentice position refers to
   a. glass prism perpendicular to visual axis

4. The purpose of Q-switching a laser is to
   b. decrease energy, increase power

5. A 50-year-old woman with aphakic glasses wants a new pair of spectacles to use when applying makeup. How much power should be added to her distance correction so that she can focus while sitting 50 cm in front of her mirror?
   c. + 1.00 D—with a plane mirror, the image is located as far behind the mirror as the object is in front of the mirror; therefore, the distance between her eye and the image of her eye is 100 cm = 1 m, and this requires +1.00 D of extra magnification

6. How far from a plano mirror must a 6-ft-tall man stand to see his whole body?
   b. 3 feet—to view one's entire body, a plane mirror need be only 1/2 one's height

7. A 33-year-old woman with a refraction of −9.00 + 3.00 × 90 OD at vertex distance 10 mm and keratometry readings of 46.00@90/43.00@180 is fit for a rigid gas-permeable (RGP) contact lens 1 D steeper than flattest *K*. What power lens is required?
   c. −7.00 D step 1: change refraction to minus cylinder form (because the tear lake negates the minus cylinder) and use this sphere (−6.00); step 2: adjust to zero vertex distance (−6 + 0.01[−6]² = −5.64); step 3: adjust for tear lens (SAM-FAP rule) (add −1.00 = −6.64)

8. What is the size of a 20/60 letter on a standard 20-ft Snellen chart (tangent of 1 minute of arc = 0.0003)?
   d. 27 mm—20/60 letter subtends 5 minutes at 60 ft (18 m); therefore, size of letter = 18 (tan 5′) = 18 (0.0015) = 0.027 m or 27 mm

9. A Galilean telescope with a +5 D objective and a −20 D eyepiece produces an image with what magnification and direction?
   a. 4 ×, erect—magnification = −(−20)/5 = + 4, meaning 4 × magnification and erect image

10. An object is placed 33 cm in front of an eye. The image formed by reflection from the front surface of the cornea (radius of curvature equals 8 mm) is located
    b. 4 mm behind cornea—reflecting power of the cornea is −2/0.008 = −250 D; thus, the focal point is 1/−250 = −4 mm, or 4 mm behind the cornea

11. A convex mirror produces what type of image?
    d. virtual, erect, minified—remember mnemonic VErMin

12. In general, the most bothersome problem associated with bifocals is
    a. image jump—therefore, choose bifocal segment type to minimize jump; flat-top segments minimize image jump because the optical center is near the top; this also reduces image displacement in myopes

13. A refraction with a stenopeic slit gives the following measurements: +1.00 at 90° and −2.00 at 180°. The corresponding spectacle prescription is
    c. −2.00 + 3.00 × 180—this is the correct spherocylindrical notation for a power cross diagram with +1.00 along the 90° meridian and −2.00 along the 180° meridian

14. A point source of light is placed 1/3 of a meter to the left of a +7 D lens. Where will its image come to focus?
    a. 25 cm to the right of the lens—the light has vergence of −3 D and encounters a +7 D lens; thus, the exiting light has vergence of +4 D, and the image will come to focus 25 cm to the right of the lens

15. What is the equivalent sphere of the following cross cylinder: − 3.00 × 180 combined with +0.50 × 90?
    b. −1.25—the cross cylinder has a spherocylindrical notation of −3.00 + 3.50 × 90, so the spherical equivalent is −3.00 + (3.50/2) = − 1.25

16. What is the size of a letter on a standard 20-ft Snellen chart if it forms an image of 0.5 mm on a patient's retina?
    d. 18 cm—using the reduced schematic eye and similar triangles, 0.5/17 mm = object size/6 m; solving for object size yields 18 cm

17. The image of a distant object is largest in which patient?
    b. hyperope with spectacles

18. What type of image is produced if an object is placed in front of a convex lens within its focal length?
    b. erect and virtual

19. What is the correct glasses prescription if retinoscopy performed at 50 cm shows neutralization with a plano lens?
    a. −2.00—remember to subtract for working distance (1/0.5 m = 2 D); thus, a plano lens minus 2 D yields a −2.00 D glasses prescription

20. An anisometropic patient experiences difficulty while reading with bifocals. Which of the following is *not* helpful for reducing the induced phoria?
    c. progressive lenses—this problem is due to the prismatic effect of the underlying lens and will occur with all bifocal styles, including progressive lenses

21. A Geneva lens clock is used to measure what?
    d. base curve

22. What is the induced prism when a 67-year-old woman reads 10 mm below the upper segment optical center of her bifocals, which measure +2.50 + 1.00 × 90 OD and −1.50 + 1.50 × 180 OS add +2.50 OU?
    c. 2.5 Δ—using Prentice's rule, the induced prism is (+2.50 × 1) OD and ([−1.50 + 1.50] × 1) OS (cylinder power acts in the vertical meridian, so it must be used in the calculation); the total is +2.5 Δ BU OD; the effect is due to the underlying lens; the power of the bifocal segment can be ignored because it is the same for both lenses (5 Δ BU OD and 2.5 Δ BU OS = 2.5 Δ BU OD)

23. The optimal size of a pinhole for measuring pinhole visual acuity is approximately
    c. 1.25 mm—limited by diffraction if smaller than 1.2 mm

24. A person looking at an object 5 m away through a 10 Δ prism placed base-in over the right eye would see the image displaced
    b. 50 cm to the right—a 10 Δ prism displaces light 10 cm/1 m or 50 cm at 5 m, and the image is displaced to the apex

25. Calculate the soft CL power for a 40-year-old hyperope who wears +14.00 D glasses at a vertex distance of 11 mm.
    b. +16.00 D—using the simplified formula, new power = $14 + 0.011\,(14)^2 = 16.156$

26. After cataract surgery, a patient's refraction is −0.75 + 1.75 × 10. In what meridian should a suture be cut to reduce the astigmatism?
    d. 10°—the steep meridian corresponds to the axis of the plus cylinder (plus cylinder acts to steepen the flat meridian, which is 90° away from the cylinder axis)

27. What is the appropriate correction in the intraocular lens (IOL) power if the A constant for the lens to be implanted is changed from 117 to 118?
    b. increase IOL power by 1.0 D—the change in A constant is equivalent to the change in IOL power

28. An IOL labeled with a power of +20 D has a refractive index of 1.5. If this lens were removed from the package and measured with a lensometer, what power would be found?
    d. +59 D—using the formula for calculating the power of a thin lens immersed in fluid $(P_{air}/P_{aqueous}) = (n_{iol} - n_{air})/(n_{iol} - n_{aqueous})$, $P_{air} = 20\,([1.5 - 1.0]/[1.5 - 1.33]) = +58.8\ D$

29. The spherical equivalent of a 0.50 D cross cylinder is
    a. plano—by definition, all cross cylinders have a spherical equivalent of zero; this is evident by writing the cross cylinder in spherocylindrical notation. **Example:** +0.50 − 1.00 × 90

30. To minimize image displacement in a hyperope, the best type of bifocal segment style is
    c. round top—to minimize image displacement, the prismatic effects of the bifocal segment and the distance lens should be in opposite directions; a round top acts like a base-down prism, and the underlying hyperopic lens acts like a base-up prism

31. The logMAR equivalent to 20/40 Snellen acuity is
    b. 0.3

32. A patient who is pseudophakic in one eye and phakic in the other eye will have what amount of aniseikonia?
    b. 2.5%

33. A patient with 20/80 vision is seen for a low-vision evaluation. What add power should be prescribed so that the patient does not have to use accommodation to read the newspaper?
    b. +4—the add power is calculated from the inverse of the distance Snellen acuity: 80/20 = 4

34. The spherical equivalent of a −2.00 + 1.50 × 90 lens is
    c. −1.25—the spherical equivalent is obtained by adding half the cylinder power to the sphere: −2.00 + 0.75 = −1.25

35. After extracapsular cataract extraction, a patient is found to have 2 D of with-the-rule astigmatism and a tight suture across the wound at 12 o'clock. Corneal topography is obtained, and the placido disc image shows an oval pattern with the mires closest together at
    a. 12 o'clock with the short axis at 90°—*WTR astigmatism* refers to steep meridian (short axis) at 90° (12 o'clock), which corresponds to the tight suture. The pattern of projected placido rings is oval in astigmatism, with the lines closest together in the steepest meridian (short axis)

36. A 57-year-old woman has a 0.25 mm macular hole in her left eye. The size of the corresponding scotoma on a tangent screen at 1 m is approximately
    b. 1.5 cm—using similar triangles and the model eye with a nodal point of 17 mm, the resulting equation is: $0.25/17 = x/1000$

37. During retinoscopy, when neutralization is reached, the light reflex is
    d. widest and fastest—at neutralization, the retinoscopic reflex is fastest, widest, and brightest

38. A patient undergoing fogged refraction with an astigmatic dial sees the 9 to 3 o'clock line clearer than all the others. At what axis should this patient's minus cylinder correcting lens be placed?
    c. 90°—with an astigmatic dial, the axis of the minus cylinder correcting lens is found by multiplying the lower number of the clearest line by 30 (i.e., for the 9 to 3 o'clock line: 3 × 30 = 90)

39. Myopia is associated with all of the following conditions, *except*
    a. nanophthalmos—nanophthalmos is associated with hyperopia.

40. What is the ratio of the magnification from a direct ophthalmoscope to the magnification from an indirect ophthalmoscope with a 20 D lens at a distance of 25 cm if the patient and examiner are both emmetropic?
    c. 5:1—the magnification for the direct is 60/4 = 15 and the magnification for the indirect is 60/20 = 3, so the ratio of the magnifications is 15:3 = 5:1

41. A patient with anisometropia wears glasses with a prescription of +5.00 OD and +1.25 OS. Which of the following actions will *not* reduce the amount of aniseikonia?
    b. decrease center thickness of left lens—this will have the opposite effect (increase the anisometropia)

42. The principal measurement determined by a Prince rule and +3 D lens in front of the patient's eye is the
    b. amplitude of accommodation—the Prince rule is primarily designed to measure the amplitude of accommodation

43. The 10 × eyepiece of the slit-lamp biomicroscope is essentially a simple magnifier. Using the standard reference distance of 25 cm, what is the dioptric power of the 10 × eyepiece?
    d. +40 D—magnification = P/4, so 10 = P/4 and P = 40

44. When refracting an astigmatic patient with a Lancaster dial, the examiner should place the
    d. entire conoid of Sturm in front of the retina—the patient must be fogged so that the entire conoid of Sturm is in front of the retina

45. To increase the magnification of the image during indirect ophthalmoscopy, the examiner should
    a. move closer to the condensing lens—this causes the image to subtend a larger angle on the examiner's retina thereby increasing the magnification

46. A patient with which of the following refractive errors is most likely to develop amblyopia?
    c. +5.00 OD, +5.00 OS

47. A 23-year-old man reports blurry vision at near and wears +1.25 D reading glasses to see clearly. Which of the following is most likely to be found on examination?
    a. latent hyperopia—a cycloplegic refraction is necessary to uncover the full amount of hyperopia, and a glasses prescription should be determined from a subsequent manifest refraction pushing plus and using trial frames to allow the patient to adapt

48. In 1 year, a diabetic 60-year-old woman has a change in refraction from −5.00 to −6.50 OU, which improves her vision to 20/20 OU. What is the most likely cause of her refractive change?
    c. increasing nuclear sclerosis—nuclear sclerosis of the crystalline lens is the most common cause of a myopic shift in adults

49. The most common cause of monocular diplopia is
    a. uncorrected astigmatism

50. A patient with a prescription of −5.50 sphere OD and −1.00 sphere OS is 20/20 in each eye but glasses cause headache and double vision. The most likely reason is
    d. aniseikonia—anisometropia of >3D results in an image size discrepancy (aniseikonia) that becomes symptomatic

51. A hyperopic refraction is most likely caused by
    c. a flat cornea and a short axial length

52. How much accommodation is needed for a patient with a distance correction of +1.50 to read without correction at 40 cm?
    c. +4.00—the amount of accommodation required = (100 cm/40 cm) + 1.50 = 2.50 + 1.50 = 4.00

53. The limbal relaxing incision for a patient with a refraction of + 0.75 − 1.50 × 180 and no lenticular astigmatism should be placed at
    b. 90°—LRI for astigmatism correction is centered on the steep meridian

54. The denominator in the Snellen visual acuity notation 20/60 represents
    d. the distance at which the letter subtends the standard visual angle

55. A 26-year-old-woman with a history of myopic LASIK complains of blurriness OD. Her uncorrected visual acuity is 20/20, but corneal topography shows a decentered ablation. Which aberration is most likely to be found on wavefront analysis?
    c. 3rd order—coma is most likely to be the etiology of her blurred vision

56. If a Snellen chart is not present, then which of the following tests is best for evaluating visual acuity?
    a. contrast sensitivity

57. A cycloplegic refraction would be most helpful for a
    a. 10-year-old who has headaches—cycloplegia should be used to prevent accommodation and reveal the true refractive error of the eyes

58. The most likely cause of a refractive surprise after uncomplicated cataract surgery is
    d. wrong keratometry readings—this is the correct choice for the options given, but wrong axial length is usually the most common cause

59. Decreased color discrimination is most likely to be caused by which type of cataract?
    a. nuclear sclerotic

60. A 3-piece acrylic IOL intended for the capsular bag is placed in the sulcus without optic capture through the capsulotomy. This patient is most likely to experience what type of refractive error?
    d. myopia—the power of an IOL placed in the sulcus instead of the capsular bag should be reduced by 1 D to achieve the same refractive outcome

61. Six weeks following manual extracapsular cataract surgery with a superior limbal incision, the patient's refraction is found to be −2.00 + 4.00 × 95. The best initial treatment for this residual refractive error is
    a. suture removal—a tight suture is the most likely cause of with-the-rule astigmatism after manual extracapsular cataract surgery with a superior incision

62. Which test is most useful for following a patient with Fuchs dystrophy?
    b. corneal pachymetry—to measure changes in corneal thickness, which occurs in Fuchs dystrophy because of progressive corneal edema

63. A 28-year-old man with anisometropia and amblyopia has a best-corrected visual acuity of 20/15 OD and 20/40 OS. His refraction is +0.25+0.25 × 75 OD and +3.75 + 0.25 × 90 OS. Which of the following is the best treatment option?
    b. +3.75 contact lens in the left eye

64. A patient with cataracts and best corrected visual acuity of 20/50 complains that glasses do not work well enough. Which is the best nonsurgical option to help this patient?
    c. increase add power

65. Which higher-order aberration has the least effect on visual quality?
    d. trefoil

CHAPTER 2 PHARMACOLOGY

1. Which antibiotic results in the highest intravitreal concentration when administered orally?
    a. ciprofloxacin

2. Which anesthetic agent would most interfere with an intraocular gas bubble?
    d. nitrous oxide

3. Which of the following is *not* an adverse effect of CAIs?
    c. iris cysts

4. Which β-blocker has the *least* effect on β_2 receptors?
    b. betaxolol—this is a cardioselective β_1-blocker

5. Which drug has the *least* effect on uveoscleral outflow?
    d. dorzolamide—this is a CAI that decreases aqueous production; Xalatan and atropine increase uveoscleral outflow, and pilocarpine decreases uveoscleral outflow.

6. Which enzyme is inhibited by steroids?
    b. phospholipase A_2

7. Which of the following steroid formulations has the best corneal penetrability?
    a. prednisolone acetate—order of corneal penetrability is acetate > alcohol > phosphate

8. Adverse effects of foscarnet include all of the following, *except*
    b. infertility

9. Which glaucoma medication is *not* effective when the IOP is >60 mm Hg?
    c. pilocarpine—because of iris ischemia, which occurs at IOP > 40 mm Hg

10. Which medicine is *not* associated with OCP-like conjunctival shrinkage?
    d. timolol

11. Which β-blocker is β_1-selective?
    c. betaxolol

12. The most appropriate treatment for neurosyphilis is
    a. penicillin G—IV penicillin is used to treat neurosyphilis

13. Which is the correct mechanism of action of botulinum toxin?
    a. it prevents the release of acetylcholine

14. Fluoroquinolones are *least* effective against
    c. anaerobic cocci

15. Hydroxychloroquine toxicity depends most on
    b. daily dose—total daily dose is the most important risk factor for developing retinal toxicity

16. Calculate the amount of cocaine in 2 mL of a 4% solution.
    d. 80 mg—a 1% solution indicates 1 g/100 mL; therefore, a 4% solution is 4000 mg/100 mL = 40 mg/mL

17. NSAIDs block the formation of all of the following substances, *except*
    b. leukotrienes—NSAIDs block the conversion of arachidonic acid by cyclooxygenase into endoperoxides (thus inhibiting the formation of prostaglandins, thromboxane, and prostacyclin); leukotrienes are formed from arachidonic acid by lipoxygenase; steroids block the formation of arachidonic acid (and therefore, all subsequent end products) by inhibiting phospholipase A_2

18. Systemic effects of steroids may include all of the following, *except*
    d. renal tubular acidosis

19. Which drug does *not* produce decreased tear production?
    a. pilocarpine

20. Natamycin is a
    c. polyene

21. Which glaucoma medicine does *not* decrease aqueous production?
    b. pilocarpine—miotics increase aqueous outflow

22. β-blockers may cause all of the following, *except*
    a. constipation

23. Idoxuridine may cause all of the following, *except*
    c. corneal hypesthesia

24. Which of the following antifungal agents has the broadest spectrum against yeast-like fungi?
    d. amphotericin

25. All of the following medications are combination antihistamine and mast cell stabilizers, *except*
    a. Alomide—is only a mast cell stabilizer

26. The antidote for atropine toxicity is
    b. physostigmine

27. Which of the following agents is contraindicated for ruptured globe repair?
    d. succinylcholine—this nicotinic receptor antagonist causes muscle contraction and is therefore contraindicated in ruptured globe repair because EOM contraction could result in extrusion of intraocular contents

28. The duration of action of one drop of proparacaine is
    b. 20 minutes—the duration of proparacaine is 10-30 minutes

29. Which of the following medications is *not* commercially available as a topical formulation?
    d. vancomycin—must be compounded; the others are available as Zirgan, AzaSite, and Restasis or Cequa, respectively

30. All of the following are complications of CAIs, *except*
    c. metabolic alkalosis—CAIs cause metabolic acidosis

31. Topiramate is associated with
    d. angle-closure glaucoma without pupillary block

32. A patient with ocular hypertension and an allergy to sulfonamides should *not* be treated with
    b. dorzolamide— CAIs are sulfa drugs and are contraindicated in patients with a sulfa allergy

33. Infectious keratitis caused by *Candida albicans* is best treated with topical
    a. amphotericin B

34. Which of the following oral agents should be used to treat a patient with ocular cicatricial pemphigoid?
    c. cyclophosphamide—this cytotoxic agent is used to treat patients with OCP

35. The glaucoma medication contraindicated in infants is
    b. brimonidine—selective α-agonists can cause death in infants

36. Which systemic antibiotic is used to treat *Chlamydia* during pregnancy?
    d. erythromycin—erythromycins are the preferred antibiotic for chlamydia infection and are safe during pregnancy

37. The local anesthetic with the longest duration of action is
    c. bupivacaine

38. A 33-year-old man has had follicular conjunctivitis with a watery discharge for 5 weeks. Elementary bodies are present on a conjunctival smear; therefore, the most appropriate treatment is
    a. oral azithromycin—the patient has chlamydial conjunctivitis and requires oral antibiotics

39. The most appropriate treatment for *Fusarium* keratitis is topical
    b. pimaricin—this antifungal, also known as *natamycin*, is used to treat fungal keratitis

40. All of the following are associated with vitamin A toxicity, *except*
    d. band keratopathy

41. Which of the following is a serious adverse effect of a long-acting cycloplegic agent?
    c. urinary retention—cycloplegic agents are anticholinergic drugs (muscarinic antagonists), and long-acting ones can have serious systemic effects, including urinary retention, particularly in elderly patients

42. An oral NSAID should *not* be used in a patient with
    a. renal insufficiency—NSAIDs can cause acute renal failure in healthy individuals and should not be administered to patients with chronic kidney disease

43. Ocular rosacea is best treated with which of the following oral medications?
    c. doxycycline

44. A patient taking which of the following medications is at increased risk for complications at the time of cataract surgery?
    c. α₁-adrenergic antagonist—these oral medications (i.e., tamsulosin [Flomax]) are associated with intraoperative floppy iris syndrome (IFIS) and cataract surgery complications

45. A patient suddenly stops breathing after administration of a peribulbar injection of anesthetic. The most likely reason is
    d. injection into the optic nerve sheath—anesthetic injected into the optic nerve sheath may result in central anesthesia with respiratory arrest

46. Which of the following anesthetic agents is most likely to increase IOP?
    d. ketamine—ketamine and succinylcholine raise IOP, chloral hydrate has no effect, and halothane and thiopental decrease IOP

47. Which of the following medications is most likely to cause hallucinations?
    b. cyclopentolate

48. A 10-year-old African American boy with a hyphema develops increased intraocular pressure. Which of the following drugs should be avoided?
    a. carbonic anhydrase inhibitors—these agents can lower the pH in the anterior chamber increasing the risk of sickling red blood cells in patients with sickle cell disease

49. General anesthesia for cataract surgery is most likely the best option in a patient with
    c. dementia—because the patient is least likely to be able to cooperate and hold still

50. All of the following medications are causes of cornea verticillata, *except*
    d. tobramycin—cornea verticillata occurs in Fabry disease and is associated with various drugs including systemic amiodarone, chloroquine, hydroxychloroquine, indomethacin, ibuprofen, naproxen, chlorpromazine, suramin, clofazimine, tamoxifen, and topical netarsudil

51. Which eye drop preservative is least toxic?
    c. sodium perborate—this oxidant preservative has reduced toxicity, it is converted to inert substances with light exposure

52. Bladder cancer is most commonly associated with which drug?
    b. cyclophosphamide

53. Regarding topical eye medications, the volume of 1 drop is approximately
    b. 50 μL

54. Which of the following statements regarding Miostat and Miochol is true?
    c. Miochol is faster acting—intracameral acetylcholine (Miochol) is faster acting than carbachol (Miostat), but Miostat is more effective, has a longer duration of action, and reduces IOP

55. Methazolamide can be used to treat all of the following except
    a. fungal keratitis—methazolamide is an oral carbonic anhydrase inhibitor, not an antifungal agent

411

CHAPTER 3 EMBRYOLOGY/PATHOLOGY

1. Which stain is the most helpful in the diagnosis of sebaceous gland carcinoma?
   c. oil-red-O–which stains lipid

2. Pagetoid spread is most commonly associated with
   c. sebaceous gland carcinoma—this is invasion of intact epithelium by nests of cells and is characteristic of sebaceous gland carcinoma; pagetoid spread can also occur in the rare superficial spreading form of melanoma that occurs on unexposed skin areas (back, legs)

3. A melanoma occurring in which of the following locations has the best prognosis?
   a. iris—often can be completely excised

4. Calcification in retinoblastoma is caused by
   a. RPE metaplasia

5. The type of organism that causes Lyme disease is a
   b. spirochete

6. Characteristics of ghost cells include all of the following, *except*
   d. biconcave

7. A gland of Moll is best categorized as
   b. apocrine

8. Which of the following is *not* a gram-positive rod?
   c. *Serratia*—this bacterium is gram-negative

9. Trantas dots are composed of what cell type?
   c. eosinophil

10. Types of collagen that can be found in the cornea include all of the following, *except*
    b. II—is found in vitreous; type I is found in normal corneal stroma, III in stromal wound healing, and IV in basement membranes

11. Lens nuclei are retained in all of the following conditions, *except*
    d. Alport syndrome

12. VKH syndrome is best described by which type of hypersensitivity reaction?
    d. IV

13. Lacy vacuolization of the iris pigment epithelium occurs in which disease?
    b. diabetes—lacy vacuolization is a pathologic finding of glycogen-filled cysts in the iris pigment epithelium

14. Antoni A and B cells occur in which tumor?
    a. neurilemmoma (schwannoma)

15. Which tumor is classically described as having a "Swiss cheese" appearance?
    b. adenoid cystic carcinoma

16. Which iris nodule is correctly paired with its pathology?
    b. Lisch nodule, neural crest hamartoma—this is correct; JXG nodules are composed of histiocytes and Touton giant cells, Koeppe nodules are collections of inflammatory cells, and Brushfield spots are stromal hyperplasia

17. Which of the following statements is true concerning immunoglobulin?
    a. IgG crosses the placenta

18. A retinal detachment caused by fixation artifact can be differentiated from a true retinal detachment by all of the following, *except*
    a. a fold at the ora serrata—is a fixation artifact found in newborn eyes called Lange's fold; it is *not* related to an artifactual or true retinal detachment.

19. Which of the following epithelial changes in the eyelid refers to thickening of the squamous cell layer?
    b. acanthosis

20. Intraocular hemorrhage may cause all of the following sequelae, *except*
    c. asteroid hyalosis—is calcium soaps suspended in the vitreous and is unrelated to hemorrhage

21. Intraocular calcification may occur in all of the following, *except*
    b. medulloepithelioma—this tumor may contain cartilage

22. The histopathology of which tumor is classically described as a storiform pattern of tumor cells?
    d. fibrous histiocytoma

23. Which of the following findings is a histologic fixation artifact?
    a. Lange's fold—is a fold at the ora serrata that is a fixation artifact in newborn eyes

24. The corneal stroma is composed of
    b. neural crest cells

25. *Neisseria* is best cultured with which media?
    d. chocolate agar

26. Which of the following stains is used to detect amyloid?
    c. crystal violet—stains used to detect amyloid are Congo red, crystal violet, and thioflavin T

27. HLA-B7 is associated with
    b. presumed ocular histoplasmosis syndrome—POHS is associated with HLA-B7; the other associations are Behçet disease with B51, iridocyclitis with B27, and sympathetic ophthalmia with DR4

28. Which of the following conjunctival lesions should be sent to the pathology lab as a fresh unfixed tissue specimen?
    a. lymphoma—fresh tissue is required for immunohistochemical staining

29. Subepithelial infiltrates in the cornea from epidemic keratoconjunctivitis are thought to be
    c. macrophages containing adenoviral particles

30. Which is the correct order of solutions for performing a Gram stain?
    d. crystal violet stain, iodine solution, ethanol, safranin

31. The iris sphincter is derived from what embryologic tissue?
    c. neural ectoderm

32. Blepharitis is most commonly associated with
    b. *Staphylococcus aureus*

33. Which type of radiation causes lens capsule scrolling?
    a. infrared—this nonionizing radiation causes true exfoliation of the crystalline lens capsule, also known as *glassblowers cataract*

34. Which of the following measures is most likely to reduce the risk of postoperative endophthalmitis following cataract surgery?
    a. preoperative povidone-iodine drops—when applied to the conjunctiva as part of the preoperative prep, povidone-iodine has been documented to reduce the rate of postop endophthalmitis

35. The most common causative organism of canaliculitis is
    c. *Actinomyces israelii*

36. The crystalline lens is formed from which embryologic tissue?
    b. ectoderm

37. Which of the following bacteria can penetrate an intact corneal epithelium?
    c. *Neisseria gonorrhoeae*—the others are *Corynebacterium diphtheriae*, *Shigella*, *Haemophilus aegyptus*, and *Listeria monocytogenes*

38. Which immunoglobulin is *not* found in the tear film?
    b. IgD

39. Where is the major arterial circle of the iris located?
    d. ciliary body

40. The zonules are formed from
    c. tertiary vitreous

CHAPTER 4 NEURO-OPHTHALMOLOGY

1. The VF defect most characteristic of optic neuritis is
   b. central—all of these may occur in optic neuritis, but a central scotoma is most characteristic

2. Which cranial nerve is most prone to injury in the cavernous sinus?
   d. 6—travels in middle of sinus and is not protected by lateral wall as are CN 3, 4, and 5

3. Which of the following agents is *least* toxic to the ON?
   b. dapsone

4. See-saw nystagmus is produced by a lesion located in which area?
   c. suprasellar—also associated with bitemporal hemianopia; chiasmal gliomas can cause spasmus nutans–like eye movements in children; lesions in the posterior fossa cause dissociated nystagmus, and those in the cervicomedullary junction cause downbeat nystagmus

5. What is the location of a lesion that causes an ipsilateral Horner syndrome and a contralateral CN 4 palsy?
   a. midbrain—this is due to a nuclear/fascicular lesion at the level of the midbrain

6. The *least* useful test for functional visual loss is
   c. HVF—the other tests can commonly be used to trick the patient

7. Optociliary shunt vessels may occur in all of the following conditions, *except*
   d. ischemic optic neuropathy

8. Which is *not* a symptom of pseudotumor cerebri?
   b. entoptic phenomena

9. A 63-year-old woman reports sudden onset of jagged lines in the right peripheral vision. She has experienced three episodes, which lasted approximately 10 to 20 minutes, in the past month. She denies headaches and any history or family history of migraines. The most likely diagnosis is
   c. migraine variant—this is a characteristic visual disturbance that occurs in acephalgic migraines and is called a *fortification phenomenon*; the other common visual alteration is a scintillating scotoma (appears as flickering colored lights that grow in the visual field)

10. A 60-year-old man with optic disc swelling in the right eye and left optic atrophy most likely has
    a. ischemic optic neuropathy—these findings are consistent with Foster-Kennedy syndrome; however, the most common cause is pseudo-Foster-Kennedy syndrome due to ION

11. Which of the following findings may *not* be present in a patient with an INO?
    c. absent convergence—this occurs only in an anterior INO, not in a posterior INO (convergence is preserved); thus if the patient has a posterior INO, then absent convergence will not be found; the other three findings occur in both anterior and posterior forms of INO

12. A paradoxical pupillary reaction is *not* found in which condition?
    b. albinism—foveal hypoplasia occurs but pupillary reactivity is normal; paradoxical pupillary response is found in CSNB, achromatopsia, Leber congenital amaurosis, optic atrophy, and optic nerve hypoplasia

13. Inheritance of Leber hereditary optic neuropathy is
    c. mitochondrial DNA

14. An OKN strip moved to the left stimulates what parts of the brain?
    a. right frontal, left occipital

15. The smooth pursuit system does *not* involve the
    d. frontal motor area—this area is involved with fast eye movements

16. Dorsal midbrain syndrome is *not* associated with
    a. absent convergence—convergence is present and results in convergence-retraction nystagmus

17. The location of Horner syndrome is best differentiated by which drug?
    b. hydroxyamphetamine (Paredrine)—distinguishes between preganglionic and postganglionic lesions

18. The blood supply to the prelaminar ON is
    c. short posterior ciliary arteries

19. ON hypoplasia is associated with all of the following, *except*
    d. spasmus nutans

20. A lesion in the pons causes
    b. miosis

21. Which of the following syndromes is characterized by abduction deficit and contralateral hemiplegia?
    c. Millard-Gubler—Foville and Gradenigo involve CN 6 but do not cause hemiparesis; Weber does cause hemiparesis but involves CN 3, not CN 6

22. All of the following are features of progressive supranuclear palsy, *except*
    b. loss of oculovestibular reflex

23. Pituitary apoplexy is characterized by all of the following, *except*
    a. nystagmus

24. Which of the following is most likely to produce a junctional scotoma?
    d. meningioma—a junctional scotoma is caused by a lesion at the junction of the optic nerve and chiasm; this is most commonly due to a meningioma

25. All of the following are characteristics of an optic tract lesion, *except*
    b. decreased vision—visual acuity is not affected

26. The saccade system does *not* involve the
    a. occipital motor area

27. A 22-year-old man sustains trauma resulting in a transected left ON. Which of the following is true regarding the right pupil?
    c. it is equal in size to the left pupil—because of the intact consensual response in the left eye

28. Characteristics of spasmus nutans include all of the following, *except*
    d. signs present during sleep—spasmus nutans disappears during sleep

29. A congenital CN 4 palsy can be distinguished from an acquired palsy by
    a. vertical fusional amplitude > 10 Δ

30. Characteristics of a diabetic CN 3 palsy may include all of the following, *except*
    d. aberrant regeneration—this does not occur with vasculopathic causes of CN 3 palsy, only with compression (aneurysm, tumor) or trauma

31. A CN 3 lesion may cause all of the following, *except*
    a. contralateral ptosis—depending on location of the lesion, the ptosis may be ipsilateral (complete or superior division CN 3 paresis) or bilateral (nuclear), or there may be no ptosis present (inferior division CN 3 palsy)

32. ON drusen is associated with all of the following, *except*
    c. cystoid macular edema

33. A lesion causing limited upgaze with an intact Bell's phenomenon is located where?
    a. supranuclear—if Bell's phenomenon is intact, then the lesion must be supranuclear

34. An acute subarachnoid hemorrhage due to a ruptured aneurysm may produce all of the following, *except*
    b. orbital hemorrhage—does not result from a subarachnoid hemorrhage, but vitreous hemorrhage (Terson syndrome), ptosis, and an efferent pupillary defect (CN 3 palsy) can occur

35. The typical length of the intracranial portion of the optic nerve is approximately
    b. 10 mm

36. Findings in ocular motor apraxia include all of the following, *except*
    b. abnormal pursuits

37. Which of the following statements is true regarding the optic chiasm?
    c. 53% of nasal retinal fibers cross to the contralateral optic tract

38. Which of the following statements is *false* regarding the LGB?
    d. P cells are important for motion detection—this is false because P cells are involved with fine spatial resolution and color vision; M cells are important for motion detection, stereoacuity, and contrast

39. A patient with a homonymous hemianopia is found to have an asymmetric OKN response. The location of the lesion is
    a. parietal lobe—this is Cogan's dictum: for homonymous hemianopia, asymmetric OKN indicates parietal lobe lesion, and symmetric OKN indicates occipital lobe lesion

40. The only intact eye movement in one-and-a-half syndrome is
    c. abduction of contralateral eye

41. A pineal tumor is most likely to cause
    d. Parinaud syndrome

42. Metastatic neuroblastoma is most likely to be associated with
    a. opsoclonus

43. Which of the following statements regarding pupillary innervation is true?
    d. sympathetic innervation of the iris dilator involves three neurons and the ciliospinal center of Budge

44. Which is the most important test to order in a patient with chronic progressive external ophthalmoplegia?
    b. EKG—to rule out heart block from Kearns-Sayre syndrome

45. Pseudotumor cerebri is most likely to cause a palsy of which cranial nerve?
    d. 6

46. A CT scan of a patient with visual loss shows a railroad-track sign. The most likely diagnosis is
    c. ON meningioma

47. The most likely etiology of homonymous hemianopia with macular sparing is
    a. vascular—the most common cause of occipital lobe lesions

48. All of the following findings can occur in optic neuritis, *except*
    d. metamorphopsia

49. Which of the following findings is *not* associated with an acoustic neuroma?
    b. light-near dissociation

50. A superior oblique muscle palsy is most commonly caused by
    d. trauma—the most common etiology of a CN 4 palsy

51. A 29-year-old obese woman with headaches, papilledema, and a normal head CT scan is diagnosed with idiopathic intracranial hypertension. All of the following findings are consistent with her diagnosis, *except*

    b. homonymous hemianopia

52. Transection of the left ON adjacent to the chiasm results in

    a. a VF defect in the right eye—junctional scotoma due to crossing fibers in knee of von Willebrand

53. The Amsler grid tests how many degrees of central vision?

    b. 10

54. Aberrant regeneration of CN 3 may cause all of the following, *except*

    c. monocular dampening of the OKN response

55. A 42-year-old woman admitted to the hospital with severe headache and neck stiffness suddenly becomes disoriented and vomits. On examination, her left pupil is dilated and does not react to light. She most likely has

    d. subarachnoid hemorrhage—this scenario represents a CN 3 palsy due to a ruptured aneurysm (posterior communicating artery)

56. A healthy 19-year-old woman presents with gradual loss of vision OD and pain when looking side to side. Her past medical history and review of systems are negative. Exam shows visual acuity of 20/50, reduced color vision, a relative afferent pupillary defect, and a normal-appearing optic nerve OD. The most important test to obtain is

    c. MRI—patients with optic neuritis without a diagnosis of MS should have an MRI of the head and orbits to detect demyelinating lesions/plaques in the periventricular white matter

57. A 68-year-old patient with diabetes reports double vision. Exam is normal *except* for a right abducens palsy. Further questioning reveals recent weight loss and scalp and jaw pain. Which of the following tests is most useful?

    b. CRP—giant cell arteritis (GCA) can present with an isolated cranial nerve palsy

58. A patient is found to have anisocoria, which is greater in a dim room. The most likely etiology is

    b. Horner syndrome—anisocoria is accentuated in dim light when the abnormal pupil is miotic (and conversely in bright light when the abnormal pupil is mydriatic)

59. A middle-aged man relates a history of double vision and hearing loss from his left ear. On exam, he has a left esotropia and facial palsy. The most likely location of his lesion is

    d. cerebellopontine angle—usually a meningioma or acoustic neuroma that causes pseudo-Gradenigo syndrome

60. A risk factor for nonarteritic anterior ischemic optic neuropathy is

    b. hypertension

61. A 73-year-old man complains of reduced vision in his right eye. His visual acuity is found to be 20/400 OD and 20/25 OS. Upon further questioning he reports recent headaches, scalp tenderness, and pain when eating. The most appropriate initial course of action is to

    a. start treatment with systemic steroids immediately—GCA must be treated immediately with systemic steroids to prevent fellow eye involvement. The workup includes STAT lab tests (ESR and CRP) and possible temporal artery biopsy

62. A. 23-year-old woman complains of transient episodes of blurred vision and sometimes double vision. She also reports frequent headaches. Fundus exam shows blurred optic disc margins in both eyes. The most likely diagnosis is

    d. increased ICP

63. The swinging flashlight test would be most helpful in diagnosing a patient with

    d. prechiasmal afferent lesion—the swinging flashlight test is used to diagnose a relative afferent pupillary defect (Marcus-Gunn Pupil)

64. Cervicomedullary junction lesions are associated with which types of nystagmus?

    b. downbeat and periodic alternating

CHAPTER 5 PEDIATRICS/STRABISMUS

1. The approximate age of onset for accommodative ET is closest to

    b. 3 years old

2. A 15-year-old girl with strabismus is examined, and the following measurements are recorded: distance deviation of 10 Δ, near deviation of 35 Δ at 20 cm, and interpupillary distance of 60 mm. Her AC/A ratio is

    a. 11:1—to calculate the AC/A ratio with this information, use the heterophoria method: $IPD + [(N - D)/Diopt] = 6 + [(35 - 10)/5] = 11$ (remember to convert IPD to cm, and 20 cm = 5 D)

3. Duane syndrome is thought to result from a developmental abnormality of the

    d. abducens nucleus

4. The most helpful test in a patient with aniridia is

    b. abdominal ultrasound—to rule out Wilms tumor in sporadic cases

5. The best test for an infant with a normal fundus and searching eye movements is

    a. VER—can be used to determine acuity

6. The most common congenital infection is

    c. CMV

7. ARC is most likely to develop in a child with

    a. congenital esotropia

8. Which of the following most accurately reflects what a patient with harmonious ARC reports when the angle of anomaly is equal to the objective angle?

    c. simultaneous macular perception

9. The inferior oblique muscle is weakened most by which procedure?

    d. anteriorization

10. The test that gives the best dissociation is
    b. Worth 4-Dot

11. The 3-step test shows a left hypertropia in primary position that worsens on right gaze and with left head tilt. The best surgical procedure is
    d. LIO weakening—this is an LSO palsy, so possible treatments include LIO weakening, RIR recession, LSO tuck, and LIR resection

12. In the treatment of a superior oblique palsy, Knapp recommended all of the following, *except*
    d. resection of the contralateral SR—the contralateral SR should be weakened with a recession, not strengthened with a resection

13. The best results of cryotherapy for ROP occur for treatment of disease in which location?
    b. anterior zone II

14. The *least* common finding of congenital ET is
    c. amblyopia

15. The contralateral antagonist of the right superior rectus
    a. passes under another muscle—the contralateral antagonist of the right superior rectus is the left superior oblique (LSO; the antagonist LSO) of the yoke muscle (left inferior oblique [LIO]) of the paretic muscle (right superior rectus [RSR]); the superior oblique (SO) passes under the superior rectus (SR), is an incyclotorter (therefore causes excyclotorsion when paretic), abducts the eye, and is innervated by CN 4

16. With respect to Panum's area, physiologic diplopia occurs at what point?
    c. in front of Panum's area—physiologic diplopia occurs in front of and behind Panum's area; within Panum's area, binocular vision occurs with fusion and stereopsis, on the horopter only fusion

17. The best treatment of an A pattern ET with muscle transposition is
    d. LR resection with downward transposition— appropriate surgery for the ET is LR resection or MR recession; to fix the A pattern, the LRs are moved toward the empty space of the pattern (down for ET) or the MRs are moved toward the apex of the pattern (up for ET)

18. A superior rectus Faden suture is used for the treatment of which condition?
    b. dissociated vertical deviation

19. Which medication should be administered to a child who develops trismus under general anesthesia?
    d. dantrolene—because trismus is a sign of malignant hyperthermia

20. Congenital superior oblique palsy is characterized by all of the following, *except*
    d. <10 D of vertical vergence amplitudes—usually, these amplitudes are >10 D

21. Which of the following statements regarding monofixation syndrome is *false*?
    c. fusional vergence amplitudes are absent

22. Iridocyclitis is most commonly associated with which form of JIA?
    d. pauciarticular

23. Congenital rubella is most commonly associated with
    a. retinal pigment epitheliopathy

24. The most common cause of proptosis in a child is
    b. orbital cellulitis

25. Which form of rhabdomyosarcoma has the worst prognosis?
    c. alveolar—is the most malignant and has the worst prognosis; embryonal is the most common, botryoid is a subtype of embryonal, and pleomorphic is the rarest and has the best prognosis

26. Which of the following conditions is the *least* common cause of childhood proptosis?
    a. cavernous hemangioma—this is the most common benign orbital tumor of adults and occurs most commonly in middle-aged women

27. A child with retinoblastoma is born to healthy parents with no family history of RB. The chance of RB occurring in a second child is approximately
    a. 5%

28. The best chronologic age to examine a baby for ROP is
    c. 36 weeks

29. All of the following are associated with trisomy 13, *except*
    c. epiblepharon

30. Paradoxical pupillary response does *not* occur in
    d. albinism

31. An infant with bilateral cataracts is diagnosed with galactosemia. Which enzyme is most likely to be defective?
    b. galactose-1-P-uridyl transferase

32. All of the following are associated with ON drusen, *except*
    c. increased risk of intracranial tumors

33. Which is the most likely etiology of torticollis and intermittent, fine, rapid, pendular nystagmus of the right eye in a 10-month-old baby?
    d. none of the above—this infant has spasmus nutans, which is usually benign and rarely caused by optic nerve glioma

34. The most common malignant tumor of the orbit in a 6-year-old boy is
    b. rhabdomyosarcoma

35. RP and deafness occur in all of the following disorders, *except*
    c. Refsum disease—there is no deafness in this retinitis pigmentosa variant

36. α-Galactosidase A deficiency is associated with
    a. cornea verticillata—this is the enzyme defect in Fabry disease

37. Congenital cataracts and glaucoma may occur in all of the following disorders, *except*
    b. Alport syndrome—glaucoma is not a finding in Alport syndrome

38. RPE degeneration and optic atrophy are found in all of the following mucopolysaccharidoses, *except*
    d. MPS type IV—findings in MPS type IV include corneal clouding and optic atrophy, not RPE degeneration

39. Which vitamin is *not* deficient in a patient with abetalipoproteinemia (Bassen-Kornzweig syndrome)?
    b. C—the fat-soluble vitamins A, D, E, and K cannot be absorbed in abetalipoproteinemia

40. Hearing loss is *not* found in
    b. Refsum disease—this is a form of retinitis pigmentosa without hearing loss

41. Pheochromocytoma may occur in all of the following phakomatoses, *except*
    a. Louis-Bar syndrome

42. Maternal ingestion of LSD is most likely to result in which congenital ON disorder?
    c. hypoplasia—optic nerve hypoplasia is associated with maternal ingestion of alcohol, LSD, quinine, and dilantin

43. A patient with strabismus wearing −6 D glasses is measured with prism and cover test. Compared to the actual amount of deviation, the measurement would find
    b. more esotropia and more exotropia—remember, minus measures more

44. Prism glasses are *least* helpful for treating
    c. sensory esotropia

45. A 4-year-old boy has bilateral lateral rectus recessions for exotropia. Two days after surgery, he has an esotropia measuring 50 Δ. The most appropriate treatment is
    d. surgery—this indicates a slipped muscle that requires surgical repair

46. The most common cause of a vitreous hemorrhage in a child is
    b. shaken baby syndrome—trauma is the most common etiology, followed by regressed ROP (which is the most common cause of a spontaneous vitreous hemorrhage)

47. A 5-year-old girl with 20/20 vision OD and 20/50 vision OS is diagnosed with an anterior polar cataract OS. Which is the most appropriate treatment?
    a. start occlusion therapy

48. Chronic iritis in a child is most commonly caused by
    a. JIA

49. All are features of ataxia-telangiectasia, *except*
    b. thymic hyperplasia—the thymus is hypoplastic

50. All of the following vitreoretinal disorders are inherited in an AD pattern, *except*
    d. Goldmann-Favre disease—this is autosomal recessive

51. The most common location for an iris coloboma is
    d. inferonasal

52. Von Hippel–Lindau disease has been mapped to which chromosome?
    a. 3

53. Which X-linked disorder is *not* associated with an ocular abnormality in the female carrier?
    c. juvenile retinoschisis—female carriers have normal fundus; in the other three disorders, female carriers have retinal changes: midperipheral pigment clusters and mottling in macula in albinism, equatorial pigment mottling in choroideremia, golden reflex in posterior pole in retinitis pigmentosa

54. Which tumor is *not* associated with von Hippel-Lindau disease?
    a. hepatocellular carcinoma

55. The most useful diagnostic test in an infant with an oil-droplet cataract is
    d. urine-reducing substances—to check for galactosemia

56. The genetics of aniridia are best summarized as
    d. 1/4 sporadic, 3/4 AD

57. A pigmentary retinopathy occurs in which mesodermal dysgenesis syndrome?
    b. Alagille syndrome

58. Which of the following laboratory tests is most commonly found in JIA-related iritis?
    c. RF−, ANA+—which occurs most commonly in pauciarticular JIA

59. The size of an esodeviation is measured with
    c. alternate prism and cover test

60. Toxoplasmosis is most likely to be acquired from
    b. undercooked meat

61. A 10-day-old infant develops an acute papillary conjunctivitis with mucoid discharge. Which of the following is the most likely cause?
    c. *Chlamydia*

62. An infant is brought to the emergency department after a fall. There is a bruise on the forehead and numerous retinal hemorrhages. There are also bruises on the back. An X-ray shows previous rib fractures. The most likely diagnosis is
    d. nonaccidental trauma—fundus hemorrhages at multiple layers in an infant are most commonly due to shaken baby syndrome, and other signs of abuse should be looked for

63. A child undergoes uncomplicated cataract surgery with phacoemulsification and insertion of an acrylic posterior chamber intraocular lens. What is the most likely complication to develop in the future?
    a. capsular opacification

64. On a routine eye exam, a 5-year-old girl is found to have mild iritis in both eyes. What is the most helpful test to order?
    a. ANA—ANA and RF are the most helpful test to diagnose JIA

65. The most common color vision defect is
    c. deuteranomaly—approximately 5% of men have this X-linked recessive congenital color deficiency

66. Corneal clouding does not occur in which mucopolysaccharidosis?
    a. Hunter

67. Which combination of findings is least likely to occur in congenital rubella syndrome
    b. glaucoma and cataract—each occurs but rarely together

68. Which is least helpful for the diagnosis of toxocariasis?
    d. stool examination—no ova or parasites are found in the stool

69. What is the chance that a child of a patient with Best disease will inherit the disorder?
    b. 50%—Best is autosomal dominant

70. The inheritance of gyrate atrophy is
    d. autosomal recessive

71. An 8-year-old boy has new onset ptosis and proptosis. His CT scan shows a superior orbital mass. The most appropriate treatment is
    d. biopsy—suspected rhabdomyosarcoma requires urgent orbital exploration and biopsy followed by radiation treatment

CHAPTER 6   ORBIT/LIDS/ADNEXA

1. Which organism is most commonly associated with angular blepharitis?
    b. *Moraxella*

2. Sequelae of a CN 7 palsy may include all of the following, *except*
    b. ptosis—CN 7 palsy causes inability to close the lid and exposure keratopathy; CN 3 palsy causes ptosis

3. Which procedure is the best treatment option for the repair of a large upper eyelid defect?
    a. Cutler-Beard—is a lid-sharing procedure for repair of large upper eyelid defects, Bick is a horizontal lid-shortening procedure, Hughes is a lid-sharing procedure for repair of large lower eyelid defects, and Fasanella-Servat is a tarsoconjunctival resection for ptosis repair

4. The extraocular muscle with the largest arc of contact is the
    b. IO—which is 15 mm; next is LR at 12 mm, then SO at 7-8 mm, and MR at 7 mm

5. The risk of systemic involvement is highest for an ocular lymphoid tumor in which location?
    b. eyelid—67% have systemic involvement; for orbit, it is 35%, and for conjunctiva, 20%

6. The rectus muscle with the shortest tendon of insertion is the
    c. MR—the IO has the shortest tendon (1 mm), but of the rectus muscles, the MR has the shortest tendon at 4.5 mm; the others are SR = 6 mm, IR = 7 mm, and LR = 7 mm

7. Which of the following bones does *not* make up the medial orbital wall?
    d. palatine—is part of the orbital floor; the medial wall is composed of the other three bones and the ethmoid

8. Which of the following clinical features is *least* commonly associated with a tripod fracture?
    a. restriction of the inferior rectus—tripod fractures include disruption of the orbital floor, but entrapment of ocular tissues is rare and is usually associated with large floor fractures (blow-out fracture); the other three findings are much more common in a tripod fracture

9. A carotid-cavernous fistula is commonly differentiated from a dural-sinus fistula by all of the following characteristics, *except*
    a. proptosis—this can occur in both types of AV fistula; (a bruit can too, but rarely); the other signs are seen with CC fistulas

10. Basal cell carcinoma is *least* likely to occur at which site?
    d. lateral canthus—the order (in decreasing frequency) is as follows: lower lid > medial canthus > upper lid > lateral canthus

11. All of the following are sites of attachment of the limbs of the medial canthal tendon, *except*
    c. orbital process of the frontal bone

12. Which muscle is most commonly responsible for vertical diplopia after four-lid blepharoplasty?
    b. inferior oblique—because it lies below the inferior rectus and is encircled by the capsulopalpebral fascia

13. Congenital and involutional ptosis can be distinguished by all of the following, *except*
    c. width of palpebral fissure

14. Congenital obstruction of the lacrimal drainage system usually occurs at the
    d. valve of Hasner

15. What is the correct order of structures that would be encountered when the upper eyelid is penetrated 14 mm above the lid margin?
    a. preseptal orbicularis muscle, orbital septum, levator aponeurosis, Müller muscle

16. What is the best treatment option for a child who develops recurrent proptosis after upper respiratory infections?
    a. observation—this scenario is common with an orbital lymphangioma, and spontaneous regression often occurs

17. All of the following are features of mucormycosis, *except*
    b. ipsilateral CN 7 palsy—mucor may cause an orbital apex syndrome, but CN 7 is not involved

18. All of the following are associated with blepharophimosis, *except*
    c. AR inheritance—blepharophimosis may be part of an AD syndrome (chromosome 3q), as well as trisomy 18; findings include blepharophimosis, ptosis, telecanthus, ectropion, and epicanthus inversus

19. Which of the following is the most important test to perform in a patient with a capillary hemangioma?
    d. bleeding time—to look for Kasabach-Merritt syndrome (consumptive coagulopathy)

20. For entropion repair, the lateral tarsal strip is sutured
    c. above and anterior to the rim

21. Staged surgery for a patient with severe thyroid eye disease is best done in what order?
    a. decompression, strabismus, lid repair—because decompression may affect ocular alignment and lid position, and strabismus surgery may affect lid position

22. Which of the following best explains why when a ptotic lid is lifted, the contralateral lid falls?
    d. Hering's law—equal and simultaneous innervation to synergistic muscles; thus, lifting a ptotic lid decreases the innervation to the levator bilaterally, so the contralateral lid will fall slightly

23. Which study is most helpful in the evaluation of a patient with opsoclonus?
    b. MRI—to rule out neuroblastoma or visceral carcinoma

24. What is the most appropriate treatment for a benign mixed tumor of the lacrimal gland?
    b. excision—must excise completely en bloc to prevent recurrence and malignant transformation

25. What is the most appropriate treatment for a biopsy-positive basal cell carcinoma of the lower eyelid?
    d. excision with frozen section control of the margins

26. Which of the following CT-enhancing lesions has a pathognomonic appearance?
    d. meningioma—produces characteristic railroad track sign

27. Which of the following factors is *least* likely to contribute to the development of entropion?
    a. preseptal orbicularis override—this can occur but is less common than the other factors

28. A 24-year-old woman presents after blunt trauma to the left orbit with enophthalmos and restriction of upgaze. Which plain-film radiographic view would be most helpful?
    c. Waters view—gives best view of orbital floor

29. All of the following may cause enophthalmos, *except*
    b. lymphoma—may cause proptosis but not enophthalmos, breast cancer can cause either, and phthisis and floor fractures may cause enophthalmos

30. All of the following nerves pass through the superior orbital fissure, *except*
    c. CN V$_2$—passes through the inferior orbital fissure

31. Blepharospasm is associated with
    d. Parkinson disease

32. The anatomic boundaries of the superior orbital fissure are
    b. the greater and lesser wings of the sphenoid

33. Which of the following is most likely to exacerbate the symptoms of thyroid eye disease
    b. cigarettes

34. A 44-year-old woman develops a left lower eyelid ectropion following a severe facial burn. The most appropriate procedure includes
    a. horizontal tightening—and revision of the cicatrix is performed for cicatricial ectropion repair, and a vertical lengthening procedure with full-thickness graft may also be required

35. All of the following are methods of treating spastic entropion, *except*
    c. Wies marginal rotation—is used to treat involutional entropion

36. The most common complication of a hydroxyapatite orbital implant is
    d. conjunctival erosion

37. Which collagen vascular disease is associated with malignancy?
    a. dermatomyositis

38. Oral antibiotics are indicated for
    b. dacryocystitis—dacryocystitis is treated with topical and systemic antibiotics, whereas dacryoadenitis may sometimes require systemic antibiotics

39. The levator muscle inserts onto all of the following structures, *except*
    d. trochlea

40. When performing a DCR, at which level is the ostium created?
    b. middle turbinate

41. An adult with a complete NLD and patent puncta and canaliculi is best treated with which procedure?
    d. dacryocystorhinostomy—acquired NLDO is treated with DCR

42. The most effective procedure for involutional ectropion is
    a. lateral tarsal strip

43. A patient presents with follicular conjunctivitis and a cluster of umbilicated papules is noted near the eyelashes of the left eye. The most effective treatment for this condition is
    c. cryotherapy—molluscum contagiosum is best treated with excision, cryotherapy, or incision and curettage

44. The most common cause of unilateral proptosis in a middle-aged woman is
    b. thyroid eye disease—this is the most common cause of proptosis in adults (unilateral and bilateral)

45. The most common cause of involutional entropion of the lower eyelid is
    b. laxity and retractor disinsertion

46. An elderly woman with chronic unilateral blepharitis, thickening of the left upper eyelid, and submandibular lymphadenopathy is most likely to have
    d. sebaceous gland carcinoma—this malignant tumor can masquerade as chronic blepharitis

47. A 56-year-old woman with diabetes presents with pain, swelling, and redness of the left upper eyelid. Orbital involvement is most likely if she also has
    d. pain with eye movement—this is a sign of orbital involvement of the infection; ptosis may occur in both preseptal and orbital cellulitis

48. A 72-year-old man has bilateral ptosis and levator function measuring 14 mm OU. The most likely diagnosis is
    c. levator aponeurotic dehiscence—this is the most common cause of ptosis with good levator function in elderly individuals

49. The sensory nerve most likely to be affected by an orbital fracture is
    c. infraorbital—which results in infraorbital hypesthesia after orbital floor and zygomatic fractures

50. Which of the following findings is most helpful for making the diagnosis in a patient with suspected thyroid eye disease?
    a. abnormal forced ductions—TED causes restrictive strabismus

51. A patient suddenly develops pain, proptosis, loss of vision, and subconjunctival hemorrhage after a retrobulbar block. The most appropriate action is immediate
    c. lateral canthotomy—retrobulbar hemorrhage with these signs and symptoms requires emergent lateral canthotomy

52. A 60-year-old man with a one-week history of tearing is found to have a tender, swollen mass in the inferior medial canthal region of the left eye. The most appropriate initial management is
    c. start oral antibiotics—this is the initial treatment for acute dacryocystitis

53. Which of the following signs is most helpful in differentiating preseptal cellulitis from orbital cellulitis?
    d. relative afferent pupillary defect—the presence of an RAPD is a serious development indicating orbital involvement; fever may occur in both preseptal and orbital cellulitis

54. What is the most likely diagnosis in a patient with right upper eyelid retraction and normal thyroid function tests?
    c. thyroid eye disease—patients with TED are usually hyperthyroid, but can be euthyroid or rarely hypothyroid

55. *Demodex* infection is associated with
    d. angular blepharitis

CHAPTER 7 CORNEA/EXTERNAL DISEASE

1. Which is the *least* desirable method for corneal graft storage?
   b. glycerin—does not preserve endothelial cells and can be used only for lamellar or patch grafts; moist chamber at 4°C preserves tissue for 48 hours, Optisol for up to 10 days, and cryopreservation potentially for years

2. Presently in the United States, phlyctenule is most commonly associated with
   c. *Staphylococcus*

3. Which blood test is most helpful in the evaluation of a patient with Schnyder corneal dystrophy?
   d. cholesterol—may be elevated

4. Which disease has never been transmitted by a corneal graft?
   a. CMV—the others have been transmitted in humans or experimentally in animals

5. Which corneal dystrophy does *not* recur in a corneal graft?
   d. posterior polymorphous

6. A conjunctival map biopsy is typically used for which malignancy?
   c. sebaceous gland carcinoma

7. All of the following may cause follicular conjunctivitis, *except*
   b. *Neisseria*

8. Which of the following tests is *least* helpful in determining the etiology of enlarged corneal nerves?
   a. electrocardiogram—the others are all helpful in detecting disorders that are associated with enlarged corneal nerves: calcitonin for medullary thyroid carcinoma (MEN 2b), urinary vanillyl mandelic acid (VMA) for pheochromocytoma (MEN 2b), acid-fast stain for atypical *Mycobacteria* (leprosy)

9. Corneal filaments are *least* likely to be present in which condition?
   b. Thygeson SPK

10. Which of the following is *not* an appropriate treatment for SLK?
    c. silver nitrate stick—may cause globe perforation; therefore, use only silver nitrate solution

11. In what level of the cornea does a Kayser-Fleischer ring occur?
    d. Descemet membrane

12. Cornea verticillata–like changes are associated with all of the following, *except*
    b. haloperidol

13. The *least* common location for a nevus is
    a. bulbar conjunctiva

14. All of the following ions move across the corneal endothelium by both active transport and passive diffusion, *except*
    a. Cl⁻—moves across endothelium only by passive diffusion

15. Which organism is associated with crystalline keratopathy?
    d. *S. viridans*

16. Which of the following conditions is associated with the best 5-year prognosis for a corneal graft?
    b. Fuchs dystrophy

17. The best strategy for loosening a tight contact lens is to
    c. decrease the diameter—decreasing the curvature will also loosen a tight lens but not as well; increasing the diameter or curvature will tighten a lens

18. The type of contact lens that causes the *least* endothelial pleomorphism is
    a. soft daily wear

19. Which of the following conditions is associated with the worst prognosis for a corneal graft?
    c. Reis-Bucklers dystrophy—this dystrophy commonly recurs in the graft

20. Which is *not* a treatment of acute hydrops?
    d. corneal transplant—eventually, this may be an option, but short-term treatment is medical only

21. Which organism *cannot* penetrate intact corneal epithelium?
    c. *P. aeruginosa*—cannot penetrate intact corneal epithelium; the others and *Listeria* can

22. Which of the following medications would be the best choice in the treatment of microsporidial keratoconjunctivitis?
    a. fumagillin

23. All of the following agents are used in the treatment of *Acanthamoeba* keratitis, *except*
    b. natamycin

24. Goblet cells are *least* abundant in which location?
    a. limbus

25. Thygeson SPK is best treated with topical
    c. loteprednol—steroids are the best treatment

26. EKC is typically contagious for how many days?
    d. 14 days

27. A shield ulcer is associated with
    c. VKC

28. Which of the following is most likely to be associated with melanoma of the uvea?
    c. nevus of Ota—increased risk of uveal melanomas in Caucasians; this is rarer for congenital melanosis oculi (ocular melanocytosis), and acquired melanosis oculi (PAM) is not associated with uveal melanoma

29. Which of the following is *not* associated with *N. gonorrhoeae* conjunctivitis?
    a. pseudomembrane—gonococcal (GC) conjunctivitis causes a true membrane

30. Even spreading of the tear film depends most on which factor?
    c. mucin

31. A neurotrophic ulcer should *not* be treated with
    b. antiviral—this can cause more toxicity

32. Which layer of the cornea can regenerate?
    c. Descemet membrane—can regenerate if endothelium is intact

33. The most appropriate treatment for a patient with scleromalacia is
    d. oral immunosuppressive agent—scleromalacia is caused by severe rheumatoid arthritis

34. The HEDS recommendation for treating stromal (disciform) keratitis is
    b. topical steroid and topical antiviral—oral acyclovir was not found to be useful

35. Feathery edges and a satellite infiltrate are most characteristic of a corneal ulcer caused by
    d. *Fusarium*—these characteristics are associated with fungal ulcers

36. PTK would be most appropriate for treating which of the following corneal disorders?
    a. superficial granular dystrophy

37. A 62-year-old woman with KCS is most likely to demonstrate corneal staining in which location?
    b. middle 1/3 (interpalpebral)—due to exposure between the eyelids

38. Which of the following findings is most commonly associated with SLK?
    a. filaments—found in 50%

39. Which lab test is most helpful to obtain in a 38-year-old man with herpes zoster ophthalmicus?
    d. HIV test—herpes zoster is rare in healthy individuals <40 years old and may indicate immunosuppression

40. A patient with conjunctival intraepithelial neoplasia is most likely to have
    d. HPV—this virus is associated with CIN, and patients who have HIV are also more likely to develop CIN

41. Which of the following disorders is most likely to be found in a patient suffering from sleep apnea?
    c. follicular conjunctivitis—secondary to floppy eyelid syndrome

42. A patient with GVH disease is most likely to have which eye finding?
    b. symblepharon—due to cicatrizing conjunctivitis

43. Topical corticosteroids should *not* be used in a patient with which form of herpes simplex keratitis?
    a. epithelial

44. What is the most appropriate management for a patient who reports recurrent foreign body sensation when waking up but does not have a discrete epithelial defect on exam?
    b. lubrication—initial management of recurrent erosion syndrome is with lubrication/Muro 128

45. A 24-year-old swimmer reports a painful, red left eye and blurry vision after sleeping with her CL for several days. Examination shows a corneal ulcer with edema and a hypopyon. The most likely diagnosis is
    c. *Acanthamoeba*—this organism is associated with corneal infections in contact lens wearers who clean their lenses with homemade saline and swim or hot tub with their contacts in

46. The best test to measure basal tear secretion is
    c. Schirmer test with anesthesia—measures basal tear secretion, Schirmer without anesthesia measures reflex and basal tear secretion, and tear breakup time is used to evaluate the stability of the tear film. The dye disappearance and Jones tests help to identify obstruction of the lacrimal drainage system.

47. Adenoviral membranous conjunctivitis is most likely to cause which of the following?
    a. symblepharon

48. After a corneal alkali burn, which of the following signs is associated with the worst prognosis?
    d. complete limbal blanching—this is a sign of limbal ischemia, which is associated with more severe injury; the larger the area of limbal involvement, the worse the prognosis

49. The most likely cause of a corneal keratometry measurement 2.5 D steeper inferiorly than superiorly at the 3 mm zone is
    c. keratoconus—one of the corneal topography parameters classically used to diagnose keratoconus is an I-S value (difference between average inferior and superior corneal powers 3 mm from the center of the cornea) of >1.4 D

50. The nasociliary branch of the trigeminal nerve innervates the tip of the nose and the
    d. cornea—this is the reason that ocular involvement should be suspected when a herpes zoster lesion is present on the nose (Hutchinson sign)

51. The most common complication of pterygium surgery is
    d. recurrence

52. The refractive effect of Intacs is titrated by the
    c. thickness of the ring segments

53. At the 4-week postop exam of a patient who underwent uncomplicated PRK for moderate myopia, the manifest refraction is −0.25 D OD and −1.25 D OS. Slit-lamp exam shows moderate anterior stromal haze OS. How would you manage this patient?
    b. increase topical steroids—this is the initial management of corneal haze in the early postop period after PRK

54. A buttonhole flap is most likely to occur with a microkeratome if the patient has
    c. keratometry > 47 D—a steep cornea is a risk factor for a buttonhole flap

55. The best surgical option for a patient with Fuchs dystrophy, corneal edema, and a visually significant cataract is
    d. phacoemulsification, IOL, and endothelial keratoplasty

56. A large epithelial defect occurs during LASIK flap creation. This patient is most at risk for
    b. diffuse lamellar keratitis —an epithelial defect is a risk factor for DLK. Epithelial sloughing has also been associated with epithelial ingrowth, particularly in patients with epithelial basement membrane dystrophy.

57. The Kamra inlay improves near vision by which of the following methods?
    b. pinhole effect—the Kamra is inserted in the nondominant eye and utilitzes the pinhole effect to improve near vision

58. Which type of contact lens is most likely to cause giant papillary conjunctivitis?
    d. soft extended wear—prolonged wear time increases the risk of GPC

59. Which method of astigmatism correction provides the best visual acuity after cataract surgery in a patient with keratoconus?
    a. rigid contact lens—although a toric IOL can provide very good vision in some patients with keratoconus, a RGP contact lens best corrects the irregular astigmatism in these patients. LRIs and LASIK are contraindicated.

60. According to the Munnerlyn equation, the depth of an excimer laser corneal ablation is most dependent upon the
    d. diameter of the optical zone—the Munnerlyn equation is: depth = (refractive error/3) × OZ^2

CHAPTER 8 UVEITIS

1. The most effective antibiotic for the treatment of *P. acnes* endophthalmitis is
   c. vancomycin—*P. acnes* is resistant to aminoglycosides

2. For the diagnosis of granulomatous inflammation, which cell type must be present?
   d. epithelioid histiocyte

3. All of the following are true concerning sarcoidosis, *except*
   a. Touton giant cells are common—sarcoidosis is characterized by Langhans giant cells

4. Which of the following is *not* characteristic of Fuchs heterochromic iridocyclitis?
   c. posterior synechiae

5. The most common organism causing endophthalmitis following cataract surgery is
   d. *S. epidermidis*

6. MEWDS can be differentiated from APMPPE by
   b. female predilection

7. All of the following disorders are correctly paired with their HLA associations, *except*
   a. presumed ocular histoplasmosis syndrome, B9—POHS is associated with HLA-B7, DR2

8. Decreased vision in a patient with intermediate uveitis is most likely a result of
   b. macular edema

9. A 71-year-old woman with a 6-month history of fatigue, anorexia, and 10-pound weight loss is found to have left-sided weakness, visual acuity of 20/80 OD and 20/60 OS, and vitreous cells. The most helpful workup is
   a. LP and vitrectomy—to rule out CNS lymphoma

10. The most common organisms causing endophthalmitis following trauma is
    b. *Bacillus* species and *S. epidermidis*

11. All of the following are features common to both sympathetic ophthalmia and VKH syndrome, *except*
    c. pathology localized to choroid—retina is also involved in VKH

12. Which disorder is more common in males?
    b. uveal effusion syndrome

13. EVS findings include all of the following, *except*
    b. intravitreal corticosteroids were helpful—intravitreal steroids were not evaluated in the EVS

14. Which of the following is *not* characteristic of MEWDS?
    b. bilaterality

15. The most common cause of posterior uveitis is
    d. toxoplasmosis

16. All of the following are causes of HLA-B27-associated uveitis, *except*
    d. psoriasis—is not associated with uveitis, but psoriatic arthritis is

17. Which of the following is *not* part of the classic triad of findings in Reiter syndrome?
    a. iritis—iritis occurs but the classic triad of reactive arthritis syndrome (Reiter syndrome) is arthritis, conjunctivitis, and urethritis

18. Phacoantigenic endophthalmitis is characterized by which pattern of granulomatous inflammation?
    a. zonal

19. A 35-year-old man with decreased vision OD is found to have optic disc edema and a macular star. The causative organism most likely is
    b. *Bartonella henselae*—which causes cat-scratch disease and a neuroretinitis; *O. volvulus* causes onchocerciasis, *T. pallidum* causes syphilis, and *B. burgdorferi* causes Lyme disease

20. A person living in which area of the US would be most likely to develop POHS?
    c. Midwest—in the US, histoplasmosis is most prevalent in the Ohio River valley and eastern states

21. All of the following are true of birdshot chorioretinopathy, *except*
    a. more common in males—birdshot chorioretinopathy is more common in females

22. Which of the following is *least* commonly associated with *T. pallidum* infection?
    d. glaucoma—is not associated with ocular involvement of syphilis

23. The HLA association for intermediate uveitis with multiple sclerosis is
    d. DR15

24. Retinal S antigen is found in
    c. photoreceptors—retinal S antigen is found in outer segments of receptor cells

25. Features of Harada disease include all of the following, *except*
    b. deafness—only eye findings are seen in Harada disease

26. Larva cause all of the following infections, *except*
    d. cat-scratch disease—is caused by the bacteria *Bartonella henselae*

27. Which of the following signs of intermediate uveitis is most associated with multiple sclerosis?
    c. periphlebitis

28. CSF abnormalities are associated with all of the following disorders, *except*
    b. ocular sarcoidosis

29. All of the following can present as uveitis, *except*
    b. choroidal hemangioma

30. Which of the following is *not* associated with inflammatory bowel disease?
    c. interstitial keratitis

31. Anterior vitreous cells are *least* likely to be found in
    a. retinitis pigmentosa

32. GI disorders associated with uveitis include all of the following, *except*
    c. diverticulitis

33. All of the following may occur in ocular sarcoidosis, *except*
    d. low serum gamma globulin—serum gamma globulin level is elevated

34. The choroid is the primary location of the pathologic process in
    d. VKH syndrome

35. Which of the following is *least* likely to be found in a patient with sympathetic ophthalmia?
    b. granulomatous nodules in the retina—nodules occur in the choroid

36. Band keratopathy is *least* likely to occur in a patient with
    c. Behçet disease

37. A patient with APMPPE is most likely to have
    c. viral prodrome

38. A patient with a mild AC reaction, increased intraocular pressure, and iris heterochromia is most likely to also exhibit which other finding?
    d. fine vessels in the angle—occur in Fuchs heterochromic iridocyclitis

39. Which of the following cell types is found in both granulomatous and nongranulomatous KPs?
    c. lymphocytes

40. All of the following are masquerade syndromes, *except*
    a. vitreous hemorrhage—this may occur in uveitis (e.g., VKH, POHS) but is not a condition that presents as uveitis

41. A false-positive VDRL test is *least* likely to occur in a patient with
    a. granulomatosis with polyangiitis

42. A 54-year-old man with chronic recurrent uveitis OS controlled with topical steroids has developed a visually significant cataract. What is the most appropriate treatment?
    d. delay cataract surgery until the eye has been quiet for at *least* 3 months

43. All of the following are risk factors for traumatic endophthalmitis, *except*
    d. double penetrating injury

44. A pseudophakic patient develops granulomatous inflammation 8 months after cataract surgery, and a white plaque is present on the posterior capsule. The organism most likely to be causing this condition is
    c. *P. acnes*—an anaerobic, gram-positive rod, is the most common organism causing delayed endophthalmitis following cataract surgery

45. A 28-year-old woman acutely develops reduced vision, pain, redness, and floaters OS. Exam shows a mild iritis with granulomatous KP and discrete patches of peripheral necrotizing retinitis. The most appropriate management is to begin treatment with
    a. acyclovir—antiviral medication, steroids, and aspirin are used to treat acute retinal necrosis

46. CNV is most likely to occur in
    d. punctate inner choroiditis—CNV develops in the majority of patients

47. A 30-year-old man with photophobia for a week is found to have 2+ AC cells and flare OU. Initial treatment should be with
    b. topical steroid and cycloplegic

48. Which of the following tests should be obtained prior to starting oral steroids for a patient with chronic noninfectious uveitis?
    b. blood pressure, electrolytes, fasting blood glucose

49. Which systemic antibiotic is not used for endophthalmitis?
    a. tobramycin

50. Which white dot syndrome has the best visual prognosis?
    a. acute retinal pigment epitheliitis

51. The neoplastic condition that most commonly masquerades as uveitis is
    b. primary vitreoretinal lymphoma

52. Iris nodule biopsy shows foamy histiocytes. The most likely diagnosis is
    d. juvenile xanthogranuloma

53. The most common cause of endogenous endophthalmitis is
    a. fungi—usually *Candida*

54. Maculopathy with foveolitis is associated with which viral infection?
    d. Dengue

55. Necrotizing scleritis is caused by
    d. *Nocardiosis*

CHAPTER 9 GLAUCOMA

1. What is the most appropriate initial treatment of pupillary block in a patient with microspherophakia?
   d. cyclopentolate—which helps pull the anteriorly displaced lens back to its normal position

2. Which of the following statements is true?
   c. uveoscleral outflow is increased by atropine—cycloplegics and prostaglandin analogues increase (and miotics decrease) uveoscleral outflow; fluorophotometry measures the rate of aqueous formation; uveoscleral outflow accounts for 15% to 20% of total outflow and is independent of pressure

3. Risk factors for angle-closure glaucoma include all of the following, *except*
   b. myopia—this is a risk factor for open-angle glaucoma, not angle-closure glaucoma

4. Which of the following would cause the greatest elevation in IOP?
   a. blinking—IOP is lowered by decreased blood cortisol levels (reduces aqueous formation) and elevation of the head (changing from supine to sitting position); darkening the room may increase IOP in patients with narrow angles

5. The most likely cause of a large filtering bleb and a shallow chamber is
   d. overfiltration—which causes both findings; a leak would cause a flat or low bleb; pupillary block and aqueous misdirection would not change the size of the blebs

6. A change in Goldmann VF stimulus from I4e to II4e is equivalent to
   a. 1 log—the Roman numeral indicates the size of the test object in mm^2 (0 = 1/16, I = 1/4, II = 1, III = 4, IV = 16, V = 64) and is a logarithmic scale; therefore, changing from size I to II is 1 log unit

7. An Amsler grid held at 33 cm measures approximately how many degrees of central vision?
   b. 10

8. The most decreased sensitivity in an arcuate scotoma occurs in which quadrant?
   c. superotemporal

9. The best gonioscopy lens for distinguishing appositional from synechial angle closure is
   b. Zeiss—this is the only lens of the four that can be used for indentation gonioscopy (indenting the cornea forces aqueous into the angle, pushing the iris backward and allowing one to view the angle)

10. Which is *not* a risk factor for POAG?
    d. central retinal artery occlusion

11. ALT would be most effective in a patient with which type of glaucoma?
    c. pigmentary—patients with pigmentary glaucoma often respond well to ALT, whereas those with inflammatory, congenital, and aphakic glaucoma do not

12. In which direction should a patient look to aid the examiner's view of the angle during Zeiss gonioscopy?
    b. toward the mirror—this allows for a better view of the portion of the angle being inspected; alternatively, tilt the lens toward the angle being inspected (away from mirror)

13. The best parameter for determining the unreliability of a Humphrey VF is
    a. fixation losses

14. Which of the following does *not* cause angle-closure glaucoma?
    c. RD—does not cause angle closure; the others do: PHPV and choroidal effusion by a posterior pushing mechanism and ICE syndrome by an anterior pulling mechanism

15. Which of the following is *least* likely to cause increased IOP 2 days postoperatively?
    d. steroid drops—steroid response usually takes at least 7-10 days to occur

16. Treatment of malignant glaucoma may include all of the following, *except*
    b. pilocarpine—miotics are contraindicated in malignant glaucoma because the aim of medical therapy is to pull the lens/iris diaphragm posteriorly (cycloplegics)

17. The most common organism associated with bleb-related endophthalmitis is
    a. *Streptococcus* species—are most common (~50%) followed by coagulase-negative *Staphylococcus* and then *H. influenzae*

18. Which VF defect is *least* characteristic of glaucoma?
    c. central scotoma—central vision is not affected until late in the disease

19. The type of tonometer most greatly affected by scleral rigidity is
    c. Schiøtz—low scleral rigidity yields falsely low readings (i.e., high myopia, thyroid disease, previous ocular surgery, miotic therapy), and high scleral rigidity yields falsely high readings (i.e., high hyperopia, vasoconstrictor therapy)

20. As compared with plasma, aqueous has a higher concentration of
    c. ascorbate—has a concentration 15 × higher in aqueous than in plasma, whereas the concentrations of sodium, calcium, and protein are lower in aqueous

21. The rate of aqueous production per minute is approximately
    b. 2.6 µL—1% of aqueous turned over per minute, 100% turnover in 100 min; AC volume = 200 µL, PC volume = 60 µL, total volume = 260 µL

22. Which location has the greatest resistance to aqueous outflow?
    c. juxtacanalicular connective tissue

23. The facility of aqueous outflow is best measured by
    a. tonography—manometry measures episcleral venous pressure, tonometry measures intraocular pressure, fluorophotometry measures rate of aqueous formation (via decreasing fluorescein concentration)

24. A patient recently had an acute angle closure attack in the right eye. What is the most appropriate treatment for her left eye?
    b. laser peripheral iridotomy—iridotomies must be performed in both eyes

25. The most likely gonioscopic finding in a patient with glaucoma and radial midperipheral spoke-like iris transillumination defects is
    a. concave peripheral iris—this is the characteristic iris configuration in pigment dispersion syndrome and pigmentary glaucoma

26. A 60-year-old myope with early cataracts and enlarged C/D ratios of 0.6 OU is found to have an abnormal Humphrey VF test OS. He has no other risk factors for glaucoma. What is the most appropriate next step for this patient?
    a. repeat VF testing—any initial abnormal glaucoma field test or interval change in field should be confirmed by repeating the test

27. Bilateral scattered PAS in an elderly hyperope with no past ocular history is most likely a result of
    c. chronic angle-closure glaucoma

28. According to the CIGTS 5-year results, initial treatment of POAG with which two methods had similar VF outcomes?
    b. medicine or trabeculectomy

29. Which of the following medications should *not* be used to treat a patient with herpes simplex virus keratouveitis and elevated IOP?
    a. pilocarpine—miotics can exacerbate the inflammation and increase the risk of the development of posterior synechiae

30. A patient undergoes multiple subconjunctival injections of 5-FU after glaucoma filtration surgery. The most common reason for discontinuing these injections is if the patient develops toxicity of which tissue?
    c. cornea—corneal epithelial toxicity (i.e., superficial punctate keratitis, epithelial defects, ulcers) is the most common complication of subconjunctival 5-FU injections

31. A patient with retinoblastoma develops glaucoma. The most common mechanism is
    c. neovascular—NVG (as a result of retinal ischemia) is the cause of ~75% of RB-associated glaucoma cases; the other mechanism is secondary angle closure as a result of anterior displacement of the lens–iris diaphragm

32. Glaucoma resulting from elevated episcleral venous pressure occurs in all of the following, *except*
    b. hyphema—glaucoma is caused by red blood cells clogging the trabecular meshwork

33. The earliest color deficit in glaucoma is the loss of the
    d. blue–yellow axis—this is the rationale for using short-wavelength automated perimetry (SWAP) visual field testing for early glaucoma

34. Blood in the Schlemm canal is *not* associated with
    a. Fuchs heterochromic iridocyclitis—there is no blood in the Schlemm canal, but fine-angle neovascularization occurs and may cause spontaneous hyphema (Amsler sign)

35. According to the OHTS conclusions, a predictive factor for the development of POAG is a central corneal thickness of less than or equal to how many microns?
    b. 555

36. Which index on Humphrey VF testing is most helpful for determining the progression of VF loss?
    c. pattern standard deviation—a measure of the change in shape of the field from the expected shape for a normal field

37. Which optic disc finding is most likely to indicate the progression of glaucoma?
    d. splinter hemorrhage—a disc hemorrhage indicates glaucomatous damage and is often followed by notching

38. The most likely risk factor for phacomorphic glaucoma in a patient with brunescent cataracts and narrow angles is
    d. hyperopia—hyperopic eyes tend to be smaller, with shorter anterior chamber depths, which are further shortened with the thickening of the lens from nuclear sclerosis

39. A patient with an anterior chamber IOL presents with ciliary block. Exam shows a patent iridectomy. Which of the following is the most appropriate treatment option?
    a. topical cycloplegic—to relax the ciliary muscle and move the lens and iris posteriorly

40. A mechanic presents 1 week after an eye injury with decreased vision, redness, and eye pain. Exam reveals a self-sealing corneal laceration, elevated IOP, and white fluffy material in the anterior chamber. The most likely diagnosis is
    b. lens-particle glaucoma

41. What visual field defect would you expect to find in a patient with POAG and cup-to-disc ratio of 0.7 OD with an inferior notch?
    c. superior arcuate—results from damage to inferior arcuate bundle

42. A 68-year-old man presents with IOP of 18 mm Hg, cup-to-disc ratio of 0.8, and nasal steps on visual field testing OU. The next test to perform is
    d. tonometry—repeat measurements of intraocular pressure to determine the maximum pressure and distinguish between POAG and NTG

43. The GLT evaluated treatment with
    b. ALT and timolol

44. POAG and NTG are best differentiated with
    d. serial tonometry—to determine if the IOP is >21 mmHg

45. Angle-closure without pupillary block is caused by
    a. aqueous misdirection—malignant glaucoma is a form of angle-closure without pupillary block caused by a posterior "pushing" mechanism with anterior displacement of the lens-iris diaphragm

CHAPTER 10 ANTERIOR SEGMENT

1. The most helpful test for evaluating macular function in a patient with advanced cataract is
    b. 2-light separation—the others test gross function

2. Ectopia lentis is *least* likely to be associated with
    a. cleft palate—is not associated with lens subluxation; the other abnormalities are pectus excavatum in Marfan syndrome; short stature in Weill-Marchesani syndrome; and mental retardation in homocystinuria, sulfite oxidase deficiency, and hyperlysinemia

3. Anterior segment signs of CB melanoma include all of the following, *except*
    a. corneal edema—does not occur; however, ciliary body melanoma can cause increased IOP from angle closure (posterior pushing mechanism) and can cause astigmatism and cataract from mechanical effects on the crystalline lens

4. Which of the following is *least* characteristic of ICE syndrome?
    b. increased IOP

5. A stellate anterior subcapsular cataract is most likely to be found in a patient with
    d. electrical injury—the other entities cause different types of cataract: atopic dermatitis (ASC), myotonic dystrophy (Christmas tree cataract), Fabry disease (spoke-like cataract)

6. Which of the following does *not* occur in siderosis bulbi?
    c. sunflower cataract—is seen in conditions with abnormal copper (not iron) deposition (i.e., Wilson disease and chalcosis)

7. A patient has a history of increased IOP with exercise; which finding is associated with this condition?
    a. Krukenberg spindle—these are both signs of pigment dispersion syndrome

8. Separation between the longitudinal and circumferential fibers of the ciliary muscle is called
    b. angle recession—this is the definition; iridoschisis is separation of the iris surface, iridodialysis is separation of the iris root from its insertion, and cyclodialysis is separation of the ciliary body from the scleral spur

9. Characteristics of pigment dispersion syndrome include all of the following, *except*
    c. phacodonesis

10. A patient with sickle cell with a hyphema develops increased IOP; which of the following treatment choices is best?
    d. timolol—is the safest medication because it does not affect sickling; miotics destabilize the blood–aqueous barrier, CAIs decrease aqueous pH (leading to sickling), and hyperosmotics cause hemoconcentration and sickling

11. Of the following causes of iris heterochromia, the involved iris is hyperchromic in
    a. ICE syndrome—pigmented iris nodules (pseudonevi) can occur; the involved iris is hypochromic in the other three conditions

12. Which of the following iris lesions is a true tumor?
    c. Lisch nodule—is an iris hamartoma associated with neurofibromatosis; Kunkmann-Wolffian body is composed of normal iris stroma, Koeppe nodule is composed of inflammatory cells, and nodules in JXG are granulomatous infiltrates

13. At which location is the lens capsule the thinnest?
    b. posterior capsule

14. Which of the following is *not* associated with sunset syndrome?
    d. hyphema—is not associated with inferior decentration of an IOL; polyopia can occur if the edge of the lens is within the pupil; asymmetric haptic placement and weak zonules (which occur in pseudoexfoliation) are risk factors

15. Lens epithelial cells differentiate into lens fibers
    a. anterior to the equator

16. Light of which wavelength is absorbed the greatest by a dense nuclear sclerotic cataract?
    d. blue—this is why patients notice that blues and purples are especially vibrant after cataract surgery

17. A patient with background diabetic retinopathy and clinically significant macular edema desires cataract surgery. The most appropriate management is
    b. focal laser treatment, then cataract surgery—it is important to treat and stabilize the preexisting macular edema prior to cataract surgery, which can exacerbate it

18. After finishing phacoemulsification on a dense cataract, the surgeon notes whitening of the clear corneal incision. The most likely cause is
    a. tight incision—causes reduced irrigation and insufficient cooling of the phaco needle, resulting in a wound burn

19. Nuclear brunescence increases with higher concentrations of which lens protein?
    d. main intrinsic protein

20. Lens fibers contain nuclei in all of the following conditions, *except*
    b. syphilis

21. The most likely cause of an intraoperative complication during cataract surgery in a patient with pseudoexfoliation syndrome is
    c. weak zonules

22. The majority of glucose metabolism in the lens is by
    a. glycolysis

23. The most appropriate systemic treatment for a patient with a sunflower cataract is
    b. penicillamine—to reduce serum copper levels

24. Which of the following is the *least* likely cause of decreased vision 2 years after cataract surgery?
    d. CME—occurs in the first 2 months after surgery

25. Which type of cataract is most closely associated with UV-B exposure?
    b. cortical

26. Which of the following strategies is *least* likely to be effective for treating IFIS?
    c. manual pupil stretching—the iris is floppy and atonic, so stretching the pupil will not improve IFIS; however, this strategy is helpful in cases of a rigid or fibrotic pupil, such as in pseudoexfoliation syndrome or chronic uveitis

27. Ocular melanoma is *least* likely to occur in which portion of the uvea?
    b. iris—this is the least likely site of developing a uveal melanoma; conjunctival melanoma is the rarest ocular melanoma (followed by eyelid melanoma, then uveal melanoma) and only accounts for 2% of ocular malignancies

28. A patient reports acute pain while hammering metal and presents with 20/20 vision, subconjunctival hemorrhage, and small hyphema OD. The most appropriate test to obtain is
    d. CT—this patient has a presumed metallic intraocular foreign body

29. A patient with a traumatic cataract requires cataract surgery. Which of the following is most helpful?
    a. laser interferometer—tests macular potential in patients with media opacities and would be the most helpful for evaluating potential visual acuity

30. Pseudoexfoliation syndrome and pigment dispersion syndrome share which of the following findings?
    b. pigmented trabecular meshwork—increased pigment on the angle structures is common to both syndromes

31. The most likely cause of monocular diplopia after blunt trauma is
    c. lens subluxation

32. Which of the following tests is most helpful in a patient with a Morgagnian cataract?
    b. HbA1c—patients with diabetes are more likely to develop cortical (and posterior subcapsular) cataracts, and the risk of cataract formation increases with elevated blood sugar levels

33. A truck driver desires the best range of vision after cataract surgery. Which IOL strategy is most appropriate?
    c. mini-monovision with accommodating lens—Crystalens with mini-monovision will achieve the best range of vision with the least risk of glare; multifocal lenses should be used with caution in professional drivers because of nighttime glare

34. One week after cataract surgery, a patient has increased AC cells and flare, IOP of 36 mm Hg, and a nuclear fragment in the inferior angle. Which is the most appropriate treatment option?
    d. remove the retained fragment—retained nuclear material in the anterior chamber is poorly tolerated (even small fragments) and must be removed if corneal edema, iritis, elevated IOP, or CME develops

35. Which of the following tools is most helpful when performing surgery on a patient with a mature cataract?
    a. Trypan blue—capsular stain to aid in the creation of the capsulorhexis

36. Glaukomflecken is caused by
    d. ischemia—elevated IOP from angle closure causes ischemia and necrosis of lens epithelial cells, appearing as central, subcapsular white dots and flecks

37. Which of the following symptoms is *least* associated with posterior subcapsular cataracts?
    b. poor blue discrimination—this is a characteristic of nuclear sclerosis

38. A piggyback IOL is most likely to be necessary in which of the following conditions?
    c. high hyperopia—a patient with high hyperopia is most likely to require a primary piggyback lens (needs IOL power > +34 D) or secondary piggyback lens (due to surprise)

39. A 77-year-old woman with cataracts and macular degeneration is interested in cataract surgery. The most helpful test for evaluating this patient is
    d. potential acuity meter (PAM)—the most useful test for evaluating the benefit of cataract surgery in this patient is the PAM, which projects the image of letter chart onto the retina to test macular potential in patients with media opacities

40. In which situation does optical biometry have the largest advantage over ultrasound biometry in determining an accurate measurement?
    c. high myopia—may have posterior staphyloma, which is more accurately measured with optical biometry; ultrasound biometry has an advantage in patients with dense posterior capsular and mature cataracts

41. During phacoemulsification a milky substance (lens milk or lens dust) appears. What is the most appropriate next step?
    a. check for tight incision—lens milk/dust is a sign of not enough irrigation, and if not corrected, a wound burn may rapidly occur, so the first step should be to check if the incision is too tight, thereby compressing the sleeve, or the phaco tip is obstructed

42. Which of the following is the most likely complication of Nd:YAG laser posterior capsulotomy?
    c. retinal detachment

43. A patient with vitreous to the wound is most at risk for which postoperative complication?
    d. cystoid macular edema

44. On postop day 1 after cataract surgery, exam shows wound gape and a flat AC. The most appropriate treatment is
    c. suture wound—a significant wound leak requires sutures or ocular sealant

45. A silicone IOL should *not* be used in a patient with
    b. proliferative diabetic retinopathy—a patient who may require silicone oil for retinal detachment repair should not have a silicone IOL because silicone oil can adhere to the IOL

46. A patient with a posterior subcapsular cataract desires surgery. What is the most appropriate reason for performing cataract surgery?
    a. patient complains of glare and difficulty reading—indication for cataract surgery is subjective and depends on patient symptoms

47. An anterior subcapsular cataract is most likely to develop in a patient with which skin condition?
    d. atopic dermatitis

48. Reduced color discrimination is most likely caused by which type of cataract?
    c. nuclear sclerotic

49. Which of the following is most likely to occur following cataract surgery in a patient with previous myopic LASIK?
    b. hyperopia—secondary to incorrect keratometry readings (true curvature is flatter than measured)

50. A patient with no visual complaints is noted to have a normal eye exam, except for chronic pupillary capture of an IOL. What is the most appropriate management?
    a. observation—if the patient is asymptomatic and there are no ocular sequelae, then the patient should be observed

51. One day after uncomplicated cataract surgery with phacoemulsification, the exam shows counting fingers vision, 3+ corneal edema with Descemet folds, and severe AC reaction with fibrinous material. The most likely diagnosis is
    c. toxic anterior segment syndrome—a form of sterile endophthalmitis

52. A patient with high hyperopia is at increased risk for which of the following complications of cataract surgery?
    d. choroidal effusion—short axial length increases the risk of choroidal effusion/hemorrhage from cataract surgery

53. The largest risk for capsule rupture during hydrodissection occurs with
    c. posterior polar cataract—hydrodissection should not be performed in the presence of a posterior polar cataract because of the high risk of a posterior capsular defect; instead, only hydrodelineation should be performed. Mature cataract increases the risk of an anterior capsular tear during capsulorhexis, and pseudoexfoliation syndrome and small pupil are risk factors for capsular rupture during phacoemulsification and I/A.

54. After hydrodissection you notice capsular block. The next step is to
    d. decompress the nucleus and lift the anterior capsule—this technique is used to reverse capsular block

55. Which of the following measures is most likely to reduce the risk of postocclusion surge during phacoemulsification?
    b. reduce the maximum vacuum setting

56. Which of the following IOL designs is most likely to be associated with a complication of laser posterior capsulotomy?
    c. silicone plate haptic—this type of IOL has been associated with posterior dislocation after laser capsulotomy, particularly if performed shortly after cataract surgery

57. A patient with previous radial keratotomy surgery undergoes uncomplicated phacoemulsification. Two weeks after the cataract surgery, the patient states that her vision is blurry and unchanged. Her refraction is +2.00 + 0.50 × 30, which improves her vision to 20/20. At this point, the most appropriate management option is
    a. observation—refraction may take over 1 month to stabilize after cataract surgery in patients with previous corneal refractive surgery, especially post-RK, where hyperopic refraction is common due to corneal edema

58. What is the most appropriate treatment for a patient with a hyphema and persistent elevated IOP for 1 week despite maximal medical therapy?
    d. AC washout—uncontrolled increased IOP is an indication for AC washout for hyphema

59. A 32-year-old man presents 1 week after blunt trauma with 20/20 visual acuity and a dilated, unresponsive pupil OD. The most appropriate next step is
    a. careful slit-lamp exam of iris—traumatic mydriasis caused by sphincter tears is the most likely diagnosis, so a careful slit-lamp exam should be performed first

60. Which of the following IOL designs is most appropriate for placement in the sulcus?
    d. 13.5 mm PMMA—the best IOL design for the ciliary sulcus is a 3-piece foldable lens or a 1-piece PMMA lens that is posteriorly vaulted with an overall length of 13.5 mm and optic diameter of at least 6 mm

61. One day after cataract surgery, a patient has an IOP of 6 mm Hg. The anterior chamber is formed and the 2.4 mm cataract incision is Seidel positive demonstrating a slow, intermittent leak. Which of the following treatment options is most appropriate?
    d. pressure patch—administration of a topical antibiotic and pressure patching the eye for a small Seidel positive wound is often effective, as is placing a bandage contact lens in conjunction with an aqueous suppressant; however, suturing the wound may be necessary

62. When performing a capsulorhexis in a patient with a mature cataract, which of the following is most helpful to prevent splitting of the anterior capsule?
    d. aspirate liquid cortex from a small capsular opening and then enlarge—this technique is most useful for decompressing an intumescent cataract to avoid a rent in the anterior capsule. Capsular stain helps to visualize the anterior capsule but does not prevent the Argentinian flag sign, and a cohesive (high viscosity at rest; zero shear rate) rather than a dispersive OVD is better at maintaining space when there is no flow

63. During phacoemulsification, the pupil is noted to suddenly dilate and the anterior chamber deepen. What is the most likely cause?
    b. posterior capsular rupture

64. Which type of IOL is best for sulcus placement?
    c. three-piece acrylic

65. The type of cataract with the least effect on visual function is
    c. sutural—these are congenital opacities in the Y sutures that do not affect vision

66. All of the following are risk factors for the progression of an iris nevus except
    a. older age—younger (not older) age is a risk factor

67. The retina is least protected from UV light by the
    d. vitreous

CHAPTER 11 POSTERIOR SEGMENT

1. Which substance does not cause crystalline deposits in the retina?
   a. thioridazine

2. The finding most predictive of VA in a patient with PDR is
   b. macular edema

3. The MPS showed the best prognosis for laser treatment of CNV in which disorder?
   d. POHS—the MPS studied laser treatment of CNV in patients with AMD, POHS, and idiopathic membranes; patients with POHS had the best response to laser treatment; patients with CNV secondary to myopia and angioid streaks were not studied

4. Which of the following is not a feature of Stickler syndrome?
   c. retinoschisis

5. Sites at which the uvea is attached to the sclera include all of the following, except
   d. ora serrata

6. A patient with multifocal choroiditis and retinal vasculitis is most likely to have
   d. sarcoidosis

7. All 3 types of retinal hemorrhage (preretinal, intraretinal, and subretinal) may occur simultaneously in all of the following conditions, except
   c. diabetes—diabetic retinopathy can cause preretinal and intraretinal hemorrhages but does not cause subretinal hemorrhage

8. Characteristics of choroidal melanoma include all of the following, except
   b. high internal reflectivity

9. Which of the following statements regarding the ETDRS is false?
   a. The ETDRS concluded that PRP reduces the risk of severe visual loss in patients with high-risk PDR—this conclusion is from the DRS

10. The DRVS found that early vitrectomy for VH was helpful in which patients?
    a. patients with type 1 diabetes

11. Which of the following treatments is a CVOS recommendation?
    c. PRP for iris or angle NV

12. Which peripheral retinal lesion has the most risk of an RD?
    d. lattice degeneration

13. The intraocular structure most commonly affected by leukemia is the
    d. optic nerve

14. Which is not a function of the RPE?
    b. concentration of taurine

15. Which of the following best describes the cellular reaction when light strikes a photoreceptor?
    c. decreased cGMP, closed Na channel

16. Prognostic factors for choroidal melanoma include all of the following, *except*
    d. pigmentation

17. Which of the following does *not* involve the outer plexiform layer of the retina?
    d. diabetic microaneurysm

18. The best test for distinguishing between a subretinal hemorrhage and a choroidal melanoma is
    a. FA—blockage occurs from the hemorrhage, and tumor circulation is visible in the melanoma

19. Which of the following is the *least* radiosensitive lesion?
    d. melanoma

20. Which of the following is *not* a complication of PRP?
    c. RD

21. A cluster of pigmented lesions is seen in the peripheral retina of a patient's left eye during routine ophthalmoscopy. Which of the following tests would be most helpful in detecting an associated hereditary disorder?
    b. colonoscopy—check for polyps (familial adenomatous polyposis, Gardner disease)

22. Which of the following is *not* associated with a typical angiographic appearance of CME?
    a. nicotinic acid—this maculopathy clinically appears like CME, but there is no fluorescein filling of the cysts; other entities that fall into this category are juvenile retinoschisis, Goldmann-Favre disease, and some types of RP

23. The *least* likely finding in a patient with a chronic detachment of the inferotemporal retina is
    c. fixed folds—may occur from PVR, whereas the other three findings are common with chronic RD

24. In a patient with AMD, which type of drusen is most associated with the development of CNV?
    a. soft

25. The ERG oscillatory potential is caused by which cell type?
    b. amacrine

26. Chloroquine retinopathy
    b. can be associated with other CNS reactions—including tinnitus

27. Proven systemic control for diabetic retinopathy include
    d. blood pressure control—shown in the UKPDS

28. Retinal artery macroaneurysms
    b. produce multilayered hemorrhages

29. The BVOS reported that
    b. focal laser photocoagulation decreased visual loss—especially when vision was < 20/40

30. True statements about ocular photodynamic therapy include all of the following, *except*
    c. often requires retreatment every 6 weeks—actually it is every 3 months; early retreatment was not shown to be beneficial

31. Cystoid macular edema
    a. does not leak fluorescein when associated with nicotinic acid

32. PDR is most likely to develop if which one of the following findings is present on fundus exam?
    d. venous beading

33. Which of the following is the biggest risk factor for AMD?
    a. smoking

34. The most important visual prognostic factor for a rhegmatogenous RD is
    c. macular involvement—macula-on has a better prognosis than macula-off

35. The earliest sign of a macular hole is
    c. yellow spot in the fovea—stage 1a hole

36. Focal laser treatment is indicated for diabetic macular edema when there is
    d. retinal edema within 500 µm of the center of the fovea

37. Reduced IOP would be most unexpected in a patient with
    b. choroidal hemorrhage—choroidal hemorrhage causes increased IOP

38. Which of the following is the correct indication for treating macular edema from a BRVO?
    d. vision < 20/40 for > 3 months

39. Which test is best for distinguishing a choroidal melanoma from a choroidal hemangioma?
    c. ultrasound

40. The etiology of vitreous hemorrhage in Terson syndrome is
    a. intracranial hypertension—from a subarachnoid or subdural hemorrhage

41. Which is the most common site of metastasis for a choroidal melanoma?
    b. liver—92% of metastases are to the liver

42. Which of the following is *least* characteristic of Eales disease?
    d. macular edema

43. Crystalline retinopathy is *not* associated with
    c. thioridazine—causes a pigmentary retinopathy

44. Combined hamartoma of the retina and RPE has been associated with all of the following, *except*
    d. Gardner syndrome

45. Which of the following statements regarding uveal metastases is *false*?
    b. the most common ocular location is the anterior choroid—usually metastasize to macula because of richest blood supply

46. The most worrisome sign in a patient with an acute PVD is
    a. pigment in the vitreous—also known as *tobacco dust* and is associated with a retinal tear

47. The most likely diagnosis in a patient with choroidal neovascular membrane in the macula, peripapillary atrophy, and punched-out chorioretinal scars is
    c. POHS

48. Which is the most common complication of an epiretinal membrane?
    b. CME—ERM most commonly causes chronic CME

49. Which is the most helpful test to obtain in a patient with a branch retinal artery occlusion?
    d. carotid ultrasound—90% of BRAO is caused by emboli, so patients should have a complete cardiovascular workup

50. Angioid streaks are associated with all of the following systemic conditions, *except*
    c. syphilis

51. An elderly hypertensive man with a sudden change in vision is found to have hemorrhages and cotton wool spots in the superior temporal retina and a reduced foveal reflex. The most appropriate initial management is to obtain a(n)
    b. FA—the patient has a BRVO and should be evaluated with an FA

52. Which of the following is not a type of visual pigment?
    c. P—the cone photopigments are designated according to the wavelength of light they are sensitivie to: L (long), M (middle), and S (short)

Additional Readings

Albert, W. M., & Jakobiec, F. A. (2008). *Principles and Practice of Ophthalmology* (3rd ed.). Philadelphia: WB Saunders.

Friedman, N. J., Kaiser, P. K., & Pineda, R., II (2021). *The Massachusetts Eye & Ear Infirmary's Illustrated Manual of Ophthalmology* (5th ed.). Philadelphia: Elsevier.

Levin, L. A., Nilsson, S. F. E., Ver Hoeve, J., et al. (2011). *Adler's Physiology of the Eye* (11th ed.). Philadelphia: Saunders.

Mannis, M. J., MacSai, M. S., & Huntley, A. C. (1996). *Eye and Skin Disease*. Philadelphia: Lippincott-Raven.

Pepose, J. S., Holland, G. N., & Wilhelmus, K. R. (1996). *Ocular Infection and Immunity*. St Louis: Mosby.

Riordan-Eva, P., & Augsburger, J. J. (2017). *Vaughan and Asbury's General Ophthalmology* (19th ed.). Columbus, OH: McGraw-Hill.

Roy, F. H. (2012). *Ocular Differential Diagnosis* (9th ed.). London: Jaypee Brothers Medical.

Salmon, J. (2021). *Kanski's Clinical Ophthalmology* (9th ed.). Philadelphia: Elsevier.

Spaeth, G. L., Danesh-Meyer, H., Goldberg, I., & Kampik, A. (2011). *Ophthalmic Surgery Principles and Practice* (4th ed.). Philadelphia: Elsevier.

Spalton, D. J., Hitchings, R. A., & Hunter, P. A. (2004). *Atlas of Clinical Ophthalmology* (3rd ed.). St Louis: Mosby.

Tabbara, K. F., Abu, El-Asrar, A., M., & Khairallah, M. (2014). *Ocular Infections*. New York: Springer.

Tasman, W., & Jaeger, E. A. (2013). *Duane's Ophthalmology*. Philadelphia: Lippincott Williams & Wilkins.

Weingeist, T. A., & Gold, D. H. (2001). *Color Atlas of the Eye in Systemic Disease*. Philadelphia: Lippincott Williams & Wilkins.

Yanoff, M., & Duker, J. S. (2019). *Ophthalmology* (5th ed.). Philadelphia: Elsevier.

Index

Note: Page numbers followed by *f* indicate figures, *t* indicate tables, and *b* indicate boxes.